2006
YEAR BOOK OF
MEDICINE®

The 2006 Year Book Series

Year Book of Allergy, Asthma, and Clinical Immunology™: Drs Rosenwasser, Boguniewicz, Milgrom, Routes, and Weber

Year Book of Anesthesiology and Pain Management™: Drs Chestnut, Abram, Black, Gravlee, Lee, Mathru, and Roizen

Year Book of Cardiology®: Drs Gersh, Cheitlin, Elliott, Graham, Sundt, and Waldo

Year Book of Critical Care Medicine®: Drs Dellinger, Parrillo, Balk, Bekes, Dorman, and Dries

Year Book of Dentistry®: Drs McIntyre, Belvedere, Buhite, Davis, Henderson, Johnson, Jureyda, Ohrbach, Olin, Scott, Spencer, and Zakariasen

Year Book of Dermatology and Dermatologic Surgery™: Drs Thiers and Lang

Year Book of Diagnostic Radiology®: Drs Osborn, Birdwell, Dalinka, Gardiner, Levy, Maynard, Oestreich, and Rosado de Christenson

Year Book of Emergency Medicine®: Drs Burdick, Hamilton, Handly, Quintana, and Werner

Year Book of Endocrinology®: Drs Mazzaferri, Bessesen, Clarke, Howard, Kennedy, Leahy, Meikle, Molitch, Rogol, and Schteingart

Year Book of Family Practice®: Drs Bowman, Apgar, Dexter, Miser, Neill, and Scherger

Year Book of Gastroenterology™: Drs Lichtenstein, Burke, Campbell, Dempsey, Drebin, Ginsberg, Katzka, Kochman, Morris, Rombeau, Shah, and Stein

Year Book of Hand and Upper Limb Surgery®: Drs Chang and Steinmann

Year Book of Medicine®: Drs Barkin, Frishman, Garrick, Loehrer, Phillips, Pillinger, and Snydman

Year Book of Neonatal and Perinatal Medicine®: Drs Fanaroff, Maisels, and Stevenson

Year Book of Neurology and Neurosurgery®: Drs Gibbs and Verma

Year Book of Nuclear Medicine®: Drs Coleman, Blaufox, Royal, Strauss, and Zubal

Year Book of Obstetrics, Gynecology, and Women's Health®: Dr Shulman

Year Book of Oncology®: Drs Loehrer, Arceci, Glatstein, Gordon, Hanna, Morrow, and Thigpen

Year Book of Ophthalmology®: Drs Rapuano, Cohen, Eagle, Flanders, Hammersmith, Myers, Nelson, Penne, Sergott, Shields, Tipperman, and Vander

Year Book of Orthopedics®: Drs Morrey, Beauchamp, Peterson, Swiontkowski, Trigg, and Yaszemski

Year Book of Otolaryngology-Head and Neck Surgery®: Drs Paparella, Gapany, and Keefe

Year Book of Pathology and Laboratory Medicine®: Drs Raab, Parwani, Bejarano, and Bissell

Year Book of Pediatrics®: Dr Stockman

Year Book of Plastic and Aesthetic Surgery™: Drs Miller, Bartlett, Garner, McKinney, Ruberg, Salisbury, and Smith

Year Book of Psychiatry and Applied Mental Health®: Drs Talbott, Ballenger, Buckley, Frances, Jensen, and Markowitz

Year Book of Pulmonary Disease®: Drs Phillips, Barker, Lewis, Maurer, Tanoue, and Willsie

Year Book of Rheumatology, Arthritis, and Musculoskeletal Disease™: Drs Panush, Furst, Hadler, Hochberg, Lahita, and Paget

Year Book of Sports Medicine®: Drs Shephard, Alexander, Cantu, Feldman, McCrory, Nieman, Rowland, Sanborn, and Shrier

Year Book of Surgery®: Drs Copeland, Bland, Cerfolio, Daly, Eberlein, Fahey, Mozingo, Pruett, and Seeger

Year Book of Urology®: Drs Andriole and Coplen

Year Book of Vascular Surgery®: Dr Moneta

2006

The Year Book of MEDICINE®

Editors

Jamie S. Barkin, MD
William H. Frishman, MD
Renee Garrick, MD
Patrick J. Loehrer, Sr, MD
Ernest L. Mazzaferri, MD
Barbara A. Phillips, MD, MSPH
Michael H. Pillinger, MD
David R. Snydman, MD

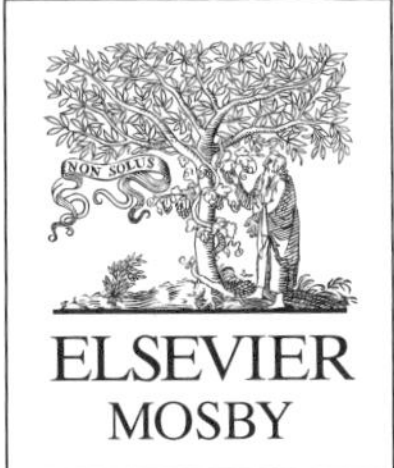

ELSEVIER
MOSBY

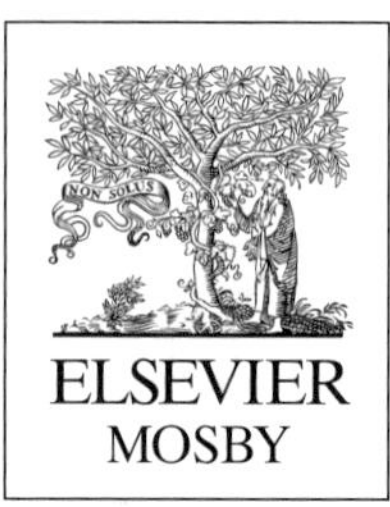

Vice President, Continuity: John A. Schrefer
Developmental Editor: Timothy Maxwell
Senior Manager, Continuity Production: Idelle L. Winer
Senior Issue Manager: Pat Costigan
Illustrations and Permissions Coordinator: Linda S. Jones

2006 EDITION

Printed in the United States of America
Composition by Thomas Technology Solutions, Inc.
Printing/binding by Sheridan Books, Inc.

Editorial Office:
Elsevier
Suite 1800
1600 John F. Kennedy Blvd
Philadelphia, PA 19103-2899

International Standard Serial Number: 0084-3873
International Standard Book Number: 1-4160-3314-9
978-1-4160-3314-1

Editorial Board

Contributors

Aryeh M. Abeles, MD

Instructor of Medicine, New York University School of Medicine, The Hospital for Joint Diseases; Co-director, Rheumatology Clinic, Department of Veterans Affairs, New York Harbor Healthcare System–New York Campus, New York, New York

Stephen Adler, MD

Professor of Medicine and Physiology, New York Medical College; West Chester Medical Center, Valhalla, New York

Robert J. Arceci, MD, PhD

King Fahd Professor of Pediatric Oncology, Johns Hopkins University School of Medicine; Director of Pediatric Oncology, Johns Hopkins Hospital, Baltimore, Maryland

Ami Ben-Artzi, MD

Instructor of Medicine, New York University School of Medicine, The Hospital for Joint Diseases, New York, New York

James A. Barker, MD

Professor of Medicine and Chief, Pulmonary and Critical Care Medicine, University of South Carolina; Medical Director, MICU, PCU, and Respiratory Therapy, Palmetto Richland Hospital, Columbia, South Carolina

Daniel H. Bessesen, MD

Associate Professor of Medicine, University of Colorado at Denver Health Sciences Center; Chief of Endocrinology, Denver Health Medical Center, Denver, Colorado

Maureen Brogan, MD

Assistant Professor of Medicine, New York Medical College; West Chester Medical Center, Valhalla, New York

Bart L. Clarke, MD

Assistant Professor of Medicine, Mayo Clinic; Consultant, St. Mary's Hospital; Consultant, Rochester Methodist Hospital, Rochester, Minnesota

Eli Glatstein, MD

Morton Kligerman Professor of Radiation Oncology, University of Pennsylvania; Hospital of the University of Pennsylvania, Philadelphia, Pennsylvania

Michael S. Gordon, MD

Clinical Associate Professor of Medicine, University of Arizona College of Medicine; Premiere Oncology of Arizona, Scottsdale, Arizona

Nasser Hanna, MD

Assistant Professor of Medicine, Indiana University, Indianapolis, Indiana

Wm. James Howard, MD

Professor of Medicine, Vice President for Academic Affairs, Washington Hospital Center, Washington, District of Columbia

Peter I. Izmirly, MD
Instructor of Medicine, New York University School of Medicine, The Hospital for Joint Diseases, New York, New York

Laurence Kennedy, MD, FRCP
Professor of Medicine, Endocrine Division, University of Florida; Chief of Endocrinology, Shands Hospital at the University of Florida, Gainesville, Florida

Michael Klein, MD, JD
Assistant Professor of Medicine, New York Medical College; West Chester Medical Center, Valhalla, New York

Svetlana Krasnokutsky, MD
Instructor of Medicine, New York University School of Medicine, The Hospital for Joint Diseases, New York, New York

John (Jack) L. Leahy, MD
Professor of Medicine, Chief, Division of Endocrinology, Diabetes, and Metabolism, University of Vermont, Burlington, Vermont

Kevin L. Lewis, MD
Chief Medical Officer, Sleep Disorders Center, Inc; Clinical Instructor, Oklahoma University College of Medicine, St John Medical Center, Tulsa, Oklahoma

Janet R. Maurer, MD
Medical Director, CIGNA HealthCare, Bloomfield, Connecticut

A. Wayne Meikle, MD
Professor of Medicine and Pathology, University of Utah School of Medicine; Director of Endocrine Testing, ARUP Laboratories, The University of Utah Hospitals, Salt Lake City, Utah

Mark E. Molitch, MD
Professor of Medicine, Northwestern University, Feinberg School of Medicine; Attending Physician, Northwestern Memorial Hospital, Chicago, Illinois

Monica Morrow, MD
G. Willing Pepper Chair in Cancer Research, Professor of Surgery; Chair, Department of Surgical Oncology, Fox Chase Cancer Center, Philadelphia, Pennsylvania

Alan D. Rogol, MD, PhD
Professor of Clinical Pediatrics, University of Virginia, Charlottesville, Virginia

David E. Schteingart, MD
Professor, Department of Internal Medicine, Division of Metabolism, Endocrinology, and Diabetes, University of Michigan Health System, Ann Arbor, Michigan

Lynn T. Tanoue, MD
Associate Professor of Medicine, Pulmonary and Critical Care Section, Department of Medicine, School of Medicine, Yale University, New Haven, Connecticut

Fasika Tedla, MD
Assistant Professor of Medicine, New York Medical College; West Chester Medical Center, Valhalla, New York

James Tate Thigpen, MD
Professor of Medicine and Director, Division of Oncology, University of Mississippi Medical Center, Jackson, Mississippi

Sandra K. Willsie, DO
Professor of Medicine, Executive Vice President for Academic Affairs, Kansas City University of Medicine and Biosciences, Kansas City, Missouri

Table of Contents

Journals Represented

Journals represented in this Year Book are listed below.

Academic Radiology
American Journal of Cardiology
American Journal of Gastroenterology
American Journal of Kidney Diseases
American Journal of Medicine
American Journal of Public Health
American Journal of Respiratory and Critical Care Medicine
American Journal of Transplantation
American Surgeon
Annals of Emergency Medicine
Annals of Internal Medicine
Annals of Rheumatic Diseases
Annals of Surgical Oncology
Antimicrobial Agents and Chemotherapy
Archives of Internal Medicine
Arthritis and Rheumatism
British Journal of Urology International (WRONG)
British Medical Journal
Canadian Medical Association Journal
Cancer Epidemiology, Biomarkers and Prevention
Chest
Circulation
Clinical Cancer Research
Clinical Endocrinology (Oxford)
Clinical Gastroenterology and Hepatology
Clinical Infectious Diseases
Critical Care Medicine
Diabetes
Diabetes Care
Diagnostic Cytopathology
Endoscopy
European Journal of Endocrinology
European Respiratory Journal
Experimental and Clinical Endocrinology and Diabetes
Gastroenterology
Gastrointestinal Endoscopy
Gut
Hypertension
Intensive Care Medicine
Journal of Acquired Immune Deficiency Syndromes
Journal of Allergy and Clinical Immunology
Journal of Bone and Mineral Research
Journal of Clinical Endocrinology and Metabolism
Journal of Clinical Investigation
Journal of Clinical Oncology
Journal of General Internal Medicine
Journal of Immunology
Journal of Infectious Diseases
Journal of Rheumatology

Journal of the American College of Cardiology
Journal of the American Geriatrics Society
Journal of the American Medical Association
Journal of the American Society of Nephrology
Journal of the National Cancer Institute
Kidney International
Lancet
Medical Care
Medicine
Nephrology, Dialysis, Transplantation
New England Journal of Medicine
Otolaryngology-Head and Neck Surgery
Pediatrics
Proceedings of the National Academy of Sciences
Radiology
Respiratory Medicine
Scandinavian Journal of Rheumatology
Science
Sleep
Urology

Standard Abbreviations

The following terms are abbreviated in this edition: acquired immunodeficiency syndrome (AIDS), cardiopulmonary resuscitation (CPR), central nervous system (CNS), cerebrospinal fluid (CSF), computed tomography (CT), deoxyribonucleic acid (DNA), electrocardiography (ECG), health maintenance organization (HMO), human immunodeficiency virus (HIV), intensive care unit (ICU), intramuscular (IM), intravenous (IV), magnetic resonance (MR) imaging (MRI), ribonucleic acid (RNA), and ultrasound (US).

Note

The Year Book of Medicine is a literature survey service providing abstracts of articles published in the professional literature. Every effort is made to assure the accuracy of the information presented in these pages. Neither the editors nor the publisher of the Year Book of Medicine can be responsible for errors in the original materials. The editors' comments are their own opinions. Mention of specific products within this publication does not constitute endorsement.

To facilitate the use of the Year Book of Medicine as a reference tool, all illustrations and tables included in this publication are now identified as they appear in the original article. This change is meant to help the reader recognize that any illustration or table appearing in the Year Book of Medicine may be only one of many in the original article. For this reason, figure and table numbers will often appear to be out of sequence within the Year Book of Medicine.

PART ONE

RHEUMATOLOGY

MICHAEL H. PILLINGER, MD

Introduction

The therapeutic revolution in rheumatology continues apace. The past year has seen the ongoing integration of tumor necrosis factor (TNF) inhibitors into the treatment of rheumatoid arthritis and seronegative spondyloarthropathies, to the point where these marvelous agents are no longer considered experimental. Additionally, 2 new therapies for rheumatoid arthritis—abatacept, which blocks costimulation, and rituximab, which attacks B cells—have been approved by the US Food and Drug Administration. In contrast to the TNF inhibitors, these agents hold promise for the treatment of lupus as well, and are currently under investigation for that application. In lupus, too, the introduction of mycophenolate mofetil and its further validation in clinical studies has given us, at the least, a backup to cyclophosphamide that appears to be much less toxic and may prove as good or even better, when all the data are in. The cyclooxygenase (COX)-2 inhibitors remain controversial, and much less used than previously; yet data are accumulating that not all COX-2's may be worse than traditional nonsteroidal anti-inflammatory drugs when it comes to cardiovascular risk, and in some situations, they may even be better. For the first time in many years, new drugs may be on the threshold for gout, and even Still's disease, of which we understand little, is appearing to respond to blockade of interleukin-1. In sum, when it comes to therapy of most rheumatic diseases (osteoarthritis remaining a notable exception), we are getting better and better and better.

With so much activity going on in the field of rheumatology, the selection of important articles to highlight for the YEAR BOOK OF MEDICINE has been a challenge. As in the past, I have followed several rules. First, I have included most of the large-scale clinical trials of agents in use or likely to enter the therapeutic arena shortly. Second, I have included large observational studies that shed light on important disease processes. Third, I have included smaller clinical studies where I felt that the results were clear-cut and appear to indicate a potentially important therapeutic approach. And finally, while readers of this YEAR BOOK are likely to be clinically oriented, I have included a small number of more basic studies that seem to me to suggest fundamentally new thoughts about the rheumatic diseases. These selections merely skim the surface; rheumatologists and their patients are fortunate to be living in such exciting and hopeful times.

Michael H. Pillinger, MD

1 Gout and Other Crystal Diseases

Serum Uric Acid Concentration as a Risk Factor for Cardiovascular Mortality: A Longterm Cohort Study of Atomic Bomb Survivors

Hakoda M, Masunari N, Yamada M, et al (Radiation Effects Research Found, Hiroshima, Japan)

J Rheumatol 32:906-912, 2005 1–1

Objective.—To elucidate the association of serum uric acid concentration with cardiovascular mortality risk.

Methods.—Serum uric acid level measured from 1966 through 1970 in 10,615 Japanese individuals from a cohort of atomic bomb survivors was analyzed for association with subsequent cardiovascular and all-cause mortality until 1999 using the Cox proportional hazard model.

Results.—During an average followup of 24.9 years, 5225 deaths occurred, of which 1984 were ascribed to cardiovascular disease. In men, after adjustment for age, elevated serum uric acid level was associated with both cardiovascular and all-cause mortality. After additional adjustment for potential cardiovascular disease risk factors including body mass index, smoking status, alcohol consumption, systolic blood pressure, cholesterol level, and histories of hypertension, diabetes and cardiovascular disease, elevated serum uric acid level in men was associated with all-cause mortality but not with cardiovascular mortality. In women, even after these adjustments, elevated serum uric acid level was significantly associated with cardiovascular and all-cause mortality.

Conclusion.—Increased serum uric acid level is a significant and independent risk factor for cardiovascular mortality in women and for all-cause mortality in both men and women.

► For many rheumatologists, gout is a bread and butter disease that takes a back seat to the more "serious" rheumatologic conditions, such as lupus and rheumatoid arthritis. "After all," goes the reasoning, "gout doesn't kill you." This, however, may be a cavalier assumption. Hyperuricemia has long been associated with risk factors, such as hypercholesterolemia and hypertension, and some evidence suggests that hyperuricemia may be a cause, rather than a consequence, of at least some of these conditions (see, for example, Richard

Johnson's studies linking hyperuricemia to gout).[1] Moreover, the signals have been present, albeit mixed, as to whether hyperuricemia may indeed affect mortality. In this manuscript, Hakoda et al took advantage of a large, well-established cohort to conclude that elevated levels of serum urate do, indeed, affect long-term survival. The database that the authors used was the Adult Health Study Cohort, established in 1958 to track individuals who were exposed to ionizing radiation from the atomic bombs on Hiroshima and Nagasaki. More than 10,000 individuals have participated, about half of whom were not felt to have been exposed to significant radiation (by dint of distance from the epicenter, or absence at the time of the explosions). From 1966 through 1970, these individuals had their serum urate checked. They were then followed up until death, or until 1999, making this the largest and longest of all studies on the association of uric acid levels and risk for cardiovascular and all-cause mortality.

The results were as follows: males in the highest quintile for uric acid (≥8.0/dL) had an age-adjusted mortality rate more than one third increased relative to those in the lowest quintile (<5.0 mg/dL), and a statistically insignificant increase in cardiovascular mortality rate (MI, stroke, other). Females with hyperuricemia (≥7.0 mg/dL) had an even higher increase in age-adjusted all-cause mortality, by about double; females with hyperuricemia also had approximately double the rate of coronary heart disease and stroke mortality, even when adjusted for confounding variables, such as hypertension. These data suggest that we may be underestimating the importance of hyperuricemia, particularly in the female population, in whom serum urates are rarely even assessed. The mechanisms of increased mortality caused by serum urate remain to be determined, but may relate, in part, to effects on the vasculature. Why the effect of hyperuricemia on women is more apparent than in men (although it is worth noting that other studies have documented both increased all-cause mortality and increased hyperuricemia in men) is another interesting question and may relate to hormonal differences, the already higher cardiovascular mortality rate in men, or undetermined factors.

Gout, and by implication hyperuricemia, continue to be epidemic in American society (compare article referenced in prior Year Book reporting a doubling of gout prevalence in Rochester Minnesota during a 20-year period).[2] Given the large number of individuals with elevated urates, and the fact that we have several effective drugs for decreasing serum urate, and at least 1 more potentially in the pipeline (see the article by Becker et al referenced in this volume of the Year Book (Abstract 1–2), it strongly behooves us to better understand the scope, and implications, of this potentially major public health question.

M. H. Pillinger, MD

References

1. 2003 Year Book of Medicine, pp 46-47.
2. 2003 Year Book of Medicine, pp 45-46.

Febuxostat, a Novel Nonpurine Selective Inhibitor of Xanthine Oxidase: A Twenty-Eight–Day, Multicenter, Phase II, Randomized, Double-blind, Placebo-controlled, Dose-Response Clinical Trial Examining Safety and Efficacy in Patients With Gout

Becker MA, Schumacher HR Jr, Wortmann RL, et al (Univ of Chicago; Univ of Pennsylvania, Philadelphia; Univ of Oklahoma, Tulsa; et al)

Arthritis Rheum 52:916-923, 2005 1–2

Objective.—Gout affects ~1-2% of the American population. Current options for treating hyperuricemia in chronic gout are limited. The purpose of this study was to assess the safety and efficacy of febuxostat, a nonpurine selective inhibitor of xanthine oxidase, in establishing normal serum urate (sUA) concentrations in gout patients with hyperuricemia (≥8.0 mg/dl).

Methods.—We conducted a phase II, randomized, double-blind, placebo-controlled trial in 153 patients (ages 23-80 years). Subjects received febuxostat (40 mg, 80 mg, 120 mg) or placebo once daily for 28 days and colchicine prophylaxis for 14 days prior to and 14 days after randomization. The primary end point was the proportion of subjects with sUA levels <6.0 mg/dl on day 28.

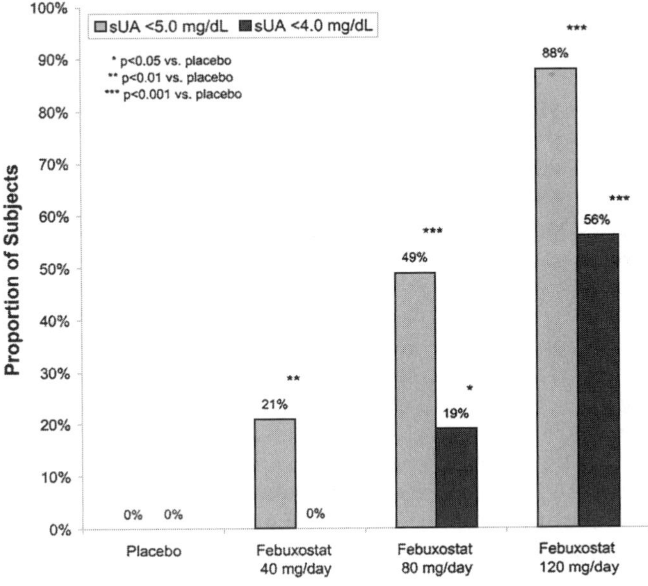

FIGURE 3.—Proportion of intent-to-treat population (140 patients with a serum urate concentration ≥8.0 mg/dl on day −2) with a serum urate (sUA) level <5.0 mg/dl or <4.0 mg/dl on day 28, by treatment group. (Courtesy of Becker MA, Schumacher HR Jr, Wortmann RL, et al: Febuxostat, a novel nonpurine selective inhibitor of xanthine oxidase: A twenty-eight–day, multicenter, phase II, randomized, double-blind, placebo-controlled, dose-response clinical trial examining safety and efficacy in patients with gout. *Arthritis Rheum* 52;916-923, 2005. Copyright 2005, American College of Rheumatology. Reprinted by permission of John Wiley & Sons, Inc.)

Results.—Greater proportions of febuxostat-treated patients than placebo-treated patients achieved an sUA level <6.0 mg/dl at each visit ($P < 0.001$ for each comparison). The targeted sUA level was attained on day 28 in 0% of those taking placebo and in 56% of those taking 40 mg, 76% taking 80 mg, and 94% taking 120 mg of febuxostat. The mean sUA reduction from baseline to day 28 was 2% in the placebo group and 37% in the 40-mg, 44% in the 80-mg, and 59% in the 120-mg febuxostat groups. Gout flares occurred with similar frequency in the placebo (37%) and 40-mg febuxostat (35%) groups and with increased frequency in the higher dosage febuxostat groups (43% taking 80 mg; 55% taking 120 mg). During colchicine prophylaxis, gout flares occurred less frequently (8-13%). Incidences of treatment-related adverse events were similar in the febuxostat and placebo groups.

Conclusion.—Treatment with febuxostat resulted in a significant reduction of sUA levels at all dosages. Febuxostat therapy was safe and well tolerated (Fig 3).

▶ From a therapeutic standpoint, not much has happened in the field of gout in 30-odd years. Recombinant human uricase became available about 2 years ago, but its prodigious expense (tens of thousands of dollars a dose) and its short half-life make it truly useful only for specific prophylaxis of tumor lysis syndrome. While the currently available therapies are adequate for most patients with gout (allopurinol and probenecid and, in Europe, benzbromarone for lowering uric acid levels; steroids, nonsteroidal anti-inflammatory drugs, and colchicine for blocking or preventing gouty inflammation), these drugs each have their own toxicities that make them inappropriate for some patients. Additional medications would be helpful.

In this study, Becker et al report on a Phase II trial of just such an additional medication: febuxostat, a nonpurine inhibitor of xanthine oxidase. The authors randomly selected 153 patients for study, all of whom had hyperuricemia (sUA, ≥8 mg/dL) and documented gout; enrollees received either placebo or febuxostat (40, 80, or 120 mg daily) for 28 days. The primary end point was a decrease in serum uric acid to less than 6.0 mg/dL by 28 days. Secondary end points included reduction in serum uric acid to less than 6.0 mg/dL at earlier time points, and reduction in serum uric acid to less than 5.0 mg/dL or 4.0 mg/dL at 28 days.

The results were impressive. At the lowest dose, 56% of patients achieved the primary end point by the end of the study. At the highest dose, 94% did. (Among placebo takers, no patients achieved the target urate.) In fact, these effects were more or less achieved at the earliest time point assessed (7 days), indicating that febuxostat acts rapidly to decrease sUA. Lower sUAs (as would be desired in treating most cases of tophaceous gout, for example) were also achievable: in patients taking 120 mg daily, 88% achieved sUAs less than 5.0, and 56% achieved sUAs less than 4.0 mg/dL. All patients were placed on colchicine during the initiation of febuxostat. When colchicine was discontinued after 2 weeks, the number of gout flares was greater in the febuxostat patients, confirming the old bias that urate lowering can transiently increase the risk for gouty attacks, and indicating that 2 weeks of prophylaxis with colchicine is too short a period during the initiation of febuxostat. Otherwise, side effects were relatively rare. A few patients got abdominal pain or diarrhea, but placebo patients had these complaints to an equal degree. A few patients had abnormal liver function tests, but these were felt to correspond with, and resolve with, the discontinuation of colchicine. Two serious adverse events were seen. One patient had a suicide attempt; this was judged unrelated to febuxostat use. And a single patient had a Guillain-Barré-like illness, whose relation to the drug use was uncertain.

Overall, it would seem likely that febuxostat will be a useful adjunct to the gout armamentarium, if and when it receives Food and Drug Administration (FDA) approval. Which patients would be most likely to benefit from febuxostat? The most likely candidates would appear to be patients who need allopurinol but are unable to tolerate it owing to rashes, cytopenias, hepatitis, vasculitis, and life-threatening hypersensitivity reactions. As a nonpurine agent, febuxostat is unlikely to cause cross-reactive hypersensitivity and less likely to cause the other side effects. Another group who may be well suited for this agent are individuals for whom allopurinol is indicated but who have renal insufficiency. At present, such patients are dosed with allopurinol cautiously; because febuxostat is metabolized by the hepatobiliary conjugation (unlike allopurinol, which is largely excreted via the kidneys), renal adjustment is likely unnecessary (confirming studies are ongoing). On the other hand, febuxostat is not likely to be any more useful and may turn out to be even more problematic than allopurinol for patients with liver disease. Most rheumatologists also have a few patients who are unexpectedly refractory to the effects of allopurinol; whether such patients will benefit from febuxostat, or perhaps a combination of febuxostat and allopurinol, remains to be determined.

M. H. Pillinger, MD

Association of Sporadic Chondrocalcinosis With a −4-Basepair G-to-A Transition in the 5'-Untranslated Region of *ANKH* That Promotes Enhanced Expression of ANKH Protein and Excess Generation of Extracellular Inorganic Pyrophosphate

Zhang Y, Johnson K, Russell RGG, et al (Univ of Oxford, England; Univ of California, San Diego)

Arthritis Rheum 52:1110-1117, 2005 1–3

Objective.—Certain mutations in *ANKH*, which encodes a multiple-pass transmembrane protein that regulates inorganic pyrophosphate (PPi) transport, are linked to autosomal-dominant familial chondrocalcinosis. This study investigated the potential for *ANKH* sequence variants to promote sporadic chondrocalcinosis.

Methods.—*ANKH* variants identified by genomic sequencing were screened for association with chondrocalcinosis in 128 patients with severe sporadic chondrocalcinosis or pseudogout and in ethnically matched healthy controls. The effects of specific variants on expression of common markers were evaluated by in vitro transcription/translation. The function of these variants was studied in transfected human immortalized CH-8 articular chondrocytes.

Results.—Sporadic chondrocalcinosis was associated with a G-to-A transition in the *ANKH* 5'-untranslated region (5'-UTR) at 4 bp upstream of the start codon (in homozygotes of the minor allele, genotype relative risk 6.0, $P = 0.0006$; overall genotype association $P = 0.02$). This −4-bp transition, as well as 2 mutations previously linked with familial and sporadic chondrocalcinosis (+14 bp C-to-T and C-terminal GAG deletion, respectively), but not the French familial chondrocalcinosis kindred 143-bp T-to-C mutation, increased reticulocyte *ANKH* transcription/ANKH translation in vitro. Transfection of complementary DNA for both the wild-type ANKH and the −4-bp ANKH protein variant promoted increased extracellular PPi in CH-8 cells, but unexpectedly, these ANKH mutants had divergent effects on the expression of extracellular PPi and the chondrocyte hypertrophy marker, type X collagen.

Conclusion.—A subset of sporadic chondrocalcinosis appears to be heritable via a −4-bp G-to-A *ANKH* 5'-UTR transition that up-regulates expression of ANKH and extracellular PPi in chondrocyte cells. Distinct *ANKH* mutations associated with heritable chondrocalcinosis may promote disease by divergent effects on extracellular PPi and chondrocyte hypertrophy, which is likely to mediate differences in the clinical phenotypes and severity of the disease.

► Our understanding of the biology of chondrocalcinosis and pseudogout remains in its infancy. One emerging theme of the past decade is that, in contrast to gout, in which the source of urate for crystals is the systemic circulation and the body's extracellular fluid, the deposition of calcium pyrophosphate in cartilage appears to be a local phenomenon and related to the enzymatic responses of chondrocytes. One such enzyme appears to be nucleotide pyrophosphatase, an ectoenzyme that liberates PPi from such molecules as adenosine triphosphate. The other enzyme is ANKH (ANK in the mouse), which plays its role by participating in the secretion of intracellular PPi to the extracellular environment. In this study, Zhang et al look for hereditary alteration in the *ANKH* gene among a group of patients with "sporadic" (ostensibly nonhereditary) chondrocalcinosis and find that some of them have a G-to-A mutation in the 5'-UTR of *ANKH*. When transfected into cells in vitro, this same variant of the gene resulted in a high level of extracellular PPi, supporting (though not proving) the idea that this gene sequence variant plays a role in chondrocalcinosis. I have included this report as a YEAR BOOK selection, not because it is clinically important at this time, but because it may become so in the future. At present we have no good therapy to address the deposition of crystals in chondrocalcinosis and pseudogout; with our incremental but steady increase in understanding the role of enzymes such as ANKH and nucleotide pyrophosphatase, we may eventually see the development of drugs that can target this disease at its source.

M. H. Pillinger, MD

2 Rheumatoid Arthritis

Very Early Treatment With Infliximab in Addition to Methotrexate in Early, Poor-Prognosis Rheumatoid Arthritis Reduces Magnetic Resonance Imaging Evidence of Synovitis and Damage, With Sustained Benefit After Infliximab Withdrawal: Results From a Twelve-Month Randomized, Double-blind, Placebo-controlled Trial

Quinn MA, Conaghan PG, O'Connor PJ, et al (Leeds Gen Infirmary, England)

Arthritis Rheum 52:27-35, 2005 2–1

Objective.—Anti–tumor necrosis factor α agents are among the most effective therapies for rheumatoid arthritis (RA). However, their optimal use is yet to be determined. This 12-month double-blind study attempted remission induction using standard therapy with or without infliximab in patients with early, poor-prognosis RA. The primary end point was synovitis (measured by magnetic resonance imaging [MRI]). Clinical observations continued to 24 months.

Methods.—All patients had fewer than 12 months of symptoms. Assessments included full metrologic evaluation, laboratory tests, radiographs, functional evaluation using the Health Assessment Questionnaire (HAQ), and quality of life measurement using the RA Quality of Life (RAQoL) questionnaire. MRI was performed at 0, 4, 14, and 54 weeks; MR images were scored blindly. Patients received methotrexate (MTX) and were randomized to receive either infliximab or placebo for 12 months.

Results.—Twenty patients were recruited (mean age 52 years, mean symptom duration 6 months, mean C-reactive protein level 42 mg/liter, and 65% rheumatoid factor positive). At 1 year, all MRI scores were significantly better, with no new erosions in the infliximab plus MTX group; a greater percentage of infliximab plus MTX–treated patients fulfilled the American College of Rheumatology (ACR) 50% and 70% improvement criteria (78% versus 40% in the placebo plus MTX group and 67% versus 30%, respectively) and had a greater functional benefit ($P < 0.05$ for all comparisons). Importantly, at 1 year after stopping induction therapy, response was sustained in 70% of the patients in the infliximab plus MTX group, with a median Disease Activity Score in 28 joints (DAS28) of 2.05 (remission range). At 2 years, there were no significant between-group differences in the DAS28, ACR response, or radiographic scores, but differences in the HAQ and RAQoL scores were maintained ($P < 0.05$).

Conclusion.—Remission induction with infliximab plus MTX provided a significant reduction in MRI evidence of synovitis and erosions at 1 year. At 2 years, functional and quality of life benefits were sustained, despite withdrawal of infliximab therapy. These data may have significant implications for the optimal use of expensive biologic therapies.

► It is becoming a commonplace in the academic arthritis literature (and there are even some data to support it!) that aggressive and maximal therapy for patients in the earliest stages of rheumatoid arthritis may be markedly more beneficial than the same therapy administered later on. Rheumatologists in practice, however, generally still adhere to a ramping-up strategy (albeit with a steeper ramp than in the past) in which standard therapy (usually MTX) is allowed to fail before fancier therapy (usually a tumor necrosis factor inhibitor) is instituted. One reason for this conservative approach is prudence: we don't have the extended experience with biologics that we have with MTX, and in any event the benefits of aggressive early therapy are not yet definitive. Another reason is cost: biologics are expensive, their use is expected to be long term, and someone (the patient, the insurance company) is going to need to agree to pay for them.

In this pilot study Quinn et al make a case for early treatment and suggest a way to keep therapeutic costs down in the bargain. The investigators recruited 20 patients with early rheumatoid arthritis (mean duration, 6 months) at high risk for future damage (eg, rheumatoid factor positive, high C-reactive protein level, high initial HAQ score, and/or shared epitope positive) and randomized them to receive either MTX alone or MTX plus infliximab. The outcomes they measured were synovitis and structural damage (using MRI and radiographs) as well as ACR 20, 50, and 70; DAS28; and the HAQ. The study was carried out for 54 weeks, and then the infliximab was stopped; for an additional 54 weeks, the investigators followed the patients to see whether early use of a tumor necrosis factor antagonist could have persistent benefit.

Some of the results might have been expected, to the extent that the patients getting infliximab plus MTX fared better while they were on the infliximab than did the MTX-alone group. At 14 weeks the infliximab group had less synovitis and less bone edema; at 54 weeks these advantages persisted, and the infliximab group also had no new erosions, which was not true for the MTX-alone group (despite the fact that, by the end of the 54-week period, the MTX-only patients tended to be taking more MTX than the infliximab plus MTX patients). The infliximab plus MTX group also had markedly greater ACR 20, 50, and 70 response rates at each interval and lower DAS28 scores. Thus, patients getting infliximab not only felt better, they were better and had less damage, making the case for not delaying aggressive therapy.

The really interesting part is what happened in the 54 weeks after the infliximab was discontinued. Strikingly, the patients who received infliximab in the first year had persistent benefit; that is, their DAS28 scores and C-reactive protein levels remained at the levels that were established in response to infliximab. During this time, patients in the MTX-alone group continued to have gradual improvement, so that by the end of the study the DAS28 scores and C-reactive protein levels of the 2 groups were comparable. However, the infliximab plus MTX group had spent more time at lower levels of disease activity (area under the curve). Perhaps because of this, or for other possible reasons (eg, the authors cite the importance of early response in helping patients avoid becoming ensnared in the sick role), the HAQ scores of the patients who received infliximab plus MTX remained markedly better at the end of 2 years compared with the MTX-alone group. Since we now understand that HAQ scores are perhaps our best measure of physical function, psychological well-being, and future prognosis, these results are not trivial.

The authors posit, quite reasonably, that what they have accomplished with early infliximab may be the equivalent of oncologic induction therapy, and that an early reduction in the synovial bulk and rheumatoid disease activity can consolidate long-term improvements in patient status (at least if MTX is continued). If confirmed (larger studies are ongoing), these observations may help guide us out of our current economic swamp, in which we are being overwhelmed by the cost of our newer, more effective agents. If the early application of a tumor necrosis factor inhibitor gives the most "bang for the buck," then even if we can't afford the routine chronic use of these important agents, it may at least be possible—and advisable—to get them on board up front for a finite period of time.

M. H. Pillinger, MD

Treatment of Rheumatoid Arthritis With the Selective Costimulation Modulator Abatacept: Twelve-Month Results of a Phase IIb, Double-blind, Randomized, Placebo-controlled Trial

Kremer JM, Dougados M, Emery P, et al (Ctr for Rheumatology, Albany, NY; Rene Descartes Univ, Paris; Leeds Gen Infirmary, England; et al)

Arthritis Rheum 52:2263-2271, 2005 2–2

Objective.—To determine the clinical efficacy, safety, and immunogenicity of abatacept (CTLA-4Ig), a selective costimulation modulator, in patients with rheumatoid arthritis (RA) that has remained active despite methotrexate (MTX) therapy.

Methods.—This was a 12-month, multicenter, randomized, double-blind, placebo-controlled study. A total of 339 patients with active RA despite MTX therapy were randomly assigned to receive 10 mg/kg abatacept (n = 115), 2 mg/kg abatacept (n = 105), or placebo (n = 119). This report focuses on the results observed at month 12 of a phase IIb trial.

Results.—A significantly greater percentage of patients treated with 10 mg/kg abatacept met the American College of Rheumatology 20% improvement criteria (achieved an ACR20 response) at 1 year compared with patients who received placebo (62.6% versus 36.1%; $P < 0.001$). Greater percentages of patients treated with 10 mg/kg abatacept also achieved ACR50 responses (41.7% versus 20.2%; $P < 0.001$) and ACR70 responses (20.9% versus 7.6%; $P = 0.003$) compared with patients who received placebo. For patients treated with 10 mg/kg abatacept, there were also statistically significant and clinically important improvements in modified Health Assessment

Questionnaire scores compared with patients who received placebo (49.6% versus 27.7%; $P < 0.001$). Abatacept at a dosage of 10 mg/kg elicited an increase in rates of remission (Disease Activity Score in 28 joints of <2.6) compared with placebo at 1 year (34.8% versus 10.1%; $P < 0.001$). The incidence of adverse events was comparable between the groups, and no significant formation of neutralizing antibodies was noted.

Conclusion.—Abatacept was associated with significant reductions in disease activity and improvements in physical function that were maintained over the course of 12 months in patients with RA that had remained active despite MTX treatment. Abatacept was found to be well tolerated and safe over the course of 1 year. Abatacept in combination with MTX has the potential to play an important role in future RA therapy.

▶ When an antigen-presenting cell encounters a T cell, several interactions need to occur for an immune response to take place. The first, of course, is the antigen presentation itself, with an antigen, ensconced in a major histocompatibility complex (MHC) molecule, being offered to the T cell's antigen receptor. But a group of side events, termed "co-stimulation," must also occur between the 2 cells, essentially to signal to the T cell that this is a serious interaction that ought to result in a response. One such costimulatory event is that between a CD80 or CD86 molecule on the antigen-presenting cell, and a CD28 molecule on the T cell surface. These interactions can be abrogated by the presence of CTLA4, a molecule that is normally expressed on T cells late in the antigen-presentation cycle and binds to CD80/CD86 with far more avidity than CD28. Like a more handsome suitor at a debutante ball, CTLA-4 "cuts in," to "dance" with CD80/CD86 and block the interaction between that molecule and CD28. Given its late appearance, it is likely that CTLA-4 in nature is intended to interrupt, or downregulate, the T cell-antigen-presenting cell relationship after it has already been established. However, investigators have now attempted to exploit the high avidity of CTLA-4, by generating a more stable, infusible form of CTLA-4 (actually, the extracellular portion of CTLA-4) complexed to the Fc portion of an IgG1 immunoglobulin, modified to prevent complement activation (CTLA-4Ig). In last year's YEAR BOOK, we included a report on the 6 month safety and efficacy of this molecule in RA patients who had failed MTX; this year, we are including the 12 month follow-up on the same study.

A total of 339 patients with RA were selected randomly to receive placebo, abatacept 2 mg/kg, or abatacept 10 mg/kg by infusion, in addition to their usual stable doses of MTX. Patients were allowed to also receive stable, but low doses of prednisone in the first 6 months of the study; in the second 6 months, some adjustments of other RA medications was permitted. The primary end point was improvement in ACR 20, with secondary end points including ACR 50, ACR 70, DAS (Disease Activity Score), mHAQ (modified Health Assessment Questionnaire), and so on. For the 10-mg/kg dose, the results were impressive early, and persisted late into the study: significant ACR 20 responses (range of about 60%, vs about 30% for placebo); significant ACR 50 and 70 responses (40 and 25%, respectively, vs 20 and 5% for placebo), and significant improvement in DAS, mHAQ and other indicators. Moreover, improvement in ACR scores was observed across all parameters measured (objective physical exam, laboratory evidence of systemic inflammation, and physician and patient assessments). Equally impressive was the fact that a significant proportion of patients achieved disease remission as measured by the DAS; given that all of these patients had previously had an inadequate response to MTX, it might have been expected that some of their symptoms were due to irremediable joint damage. The benefits of abatacept did not decline over the course of the study, and in some cases actually appeared to continue to improve. Moreover, abatacept, at least in this relatively small cohort, appeared to be safe, with no more serious adverse events than were seen in the placebo group. However, the 2-mg/kg dose, identified in a previous study as potentially useful, turned out to be not significantly different than placebo in treating RA. Moreover, this study did not address whether structural integrity of the joints was preserved by abatacept, which will be an important question for future studies to address.

Despite the tremendous advances in RA therapy achieved through TNF inhibition, new therapies continue to be badly needed. Some patients simply do not respond adequately to TNF blockade, while others cannot tolerate it, or have serious adverse events. The use of costimulatory blockade via CTLA-4Ig is showing true promise, and CTLA-4Ig may well be the next RA biological to come to market. Many questions remain, of course, for example about the long-term efficacy, the potential long-term side effects, and whether CTLA-4IG ought to be given instead of, or perhaps even in conjunction with, a TNF inhibitor. These questions should all be answerable in time, and our patients may find themselves with a better, or at least, a useful new option, for the management of their RA.

M. H. Pillinger, MD

Abatacept for Rheumatoid Arthritis Refractory to Tumor Necrosis Factor α Inhibition

Genovese MC, Becker J-C, Schiff M, et al (Stanford Univ, Calif; Bristol-Myers Squibb, Princeton, NJ; Denver Arthritis Clinic; et al)

N Engl J Med 353:1114-1123, 2005 2–3

Background.—A substantial number of patients with rheumatoid arthritis have an inadequate or unsustained response to tumor necrosis factor α (TNF-α) inhibitors. We conducted a randomized, double-blind, phase 3 trial to evaluate the efficacy and safety of abatacept, a selective costimulation modulator, in patients with active rheumatoid arthritis and an inadequate response to at least three months of anti–TNF-αtherapy.

Methods.—Patients with active rheumatoid arthritis and an inadequate response to anti–TNF-αtherapy were randomly assigned in a 2:1 ratio to receive abatacept or placebo on days 1, 15, and 29 and every 28 days thereafter for 6 months, in addition to at least one disease-modifying antirheumatic drug. Patients discontinued anti–TNF-αtherapy before randomization. The rates of American College of Rheumatology (ACR) 20 responses (indicating a clinical improvement of 20 percent or greater) and improvement in functional disability, as reflected by scores for the Health Assessment Questionnaire (HAQ) disability index, were assessed.

Results.—After six months, the rates of ACR 20 responses were 50.4 percent in the abatacept group and 19.5 percent in the placebo group ($P<0.001$); the respective rates of ACR 50 and ACR 70 responses were also significantly higher in the abatacept group than in the placebo group (20.3 percent vs. 3.8 percent, $P<0.001$; and 10.2 percent vs. 1.5 percent, $P=0.003$). At six months, significantly more patients in the abatacept group than in the placebo group had a clinically meaningful improvement in physical function, as reflected by an improvement from baseline of at least 0.3 in the HAQ disability index (47.3 percent vs. 23.3 percent, $P<0.001$). The incidence of adverse events and peri-infusional adverse events was 79.5 percent and 5.0 percent, respectively, in the abatacept group and 71.4 percent and 3.0 percent, respectively, in the placebo group. The incidence of serious infections was 2.3 percent in each group.

Conclusions.—Abatacept produced significant clinical and functional benefits in patients who had had an inadequate response to anti–TNF-αtherapy.

► If abatacept works about as well as TNF inhibitors, one question that comes up is, "when should we use abatacept in our patients with rheumatoid arthritis?" The cautious approach that many physicians take to new drugs is to reserve the new agent for those patients who have failed more standard therapy. In this case, that would imply using abatacept in the setting of anti–TNF-α failure. But will abatacept work in such patients? Genovese et al studied 738 patients with an eye to finding out. All patients had failed 1, or possibly 2 anti–TNF-α agents, though the patients varied between those who were still on their anti–TNF-α agent at the time of entry to the study (a washout period was then required) and those who had already discontinued it. Abatacept proved somewhat to very efficacious in a meaningful proportion of those patients, as measured by ACR 20, 50, and 70 scores, as well as by disease activity score. While the numbers were meaningful, the degree of response was roughly the same as could be obtained by switching patients from one anti–TNF-α agent (that they had failed) to another.

Abatacept also worked about as well in patients who had failed 2 anti–TNF-α agents as in those who had only failed 1. These data give us important information. First, they offer us a possible alternative for patients for whom anti–TNF-α therapy does not work. We also learn from this study that as we begin to use abatacept on our patients, a cautious approach, while warranted, may yield less-impressive results than we will see later on as we begin to consider abatacept for first-line therapy. Finally, these results tell us that, however useful abatacept proves to be, it is unlikely to solve all our rheumatoid arthritis treatment problems. There is much more work still to be done.

M. H. Pillinger, MD

Preclinical Carotid Atherosclerosis in Patients With Rheumatoid Arthritis

Roman MJ, Moeller E, Davis A, et al (Cornell Univ, New York; Rogosin Inst, New York; SUNY–Stony Brook, NY)

Ann Intern Med 144:249-256, 2006 2–4

Background.—Rheumatoid arthritis is associated with increased morbidity and mortality because of cardiovascular disease, independent of traditional risk factors.

Objective.—To determine the prevalence of preclinical atherosclerosis in patients with rheumatoid arthritis and to identify clinical and biological markers for atherosclerotic disease in this patient population.

Design.—Matched, cross-sectional study.

Setting.—Hospital for Special Surgery in New York City.

Patients.—98 consecutive outpatients with rheumatoid arthritis who were followed by rheumatologists and 98 controls matched on age, sex, and ethnicity.

Measurements.—Cardiovascular risk factor ascertainment and carotid ultrasonography in all participants; disease severity, disease treatment, and inflammatory markers in patients with rheumatoid arthritis.

Results.—Despite a more favorable risk factor profile, patients with rheumatoid arthritis had a 3-fold increase in carotid atherosclerotic plaque (44% vs. 15%; $P < 0.001$). The relationship between rheumatoid arthritis and carotid atherosclerotic plaque remained after accounting for age, serum cholesterol levels, smoking history, and hypertensive status; adjusted predicted prevalence was 7.4% (95% CI, 3.4% to 15.2%) for the control group and 38.5% (CI, 25.4% to 53.5%) for patients with rheumatoid arthritis. Age ($P < 0.001$) and current cigarette use ($P < 0.014$) were also significantly associated with carotid atherosclerotic plaque. Among patients with rheumatoid arthritis, atherosclerosis was related to age, hypertension status, and use of tumor necrosis factor-α inhibitors (a possible marker of disease severity).

Limitations.—The study had a cross-sectional design, and inflammatory markers were determined only once.

Conclusions.—Patients with rheumatoid arthritis have a high prevalence of preclinical atherosclerosis independent of traditional risk factors, suggesting that chronic inflammation and, possibly, disease severity are atherogenic in this population.

► It is now appreciated that, even setting aside traditional risk factors, patients with rheumatoid arthritis are at increased risk of dying of cardiovascular disease when compared with the general population. Other rheumatologic diseases, including lupus and antiphospholipid syndrome, carry similar or even greater increases in risk, suggesting that chronic inflammation plays a role in the progression to occluded arteries. However, the characteristics of the risk, as well as the nature of the process leading to occlusion, remain poorly established.

Roman et al studied 98 patients with rheumatoid arthritis, compared with 98 age-matched, sex-matched, and ethnically matched historical controls selected from a previously conducted hypertension study. Data were collected on the prevalence of carotid artherosclerosis, detected by carotid US. Both the presence of plaque and the degree of intimal medial thickening were determined. Select clinical and biologic markers were also measured, to determine their predictive value. The control population was not a perfect match for the rheumatoid patients, since the control group at baseline was enriched in both smoking history and hypertension. Nonetheless, patients with rheumatoid arthritis more frequently demonstrated carotid plaque (44% vs 15%), supporting that rheumatoid arthritis is a risk factor for vascular disease. Using a multivariate logistic regression analysis incorporating disease status, age, hypertension, current cigarette use, and total serum cholesterol, the authors confirmed rheumatoid arthritis as an independent risk factor for the presence of carotid plaque.

The authors next compared rheumatoid arthritis patients with and without plaque in an attempt to identify class differences between the 2 subgroups. Rheumatoid patients with plaque were older, had higher systolic blood pressure, and had higher total cholesterol, low-density lipoprotein cholesterol, and serum homocysteine levels compared with rheumatoid patients without plaque. After adjusting for all of these factors, the only parameter that remained statistically significant between rheumatoid patients with and without plaque was use of a tumor necrosis factor (TNF) inhibitor, which was more frequent in the patients with plaque. Whether anti-TNF use represents an independent risk factor, or is itself simply a marker of more severe disease, was not determined.

It is interesting to compare the findings of this report with those of a previous study by the same authors,[1] measuring carotid plaque in patients with systemic lupus. Both studies confirmed an increase in plaque concordant with the presence of disease, but both also revealed a decrease in intimal-medial thickening in patients with active disease compared with controls. Since intimal-medial thickening typically precedes plaque in the genesis of atherosclerosis, one would have expected that intimal-medial thickening should be present in most patients with plaque. Does the inverse relationship between plaque and intimal-medial thickening tell us that the process of atherosclerosis is different in rheumatic diseases than in other situations? Another interesting finding in both studies was that inflammatory markers did not correlate with the presence of plaque, suggesting that it may not be the inflammatory processes in rheumatic diseases that cause atherosclerosis. These studies remind us of the importance of screening for atherosclerosis in patients with rheumatic diseases. They also remind us of how little we know about the processes that cause atherosclerosis to develop.

P. I. Izmirly, MD

Reference

1. Roman MJ, Shanker BA, Davis A, et al: Prevalence and correlates of accelerated atherosclerosis in systemic lupus erythematosus. *N Engl J Med* 349:2399-2406, 2003.

Leflunomide or Methotrexate for Juvenile Rheumatoid Arthritis

Silverman E, for the Leflunomide in Juvenile Rheumatoid Arthritis (JRA) Investigator Group (Univ of Toronto; et al)

N Engl J Med 352:1655-1666, 2005 2–5

Background.—We compared the safety and efficacy of leflunomide with that of methotrexate in the treatment of polyarticular juvenile rheumatoid arthritis in a multinational, randomized, controlled trial.

Methods.—Patients 3 to 17 years of age received leflunomide or methotrexate for 16 weeks in a double-dummy, blinded fashion, followed by a 32-week blinded extension. The rates of American College of Rheumatology Pediatric 30 percent responses (ACR Pedi 30) and the Percent Improvement Index were assessed at baseline and every 4 weeks for 16 weeks and every 8 weeks during the 32-week extension study.

Results.—Of 94 patients randomized, 86 completed 16 weeks of treatment, 70 of whom entered the extension study. At week 16, more patients in the methotrexate group than in the leflunomide group had an ACR Pedi 30 response (89 percent vs. 68 percent, $P=0.02$), whereas the values for the Percent Improvement Index did not differ significantly (−52.87 percent vs. −44.41 percent, $P=0.18$). In both groups, the improvements achieved at week 16 were maintained at week 48. The most common adverse events in both groups included gastrointestinal symptoms, headache, and nasopharyngeal symptoms. Aminotransferase elevations were more frequent with methotrexate than with leflunomide during the initial study and the extension study.

Conclusions.—In patients with polyarticular juvenile rheumatoid arthritis, methotrexate and leflunomide both resulted in high rates of clinical improvement, but the rate was slightly greater for methotrexate. At the doses used in this study, methotrexate was more effective than leflunomide.

▶ The treatment of inflammatory arthritis in children invokes a unique set of questions, problems and limitations. As a result, new treatments often trickle down to children only after they have been deemed safe and effective in the adult population. Even then, questions about pediatric toxicity, and pediatric usefulness (including the fact that juvenile arthritis comes with a different set of categories, and clinical pictures, than adult RA), lead most pediatric rheumatologists to be appropriately conservative and cautious in their use of the drugs. In this study, Silverman et al provide important and useful information on the pediatric use of 2 of the mainstays of therapy of adult RA. They performed a 16-week, double-blinded trial of methotrexate vs leflunomide for juvenile polyarticular arthritis, followed by a 32-week blinded extension. Both drugs were dosed according to body weight (methotrexate on a continuous scale, leflunomide by categories), with the outcomes being standard ones for pediatric arthritis (ACR Pedi 30 and Percent Improvement Index as primary outcomes, and ACR Pedi 50, 70 and others as secondary outcomes). The results were encouraging: children in both groups did extremely well. At 16 weeks, the Percent Improvement Index was similar in both groups (44 ± 4% for leflunomide, 53 ± 4% improvement for methotrexate). Both groups of patients also did well as measured by ACR Pedi 30, with the methotrexate group having a slightly but significantly better response (89% vs 68%); on this latter basis, the authors conclude that methotrexate was more efficacious than leflunomide. Even more impressive were the ACR Pedi 50 and 70 responses, which were 60% and 75% (leflunomide vs methotrexate), and 43% and 60% (leflunomide vs methotrexate), respectively. At the end of the 32-week extension, the benefits of both drugs persisted, though the differences between methotrexate and leflunomide were ablated. Both drugs were about equally safe, though there were more liver function test (LFT) abnormalities in the methotrexate group, and more serious adverse events in the leflunomide group (1 case of salmonellosis, 1 case of seriously elevated LFTs, 1 case of parapsoriasis).

This study provides important and useful information, supporting that both drugs are generally safe, and generally effective in juvenile arthritis, at least during a period of 48 weeks. That methotrexate appeared to have some efficacy advantage over leflunomide will need to be confirmed in future studies, since the dosing of the 2 drugs was slightly different (methotrexate was probably dosed a bit more aggressively), and the longer-term (48-week performance) of the 2 drugs was roughly comparable. Because this study was a study of early arthritis, the efficacy of leflunomide in more established arthritis will need to be confirmed (at least 1 study with methotrexate already suggests that it is useful in established arthritis, though probably less efficacious than was seen in the current report). Finally, it is worth noting that this study included patients with all of the categories of juvenile arthritis (ANA-positive, pauciarticular, polyarticular (both RF-positive and negative), and systemic), as well as children in a variety of different age ranges (3-17 years). Whether optimizing therapy with either methotrexate or leflunomide (or another agent entirely) will require that we stratify the patients, before deciding on 1 drug or another, remains to be determined.

M. H. Pillinger, MD

Cell-based Immunotherapy With Suppressor CD8$^+$ T Cells in Rheumatoid Arthritis

Davila E, Kang YM, Park YW, et al (Emory Univ, Atlanta, Ga)
J Immunol 174:7292-7301, 2005 2–6

Introduction.—The chronic persistence of rheumatoid synovitis, an inflammation driven by activated T cells, macrophages, and fibroblasts causing irreversible joint damage, suggests a failure in physiologic mechanisms that down-regulate and terminate chronic immune responses. In vitro $CD8^+CD28^-CD56^+$ T cells tolerize APCs, prevent the priming of naive $CD4^+$ T cells, and suppress memory $CD4^+$ T cell responses. Therefore, we generated $CD8^+CD28^-CD56^+$ T cell clones from synovial tissues, expanded them in vitro, and adoptively transferred them into NOD-SCID mice engrafted with synovial tissues from patients with rheumatoid arthritis. Adoptively transferred $CD8^+CD28^-CD56^+$ T cells displayed strong anti-inflammatory activity. They inhibited production of IFN-γ, TNF-α, and chemokines in autologous and HLA class I-matched heterologous synovitis. Down-regulation of costimulatory ligands CD80 and CD86 on synovial fibroblasts was identified as one mechanism of immunosuppression. We propose that rheumatoid synovitis can be suppressed by cell-based immunotherapy with immunoregulatory $CD8^+$ T cells.

► I've included this very basic research article as a YEAR BOOK selection for 2 reasons. First, it provides some very interesting insights into the regulation of immune response, and second, it uses an interesting, and highly relevant, model of rheumatoid arthritis (RA) to test the potential efficacy of a cell-based immunomodulatory therapy that may well be the first step in applying such therapies to clinical use.

The authors first used classic, in vitro immunology techniques to isolate and culture a specific class of CD8 T cells with immunosuppressive capacity. The literature is replete, at present, with articles documenting that CD8 cells may both stimulate and inhibit immune responses; the current study would seem to settle that question, by showing that while most CD8 cells are proimmune, this particular subset, characterized by the presence of CD56 but a lack of CD28, are capable of potently downregulating the antigen-stimulated proliferation of CD4 cells. The effect of these T suppressor (Ts) cells on the CD4 cells is antigen-specific, and depends upon both the CD4 cells and the Ts cells undergoing exposure to antigen. Moreover, the CD4 and Ts cells must match as regards major histocompatibility complex (MHC) class I (but not MHC class II), and must make contact, indicating that the suppressive effect of the Ts cells is quite specific, and suggesting that it might be possible to generate a Ts-based therapy that would affect only the desired target without generally inhibiting the immune response.

The authors next turn to a unique RA animal model, in which human RA synovium is engrafted into immunodeficient mice. Thus, the authors can perform "human" trials in an animal model, without the risk to their human subjects. When the appropriate, MHC class I-matched Ts cells were infused, there was a significant improvement in the rheumatoid lesion, including loss of T-cell infiltrates, as well as loss of cytokine and chemokine production. In addition, interesting effects were observed on fibroblast-like synovial cells (FLS), which have been shown by some authors to have antigen-presenting capacity in RA. In these studies, the infusion of the Ts cells led to a downregulation of costimulatory molecules on FLS, suggesting the possibility that Ts cells may actually lead, not merely to suppression of immunity, but to tolerance.

The take-home message? The human organism is possessed of the capacity to regulate its own immunity and inflammation. If we can find appropriate targets and technologies to exploit these innate suppressive capacities, we may find better, and more specific, ways to treat our patients with autoimmune diseases. This study by Davila et al appears to be a step in the right direction.

M. H. Pillinger, MD

3 Systemic Lupus Erythematosus

Mycophenolate Mofetil or Intravenous Cyclophosphamide for Lupus Nephritis

Ginzler EM, Dooley MA, Aranow C, et al (State Univ of New York, Brooklyn; Univ of North Carolina, Chapel Hill; Albert Einstein College of Medicine, Bronx, NY; et al)

N Engl J Med 353:2219-2228, 2005 3–1

Background.—Since anecdotal series and small, prospective, controlled trials suggest that mycophenolate mofetil may be effective for treating lupus nephritis, larger trials are desirable.

Methods.—We conducted a 24-week randomized, open-label, noninferiority trial comparing oral mycophenolate mofetil (initial dose, 1000 mg per day, increased to 3000 mg per day) with monthly intravenous cyclophosphamide (0.5 g per square meter of body-surface area, increased to 1.0 g per square meter) as induction therapy for active lupus nephritis. A change to the alternative regimen was allowed at 12 weeks in patients who did not have an early response. The study protocol specified adjunctive care and the use and tapering of corticosteroids. The primary end point was complete remission at 24 weeks (normalization of abnormal renal measurements and maintenance of baseline normal measurements). A secondary end point was partial remission at 24 weeks.

Results.—Of 140 patients recruited, 71 were randomly assigned to receive mycophenolate mofetil and 69 were randomly assigned to receive cyclophosphamide. At 12 weeks, 56 patients receiving mycophenolate mofetil and 42 receiving cyclophosphamide had satisfactory early responses. In the intention-to-treat analysis, 16 of the 71 patients (22.5 percent) receiving mycophenolate mofetil and 4 of the 69 patients receiving cyclophosphamide (5.8 percent) had complete remission, for an absolute difference of 16.7 percentage points (95 percent confidence interval, 5.6 to 27.9 percentage points; P=0.005), meeting the prespecified criteria for noninferiority and demonstrating the superiority of mycophenolate mofetil to cyclophosphamide. Partial remission occurred in 21 of the 71 patients (29.6 percent) and 17 of the 69 patients (24.6 percent), respectively (P=0.51). Three patients assigned to cyclophosphamide died, two during protocol therapy. Fewer severe infections and hospitalizations but more diarrhea occurred among those receiving mycophenolate.

Conclusions.—In this 24-week trial, mycophenolate mofetil was more effective than intravenous cyclophosphamide in inducing remission of lupus nephritis and had a more favorable safety profile.

▶ To paraphrase Franklin Roosevelt, the only thing we have to fear more than cyclophosphamide for lupus nephritis is lupus nephritis itself. This alkylating agent, which has been the gold standard for lupus nephritis therapy for more than a decade, is neither universally efficacious nor benign. Toxicities of cyclophosphamide include nausea, vomiting, alopecia, infertility, cystitis, bladder cancer, marrow suppression, hematologic malignancy, and infection, including potentially life-threatening infections. No one would use ever use cyclophosphamide if there were any better alternative. Now, at last, it begins to appear that there might be.

Based on some small but encouraging studies, Ginzler et al set out to test the hypothesis that mycophenolate mofetil, an antipurinergic drug used commonly to prevent transplant rejection, would be at least as good as cyclophosphamide in lupus nephritis. Working as an investigator-initiated study, the Ginzler group recruited 140 patients with active and usually severe lupus nephritis, and treated either with a standard cyclophosphamide regimen (0.5 g/m^2 of body surface area, advancing to 1 g/m^2) or mycophenolate mofetil (1000 mg/d, advancing as tolerated to 3 g/d). All patients also received oral prednisone at 1 mg/kg. The results were impressive. After 12 weeks, 79% in the mycophenolate mofetil group, but only 61% in the cyclophosphamide group, met the criteria for early response to therapy. Moreover, 23% of the mycophenolate mofetil patients, but only 6% of the cyclophosphamide therapy patients, met the preestablished criteria for complete remission. After 24 weeks, the treatment failure rates (neither partial or complete remission, nor failure to complete the study) were 49% for the mycophenolate mofetil group versus 70% for the cyclophosphamide group. The authors thus concluded that mycophenolate mofetil was not only not inferior to cyclophosphamide in these studies, it was actually superior. Moreover, it was also much less toxic. Severe infections were seen almost exclusively in the cyclophosphamide group, where they were common (12 severe infections in the cyclophosphamide group vs 1 in the mycophenolate mofetil group). Cytopenias, alopecia, and menstrual irregularities were also much more common in the cyclophosphamide group. Ominously, 2 deaths occurred in the cyclophosphamide group but none in the mycophenolate mofetil group.

These results have all the earmarks of a major breakthrough in lupus treatment. True, the study has limitations, as the authors readily admit; these include the fact that the trial was not blinded to therapy, and that the duration of the study doesn't permit us to draw any conclusions about the long-term outcome (clearly the most important end point) of mycophenolate mofetil therapy. We also don't yet reliably know whether mycophenolate mofetil will be as efficacious as cyclophosphamide for other aspects of lupus (eg, CNS lupus). And while mycophenolate mofetil was better than cyclophosphamide, it was far from perfectly effective, with many patients failing treatment. Still, if this drug is even nearly as good as cyclophosphamide, its apparently improved safety profile will make it the therapy of choice for most cases. For now, I suspect many rheumatologists will begin to use mycophenolate mofetil in patients who have failed, or failed to tolerate cyclophosphamide; academic rheumatologists who have already been using the drug in that manner may find they have a lower threshold for embracing such a strategy. But if even a few more studies come out in favor of mycophenolate mofetil, the day may not be far off when it, rather than cyclophosphamide, is the first-line therapy for our patients with severe and active lupus.

M. H. Pillinger, MD

The Effect of Combined Estrogen and Progesterone Hormone Replacement Therapy on Disease Activity in Systemic Lupus Erythematosus: A Randomized Trial

Buyon JP, Petri MA, Kim MY, et al (New York Univ; Johns Hopkins Univ, Baltimore, Md)

Ann Intern Med 142:953-962, 2005 3–2

Background.—There is concern that exogenous female hormones may worsen disease activity in women with systemic lupus erythematosus (SLE).

Objective.—To evaluate the effect of hormone replacement therapy (HRT) on disease activity in postmenopausal women with SLE.

Design.—Randomized, double-blind, placebo-controlled noninferiority trial conducted from March 1996 to June 2002.

Setting.—16 university-affiliated rheumatology clinics or practices in 11 U.S. states.

Patients.—351 menopausal patients (mean age, 50 years) with inactive (81.5%) or stable-active (18.5%) SLE. Interventions: 12 months of treatment with active drug (0.625 mg of conjugated estrogen daily, plus 5 mg of medroxyprogesterone for 12 days per month) or placebo. The 12-month follow-up rate was 82% for the HRT group and 87% for the placebo group.

Measurements.—The primary end point was occurrence of a severe flare as defined by Safety of Estrogens in Lupus Erythematosus, National Assessment-Systemic Lupus Erythematosus Disease Activity Index composite.

Results.—Severe flare was rare in both treatment groups: The 12-month severe flare rate was 0.081 for the HRT group and 0.049 for the placebo group, yielding an estimated difference of 0.033 ($P = 0.23$). The upper limit of the 1-sided 95% CI for the treatment difference was 0.078, within the prespecified margin of 9% for noninferiority. Mild to moderate flares were significantly increased in the HRT group: 1.14 flares/person-year for HRT and 0.86 flare/person-year for placebo (relative risk, 1.34; $P = 0.01$). The probability of any type of flare by 12 months was 0.64 for the HRT group and 0.51 for the placebo group ($P = 0.01$). In the HRT group, there were 1 death, 1 stroke, 2 cases of deep venous thrombosis, and 1 case of thrombosis

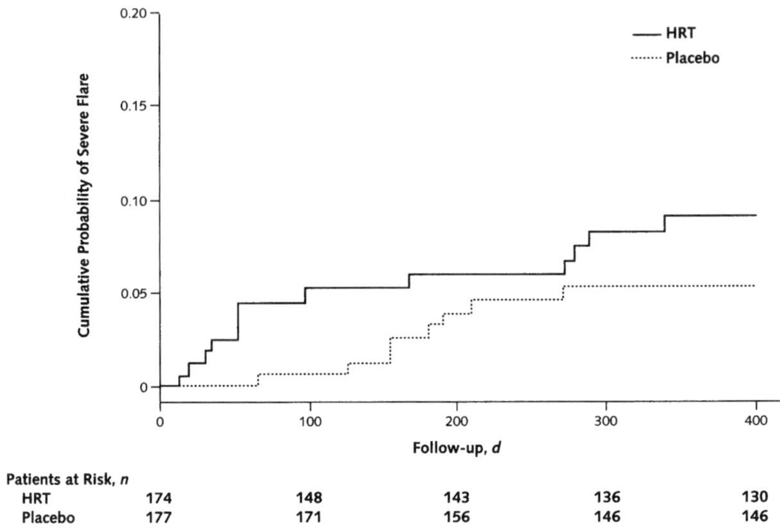

FIGURE 2.—Kaplan-Meier estimates of the cumulative probability of severe flare for patients in the hormone replacement therapy (*HRT*) and placebo groups. *Note:* The difference between treatment groups in the 12-month severe flare rate is 0.033 $P = 0.023$). (Courtesy of Buyon JP, Petri MA, Kim MY, et al: The effect of combined estrogen and progesterone hormone replacement therapy on disease activity in systemic lupus erythematosus: A randomized trial. *Ann Intern Med* 142:953-962, 2005.)

in an arteriovenous graft; in the placebo group, 1 patient developed deep venous thrombosis.

Limitations.—Findings are not generalizable to women with high-titer anticardiolipin antibodies, lupus anticoagulant, or previous thrombosis.

Conclusions.—Adding a short course of HRT is associated with a small risk for increasing the natural flare rate of lupus. Most of these flares are mild to moderate. The benefits of HRT can be balanced against the risk for flare because HRT did not significantly increase the risk for severe flare compared with placebo (Fig 2).

► The striking female predominance of SLE has led to the inevitable assumption that estrogenic hormones may play a role in either the pathogenesis or the exacerbation of SLE, and multiple studies have tended to support this position. That SLE onset is typically after onset of menarche; that oophorectomy reduces SLE severity in mouse models; and that estrogens augment B-cell survival and autoreactivity—all are consistent with this point of view. The human data, however, are not sufficient to be entirely convincing. And if estrogen plays a role in SLE, how big a role is it? Are all levels of estrogen potentially harmful in SLE, or are some levels safe? And what effect would the use of progesterone have on any specific estrogen effect?

Set against the potential harm of estrogen is its potential benefit to patients with SLE. SLE patients often have premature menopause, relating to disease and/or therapy with cyclophosphamide. The vasomotor symptoms of menopause can be particularly distressing in young women who are already psychologically stressed by both their illness and their loss of fertility. Moreover, SLE patients are at increased risk for osteoporosis, a disease particularly remediable to HRT. We are all aware, by now of the recent studies that indicate that long-term hormone supplementation may increase cardiovascular risk. Whether short-term perimenopausal use (which may both ameliorate vasomotor signals and have potentially durable benefit for bone density) is equally harmful is not yet clear. If SLE patients could take HRT without exacerbating their disease, many might benefit from short-term HRT.

In this exceptionally elegant, exceptionally rigorous study, Buyon et al provide the most complete clinical information to date on HRT and SLE. They enrolled 153 female patients with SLE in a double-blind placebo-controlled trial of daily conjugated estrogen (0.625 mg), together with medroxyprogesterone (5 mg) on days 1 to 12 of the month. The end points—severe flares (primary end point), and mild to moderate flares (secondary end points)—were carefully defined, and rigorously documented (interinstitutional consistency on the scoring instruments used was tested repeatedly, as was the success of the blinding process.) Patients at high risk for thrombosis, except those with anticardiolipin syndrome, were excluded.

The results were generally heartening. Severe flares were rare in both groups, and although the HRT group had a higher number of severe flares than the placebo group (7.5% vs 4.5%), the difference did not reach statistical significance. Patients getting HRT did have a significantly greater rate of mild to moderate flares, though again the difference was not large (59% vs 50% of patients). And the overall disease activity index did not differ between the 2 groups.

These data tell us something about biology: that low to moderate doses of estrogen may not induce SLE activity (though the data also suggest that higher doses may be a different question, and one that these same authors are addressing by looking at the effects of birth control pills in a separate study). The data also tell us something about our clinical practice: that it is probably relatively safe to go ahead carefully with HRT in stable, perimenopausal SLE patients, when such therapy is strongly indicated. Whether such a strategy is advisable will be up to individual physicians. Perhaps future studies will determine its utility, particularly, because the current study was not designed to assess cardiovascular disease, the major bad outcome of HRT.

M. H. Pillinger, MD

4 Fibromyalgia and Other Soft Tissue Musculoskeletal Problems

A Randomized Clinical Trial of Acupuncture Compared With Sham Acupuncture in Fibromyalgia

Assefi NP, Sherman KJ, Jacobsen C, et al (Univ of Washington, Seattle)

Ann Intern Med 143:10-19, 2005 4–1

Background.—Fibromyalgia is a common chronic pain condition for which patients frequently use acupuncture.

Objective.—To determine whether acupuncture relieves pain in fibromyalgia.

Design.—Randomized, sham-controlled trial in which participants, data collection staff, and data analysts were blinded to treatment group.

Setting.—Private acupuncture offices in the greater Seattle, Washington, metropolitan area.

Patients.—100 adults with fibromyalgia.

Intervention.—Twice-weekly treatment for 12 weeks with an acupuncture program that was specifically designed to treat fibromyalgia, or 1 of 3 sham acupuncture treatments: acupuncture for an unrelated condition, needle insertion at nonacupoint locations, or noninsertive simulated acupuncture.

Measurements.—The primary outcome was subjective pain as measured by a 10-cm visual analogue scale ranging from 0 (no pain) to 10 (worst pain ever). Measurements were obtained at baseline; 1, 4, 8, and 12 weeks of treatment; and 3 and 6 months after completion of treatment. Participant blinding and adverse effects were ascertained by self-report. The primary outcomes were evaluated by pooling the 3 sham-control groups and comparing them with the group that received acupuncture to treat fibromyalgia.

Results.—The mean subjective pain rating among patients who received acupuncture for fibromyalgia did not differ from that in the pooled sham acupuncture group (mean between-group difference, 0.5 cm [95% CI, −0.3 cm to 1.2 cm]). Participant blinding was adequate throughout the trial, and no serious adverse effects were noted.

Limitations.—A prescription of acupuncture at fixed points may differ from acupuncture administered in clinical settings, in which therapy is individualized and often combined with herbal supplementation and other adjunctive measures. A usual-care comparison group was not studied.

Conclusion.—Acupuncture was no better than sham acupuncture at relieving pain in fibromyalgia.

► Does acupuncture work for anything? Does anything work for fibromyalgia? Regular readers of the YEAR BOOK will note that we have reviewed both of these questions in prior volumes, often with conflicting results. In this case, Assefi et al have conducted an excellent, rigorous study of the use of acupuncture for fibromyalgia. They compared acupuncture for fibromyalgia against 3 control techniques. In one, the control patients received real acupuncture but in a distribution ostensibly suitable for a different medical problem (irregular menses). In another, the control patients received sham acupuncture, that is, needle insertion, but at points that do not correspond to any known acupuncture sites. A third group of control patients received toothpick pricks, without needle insertions, at the sites deemed appropriate for actual acupuncture. Extensive care was taken to blind the patients to the treatment they received, and to confirm successful blinding. In this setting, a study of 100 patients revealed no differences in pain, fatigue, and functional scales between the true acupuncture and control groups. Thus, it would appear that the specific placing of acupuncture needles has no benefit in fibromyalgia.

There are several limitations to this study, including the fact that the control groups were analyzed collectively, rather than separately, in comparison with the treatment group. One would like to know, for instance, whether the treatment group was, in fact, better than any one of the control groups (the nonacupuncture group, for example, or the group getting needles in all the wrong places). Also, it must be noted that the study was probably too small to detect subtle differences in response. Still, the study is convincing: acupuncture, per se, does not seem any better than its placebo equivalents. Acupuncture advocates may argue that this study was suboptimal, to the extent that acupuncture must be individualized to every patient, rather than using a standard regimen. Such an objection, even if legitimate, would be almost unanswerable in a scientific study, because it would be virtually impossible to control for a procedure that was different in every patient. What may be most interesting in the current study, though, is the value of placebo, because patients in all groups actually had some improvement in pain, fatigue, and functional scores early in the study. Because these effects did not depend upon the placement of the needles, they may have related to patient expectations, the relaxing and/or reassuring effect of the experience per se, or some other intangible. Because acupuncture is rarely harmful, rheumatologists may or may not elect to refer their fibromyalgia patients, if only for the placebo effect; but we would probably do at least as well, if not better, to pay attention to the ways in which we provide emotional support, encouragement, and hope to sufferers of this difficult-to-manage syndrome.

M. H. Pillinger, MD

Pregabalin for the Treatment of Fibromyalgia Syndrome: Results of a Randomized, Double-blind, Placebo-controlled Trial

Crofford LJ, for the Pregabalin 1008-105 Study Group (Univ of Michigan, Ann Arbor; et al)

Arthritis Rheum 52:1264-1273, 2005 4–2

Objective.—Fibromyalgia syndrome (FMS) is characterized by widespread musculoskeletal pain and lowered pain threshold. Other prominent symptoms include disordered sleep and fatigue. FMS affects an estimated 2% of the population, predominantly women. This trial was designed to evaluate the efficacy and safety of pregabalin, a novel α_2-δ ligand, for treatment of symptoms associated with FMS.

Methods.—This multicenter, double-blind, 8-week, randomized clinical trial compared the effects of placebo with those of 150, 300, and 450 mg/day pregabalin on pain, sleep, fatigue, and health-related quality of life in 529 patients with FMS. The primary outcome variable was the comparison of end point mean pain scores, derived from daily diary ratings of pain intensity, between each of the pregabalin treatment groups and the placebo group.

Results.—Pregabalin at 450 mg/day significantly reduced the average severity of pain in the primary analysis compared with placebo (−0.93 on a 0-10 scale) ($P \leq 0.001$), and significantly more patients in this group had ≥50% improvement in pain at the end point (29%, versus 13% in the placebo group; $P = 0.003$). Pregabalin at 300 and 450 mg/day was associated with significant improvements in sleep quality, fatigue, and global measures of change. Pregabalin at 450 mg/day improved several domains of health-related quality of life. Dizziness and somnolence were the most frequent adverse events. Rates of discontinuation due to adverse events were similar across all 4 treatment groups.

Conclusion.—Pregabalin at 450 mg/day was efficacious for the treatment of FMS, reducing symptoms of pain, disturbed sleep, and fatigue compared with placebo. Pregabalin was well tolerated and improved global measures and health-related quality of life.

► The care of patients with fibromyalgia is as much a matter of management as it is of treatment. Exercise, behavior modification, and psychotherapeutic support all have a major role, as does the use of medications. But, as many rheumatologists will confirm, the use of medications to date has been a story of relative disappointment. Most medications have modest effects at best, and often lose their efficacy over time, requiring rheumatologists to rotate medications regularly or resort to polypharmacy to try to maintain patient well-being. Newer, better medications are very much needed.

Rheumatologists who regularly care for patients with fibromyalgia have been waiting for some time, and with some anticipation, for the outcome of a study testing a relatively new drug, pregabalin, for its usefulness in fibromyalgia. Pregabalin acts at α_2-δ sites on presynaptic calcium channels, reducing the release of several neurotransmitters, including glutamate, noradrenaline, and substance P (the antiepileptic gabapentin also has activity at these receptors). Because all of these neurotransmitters, particularly glutamate, have been implicated in fibromyalgia, a drug that can inhibit their release might hold promise for fibromyalgia patients.

This study by Crofford et al offers the first solid data that pregabalin may be useful, though not by any stretch is it a miracle cure. A total of 529 patients were enrolled to receive placebo or 150, 300 or 450 mg of pregabalin a day (in 3 divided doses). Patients were followed up for 8 weeks, for end points that included pain, sleep quality, fatigue, and health-related quality of life. In all of these categories, patients on the 450-mg dose showed statistically significant improvement up until week 7. In overall response, approximately 30% of patients on the 450-mg dose reported a 50% or better improvement, compared with that of 13% in the placebo group. A self-reported 50% response in patients with fibromyalgia is quite impressive, and for this smaller group of responsive patients, pregabalin must have seemed like manna from heaven. Patients in the lower-dose groups experienced lesser responses that did not always achieve statistical significance. Pregabalin was generally well tolerated, with mostly minor side effects like dizziness and drowsiness; these tended to resolve with continued use, although more people in the 450-mg group dropped out of the study owing to adverse effects. Of some concern is the fact that the effectiveness of pregabalin waned at 8 weeks, although the authors point out that this may be due to a variety of factors other than loss of efficacy, including issues relating to study design and general fluctuation of the disease.

Overall, these results are encouraging, and if they are supported by other studies, pregabalin may turn out to be about as good as, or perhaps even better than our currently available medications for fibromyalgia. Time and additional clinical trials will tell.

M. H. Pillinger, MD

Comparing Yoga, Exercise, and a Self-care Book for Chronic Low Back Pain: A Randomized, Controlled Trial

Sherman KJ, Cherkin DC, Erro J, et al (Group Health Cooperative, Seattle; Univ of Washington, Seattle)

Ann Intern Med 143:849-856, 2005 4–3

Background.—Chronic low back pain is a common problem that has only modestly effective treatment options.

Objective.—To determine whether yoga is more effective than conventional therapeutic exercise or a self-care book for patients with chronic low back pain.

Design.—Randomized, controlled trial.

Setting.—A nonprofit, integrated health care system.

Patients.—101 adults with chronic low back pain.

Intervention.—12-week sessions of yoga or conventional therapeutic exercise classes or a self-care book.

Measurements.—Primary outcomes were back-related functional status (modified 24-point Roland Disability Scale) and "bothersomeness" of pain (11-point numerical scale). The primary time point was 12 weeks. Clinically significant change was considered to be 2.5 points on the functional status scale and 1.5 points on the bothersomeness scale. Secondary outcomes were days of restricted activity, general health status, and medication use.

Results.—After adjustment for baseline values, back-related function in the yoga group was superior to the book and exercise groups at 12 weeks (yoga vs. book: mean difference, −3.4 [95% CI, −5.1 to −1.6] [$P < 0.001$]; yoga vs. exercise: mean difference, −1.8 [CI, −3.5 to −0.1] [$P = 0.034$]). No significant differences in symptom bothersomeness were found between any 2 groups at 12 weeks; at 26 weeks, the yoga group was superior to the book group with respect to this measure (mean difference, −2.2 [CI, −3.2 to −1.2]; $P < 0.001$). At 26 weeks, back-related function in the yoga group was superior to the book group (mean difference, −3.6 [CI, −5.4 to −1.8]; $P < 0.001$) (Fig 2).

Limitations.—Participants in this study were followed for only 26 weeks after randomization. Only 1 instructor delivered each intervention.

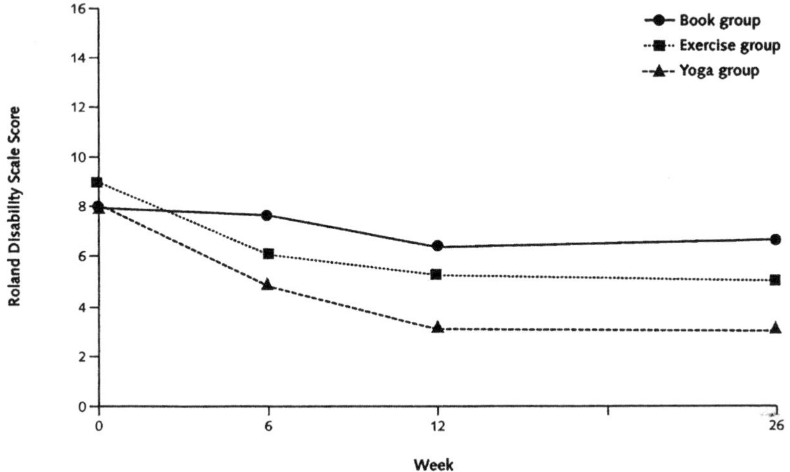

FIGURE 2.—Mean Roland Disability Scale scores at baseline, 12, and 26 weeks by treatment group. Classes ended at week 12. The x-axis signifies week after starting treatment. Higher scores signify greater disability. The *P* values for the omnibus *F* tests of any differences in mean Roland scores among the 3 treatment groups (derived from a linear regression model that was fitted to all follow-up time points, adjusting for baseline Roland score by using generalized estimating equations) are 0.046 at 6 weeks, 0.002 at 12 weeks, and 0.002 at 26 weeks. (Courtesy of Sherman KJ, Cherkin DC, Erro J, et al: Comparing yoga, exercise, and a self-care book for chronic low back pain: A randomized, controlled trial. *Ann Intern Med* 143:849-856, 2005.)

Conclusions.—Yoga was more effective than a self-care book for improving function and reducing chronic low back pain, and the benefits persisted for at least several months.

► Low back pain is a common, often chronic and disabling problem that frequently tests the patience, capacities, and good intentions of the physician. Whether because the problem is commonly multifactorial, or because physicians (with the possible exception of surgeons) have only limited capacity to improve structural damage, low back pain rarely brooks a simple solution. Analgesics, anti-inflammatories, exercise, and education all have their place, but none seems completely satisfying, and successful therapy often involves a mix of approaches. In that regard, yoga would seem to have a number of attractive features. An integrative approach, yoga emphasizes muscle strengthening, stretching, relaxation, and control, as well as the importance of breathing; but yoga is also a mental discipline, that encourages simultaneous mental discipline and relaxation in a kind of meditative state. And as anyone who has seriously practiced yoga knows, the end of a yoga session is often characterized by a sense of well-being that persists for some time after the session. Thus, yoga may represent the complete package (excluding medications) for back problems, particularly functional back problems that are not accompanied by serious anatomic limitations.

In this report, Sherman et al describe a well-done study comparing yoga with a more standard exercise class, or with a generic educational program (giving out a self-care book for back pain) in relatively well patients with chronic back pain. The yoga style taught, viniyoga, was selected for its safety and simplicity. After 12 weeks of class, the group taking yoga had significant improvement in disability and symptom bothersomeness, compared with the education-only group. Not surprisingly, the exercise group fell somewhere in-between; the efficacy of standard exercise could be distinguished from neither group. Twelve weeks after the classes ended, the yoga group continued to do better than the other groups; in fact, the yoga group was the only one to demonstrate ongoing improvement in the symptom bothersomeness score. Individuals in the yoga group also reported making fewer health care visits, having fewer adverse events, and taking fewer medications (21% medication use in the yoga group, compared with 50% in the exercise group and 59% in the education group) than the other participants.

Previous readers of the YEAR BOOK may realize that this editor expresses a healthy skepticism for nontraditional therapies, and that the inability to study such therapies in a double-blind manner is one of my common criticisms. However, back pain is a unique problem. Unless the goal to remediate the structural abnormalities of the back is the treatment aim, study blinding is practically irrelevant. In the realm of back pain, if a therapy feels like it works, then it does work; and our only concern should be whether it is also safe. Yoga, properly done under the right teacher, is safe and has numerous potential effects that could benefit the back pain sufferer. If this study is correct, those benefits are more than theoretic. Still, the study has limitations, not the least of which is that the typical participant was white, female, English-speaking, college educated, 40 to 50 years of age, and gainfully employed (affluent?). These sorts of people tend to be insightful, compliant, and aggressively involved in their self-care, and may need help less desperately than my own patients, who tend to be blue-collar or impoverished, minority or immigrant, limited in education or language skills or both, and perhaps more seriously harmed by their lack of back health. Whether yoga is a viable option for these equally, if not more deserving folks, would require its own study.

M. H. Pillinger, MD

Treatment of Lateral Epicondylitis With Botulinum Toxin: A Randomized, Double-blind, Placebo-controlled Trial

Wong SM, Hui ACF, Tong P-Y, et al (North District Hosp, Hong Kong, China; Chinese Univ of Hong Kong, China; Prince of Wales Hosp, Hong Kong, China)

Ann Intern Med 143:793-797, 2005 4–4

Background.—Lateral epicondylitis is a common condition for which botulinum toxin has been reported to have a therapeutic role in uncontrolled studies.

Objective.—To determine if an injection of botulinum toxin is more effective than placebo for reducing pain in adults with lateral epicondylitis.

Design.—Randomized, double-blind, placebo-controlled trial conducted from September 2002 to December 2004.

Setting.—Outpatient clinics at a university hospital and a district hospital in Hong Kong.

Participants.—60 patients with lateral epicondylitis.

Measurements.—The primary outcome was change in subjective pain as measured by a 100-mm visual analogue scale (VAS) ranging from 0 (no pain) to 10 (worst pain ever) at 4 weeks and 12 weeks. All patients completed post-treatment follow-up.

Interventions.—A single injection of 60 units of botulinum toxin type A or normal saline placebo.

Results.—Mean VAS scores for the botulinum group at baseline and at 4 weeks were 65.5 mm and 25.3 mm, respectively; respective scores for the placebo group were 66.2 mm and 50.5 mm (between-group difference of changes, 24.4 mm [95% CI, 13.0 to 35.8 mm]; $P < 0.001$). At week 12, mean VAS scores were 23.5 mm for the botulinum group and 43.5 mm for the placebo group (between-group difference of changes, 19.3 mm [CI, 5.6 to 32.9 mm]; $P = 0.006$). Grip strength was not statistically significantly different between groups at any time. Mild paresis of the fingers occurred in 4 patients in the botulinum group at 4 weeks. One patient's symptoms persisted until week 12, whereas none of the patients receiving placebo had the same complaint. At 4 weeks, 10 patients in the botulinum group and 6 patients in the placebo group experienced weak finger extension on the same side as the injection site.

Limitations.—The trial was small, and most participants were women. The blinding protocol may have been ineffective because the 4 participants who experienced paresis of the fingers could have correctly assumed that they received an active treatment.

Conclusions.—Botulinum toxin injection may improve pain over a 3-month period in some patients with lateral epicondylitis, but injections may be associated with digit paresis and weakness of finger extension.

► As a rheumatologist, I've always considered it a matter of time before botulinum toxin came into rheumatologic practice. Botulinum toxin (possibly the most potent neurotoxin known to man!) acts by blocking acetylcholine release at neuromuscular junctions, causing reversible muscle paralysis. As an effective inhibitor of muscular contraction, one could imagine that botulinum toxin would be useful in a variety of musculoskeletal problems that involve muscle spasm, including low back pain and trapezius spasm. There would appear to be less rationale for its use in inflammatory conditions, including enthesitis. Nonetheless, Wong et al tested the efficacy of botulinum toxin for the treatment of lateral epicondylitis. They identified 60 patients with epicondylitis not previously treated with steroid injections and administered either botulinum toxin or placebo IM. The individuals who received botulinum toxin did significantly better than those who received placebo, as regarded patient-reported pain intensity. (No objective measures of response, for example, dolorimetry at the epicondyle, were obtained—a serious deficiency in the study). Grip strength was unchanged with treatment in both groups. Not surprisingly, however (since the treatment was directed at the extensor bundle of the arm), some patients who received botulinum toxin experienced weakness in finger extension and even paresis; these effects were mostly transient, in keeping with the kinetics of botulinum toxin.

What did botulinum toxin actually do to the patients? That remains unclear, though the authors propose that the toxin may have acted to induce rest in the affected enthesis. That explanation seems as good as any other, especially given that the investigators actually injected the botulinum toxin not at the enthesis, but about an inch distal, in the adjoining muscle bundle. Regardless of the mechanism, these studies suggest that botulinum toxin may be a useful adjunct to other therapies for lateral epicondylitis. On the other hand, given the general efficacy, safety, and lengthy experience with older therapies (bracing, rehab, nonsteroidal anti-inflammatory drugs, and steroid/lidocaine injections), the use of botulinum toxin will need to remain a salvage therapy for the foreseeable future, to be used only in difficult or resistant cases.

M. H. Pillinger, MD

5 Vasculitis

Etanercept Plus Standard Therapy for Wegener's Granulomatosis

Stone JH, for the Wegener's Granulomatosis Etanercept Trial (WGET) Research Group (Johns Hopkins Vasculitis Ctr, Baltimore, Md)

N Engl J Med 352:351-361, 2005 5–1

Background.—The majority of patients with Wegener's granulomatosis have disease flares after conventional medications are tapered. There is no consistently safe, effective treatment for the maintenance of remission.

Methods.—We conducted a randomized, placebo-controlled trial at eight centers to evaluate etanercept for the maintenance of remission in 180 patients with Wegener's granulomatosis. The primary outcome was sustained remission, defined as a Birmingham Vasculitis Activity Score for Wegener's Granulomatosis of 0 for at least six months (scores can range from 0 to 67, with higher scores indicating more active disease). In addition to etanercept or placebo, patients received standard therapy (glucocorticoids plus cyclophosphamide or methotrexate). After remission, standard medications were tapered according to the protocol.

Results.—The mean follow-up for the overall cohort was 27 months. Of the 174 patients who could be evaluated, 126 (72.4 percent) had a sustained remission, but only 86 (49.4 percent) remained in remission for the remainder of the trial. There were no significant differences between the etanercept and control groups in the rates of sustained remission (69.7 percent vs. 75.3 percent, P=0.39), sustained periods of low-level disease activity (86.5 percent vs. 90.6 percent, P=0.32), or the time required to achieve those measures. Disease flares were common in both groups, with 118 flares in the etanercept group (23 severe and 95 limited) and 134 in the control group (25 severe and 109 limited). There was no significant difference between the etanercept and control groups in the relative risk of disease flares per 100 person-years of follow-up (0.89, P=0.54). During the study, 56.2 percent of patients in the etanercept group and 57.1 percent of those in the control group had at least one severe or life-threatening adverse event or died (P=0.90). Solid cancers developed in six patients in the etanercept group, as compared with none in the control group (P=0.01).

Conclusions.—Etanercept is not effective for the maintenance of remission in patients with Wegener's granulomatosis. Durable remissions were achieved in only a minority of the patients, and there was a high rate of treatment-related complications.

► Wegener's granulomatosis (WG), one of the antineutrophilic cytoplasmic antibody (ANCA)-associated vasculitides, is a relatively rare multisystem disease primarily affecting the kidneys and respiratory tract. Whereas the 2-year mortality rate is 85% without treatment, therapy with steroids and cyclophosphamide induces disease remission in up to 90% of patients by 12 months. However, considerable toxicity attends the use of these drugs, and despite their efficacy, a majority of patients go on to experience disease relapse. For these reasons, other therapeutic options are being explored. Among the drugs that have been considered for treating WG are the antitumor necrosis factor (TNF) agents.

TNF is a cytokine implicated in a number of inflammatory and autoimmune diseases. It is produced by activated immune cells, chiefly by tissue macrophages, and augments inflammation though a number of effects, including monocyte and neutrophil activation and upregulation of endothelial adhesion molecules; it also increases the production of proinflammatory cytokines and matrix metalloproteinases. TNF is implicated in the pathogenesis of WG through several lines of indirect evidence. TNF is overexpressed at sites of vasculitic injury, and active WG is associated with increased circulating levels of TNF that normalize with disease remission. Data from animal models and in vitro studies in humans also suggest that TNF plays a prominent role in the pathogenesis of ANCA-associated vasculitis.

Antagonizing TNF has already proven efficacious for inflammatory diseases such as rheumatoid arthritis, Crohn's disease, ankylosing spondylitis, and psoriatic arthritis. The WG etanercept trial explored the possibility of using etanercept as add-on therapy to standard treatment (glucocorticoids plus cyclophosphamide or methotrexate) for WG. Unfortunately, the dose and schedule of etanercept (25 mg twice a week) did not improve the efficacy of standard therapy; both the etanercept and the placebo groups experienced similar relapse rates. More worrisome is that there was an increased incidence of solid tumors in the etanercept group (6 in the etanercept group versus none in the standard treatment group), suggesting that the combination of cyclophosphamide and etanercept may dramatically increase the risk of developing solid tumors.

The failure of this study, while disappointing, does not imply that targeting TNF in medium-sized vasculitis should be abandoned. All means of TNF inhibition are not equal. Whereas the monoclonal antibodies infliximab and adalimumab target both soluble and membrane-bound TNF, the synthetic fusion TNF- receptor etanercept neutralizes only soluble TNF. Membrane-bound TNF may play a more central role in some diseases than in others, which could explain, for example, why Crohn's disease responds to both adalimumab and infliximab, but not etanercept. For the same reason, this negative study of etanercept for WG does not rule out all anti-TNF therapy for the ANCA-associated vasculitides. Future anti-TNF studies for vasculitis should, perhaps, consider focusing on monoclonal antibody therapy.

A. M. Abeles, MD

High Incidence of Venous Thrombotic Events Among Patients With Wegener Granulomatosis: The Wegener's Clinical Occurrence of Thrombosis (WeCLOT) Study

Merkel PA, for the Wegener's Granulomatosis Etanercept Trial Research Group (Boston Univ; et al)

Ann Intern Med 142:620-626, 2005 5–2

Background.—Venous thrombotic events (VTEs) have been observed in Wegener granulomatosis, but the incidence rate is not known.

Objective.—To measure the incidence of VTEs in patients with Wegener granulomatosis.

Design.—Prospective, observational cohort study.

Setting.—A multicenter, randomized, double-blind, placebo-controlled treatment trial for Wegener granulomatosis.

Patients.—180 patients with Wegener granulomatosis enrolled during periods of active disease.

Measurements.—Venous thrombotic events (deep venous thromboses or pulmonary emboli) were documented and confirmed prospectively. Incidence rates were calculated on the basis of time to first VTE.

Results.—Thirteen patients had VTEs before enrollment. During 228 person-years of prospective follow-up, 16 VTEs occurred in 167 patients

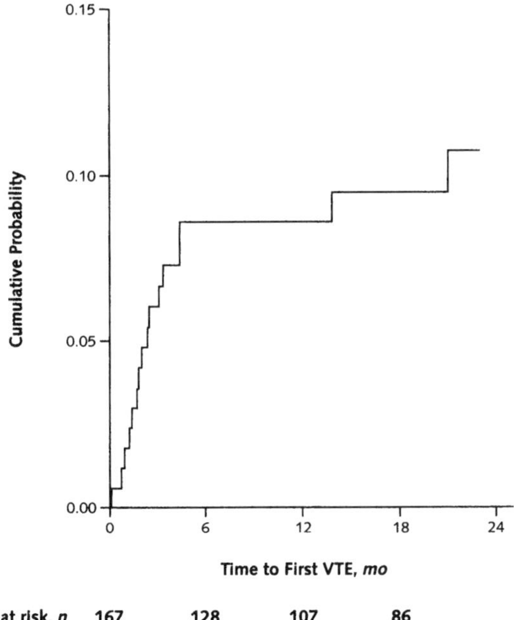

FIGURE.—Time to first venous thrombotic event (*VTE*) among patients with Wegener granulomatosis. *Note*: All patients had active disease at time 0. (Courtesy of Merkel PA, for the Wegener's Granulomatosis Etanercept Trial Research Group: High incidence of venous thrombotic events among patients with Wegener granulomatosis: The Wegener's Clinical Occurrence of Thrombosis [WEclot] study. *Ann Intern Med* 142:620-626, 2005.)

with no history of VTE. Median time from enrollment to VTE for patients with an event was 2.1 months. The incidence of VTE among patients with Wegener granulomatosis was 7.0 per 100 person-years (95% CI, 4.0 to 11.4).

Limitations.—Although prospectively recorded, screening for VTEs did not occur.

Conclusions.—The incidence rate of VTEs in Wegener granulomatosis is high when compared with available rates in the general population, patients with lupus, and patients with rheumatoid arthritis. These results have important implications for clinical care of patients with Wegener granulomatosis (Fig).

► Wegener's granulomatosis (WG) is among the most common of the primary vasculitides, which nonetheless, means that it is quite rare. Accordingly, even most rheumatologists take care of relatively few WG patients, making it difficult to identify or appreciate the more nuanced patterns of the disease. In this article, a group of investigators studying the clinical efficacy of etanercept in WG took advantage of their relatively large cohort to investigate the question of whether patients with WG might have an increased incidence of thrombotic events, given the highly activated state of their immune system, as well as their vascular endothelium.

A total of 180 patients with WG, all fulfilling American College of Rheumatology Classification Criteria for the disease, were followed up for a median of 27 months. Of these, 167 patients had no prior history of thromboembolism. As noted in the abstract, the incidence of thromboembolism for the group overall was 7.0 per 100 person-years. There were no differences between the etanercept group and the placebo group, indicating that the rate of thromboembolism was not affected by etanercept. Was this a high rate of thromboembolism? One weakness of the study is that there was no comparator group of patients who did not have WG against which to assess thrombotic rate. However, on the basis of historical controls, the thromboembolic rate in the patients with WG would appear to be quite high. Studies among the general population, among patients with lupus, and among patients who use etanercept for other reasons, would set the incidence at less than or equal to 1.0 per 100 person-years. In fact, the only historical control group that had a rate of thromboembolism equal to the rate seen in the WG patients were patients who themselves had previous thromboembolic disease, a group known to have a high incidence of reoccurrence.

What are we to do with these data? Be vigilant, certainly, and evaluate and treat our WG patients aggressively at the first suspicion of clot. If these data hold up in additional studies, then clinical studies may also be needed to address whether patients with WG should have prophylactic treatment for thrombosis, either with aspirin or anticoagulants directed at the clotting cascade. A better understanding of the mechanism of increased clotting in patients with WG is currently lacking, and may also help lead us to informed recommendations about the management of this previously unrecognized problem.

M. H. Pillinger, MD

Antineutrophil Cytoplasmic Antibodies and the Churg–Strauss Syndrome

Sablé-Fourtassou R, for the French Vasculitis Study Group (Hôpital Cochin, Paris; et al)

Ann Intern Med 143:632-638, 2005 5–3

Background.—Since testing for antineutrophil cytoplasmic antibodies (ANCA) became available for routine evaluation, no large homogeneous cohort of patients with the Churg–Strauss syndrome has been studied.

Objective.—To define the clinical and biological characteristics of newly diagnosed Churg–Strauss syndrome, according to the presence or absence of ANCA.

Design.—Cross-sectional analysis of manifestations of participants who were enrolled in treatment trials between December 1995 and December 2002.

Setting.—Multicenter study in 63 clinical centers in France, Belgium, Latvia, and the United Kingdom, coordinated by the French Vasculitis Study Group.

Participants.—112 patients with Churg–Strauss syndrome that was recently diagnosed on the basis of current classifications.

Measurements.—The authors compared principal demographic, clinical, and laboratory features according to ANCA status at diagnosis.

Results.—The authors detected ANCA in 43 (38%) patients. Positive ANCA status at diagnosis was associated with renal involvement, peripheral neuropathy, and biopsy-proven vasculitis, whereas negative ANCA status was associated with heart disease and fever.

Limitations.—The authors assessed ANCA by immunofluorescence, but they did not assess ANCA centrally or systematically retest if ANCA was undetected at diagnosis.

Conclusions.—Phenotypically, ANCA-positive and ANCA-negative Churg–Strauss syndrome might differ. The association of ANCA positivity with clinical symptoms that indicate inflammation and necrosis of small vessels might characterize a predominantly vasculitic pattern of the Churg–Strauss syndrome.

► When it comes to studying the ANCA-positive vasculitides (Wegener's granulomatosis, microscopic polyangiitis, ANCA-associated glomerulonephritis, and Churg-Strauss syndrome), Churg-Strauss usually gets the short end of the stick. Perhaps because of its relative rarity, few prospective studies of the natural history of Churg-Strauss syndrome have been performed. Therapeutic trials for Churg-Strauss almost always consist of including a few such patients in a larger study of other ANCA-positive vasculitides, on the presumption that the diseases are more or less equivalent. That's a bad strategy since Churg-Strauss syndrome is clearly not equivalent to other vasculitides. The involvement of asthma, and particularly eosinophilia, suggests that Churg-Strauss has a unique pathogenesis, and that its optimal treatment is therefore not likely to be identical to the other diseases. The significance of ANCA may also be less clear than in the other diseases, since at least a few reports suggest that a majority of Churg-Strauss patients lack demonstrable ANCA titers.

The very large French Vasculitis Study Group have now initiated what may well be the first rational, prospective clinical study of Churg-Strauss syndrome since the discovery of ANCAs. In this early report from that study, the authors report on the role of ANCA in Churg-Strauss, and the data are provocative. A total of 112 patients with Churg-Strauss were enrolled, their diseases characterized, and disease severity scored. ANCAs were obtained (enzyme-linked immunosorbent assays for anti-PR3 and anti-MPO were not universally performed, unfortunately), and the presence of ANCA positivity was evaluated alongside specific patient characteristics. Strikingly, only 38% of the patients studied had a positive ANCA; thus, ANCA is not particularly sensitive for making a Churg-Strauss diagnosis and not necessary for the development of the disease. Most of the patients (approximately 90%) who did have a positive ANCA demonstrated a pANCA pattern, as would be expected historically. The 4 patients whose ANCA showed a cytosolic pattern tested negative on anti-PR3 enzyme-linked immunosorbent assay, which is surprising since cANCA positivity is generally thought to reflect the presence of an anti-PR3 antibody.

Perhaps most interesting was the fact that ANCA-positivity appeared to define a clinically different class of Churg-Strauss patients than those who were ANCA-negative. The ANCA-positive patients had more glomerulonephritis, peripheral neuropathy, and histologically documented vasculitis than the patients who were ANCA negative. It is possible, perhaps likely, that the presence of antibodies resulted in vasculitis, which in turn affected the kidneys and nerves; but the mechanism of ANCA-positive organ involvement in Churg-Strauss remains to be ascertained. Patients who were ANCA negative had less vasculitis but had their own unique collection of problems, including an increased incidence of pleural and pericardial effusion with eosinophilic infiltrates (5 of 13 patients with pericardial effusion had tamponade!), cardiomyopathy with congestive heart failure (33% vs 9% in the ANCA-positive group), and fever. While the clinical profiles of the ANCA-positive and -negative groups were different, there was naturally overlap between the two. Moreover, the absence or presence of ANCA was not associated with differences in severity, prognosis, or outcome of the disease, and patients with and without ANCA relapsed at about the same rate.

These results are fascinating and, if confirmed, represent new and striking knowledge about this disease. From a scientific point of view, these data suggest new questions and new hypotheses to be studied about the mechanisms behind Churg-Strauss, not the least of which is whether it ought to be considered 2 separate diseases. From a clinical point of view, we can begin to use this information even now by allowing the presence or absence of ANCA to direct our vigilance for specific organ system involvement. Although the methodology behind this study had several important limitations, I believe that the strengths of the study suggest that the results will hold.

M. H. Pillinger, MD

Immunosuppressive Treatment of Chronic Periaortitis: A Retrospective Study of 20 Patients With Chronic Periaortitis and a Review of the Literature

Warnatz K, Keskin AG, Uhl M, et al (Albert-Ludwigs Univ, Freiburg, Germany)

Ann Rheum Dis 64:828-833, 2005 5–4

Background.—Retroperitoneal fibrosis (RPF) and inflammatory aneurysm of the abdominal aorta (IAAA) are regarded as two manifestations of the same disease, termed "chronic periaortitis".

Objective.—To determine the optimal therapeutic and diagnostic approaches to IAAA.

Methods.—The outcome of medical immunosuppressive and surgical treatment of 20 patients was examined. Measurements of the C reactive protein (CRP) were compared with contrast enhanced imaging studies in the follow up of the patients.

Results.—The diameter of the periaortic mantle and its contrast enhancement improved in 13/15 (87%) patients given immunosuppressive treatment for a period of more than 6 months. Strong contrast enhancement was associated with a substantial rise in CRP, but no correlation between the CRP value and thickness of the fibrotic mass was found, even at intraindividual follow up.

Conclusions.—Immunosuppressive treatment should be included in the first line treatment of patients with RPF and should be maintained long term. Imaging studies are better than CRP measurements in the evaluation of response to treatment.

► I've chosen to include this selection, not because it is a definitive report, but because it calls attention to a disease that we don't think about often and that many of us may not realize is treatable. Many physicians are not aware that IAAA and idiopathic RPF are 2 aspects of the same disease whose unifying name is chronic periaortitis. Chronic periaortitis is both an inflammatory and fibrosing disease whose causes are unknown but whose risk factors may include smoking, asbestos, and ergot exposure. Prior autoimmunity may also be a concern. The signs and symptoms of chronic periaortitis depend on where, and to what extent, the "rind" of inflammation and fibrosis occurs and may include pain in the lower back, flanks, and scrotum as well as weight loss. The most common of the dreaded complications include aortic rupture and renal failure caused by ureteral constriction by the fibrotic mass.

Since this disease is rare and probably underdiagnosed, prospective therapeutic trials are not likely to be performed. To gain insight into the treatment of chronic periaortitis, Warnatz et al scanned the records of their hospital in Freiburg, Germany, and identified 20 cases of chronic periaortitis. (Two other patients were identified but were excluded from review because they died of malignancies within 6 months of diagnosis; the authors do not discuss the possibility that the malignancies might have been associated with the disease.) Of the 20, 14 were male and 6 female; the average age at diagnosis was 51 years. Although RPF and IAAA are considered a single condition, three quarters of these patients had retroperitoneal disease and one quarter had aortic disease, without overlap; one wonders if they are really the same disease.

The good news appears to be that, in spite of the fact that chronic periaortitis has a reputation as being a relatively hopeless condition, immunosuppressive therapy helped nearly every patient who received it. Treatments used included cyclophosphamide, which seemed to work best, and mycophenolate mofetil, which seemed to work least. Azathioprine and steroids were intermediate (steroids remain controversial in treating periaortitis because of the hypothetical risk of weakening the aortic wall). Patients getting immunosuppression experienced partial or complete shrinking of the fibrotic mantle as well as improvement in renal function. (Tamoxifen has also been reported to improve periaortitis but was not used in any of the patients reported on here.) Both IAAA and RPF improved during treatment. Patients who were treated surgically, without immunosuppression, experienced improvement in the function to which surgery was addressed (eg, improvement of renal function after ureteral stenting or ureterolysis). Of the 5 such cases identified, 3 were not assessed for systemic progression, 1 experienced worsening fibrosis, and 1 experienced worsening renal failure. Thus, surgery may be useful in this disease but may not replace immunosuppression.

Although this study is unblinded, retrospective, and limited to 1 hospital, it does suggest that we should not take a nihilistic approach to periaortitis. Rather, given the potential consequences of periaortitis to the patient, it would appear that, based on the available data, a risk-benefit analysis would favor the use of immunosuppression, up to and including the use of cyclophosphamide. Whether glucocorticoids should also be used will need to be a personal decision based on the distribution of the problem and the degree of concern for aortic wall weakening.

M. H. Pillinger, MD

6 Seronegative Spondyloarthropathies

MRI Abnormalities of Sacroiliac Joints in Early Spondylarthropathy: A 1-Year Follow-up Study

Puhakka KB, Jurik AG, Schieøttz-Christensen B, et al (Aarhus Univ, Denmark; Rheumatological Hosp, Graasten, Denmark; Sønderborg Hosp, Denmark)

Scand J Rheumatol 33:332-338, 2004 6–1

Objective.—To describe changes in chronic and acute magnetic resonance imaging (MRI) abnormalities of the sacroiliac joints (SIJs) in early spondylarthropathy (SpA), and to associate these findings with computed tomography (CT), X-ray, and clinical findings during a 1-year follow-up.

Methods.—Thirty-four patients, 20 males and 14 females, median age 27 years, with inflammatory low back pain (median 23 months) were included. MRI, CT, and X-ray, as well as clinical and laboratory tests were performed. After a follow-up period of 1 year (median 377 days) the examinations were repeated, and the findings were correlated.

Results.—MRI and CT changes resulting from SIJ destruction increased significantly during follow-up, and the two modalities were significantly correlated. For the MRI findings of inflammatory activity, only bone marrow oedema decreased significantly. An increase in the Schober test was the only clinical examination that changed significantly.

Conclusion.—In early SpA, MRI can detect significant inflammatory and destructive changes of the SIJs over a 1-year follow-up period, in spite of minimal changes in the clinical parameters. The MRI changes in inflammatory activity are not detectable by CT and X-ray examinations. Thus, MRI may be a sensitive method, without known risks, for early diagnosis and for following disease progression in SpA.

► Although MRI technology is now almost 20 years old, controversy continues to exist as to how to best utilize this important tool in rheumatology. One area of ongoing uncertainty is in the assessment of sacroiliitis. Is MRI the optimal approach for diagnosing sacroiliitis, or is it too sensitive and prone to artifact? How does MRI compare with CT? With this study Puhakka et al help put our minds at ease. They subjected 34 patients with inflammatory back pain to serial MRI, CT, and radiography of the SIJ and evaluated the course of disease.

Most of those studied already had some sacroiliac bone damage at entry, and this disease progressed over the course of 1 year. Both CT and MRI were effective at identifying and showing the course of joint destruction, so practitioners should feel free to use the modality they like or have available. However, the authors did conclude that MRI can show the presence of inflammatory soft tissue, which was not visible on CT. Moreover, the presence of inflammation correlated with future joint destruction. Thus, MRI may have more utility in diagnosing the earliest (non–bone-destructive) phases of sacroiliitis. Moreover, these data suggest that MRI may also be useful to assess disease activity (or more specifically, the utility of treatment) in a patient with preexisting bone damage who has received an immunosuppressive agent; the absence of inflammation may indicate a positive response.

M. H. Pillinger, MD

7 Osteoporosis and Other Metabolic Diseases of Bone

Denosumab in Postmenopausal Women With Low Bone Mineral Density
McClung MR, for the AMG 162 Bone Loss Study Group (Providence Portland Med Ctr, Ore; et al)
N Engl J Med 354:821-831, 2006 7–1

Background.—Receptor activator of nuclear factor-κB ligand (RANKL) is essential for osteoclast differentiation, activation, and survival. The fully human monoclonal antibody denosumab (formerly known as AMG 162) binds RANKL with high affinity and specificity and inhibits RANKL action.

Methods.—The efficacy and safety of subcutaneously administered denosumab were evaluated over a period of 12 months in 412 postmenopausal women with low bone mineral density (T score of −1.8 to −4.0 at the lumbar spine or −1.8 to −3.5 at the proximal femur). Subjects were randomly assigned to receive denosumab either every three months (at a dose of 6, 14, or 30 mg) or every six months (at a dose of 14, 60, 100, or 210 mg), open-label oral alendronate once weekly (at a dose of 70 mg), or placebo. The primary end point was the percentage change from baseline in bone mineral density at the lumbar spine at 12 months. Changes in bone turnover were assessed by measurement of serum and urine telopeptides and bone-specific alkaline phosphatase.

Results.—Denosumab treatment for 12 months resulted in an increase in bone mineral density at the lumbar spine of 3.0 to 6.7 percent (as compared with an increase of 4.6 percent with alendronate and a loss of 0.8 percent with placebo), at the total hip of 1.9 to 3.6 percent (as compared with an increase of 2.1 percent with alendronate and a loss of 0.6 percent with placebo), and at the distal third of the radius of 0.4 to 1.3 percent (as compared with decreases of 0.5 percent with alendronate and 2.0 percent with placebo). Near-maximal reductions in mean levels of serum C-telopeptide from baseline were evident three days after the administration of denosumab. The duration of the suppression of bone turnover appeared to be dose-dependent.

Conclusions.—In postmenopausal women with low bone mass, denosumab increased bone mineral density and decreased bone resorption. These preliminary data suggest that denosumab might be an effective treatment for osteoporosis. (ClinicalTrials.gov number, NCT00043186.).

► Osteoporosis is a problem that affects many millions of individuals, but that is slowly starting to yield to the efforts of scientists and clinicians. The availability of bisphosphonates, parthyroid hormone–based treatments, and calcitonin have made an untreatable problem into a treatable one. Nonetheless, new therapies are needed. Since our knowledge of the pathophysiology has improved along with our therapy, we are now in a position to identify additional therapeutic targets. As it turns out, one of the most important pairs of molecules in osteoporosis is the RANK (receptor activator of nuclear factor-κB)/RANK ligand (RANKL) pair. RANK is a receptor—perhaps the key receptor—found on osteoclasts and their monocyte precursors. Engagement of RANK by RANK ligand leads to influx of monocytes, their differentiation into mature osteoclasts, and the subsequent activation and survival of those osteoclasts. Thus, blockade of the RANK/RANKL interaction would be expected to have a salutary effect on osteoporosis. In this study, McClung et al report on the effects of treating patients with denosumab, a monoclonal antibody that binds to RANKL and blocks the RANK/RANKL interaction.

The study group consisted of 412 postmenopausal women with osteopenia or osteoporosis, defined as a dual-energy x-ray absorptiometry (DEXA) T score of less than −1.8 in the spine or femoral neck. Participants were assigned to 1 of 9 different groups: placebo, denosumab at various doses every 3 months, denosumab at various doses every 6 months, or alendronate 70 mg weekly. Denosumab at most doses caused a rapid reduction in markers of bone turnover, including serum C-telopeptide, bone-specific alkaline phosphatase, and parathyroid hormone. More importantly, denosumab at various doses resulted in increased bone mineral density at the lumbar spine and at the hip that was equal or superior to the effects seen with alendronate. The response at the distal third of the radius was superior to that with alendronate, which may have to do with the ability of denosumab to modulate resorption from cortical bone. The optimal dose of denosumab appeared to be either 30 mg every 3 months or 60 mg every 6 months. There were no significant side effects in any group, except for dyspepsia in the alendronate group.

Questions remain to be answered, including whether denosumab will be appropriately efficacious in preventing fractures. The authors point out that bisphosphonates, even on a weekly basis, are relatively hard to take, leading to compliance rates of less than 70%. They suggest that an occasional subcutaneous injection, perhaps administered by a physician, would be more likely to lead to compliance. Time will tell whether they are right, and whether denosumab makes it past these phase II trials into actual use. Whatever the outcome, the fact that another biologic agent, based on knowledge and reason, has advanced into the therapeutic arena is cause for optimism and an opportunity to celebrate the power of science.

M. H. Pillinger, MD

Calcium Plus Vitamin D Supplementation and the Risk of Fractures

Jackson RD, for the Women's Health Initiative Investigators (Ohio State Univ, Columbus; et al)

N Engl J Med 354:669-683, 2006 7–2

Background.—The efficacy of calcium with vitamin D supplementation for preventing hip and other fractures in healthy postmenopausal women remains equivocal.

Methods.—We recruited 36,282 postmenopausal women, 50 to 79 years of age, who were already enrolled in a Women's Health Initiative (WHI) clinical trial. We randomly assigned participants to receive 1000 mg of elemental [corrected] calcium as calcium carbonate with 400 IU of vitamin D_3 daily or placebo. Fractures were ascertained for an average follow-up period of 7.0 years. Bone density was measured at three WHI centers.

Results.—Hip bone density was 1.06 percent higher in the calcium plus vitamin D group than in the placebo group ($P<0.01$). Intention-to-treat analysis indicated that participants receiving calcium plus vitamin D supplementation had a hazard ratio of 0.88 for hip fracture (95 percent confidence interval, 0.72 to 1.08), 0.90 for clinical spine fracture (0.74 to 1.10), and 0.96 for total fractures (0.91 to 1.02). The risk of renal calculi increased with calcium plus vitamin D (hazard ratio, 1.17; 95 percent confidence interval, 1.02 to 1.34). Censoring data from women when they ceased to adhere to the study medication reduced the hazard ratio for hip fracture to 0.71 (95 percent confidence interval, 0.52 to 0.97). Effects did not vary significantly according to prerandomization serum vitamin D levels.

Conclusions.—Among healthy postmenopausal women, calcium with vitamin D supplementation resulted in a small but significant improvement in hip bone density, did not significantly reduce hip fracture, and increased the risk of kidney stones. (ClinicalTrials.gov number, NCT00000611.).

► The WHI calcium plus vitamin D trial set out to investigate whether calcium and vitamin D supplementation prevents hip and other fractures in healthy postmenopausal women. The efficacy of calcium and vitamin D for fracture prevention was unclear before this trial began, and despite an ambitious effort by the WHI, remains unclear at the trials' conclusion. The investigators report that calcium and vitamin D supplements did not significantly affect any fracture endpoints, though it did have a small and statistically significant positive effect on total hip bone mineral density (1 % increase) compared with placebo. When the investigators analyzed, post hoc, those patients who were more than 80% adherent to therapy, the risk of hip fractures was significantly reduced by 29%.

It is likely that the methodology and characteristics of the study population reduced the chances of detecting an unequivocal benefit in the treatment group. With a mean age of 62 years, a mean body mass index of 29, and a mean bone mineral density hip T score that was above −1.0 at baseline, the subjects began the study at low risk for fragility fractures. In addition, more than 50% of all subjects were current users of hormone replacement therapy; more than

60% in the placebo group had a daily calcium intake of at least 800 mg, and more than 40% in the placebo group had a daily vitamin D intake of at least 400 IU. These factors skew the study towards a likely negative result. In addition, the use of osteoporosis medications increased more than 10-fold during follow-up (ie, both control and treatment patients were permitted to go on bisphonates, calcitonin, or selective estrogen receptor modulators), making it more difficult to detect an additional benefit of reduced fractures with calcium and vitamin D supplements. In fact, the observed hip fracture rate in the placebo group was about half the predicted, and as reported by the authors in the article itself, this reduced the power of the study to about 48%.

At best, this study suggests that calcium and vitamin D supplementation alone is insufficient to prevent fractures in postmenopausal women with "real-world" medication intake practices. It tells us nothing, however, about patients who otherwise have a low intake of calcium and vitamin D, who strictly adhere to prescribed doses, or who start off at a higher risk for fracture. Since this was, in effect, a treatment and not a prevention study, it also tells us nothing about the utility of premenopausal supplementation to prevent osteoporosis in later years. With the current use of hormone replacement therapy declining, further studies are warranted to see which specific groups of patients may benefit from calcium and vitamin D supplementation.

S. Krasnokutsky, MD

Daily and Cyclic Parathyroid Hormone in Women Receiving Alendronate

Cosman F, Nieves J, Zion M, et al (Helen Hayes Hosp, West Haverstraw, NY; Columbia Univ, New York; Saint Barnabas Osteoporosis and Metabolic Bone Disease Ctr, Livingston, NJ; et al)

N Engl J Med 353:566-575, 2005 7–3

Background.—We evaluated whether patients with osteoporosis treated with long-term alendronate have a response to parathyroid hormone treatment and whether short, three-month cycles of parathyroid hormone therapy could be as effective as daily administration.

Methods.—We randomly assigned 126 women with osteoporosis who had been taking alendronate for at least 1 year to continued alendronate plus parathyroid hormone (1-34) subcutaneously daily, continued alendronate plus parathyroid hormone (1-34) subcutaneously daily for three 3-month cycles alternating with 3-month periods without parathyroid hormone, or alendronate alone for 15 months.

Results.—In both parathyroid hormone groups, bone formation indexes rose swiftly. Among the women who were receiving cyclic parathyroid hormone, bone formation declined during cycles without parathyroid hormone and increased again during cycles with parathyroid hormone. Bone resorption increased in both parathyroid hormone groups but increased progressively more in the daily-treatment group than in the cyclic-therapy group. Spinal bone mineral density rose 6.1 percent in the daily-treatment group and 5.4 percent in the cyclic-therapy group ($P<0.001$ for each parathyroid hormone group as compared with the alendronate group and no significant difference between parathyroid hormone groups). One woman in the daily-treatment group, two in the cyclic-therapy group, and four in the alendronate group had new or worsening vertebral deformities.

Conclusions.—This study suggests that a regimen of three-month cycles of parathyroid hormone alternating with three-month cycles without parathyroid hormone causes the early phase of action of parathyroid hormone (characterized by pure stimulation of bone formation) to be dissociated from the later phase (activation of bone remodeling). The early phase may be more important to the increase in spinal bone mineral density. In patients with persistent osteoporosis after prior alendronate treatment, both daily treatment and cyclic treatment with parathyroid hormone increase spinal bone mineral density.

► The availability of both bisphosphonates and parathyroid hormone (PTH) has raised questions about whether these agents ought to be coadministered. Several reports suggest that initial coadministration of a bisphosphonate and PTH for osteoporosis may be no better than administration of the bisphosphonate alone, possibly because bone resorption (inhibited by bisphosphonates) is a necessary prerequisite to new bone deposition in response to PTH. However, physicians in 2005 rarely initiate osteoporosis treatment with PTH, owing to expense, as well as inconvenience of administration. More commonly, physicians treating osteoporosis prescribe a bisphosphonate and then, should bisphosphonate treatment prove ineffective, add PTH to the regimen.[1] But will PTH help in such a circumstance, or will previous bisphosphonate use block the PTH effect?

Cosman et al assigned 126 women with osteoporosis, all previously treated with alendronate, to receive placebo or teriparetide, (the Food and Drug Administration-approved formulation of PTH, consisting of the first 34 amino acids of the molecule). Alendronate was continued in all cases, and bone mineral density, as well as markers of bone turnover, were assessed. Patients receiving PTH had significant increases in bone density compared with the alendronate-alone group. Patients in a third study arm, who received PTH but on a cyclical basis, did about as well as the patients taking it continuously.

These results appear to be good news, because they suggest that patients who have not responded adequately to a bisphosphonate will benefit from add-on PTH therapy. But wait; there appears to be some dissonance between this report and the above-referenced report by Black et al.[1] How is it possible, for example, that addition of PTH enhances preexisting alendronate therapy, whereas starting alendronate and PTH simultaneously (as in the study by Black et al) is no better than alendronate alone? Perhaps there are genuine differences between long-term, prior alendronate therapy, and recent initiation of alendronate. Differences between the studies (excepting a different PTH formulation) may be part of the explanation, though, and we should reserve final judgment until more studies are available. In the meantime, the most prudent strategy is probably to act according to the data, wherever it most closely matches the patient's situation. For me, this means adding PTH to a bisphosphonate where the bisphosphonate has failed, but not using a combination of a bisphosphonate and PTH as initial therapy. One question that remains unanswered by these studies is whether, when initiating PTH after bisphosphonate failure, we should continue or discontinue the bisphosphonate. A case could be made for either approach at this point, with no data yet available to clarify the issue.

M. H. Pillinger, MD

Reference

1. Black DM, Greenspan SL, Ensrud KE, et al: The effects of parathyroid hormone and alendronate alone or in combination in postmenopausal osteoporosis. *N Engl J Med* 349:1207-1215, 2003.

8 Osteoarthritis

Glucosamine, Chondroitin Sulfate, and the Two in Combination for Painful Knee Osteoarthritis

Clegg DO, Reda DJ, Harris CL, et al (Univ of Utah, Salt Lake City; Hines Veterans Affairs Cooperative Studies Program Coordinating Ctr, Ill; Clinical Research Pharmacy Coordinating Ctr, Albuquerque, NM; et al)

N Engl J Med 354:795-808, 2006 8–1

Background.—Glucosamine and chondroitin sulfate are used to treat osteoarthritis. The multicenter, double-blind, placebo- and celecoxib-controlled Glucosamine/chondroitin Arthritis Intervention Trial (GAIT) evaluated their efficacy and safety as a treatment for knee pain from osteoarthritis.

Methods.—We randomly assigned 1583 patients with symptomatic knee osteoarthritis to receive 1500 mg of glucosamine daily, 1200 mg of chondroitin sulfate daily, both glucosamine and chondroitin sulfate, 200 mg of celecoxib daily, or placebo for 24 weeks. Up to 4000 mg of acetaminophen daily was allowed as rescue analgesia. Assignment was stratified according to the severity of knee pain (mild [N=1229] vs. moderate to severe [N=354]). The primary outcome measure was a 20 percent decrease in knee pain from baseline to week 24.

Results.—The mean age of the patients was 59 years, and 64 percent were women. Overall, glucosamine and chondroitin sulfate were not significantly better than placebo in reducing knee pain by 20 percent. As compared with the rate of response to placebo (60.1 percent), the rate of response to glucosamine was 3.9 percentage points higher (P=0.30), the rate of response to chondroitin sulfate was 5.3 percentage points higher (P=0.17), and the rate of response to combined treatment was 6.5 percentage points higher (P=0.09). The rate of response in the celecoxib control group was 10.0 percentage points higher than that in the placebo control group (P=0.008). For patients with moderate-to-severe pain at baseline, the rate of response was significantly higher with combined therapy than with placebo (79.2 percent vs. 54.3 percent, P=0.002). Adverse events were mild, infrequent, and evenly distributed among the groups.

Conclusions.—Glucosamine and chondroitin sulfate alone or in combination did not reduce pain effectively in the overall group of patients with osteoarthritis of the knee. Exploratory analyses suggest that the combination of glucosamine and chondroitin sulfate may be effective in the subgroup of patients with moderate-to-severe knee pain. (ClinicalTrials.gov number, NCT00032890.).

▶ The current standard of care for osteoarthritis treatment aims to improve patients' quality of life by reducing joint pain. Until last year, physicians felt quite comfortable prescribing a variety of nonsteroidal anti-inflammatory drugs (NSAIDs) and cyclooxygenase-2 (COX-2) inhibitors to treat patients with osteoarthritis. COX-2 inhibitors in particular, by virtue of their gastrointestinal safety profile, were assuming an ever-increasing role. However, in 2005, the increased emphasis on cardiovascular toxicities of the COX-2 inhibitors dropped them out of favor as a class, and also raised questions about the safety of the nonselective COX inhibitors. With attention being focused on the potential hazards of all NSAIDs, alternative therapies for osteoarthritis have become more attractive to patients and physicians alike. In this vein, there are reports that glucosamine, an amino-monosaccharide derived from bovine trachea cartilage, and chondroitin, a glycosaminoglycan extracted from the chitin of aquatic arthropod shells, may effectively treat osteoarthritis pain.[1,2] Previous clinical trials of these nutritional supplements were criticized for their methodology, and produced conflicting results. This article outlines the results of a National Institutes of Health–funded study that strived to address many of the shortcomings of previous trials assessing the efficacy of these nutritional supplements.[3]

A total of 1583 patients were randomized to receive placebo, glucosamine, chondroitin, glucosamine and chondroitin, or celecoxib. The patients were allowed to take up to 4 g of acetaminophen per day in addition to the study drugs. The primary outcome of the study was a 20% decrease in the West Ontario and McMaster Universities Osteoarthritis Index (WOMAC) pain subscore. Dozens of secondary outcomes were also predefined. Permuted block randomization was used to ensure that a valid subgroup analysis could be carried out comparing patients with more severe disease to those with mild disease (as defined by pain). The investigators decided a priori that a treatment response rate of 15% above the placebo response rate would be clinically significant. Most studies that use a graded scale to measure drug efficacy would define response by a statistically significant difference in scores among different treatment groups. By defining the response as a binary variable (greater than or less than a 20% decrease in pain score) and then requiring that 15% of the treated patients achieve this response, the investigators set a high threshold for positive outcome. The high threshold, however, may be valid when one considers how often a statistically significant response does not translate to a clinically significant response.

The most surprising result of the trial was the high rate of responders to placebo. About 45% of patients receiving placebo had a 20% decrease in their WOMAC score after 4 weeks, and an additional 15% achieved this primary outcome by week 24. None of the 4 treatment groups exceeded this response rate by 15%, which translates to negative results across all groups, even the group taking celecoxib, 200 mg once a day. However, a closer look at the subgroup analysis and secondary endpoints reveals that some positive results may be extracted.

Of the patients receiving celecoxib, 70.1% did achieve the primary outcome. While this was only a 10% higher response rate than placebo and did not cross the 15% threshold set earlier for clinical significance, the difference was nonetheless statistically significant. In addition, 66.6% of the patients receiving glucosamine plus chondroitin, and 70.1% of the patients receiving celecoxib achieved an Outcome Measures in Rheumatology Clinical Trials and Osteoarthritis Research Society International task force (OMERACT-OARSI) response, a recently adopted definition of reponse to osteoarthritis treatment. This was also a statistically significant increased response rate with respect to placebo. In the moderate-severe pain subgroup, the glucosamine plus chondroitin group did achieve the primary outcome (meeting the clinically significant outcome goal) and numerous statistically significant secondary outcomes. Surprisingly, the response rate to glucosamine plus chondroitin often exceeded the response rate to celecoxib in these patients with more severe disease. Seventy-five percent of the patients in the glucosamine plus chondroitin group had a 50% decrease in their WOMAC scores, while only 48.6% of the placebo group and 66.7% of the celecoxib group reported this dramatic response. Because these results derive from a post hoc subgroup analysis, however, the authors were rightly cautious about not overinterpreting their results.

The above study demonstrated that osteoarthritis produces a pain syndrome that is highly susceptible to nonpharmacologic interventions (eg, placebo). Future trials should take into account the effects of supportive care provided to study patients and expect a high placebo response rate. In addition, assuming the response to treatment is more durable than the response to placebo, allowing a longer follow-up period may help distinguish placebo effect from treatment effect. Glucosamine and chondroitin did appear to have some therapeutic benefit, but it is not clear if this benefit is clinically significant, especially in patients with milder disease.

A. B. Artzi, MD

References

1. McAlindton TE, Lavalley MP, Gulin JP, et al: Glucosamine and chondroitin for treatment of osteoarthritis: A systematic quality assessment and meta-analysis. *JAMA* 283:1469-1475, 2000.
2. Tetracyclins and alternative theapies, in Koopman WJ, Moreland LW (eds): *Arthritis and Allied Conditions, A Textbook of Rheumatology*, ed 15. Philadelphia, Lippincott Williams & Wilkins, 2005, pp 945-960.
3. Clegg DO, Reda DF, Harris CL, el al: Glucosamine, chondroitin sulfate, and the two in combination for painful knee ostearthritis. *N Engl J Med* 354:795-808, 2006.

Safety Study of Intraarticular Injection of Interleukin 1 Receptor Antagonist in Patients With Painful Knee Osteoarthritis: A Multicenter Study

Chevalier X, Giraudeau B, Conrozier T, et al (Univ Paris XII; Univ of Tours, France; Lyon-Sud Univ, Pierre Bénite, France; et al)

J Rheumatol 32:1317-1323, 2005 8–2

Objective.—Interleukin 1 (IL-1) plays a pivotal role in the pathogenesis of osteoarthritis (OA). In animal models of OA, IL-1 blockade by IL-1 receptor antagonist (IL-1Ra) can slow the progression of disease. We examined the safety of intraarticular (IA) injections of recombinant human IL-1Ra in patients with knee OA.

Methods.—A prospective multicenter trial was conducted using the continual reassessment method. Six doses were considered, 0.05 mg up to 150 mg IL-1Ra, and the trial was double-blind regarding the dose administered. Patients with symptomatic knee OA and without synovial fluid effusion were included. Acute inflammatory reaction (the primary endpoint defining intolerance) was recorded if pain increase over 30 mm on 100 mm visual analog scale and synovial fluid effusion occurred within 72 h after the IA injection. As a secondary aim, efficacy was estimated (by total pain and Western Ontario and McMaster University OA functional index) until Month 3.

Results.—One patient received 0.05 mg and 13 patients received 150 mg of IL-1Ra. No acute reaction occurred (one patient experienced postinjection joint swelling with no pain) and the 150 mg dose was considered the maximum tolerated dose (intolerance level 0%; confidence interval 0, 9.1%). A significant improvement was still observed until Month 3 in the 13 patients who received 150 mg IL-1Ra: pain improved by -20.4 ± 23.3 mm ($p = 0.008$) and WOMAC global score by -19.5 ± 20.1 ($p = 0.005$).

Conclusion.—IA injection of IL-1Ra in patients with knee OA was well tolerated and did not induce any acute inflammatory reaction. The feasibility of such IA injections of IL-1Ra opens a promising therapeutic perspective for patients with OA.

► As we have highlighted in previous editions of the YEAR BOOK OF MEDICINE, OA is actually an inflammatory disease in which cytokines and other mediators interact with chondrocytes and synovial fibroblasts to hasten the degradation of cartilage that is typically initiated by mechanical damage and/or strain. Such a view of OA is hopeful, in that it suggests that we may have points of intervention through which we can slow, or perhaps even reverse, OA cartilage destruction. One possible target for therapy is IL-1, which is expressed in OA joints and appears to contribute to the arthritic process. Anakinra is a soluble, recombinant version of human IL-1Ra, a naturally occurring inhibitor of IL-1 activity. Subcutaneous, daily anakinra injection is an FDA-approved therapy for rheumatoid arthritis, and it has been suggested that anakinra therapy might be helpful for OA as well. However, daily injection of anakinra is inconvenient, expensive, and may be less than efficacious for OA, since OA chondrocytes are embedded in avascular cartilage and get most of their nutrients by diffusion from the joint fluid. It makes at least hypothetical sense that direct anakinra injection into the joint space might provide a larger and more persistent (and cheaper!) IL-1Ra effect than systemic therapy. Moreover, since OA is most commonly a disease of one or a few joints (in contrast to multijoint involvement in rheumatoid arthritis), directing therapy to the affected joint(s) may represent a feasible strategy and one that is already in use with intraarticular glucocorticoid and hyaluronic acid injections.

With those thoughts in mind, Chevalier et al conducted a phase II safety study of the use of intraarticular anakinra in OA knees. Thirteen patients with knee osteoarthritis received the predicted maximum tolerated dose (150 mg) in a single intraarticular injection in the knee (a fourteenth patient received a pilot dose of 0.05 mg). With the exception of a single individual who had transient painless joint swelling 3 days after the injection, there were no side effects seen over a 3-month observation period. Although the study was neither blinded, controlled, nor designed to evaluate efficacy, it is interesting to note that about half the patients experienced marked improvement (roughly 50% decrease) in their knee pain and dysfunction, as measured by both a visual analog pain scale and the WOMAC score, and that in most patients these improvements were persistent over 3 months. Of further interest is the fact that none of the patients began the study with a joint effusion; most clinicians would agree that "dry" joints are less responsive to intraarticular steroids, but no such limitation appeared to be the case here. Improvement was also not affected by the degree of joint pathology, suggesting that anakinra injection may help even severely damaged knees. Whether higher doses, or more frequent dosing, would have been safe and/or even more effective was not addressed by the study design.

These data are surely preliminary, but they suggest the possibility that IL-1 receptor antagonism may turn out to be a useful, as well as practical, strategy in treating OA patients. Phase III trials will surely follow, at which point the real answers will begin to emerge.

M. H. Pillinger, MD

9 Miscellaneous Rheumatic Diseases and Therapies

Rapid Responses to Anakinra in Patients With Refractory Adult-Onset Still's Disease

Fitzgerald AA, LeClercq SA, Yan A, et al (Univ of Caligary, Alta, Canada; Royal Alexandra Hosp, Edmonton, Alta, Canada; Univ of Alberta, Edmonton, Canada; et al)

Arthritis Rheum 52:1794-1803, 2005 9–1

Objective.—To assess the efficacy of anakinra treatment in patients with adult-onset Still's disease (AOSD) that is refractory to corticosteroids, methotrexate (MTX), and etanercept.

Methods.—Four patients with AOSD were treated with prednisone and MTX and 2 patients were also treated with etanercept for worsening symptoms and indicators of systemic inflammation. White blood cells (WBCs), C-reactive protein (CRP) levels and/or erythrocyte sedimentation rate, and ferritin levels were measured and, in 1 patient, serum creatinine levels were determined. Treatment with anakinra at 100 mg/day was initiated.

Results.—The index patient's disease was refractory to treatment with prednisone (30 mg/day) and MTX, with spiking fevers, rash, synovitis, a serum ferritin level of 8,400 ng/ml (normal ≤200), and a CRP level of 86 mg/liter (normal <8). Levels of interleukin-1β (IL-1β), IL-1α, IL-6, IL-1 receptor antagonist, and IL-18 were elevated. Just prior to anakinra treatment, the WBC count was 14,600/mm^3, the CRP level was 86 mg/liter, and the ferritin level was 573 ng/ml, with daily spiking fevers to 104°F, rash, and swollen joints. Within hours of the first injection, the patient was afebrile and asymptomatic; within days, the WBC count, ferritin level, and CRP level decreased into the normal range. On 2 occasions, anakinra was withheld. Within a few days, the WBC count rose to >20,000/mm^3 with prominent neutrophilia, the CRP level rose to >200 mg/liter, and the ferritin level rose to >3,000 ng/ml. Upon restarting anakinra, the patient became afebrile, the WBC count fell to 8,000/mm^3, the CRP level fell to <3 mg/liter, and the ferritin level fell to <300 ng/ml. Three additional patients with refractory AOSD who experienced rapid reductions in fever, symptoms, and markers of inflammation when treated with anakinra are reported.

Conclusion.—Refractory AOSD appears to be IL-1-mediated since anakinra decreases hematologic, biochemical, and cytokine markers and also produces rapid reductions in systemic and local inflammation. Reported efficacy of tumor necrosis factor-blocking therapies in AOSD may be due to a reduction in IL-1.

► Still's Disease can be difficult to diagnose, but it can also be difficult to treat. The classical therapy, salicylates, can be useful but fails often. Steroids are often helpful, though not always completely so, and are accompanied by well-known toxicities. Disease-modifying antirheumatic drugs (DMARDs) have also been variously used, with intermittent success. The fact that Still's is clearly a highly inflammatory disease, accompanied by fever and terrifically high levels of acute phase reactants, such as ferritin, has suggested that cytokines, such as tumor-necrosis factor-α (TNF-α), might play an important role in the disease, but anti-TNF therapies have not been uniformly successful. More, and better therapeutic alternatives are badly needed.

In this ground-breaking report, Fitzgerald et al provide the first reported evidence that anti-IL-1 therapy may be an important advance. Four patients, each with severe Still's that had responded inadequately to prednisone, methotrexate and/or anti-TNF therapy, were treated with anakinra, the Food and Drug Administration (FDA)-approved soluble IL-1 receptor antagonist. In each case, fever broke within 48 hours, rash and other joint symptoms abated, and inflammatory markers returned to normal. In our own institution, we have seen a similarly rapid response in 4 additional Still's patients who had failed conventional therapy (Izmirly et al, manuscript in preparation). The rapidity of the response, together with the fact that, to our knowledge, 8 of 8 patients have responded nearly completely, suggests that IL-1 is an important mediator of Still's disease and tells us something about the pathophysiology of the disease. It also gives us a valuable alternative, or perhaps even a new first-line therapy, for this frightening and poorly understood condition.

M. H. Pillinger, MD

Sildenafil Citrate Therapy for Pulmonary Arterial Hypertension

Galiè N, for the Sildenafil Use in Pulmonary Arterial Hypertension (SUPER) Study Group (Univ of Bologna, Italy; et al)

N Engl J Med 353:2148-2157, 2005 9–2

Background.—Sildenafil inhibits phosphodiesterase type 5, an enzyme that metabolizes cyclic guanosine monophosphate, thereby enhancing the cyclic guanosine monophosphate–mediated relaxation and growth inhibition of vascular smooth-muscle cells, including those in the lung.

Methods.—In this double-blind, placebo-controlled study, we randomly assigned 278 patients with symptomatic pulmonary arterial hypertension (either idiopathic or associated with connective-tissue disease or with repaired congenital systemic-to-pulmonary shunts) to placebo or sildenafil (20, 40, or 80 mg) orally three times daily for 12 weeks. The primary end point was the change from baseline to week 12 in the distance walked in six minutes. The change in mean pulmonary-artery pressure and World Health Organization (WHO) functional class and the incidence of clinical worsening were also assessed, but the study was not powered to assess mortality. Patients completing the 12-week randomized study could enter a long-term extension study.

Results.—The distance walked in six minutes increased from baseline in all sildenafil groups; the mean placebo-corrected treatment effects were 45 m (+13.0 percent), 46 m (+13.3 percent), and 50 m (+14.7 percent) for 20, 40, and 80 mg of sildenafil, respectively ($P<0.001$ for all comparisons). All sildenafil doses reduced the mean pulmonary-artery pressure ($P=0.04$, $P=0.01$, and $P<0.001$, respectively), improved the WHO functional class ($P=0.003$, $P<0.001$, and $P<0.001$, respectively), and were associated with side effects such as flushing, dyspepsia, and diarrhea. The incidence of clinical worsening did not differ significantly between the patients treated with sildenafil and those treated with placebo. Among the 222 patients completing one year of treatment with sildenafil monotherapy, the improvement from baseline at one year in the distance walked in six minutes was 51 m.

Conclusions.—Sildenafil improves exercise capacity, WHO functional class, and hemodynamics in patients with symptomatic pulmonary arterial hypertension.

► Ever since the use of angiotensin-converting enzyme inhibitors turned scleroderma renal crisis into a (usually) manageable problem, the biggest cause of morbidity and mortality in scleroderma has been pulmonary disease. In generalized scleroderma (systemic sclerosis), the problem most commonly takes the form of lung inflammation and fibrosis. In the limited variants (CREST variant), the problem is more typically pulmonary hypertension.

The management of pulmonary hypertension has experienced a slow but noticeable advancement over the past 5 or 10 years. The previously most commonly used treatment, calcium channel blockers, has been discarded as ineffective in all but a limited subset of patients whose pulmonary pressures respond to vasodilators as measured during right heart catheterization. On the other hand, prostacyclin and its analogs, as well as the antiendothelin agent bosentan, have been shown to produce symptomatic improvement in patients with both primary pulmonary hypertension as well as those with hypertension related to connective tissue disease. However, all these current therapies have their drawbacks—they are either difficult to administer, have significant side effects, or come with a very hefty price tag (usually all 3). New therapies are desperately needed.

One potential approach to treating pulmonary hypertension is to increase local concentrations of nitric oxide (NO), also known as endothelial-derived relaxation factor. NO increases the levels of cyclic guanosine monophosphate (cGMP) in vascular cells, inducing vasodilation and possibly regulating tissue remodeling. However, NO is a gas and therefore must be administered as an inhalational agent—a cumbersome process, to say the least. An alternative approach to raising cGMP levels in the pulmonary vasculature would be to inhibit phosphodiesterase type 5, the enzyme that degrades cGMP. Sildenafil, better known by its trade name Viagra, is an FDA-approved drug that does just that.

Galiè et al enrolled 278 patients with various forms of pulmonary hypertension and treated them with placebo, 20 mg, 40 mg, or 80 mg of sildenafil 3 times daily for 12 weeks, followed by a long-term extension study. The parameters they measured were physiologic (pulmonary artery pressure) and functional (distance walked in 6 minutes, World Health Organization functional class). All doses of sildenafil tested improved all parameters, although the higher doses of sildenafil had more efficacy for dyspnea per se. Importantly for rheumatologists, sildenafil at all doses was effective for the subgroup of patients whose pulmonary hypertension was secondary to connective tissue disease. Patients also experienced benefit whether their pulmonary artery hypertension was mild, moderate, or severe. Moreover, benefit persisted in the open-label portion of the study (1 year). Side effects were generally mild.

This is good news for a difficult problem. Sildenafil is a drug that is easy to take, and although its more common use for erectile dysfunction does not necessitate daily consumption, at least we have some fairly long-term experience with its administration. In this relatively short-term study, the authors did not examine mortality rate, although they do note that walk distance has generally correlated with mortality rate in the past. One question still to be addressed with sildenafil is whether genuine remodeling of the vasculature takes place—that is, is sildenafil simply a management agent, or does it actually help improve the condition? Either way, sildenafil is a welcome addition to our armamentarium of drugs for scleroderma and other forms of pulmonary hypertension.

M. H. Pillinger, MD

PART TWO

INFECTIOUS DISEASES

DAVID R. SNYDMAN, MD

Introduction

This past year had a number of new developments within the field of infectious diseases. The theme of the past year in infectious diseases has been the renewed significance of infections due to pathogens that have been well characterized and important in the past, namely methicillin-resistant *Staphylococcus aureus*, and *Clostridium difficile*. Community-acquired methicillin-resistant *Staphylococcus aureus* (CMRSA) has become more a very common clinical entity. The pathogenesis and epidemiology is described in this volume. The emergence of CMRSA will require physicians to be increasingly vigilant and thoughtful when treating skin and soft tissue infections. The emergence of binary toxin producing *C difficile* associated with the development of very severe disease and increased mortality is another example of the changing epidemiology in which an "old disease" has now evolved into an "emerging" infectious disease. The proportion of cases of *C difficile* associated with colectomy has been noted worldwide. Steps to control this strain will need to be explored. In addition, we are seeing community acquired *C difficle* without apparent exposure to antibiotics and physicians will have to be more vigilant for this cause of community acquired diarrhea. New diagnostic methods and better recognition and treatment will be necessary to improve the outcome and reduce cases. We have seen many such cases in Boston.

In addition to the reemergence of "old diseases" as emerging infections, avian influenza continues to become a cause for concern. Articles highlighting new information on avian influenza have been cited. This virus has spread from Southeast Asia to the Middle East and Europe. The world is concerned about the potential for pandemic avian influenza virus and is taking steps to prepare for such an outbreak. But as indicated in this volume, treatment with neuraminidase inhibitors has not been shown to be effective, and, in fact, in vitro resistance with clinical failure has been documented.

A series of fungal studies were also selected. The most notable is the comparison of caspofungin to amphotericin for candidemia. It has established caspofungin as an equivalent if not superior treatment.

For HIV research in the past year, the clinical importance of low-level HIV viral replication is reported, as is a failed vaccine trial. In addition, I have selected an article on the cost effectiveness of expanded HIV screening. I acknowledge some assistance from both David Stone, MD, and Jim Hellinger, MD, MPH, for suggesting certain HIV articles for selection and for giving me their insights on these studies.

There are important selections on 2 relatively new antibiotics, ertapenem and tigecycline, as well as several important studies on antifungals. As in past years, I have tried to include articles that general internists would find useful for their practices, including some information on new vaccines that should have practical impact.

David R. Snydman, MD

10 Viral Infections

Probable Person-to-Person Transmission of Avian Influenza A (H5N1)

Ungchusak K, Auewarakul P, Dowell SF, et al (Thai Ministry of Public Health, Nonthaburi, Thailand; Mahidol Univ, Bangkok, Thailand; Ctrs for Disease Control and Prevention, Atlanta, Ga)

N Engl J Med 352:333-340, 2005 10–1

Background.—During 2004, a highly pathogenic avian influenza A (H5N1) virus caused poultry disease in eight Asian countries and infected at least 44 persons, killing 32; most of these persons had had close contact with poultry. No evidence of efficient person-to-person transmission has yet been reported. We investigated possible person-to-person transmission in a family cluster of the disease in Thailand.

Methods.—For each of the three involved patients, we reviewed the circumstances and timing of exposures to poultry and to other ill persons. Field teams isolated and treated the surviving patient, instituted active surveillance for disease and prophylaxis among exposed contacts, and culled the remaining poultry surrounding the affected village. Specimens from family members were tested by viral culture, microneutralization serologic analysis, immunohistochemical assay, reverse-transcriptase–polymerase-chain-reaction (RT-PCR) analysis, and genetic sequencing.

Results.—The index patient became ill three to four days after her last exposure to dying household chickens. Her mother came from a distant city to care for her in the hospital, had no recognized exposure to poultry, and died from pneumonia after providing 16 to 18 hours of unprotected nursing care. The aunt also provided unprotected nursing care; she had fever five days after the mother first had fever, followed by pneumonia seven days later. Autopsy tissue from the mother and nasopharyngeal and throat swabs from the aunt were positive for influenza A (H5N1) by RT-PCR. No additional chains of transmission were identified, and sequencing of the viral genes identified no change in the receptor-binding site of hemagglutinin or other key features of the virus. The sequences of all eight viral gene segments clustered closely with other H5N1 sequences from recent avian isolates in Thailand.

Conclusions.—Disease in the mother and aunt probably resulted from person-to-person transmission of this lethal avian influenzavirus during unprotected exposure to the critically ill index patient.

► Last year, I selected the report of the 14 avian influenza cases in humans from Vietnam reported in *The New England Journal of Medicine*.[1] The spread of this disease in humans from birds has been significant in Southeast Asia, with more than 100 cases reported and over 60 deaths. Essentially all the cases have arisen from bird-to-human transmission, but the world is appropriately concerned about a pandemic, with the potential emergence of human-to-human transmission from a new strain that has become more adapted to humans. Concern is raised, of course, that this pandemic might kill as many as 50 million people worldwide, like the pandemic of 1918.

The cases reported here would appear to result from human-to-human transmission, at least based on epidemiologic details able to be gleaned and from molecular studies performed on the influenza viruses isolated from the mother, the aunt, and the index case. There are some pitfalls in the report, namely, influenza A could not be documented in the index case. However, the clinical findings are consistent, especially since she was handling dead poultry, then came down with the disease shortly thereafter. Since the mother lived in a distant province, her exposure presumably came from the daughter. Although not present in the strain of influenza A isolated here, the authors point out that only one amino acid substitution can change the binding from an avian-specific sialic acid residue to a human-specific sialic acid. This is believed to be the epitope responsible for host range.

The World Health Organization and major governments are developing general influenza vaccine production capabilities, trying to develop new technology. The National Institutes of Health has developed an avian flu vaccine that is reportedly safe and immunogenic but not yet available for production or use. The manufacturer of the neuraminidase inhibitor, oseltamivir, is also increasing production, although a resistant strain has been described already (see Abstract 10–3). It is not clear yet how effective this medication will be for prophylaxis or treatment.

D. R. Snydman, MD

Reference

1. Hien TT, for the World Health Organization International Avian Influenza Investigative Team: Avian influenza A (H5N1) in 10 patients in Vietnam. *N Engl J Med* 350:1179-1188, 2004. (2005 YEAR BOOK OF MEDICINE, pp 88-91.

Characterization of the Reconstructed 1918 Spanish Influenza Pandemic Virus

Tumpey TM, Basler CF, Aguilar PV, et al (Centers for Disease Control and Prevention, Atlanta, Ga; Mount Sinai School of Medicine, New York; Armed Forces Inst of Pathology, Rockville, Md; et al)

Science 310:77-82, 2005 10–2

Background.—The influenza pandemic of 1918 was responsible for the deaths of up 50 million people throughout the world, including approximately 675,000 persons in the United States. The most remarkable feature of this pandemic was the unusually high rate of death among healthy adults age 15 to 34 years, which lowered the average life expectancy in the United

States by more than 10 years. There has been no similarly high death rate in this age group in any prior of subsequent pandemics or epidemics involving influenza A. Genomic RNA of the 1918 virus was recovered from archived formalin-fixed lung autopsy material and from frozen, unfixed lung tissues from an Alaskan influenza victim who had been buried in the permafrost in 1918. The complete coding sequences of all 8 viral RNA segments have now been determined. This study was conducted to study the properties associated with the extraordinary virulence of the 1918 virus.

Methods.—A virus containing the complete coding sequences of the 8 viral gene segments from the 1918 influenza virus was reconstructed using reverse genetics. Characteristics of this reconstructed Spanish flu virus were compared with those of several control viruses, including 2 contemporary H1N1 viruses.

Results.—Unlike the contemporary human H1N1 viruses, the 1918 pandemic virus had the ability to replicate in the absence of trypsin, caused death in mice and in embryonated chicken eggs, and showed a high-growth phenotype in human bronchial epithelial cells. A comparison of the 1918 virus with recombinant viruses expressing one or more 1918 virus genes demonstrated that the 1918 HA and polymerase genes are necessary for optimal virulence and that the constellation of all 8 genes together form a particularly virulent virus. These features provide a partial explanation for the exceptional lethality of the 1918 virus.

Conclusions.—The exceptional virulence of the 1918 pandemic influenza virus had until recently been a matter of historical curiosity. However, the emergence of another pandemic is now considered likely, if not inevitable. The characterization of the 1918 virus may provide insight into the potential threat posed by new influenza virus strains and the prophylactic and therapeutic countermeasures that will be needed to control pandemic viruses in the future.

► It is truly remarkable that the 1918 strain of influenza, which was associated with 50 million deaths worldwide and which perhaps killed 670,000 people in the United States, could be recovered from archived tissues from an Alaskan influenza victim and that genetic regulatory proteins and coding sequences could be determined and created. The authors have reconstructed this isolate under the most stringent conditions and have demonstrated a high degree of virulence in this particular virus. Remarkably, they report in a note added to the proof that the research was done by staff taking antiviral prophylaxis and in stringent biosafety conditions, probably because this work has come under some criticism as a potentially prohibited experiment. The authors nicely demonstrate the potential increased lethality of this particular strain, and by reconstructing this strain and making mutants and examining virulence properties they may provide a better understanding of the pathogenesis of influenza virus and virulence genes that have the potential to cause more severe disease.

D. R. Snydman, MD

Oseltamivir Resistance During Treatment of Influenza A (H5N1) Infection

de Jong MD, Thanh TT, Khanh TH, et al (Hosp for Tropical Diseases, Ho Chi Minh City, Vietnam; Pediatric Hosp Number One, Ho Chi Minh City, Vietnam; Hosp for Tropical Diseases, Ho Chi Minh City, Vietnam; et al)

N Engl J Med 353:2667-2672, 2005 10–3

Background.—Influenza A (H5N1) virus is a cause of severe disease in humans and is now a major pandemic threat. Oseltamivir, a neuraminidase inhibitor, is an important treatment option, and the stockpiling of this drug is part of the preparation for a pandemic. However, there are few data on the efficacy of oseltamivir and on the development of drug resistance in human influenza A (H5N1) virus. The isolation of oseltamivir-resistant influenza A (H5N1) variants from 2 patients who died of the infection, despite early initiation of treatment in 1 patient, was reported. Evidence that the presence of detectable virus after the completion of treatment is associated with a poor outcome was presented.

Case Report.—Girl, 13 years, from Viet Nam, who was previously healthy (weight, 28 kg) presented to a hospital in Vietnam with a 1-day history of fever and cough. The day before, her mother had died of influenza A (H5N1) virus infection after 1 day of oseltamivir treatment. The child received an initial 75-mg dose of oseltamivir because influenza A (H5N1) virus infection was suspected, and she was transferred to a pediatric referral hospital. At admission, the girl had a temperature of 40.3°C, a pulse of 106 beats/min, a respiratory rate of 36 breaths/min, and a normal blood pressure. Physical examination and routine biochemical measurements yielded unremarkable findings. Her white blood cell count was 4800 cells/mm^3 (normal range, 5500-15,500) with 12% lymphocytes and a platelet count of 183,000 cells/mm^3 (normal range, 250,000-550,000). A blood culture showed no growth. A chest radiograph showed a small focal pulmonary infiltrate in the right middle lobe. The patient received a second 75-mg dose of oseltamivir within 6 hours of the first, and a third dose at 24 hours after admission. Treatment was continued for 4 days with two 75-mg doses daily. The patient remained stable during the first 3 days after admission and did not require supplemental oxygen. Chest radiographs showed minimal progression of the infiltrate. On the fourth day of oseltamivir treatment, the girl's respiratory condition worsened. Supplemental high-dose oxygen was given by nasal cannula and then by continuous positive airway pressure. Antibiotic treatment was switched to vancomycin, ciprofloxacin, and amikacin. Further progression of the infiltrate was observed on radiography on the fifth day. Her white blood cell count continued to decline, to 1800 cells/mm^3 with 41% lymphocytes. Her respiratory condition worsened, and she was intubated and ventilation was initiated on the sixth day. A chest radiograph on the seventh day showed pneumonia involving the entire right lung and extension to the left lung. The patient died the same day. No autopsy was performed.

Discussion.—Influenza A (H5N1) virus with an H274Y substitution in the neuraminidase gene, which confers high-level resistance to oseltamivir, was isolated from this patient and another Vietnamese patient. These 2 patients were among 13 patients with influenza A (H5N1) virus infection confirmed with reverse transcriptase–polymerase chain reaction who were hospitalized in Vietnam between January 2004 and February 2005. Surviving patients had rapid declines in the viral load to undetectable levels during treatment. Resistance may emerge during the currently recommended regimen of oseltamivir therapy and may be associated with clinical deterioration. The strategy for treatment of influenza A (H5N1) virus infection should include the use of additional antiviral agents.

► This is the first published report of oseltamivir resistance associated with treatment failure in children with avian influenza. Of the 8 children treated, 4 died, and in 2 of the patients, resistance was detected with a change in the H274Y substitution of the neuraminidase gene, which confers high-level resistance. The isolation of resistant virus occurred in the setting of therapeutic doses of oseltamivir. In one of the patients who died, the viral load increased in the setting of resistance. In several other cases studied, the viral load did not fully decline, although the isolates remained sensitive. That resistance should occur should not be surprising, since it is known that oseltamivir resistance can occur. However, the fact that early treatment was initiated, at standard doses, is worrisome and means that additional drug targets are necessary. The use of higher doses, a longer treatment duration, or even combinations of drugs may be necessary in the future.

D. R. Snydman, MD

Incidence of Adamantane Resistance Among Influenza A (H3N2) Viruses Isolated Worldwide From 1994 to 2005: A Cause for Concern

Bright RA, Medina M-j, Xu X, et al (Centers for Disease Control and Prevention, Atlanta, Ga; Wisconsin State Laboratory of Hygiene, Madison)

Lancet 366:1175-1181, 2005 10–4

Background.—Adamantanes have been used to treat influenza A virus infections for many years. Studies have shown a low incidence of resistance to these drugs among circulating influenza viruses; however, their use is rising worldwide and drug resistance has been reported among influenza A (H5N1) viruses isolated from poultry and human beings in Asia. We sought to assess adamantane resistance among influenza A viruses isolated during the past decade from countries participating in WHO's global influenza surveillance network.

Methods.—We analysed data for influenza field isolates that were obtained worldwide and submitted to the WHO Collaborating Center for Influenza at the US Centers for Disease Control and Prevention between Oct 1, 1994, and Mar 31, 2005. We used pyrosequencing, confirmatory sequence analysis, and phenotypic testing to detect drug resistance among circulating influenza A H3N2 (n=6524), H1N1 (n=589), and H1N2 (n=83) viruses.

Findings.—More than 7000 influenza A field isolates were screened for specific aminoacid substitutions in the M2 gene known to confer drug resistance. During the decade of surveillance a significant increase in drug resistance was noted, from 0.4% in 1994-1995 to 12.3% in 2003-2004. This increase in the proportion of resistant viruses was weighted heavily by those obtained from Asia with 61% of resistant viruses isolated since 2003 being from people in Asia.

Interpretation.—Our data raise concerns about the appropriate use of adamantanes and draw attention to the importance of tracking the emergence and spread of drug-resistant influenza A viruses.

▶ While we worry about pandemic avian influenza, one cannot ignore current influenza disease and the use of antiviral agents as well as vaccine. Amantadine has been one of the primary drugs of choice for the treatment or prevention of influenza A virus infection. Drug-resistant isolates can be pathogenic, and the emergence of resistance to amantadine would essentially eliminate one of the few agents available. This analysis shows that in Asia, almost 75% of isolates are now resistant to amantadine. These data have obvious implications for public health authorities with respect to stockpiling and drug availability for prophylaxis or treatment of influenza A. Interestingly, up until 2004, the rates of amantadine-resistant influenza A isolated in the United States were quite low, that is, about 2%. However, in the first 6 months of 2005, the rate of amantadine-resistant influenza A in the United States rose to 14.5%. Thus, the circulation of these resistant viruses is cause for concern here in the United States. It is presumed that one reason for the higher rates of amantadine resistance in other parts of the world may be because of the availability of over-the-counter (or nonprescription) use of amantadine.

D. R. Snydman, MD

11 Bacterial Infection

Methicillin-Resistant *Staphylococcus aureus* Disease in Three Communities

Fridkin SK, for the Active Bacterial Core Surveillance Program of the Emerging Infections Program Network (Ctrs for Disease Control and Prevention, Atlanta, Ga; et al)

N Engl J Med 352:1436-1444, 2005 11–1

Background.—Methicillin-resistant *Staphylococcus aureus* (MRSA) infection has emerged in patients who do not have the established risk factors. The national burden and clinical effect of this novel presentation of MRSA disease are unclear.

Methods.—We evaluated MRSA infections in patients identified from population-based surveillance in Baltimore and Atlanta and from hospital-laboratory-based sentinel surveillance of 12 hospitals in Minnesota. Information was obtained by interviewing patients and by reviewing their medical records. Infections were classified as community-associated MRSA disease if no established risk factors were identified.

Results.—From 2001 through 2002, 1647 cases of community-associated MRSA infection were reported, representing between 8 and 20 percent of all MRSA isolates. The annual disease incidence varied according to site (25.7 cases per 100,000 population in Atlanta vs. 18.0 per 100,000 in Baltimore) and was significantly higher among persons less than two years old than among those who were two years of age or older (relative risk, 1.51; 95 percent confidence interval, 1.19 to 1.92) and among blacks than among whites in Atlanta (age-adjusted relative risk, 2.74; 95 percent confidence interval, 2.44 to 3.07). Six percent of cases were invasive, and 77 percent involved skin and soft tissue. The infecting strain of MRSA was often (73 percent) resistant to prescribed antimicrobial agents. Among patients with skin or soft-tissue infections, therapy to which the infecting strain was resistant did not appear to be associated with adverse patient-reported outcomes. Overall, 23 percent of patients were hospitalized for the MRSA infection.

Conclusions.—Community-associated MRSA infections are now a common and serious problem. These infections usually involve the skin, especially among children, and hospitalization is common.

► This is the first population-based study of the emergence of community-associated MRSA infections. Of interest, even if antibiotics were selected to which the isolate was not susceptible, there was no difference in outcome. Since most of these patients had skin and soft tissue infections, simple drainage may have been all that is necessary. However, we know that many of these infections and strains will have a much more virulent presentation, so I am not advocating inappropriate antibiotic therapy. In fact, current recommendations include obtaining a culture when draining an abscess, and then employing appropriate therapy operating on the assumption that one is dealing with MRSA until proven otherwise.

D. R. Snydman, MD

A Clone of Methicillin-Resistant *Staphylococcus aureus* Among Professional Football Players

Kazakova SV, Hageman JC, Matava M, et al (Ctrs for Disease Control and Prevention, Atlanta, Ga; Washington Univ, St Louis; Missouri Dept of Health and Senior Services, St Louis)

N Engl J Med 352:468-475, 2005 11–2

Background.—Methicillin-resistant *Staphylococcus aureus* (MRSA) is an emerging cause of infections outside of health care settings. We investigated an outbreak of abscesses due to MRSA among members of a professional football team and examined the transmission and microbiologic characteristics of the outbreak strain.

Methods.—We conducted a retrospective cohort study and nasal-swab survey of 84 St. Louis Rams football players and staff members. *S. aureus* recovered from wound, nasal, and environmental cultures was analyzed by means of pulsed-field gel electrophoresis (PFGE) and typing for resistance and toxin genes. MRSA from the team was compared with other community isolates and hospital isolates.

Results.—During the 2003 football season, eight MRSA infections occurred among 5 of the 58 Rams players (9 percent); all of the infections developed at turf-abrasion sites. MRSA infection was significantly associated with the lineman or linebacker position and a higher body-mass index. No MRSA was found in nasal or environmental samples; however, methicillin-susceptible *S. aureus* was recovered from whirlpools and taping gel and from 35 of the 84 nasal swabs from players and staff members (42 percent). MRSA from a competing football team and from other community clusters and sporadic cases had PFGE patterns that were indistinguishable from those of the Rams' MRSA; all carried the gene for Panton–Valentine leukocidin and the gene complex for staphylococcal-cassette-chromosome *mec* type IVa resistance (clone USA300-0114).

Conclusions.—We describe a highly conserved, community-associated MRSA clone that caused abscesses among professional football players and that was indistinguishable from isolates from various other regions of the United States.

▶ At the time this outbreak took place, it received a lot of national attention because it involved a professional football team. This outbreak, however, was only the tip of the iceberg with respect to football-associated outbreaks. Generally, only skin abscesses occurred, but in other outbreaks with less healthy individuals on college teams, more significant disease, including pneumonia, has occurred. The authors used rifampin to eradicate the carrier state and also treated players and used antimicrobial soaps in the locker room. Of interest is that types of methicillin-susceptible *S aureus* were found in the environment and in player nares, which suggests environmental–player transmission of *S aureus*.

D. R. Snydman, MD

Necrotizing Fasciitis Caused by Community-Associated Methicillin-Resistant *Staphylococcus aureus* in Los Angeles

Miller LG, Perdreau-Remington F, Rieg G, et al (Harbor-UCLA, Torrance, Calif; Univ of California, San Francisco; St Mary Med Ctr, Long Beach, Calif)

N Engl J Med 352:1445-1453, 2005 11–3

Background.—Necrotizing fasciitis is a life-threatening infection requiring urgent surgical and medical therapy. *Staphylococcus aureus* has been a very uncommon cause of necrotizing fasciitis, but we have recently noted an alarming number of these infections caused by community-associated methicillin-resistant *S. aureus* (MRSA).

Methods.—We reviewed the records of 843 patients whose wound cultures grew MRSA at our center from January 15, 2003, to April 15, 2004. Among this cohort, 14 were identified as patients presenting from the community with clinical and intraoperative findings of necrotizing fasciitis, necrotizing myositis, or both.

Results.—The median age of the patients was 46 years (range, 28 to 68), and 71 percent were men. Coexisting conditions or risk factors included current or past injection-drug use (43 percent); previous MRSA infection, diabetes, and chronic hepatitis C (21 percent each); and cancer and human immunodeficiency virus infection or the acquired immunodeficiency syndrome (7 percent each). Four patients (29 percent) had no serious coexisting conditions or risk factors. All patients received combined medical and surgical therapy, and none died, but they had serious complications, including the need for reconstructive surgery and prolonged stay in the intensive care unit. Wound cultures were monomicrobial for MRSA in 86 percent, and 40 percent of patients (4 of 10) for whom blood cultures were obtained had positive results. All MRSA isolates were susceptible in vitro to clindamycin, trimethoprim–sulfamethoxazole, and rifampin. All recovered isolates belonged to the same genotype (multilocus sequence type ST8, pulsed-field type USA300, and staphylococcal cassette chromosome *mec* type IV [SCC*mec*IV]) and carried the Panton–Valentine leukocidin (*pvl)*, *luk*D, and *luk*E genes, but no other toxin genes were detected.

Conclusions.—Necrotizing fasciitis caused by community-associated MRSA is an emerging clinical entity. In areas in which community-associated MRSA infection is endemic, empirical treatment of suspected necrotizing fasciitis should include antibiotics predictably active against this pathogen.

► In the past few years, community-acquired MRSA infections have become commonplace, and the clinical presentation is that of a more aggressive and more virulent type. This case series describes 14 such cases from the Los Angeles area. The authors note that 62% of community-acquired *S aureus* infections are now MRSA. This obviously makes clinical decision making in the offices and emergency departments more problematic because, in the past, we assumed MRSA was a nosocomial pathogen. Of interest in this article is that MRSA has rarely been reported as a cause of necrotizing fasciitis, yet this cluster illustrates a more virulent form. A number of genetic elements are common to these strains and include (*pvl*), *luk*D, and *luk*E genes. There is also a regulatory gene, *agr*, which was of a type different from others previously seen in some communities. The *agr* gene regulates some toxin production and adhesion.

This article has some limitations in that the strain represented a single clone; therefore, the clinical findings may not be generalizable to those seen in other strains circulating in different communities. However, on the basis of my own experience in Boston, we are seeing similar problems with community-acquired MRSA.

One way the clinician can recognize these strains is by their general susceptibility to bactrim, clindamycin, gentamicin, and rifampin. Many strains are also sensitive to the quinolones. This would be in marked contrast to what we usually see with health care–associated MRSA.

D. R. Snydman, MD

Severe Community-Onset Pneumonia in Healthy Adults Caused by Methicillin-Resistant *Staphylococcus aureus* Carrying the Panton-Valentine Leukocidin Genes

Francis JS, Doherty MC, Lopatin U, et al (Johns Hopkins Med Institutions, Baltimore, Md; NIH, Bethesda, Md)
Clin Infect Dis 40:100-107, 2005 11–4

Background.—Recent worldwide reports of community-onset skin abscesses, outbreaks of furunculosis, and severe pneumonia associated with methicillin-resistant *Staphylococcus aureus* (MRSA) carrying Panton-Valentine leukocidin (PVL) genes and the staphylococcal cassette chromosome *mec* (SCC*mec*) type IV indicate that MRSA infections are evolving into a community-related problem. The majority of cases reported to date involve skin and soft-tissue infections, with severe pneumonia representing a relatively rare phenomenon. During a 2-month period in the winter of 2003-2004, four healthy adults presented to 1 of 2 Baltimore hospitals with severe necrotizing MRSA pneumonia in the absence of typical risk factors for MRSA infection.

Methods.—Patients' MRSA isolates were characterized by strain typing with use of pulsed-field gel electrophoresis and SCC*mec* typing with use of a multiplex polymerase chain reaction (PCR) assay and detection of PVL genes by PCR.

Results.—All 4 patients' MRSA isolates carried the PVL genes and the SCC*mec* type IV element and belonged to the USA300 pulsed-field type. These 3 findings are among the typical characteristics of community-onset MRSA strains. In addition, 2 of our patients had concomitant influenza A diagnosed, which likely contributed to the severity of their presentation.

Conclusions.—To our knowledge, these patients represent the first reported North American adults with severe community-onset MRSA pneumonia caused by strains carrying the PVL genes.

► The change in the epidemiology of *S aureus* infection is quite extraordinary. As noted in selections to this year's YEAR BOOK, several outbreaks of skin and soft tissue infection have been well documented. These cases document community-acquired MRSA causing pneumonia, sometimes following influenza infection, and, in other cases, without any apparent risk factors. Clinicians need to be aware of the increasing likelihood of encountering these very virulent organisms, which have factors, such as the PVL gene that appear to lead to increased necrosis in the lung. Hemoptysis, shock, and cavitation are common. The best treatment regimen has not been worked out, but the isolates are susceptible typically to the quinolones, trimethoprim sulfamethoxazole, vancomycin, and linezolid. Whether more than 1 antibiotic would be useful or what the optimal regimen is remains undetermined. In the cases discussed in this article, 1 patient died, and the rest received combinations of agents empirically.

D. R. Snydman, MD

Staphylococcus aureus Native Valve Infective Endocarditis: Report of 566 Episodes From the International Collaboration on Endocarditis Merged Database

Miro JM, and the International Collaboration on Endocarditis Merged Database Study Group (Univ of Barcelona; et al)

Clin Infect Dis 41:507-514, 2005 11–5

Background.—*Staphylococcus aureus* native valve infective endocarditis (SA-NVIE) is not completely understood. The objective of this investigation was to describe the characteristics of a large, international cohort of patients with SA-NVIE.

Methods.—The International Collaboration on Endocarditis Merged Database (ICE-MD) is a combination of 7 existing electronic databases from 5 countries that contains data on 2212 cases of definite infective endocarditis (IE).

Results.—Of patients with native valve IE, 566 patients (34%) had IE due to *S. aureus*, and 1074 patients had IE due to pathogens other than *S. aureus* (non-SA-NVIE). Patients with *S. aureus* IE were more likely to die (20% vs. 12%; $P < .001$), to experience an embolic event (60% vs. 31%; $P < .001$), or to have a central nervous system event (20% vs. 13%; $P < .001$) and were less likely to undergo surgery (26% vs. 39%; $P <$ 001) than were patients with non-SA-NVIE. Multivariate analysis of prognostic factors of mortality identified age (odds ratio [OR], 1.4; 95% confidence interval [CI], 1.1-1.7), periannular abscess (OR, 2.4; 95% CI, 1.1-5.6), heart failure (OR, 3.9; 95% CI, 2.3-6.7), and absence of surgical therapy (OR, 2.3; 95% CI, 1.3-4.2) as variables that were independently associated with mortality in patients with SA-NVIE. After adjusting for patient-, pathogen-, and treatment-specific characteristics by multivariate analysis, geographical region was also found to be associated with mortality in patients with SA-NVIE ($P < .001$).

Conclusions.—*S. aureus* is an important and common cause of IE. The outcome of SA-NVIE is worse than that of non-SA-NVIE. Several clinical parameters are independently associated with mortality for patients with SA-NVIE. The clinical characteristics and outcome of SA-NVIE vary significantly by geographic region, although the reasons for such regional variations in outcomes of SA-NVIE are unknown and are probably multifactorial. A large, prospective, multinational cohort study of patients with IE is now under way to further investigate these observations.

► Although these data have limitations, such as the use of different data collection instruments and, possibly, a referral bias, the duration of the data (ie, during a 20-year period) with the changes in diagnostic and therapeutic approaches and the importance of the findings seem to be generalizable. *S aureus* endocarditis is a significant problem, annular abscess is a very poor prognostic category, and the need for surgery is apparent. However, it is not surprising that the mortality rate without surgery in left-sided disease is high, since some patients may be "too sick" to go to surgery. The findings should be considered hypothesis generating, and future prospective studies will be important to increase our understanding of SA-NVIE

D. R. Snydman, MD

Re-emergence of Early Pandemic *Staphylococcus aureus* as a Community-acquired Meticillin-Resistant Clone

Robinson DA, Kearns AM, Holmes A, et al (Univ of Bath, England; Health Protection Agency, London; Stobhill Hosp, Glasgow, Scotland; et al)

Lancet 365:1256-1258, 2005 11–6

Background.—*Staphylococcus aureus*, which has a particular phage lysis pattern known as phage type 80, was first isolated from neonatal infections in Australia in 1953. Similar isolates, known as phage type 81, were also isolated in Canada in that year. The Australian and Canadian isolates could be lysed by both phages and were thus thought to be members of the same clone, called phage type 80/81. This phage type became pandemic in the 1950s, causing skin lesions, sepsis, and pneumonia in children and young adults in hospitals and in the community. The pandemic waned throughout the 1960s as methicillin and its derivatives were used to treat penicillin-resistant staphylococcal infections. The genetic background of phage type 80/81 was determined by sequencing portions of 7 housekeeping genes from isolates of 80/81 isolated between 1955 and 1969.

Overview.—Portions of 7 housekeeping genes (*arc, aro, glp, gmk, pta, tpi,* and *yqi*) from 26 isolates of phage type 80/81, isolated between 1955 and 1969 in Australia, England, and the United States were sequenced. These sequences were compared with those of more than 1000 isolates in the multilocus sequence type (ST) 30 (ST30), a very common genotype that can both colonize and cause disease in patients in hospital and in healthy people in the community. Community-acquired methicillin-resistant *S aureus* (MRSA) is known for carrying both the phage-borne Panton-Valentine leucocidin (PVL) toxin and a particular allele of the staphylococcal chromosomal cassette *mec* (SCC*mec* type IV), a toxin associated with virulence in young healthy people. ST30 is 1 of 6 different genotypes of community-acquired PVL-positive MRSA. Such isolates are known as the southwest Pacific (SWP) clone. Data suggest that the 80/81 clone is closely related to the SWP clone.

Conclusions.—Results of multilocus sequence analysis suggested that descendants of phage type 80/81 have acquired methicillin resistance and are reemerging as a community-acquired MRSA clone. These descendants are representative of a sister lineage to pandemic hospital-acquired MRSA.

► I chose this article to underscore the potential origin of the epidemic strains of *S aureus* we are seeing today. The infamous 80/81 strain (based on phage typing) that was pandemic in the 1950s and 1960s caused very serious necrotizing infections in children. The genetic studies detailed here suggest that the strains are closely related to the clone found in the southwest Pacific (SWP clone) and the one found in the United Kingdom (ST36 MRSA-II). Thus, we may see the presage of this 80/81 clone in hospitals and the community yet again.

D. R. Snydman, MD

Changing Epidemiology of Invasive Pneumococcal Disease Among Older Adults in the Era of Pediatric Pneumococcal Conjugate Vaccine

Lexau CA, for the Active Bacterial Core Surveillance Team (Minnesota Dept of Health, Minneapolis; et al)

JAMA 294:2043-2051, 2005 11–7

Context.—A conjugate vaccine targeting 7 pneumococcal serotypes was licensed for young children in 2000. In contrast to the 23-valent polysaccharide vaccine used in adults, the 7-valent conjugate vaccine affects pneumococcal carriage and transmission. Early after its introduction, incidence of invasive pneumococcal disease declined among older adults, a group at high risk for pneumococcal disease.

Objective.—To determine among adults aged 50 years or older whether incidence of invasive pneumococcal disease, disease characteristics, or the spectrum of patients acquiring these illnesses have changed over the 4 years since pneumococcal conjugate vaccine licensure.

Design, Setting, and Population.—Population-based surveillance of invasive pneumococcal disease in 8 US geographic areas (total population, 18,813,000), 1998-2003.

Main Outcome Measures.—Incidence of invasive pneumococcal disease by pneumococcal serotype and other characteristics; frequency among case patients of comorbid conditions and other factors influencing mortality.

Results.—Incidence of invasive pneumococcal disease among adults aged 50 years or older declined 28% (95% confidence interval [CI], −31% to −24%), from 40.8 cases/100,000 in 1998-1999 to 29.4 in 2002-2003. Among those aged 65 years or older, the 2002-2003 rate (41.7 cases/100,000) was lower than the Healthy People 2010 goal (42 cases/100,000). Among adults aged 50 years or older, incidence of disease caused by the 7 conjugate vaccine serotypes declined 55% (95% CI, −58% to −51%) from 22.4 to 10.2 cases/100,000. In contrast, disease caused by any of the 16 serotypes only in polysaccharide vaccine did not change, and disease caused by serotypes not in either vaccine increased somewhat, from 6.0 to 6.8 cases/100,000 (13%; 95% CI, 1% to 27%). Between 1998-1999 and 2002-2003, the proportion of case-patients with human immunodeficiency virus infection increased from 1.7% (47/2737) to 5.6% (124/2231) ($P<.001$), and those with any comorbid condition that is an indication for pneumococcal polysaccharide vaccination increased from 62.3% (1842/2955) to 72.0% (1721/2390) ($P<.001$).

Conclusions.—Our findings indicate that use of conjugate vaccine in children has substantially benefited older adults. However, persons with certain comorbid conditions may benefit less than healthier persons from the indirect effects of the new vaccine.

► The pediatric conjugate pneumococcal vaccine licensed in 2000 has had a dramatic impact on reducing invasive pediatric pneumococcal disease. This report examines the impact on adult populations and has a number of strengths, including a large population-based surveillance system, serotyping of invasive isolates, and a standardized methodology. The authors also acknowledge a few limitations, including possible misclassification of some comorbid conditions and absence of data on polysaccharide vaccine usage among adults. Nevertheless, the facts are clear. A very significant reduction in invasive pneumococcal vaccine serotypes used in the conjugate vaccine was seen in adults, suggesting decreased circulation of such serotypes in the population because of decreased colonization and transmission among children. There is a note of caution, however. Non–vaccine serotype disease did increase slightly, and the preventive effects of herd immunity were reduced in some patients with comorbid conditions such as HIV, and in others for whom pneumococcal vaccine is indicated. One awaits the licensure of a conjugate vaccine for adults, which presumably will have increased immunogenicity, especially among those at highest risk.

D. R. Snydman, MD

Use of Gastric Acid–Suppressive Agents and the Risk of Community-Acquired *Clostridium difficile*–Associated Disease

Dial S, Delaney JAC, Barkun AN, et al (McGill Univ, Montreal)

JAMA 294:2989-2995, 2005 11–8

Context.—Recent reports suggest an increasing occurrence and severity of *Clostridium difficile*–associated disease. We assessed whether the use of gastric acid–suppressive agents is associated with an increased risk in the community.

Objective.—To determine whether the use of gastric acid–suppressive agents increases the risk of *C difficile*–associated disease in a community population.

Design, Setting, and Patients.—We conducted 2 population-based case-control studies using the United Kingdom General Practice Research Database (GPRD). In the first study, we identified all 1672 cases of *C difficile* recorded between 1994 and 2004 among all patients registered for at least 2 years in each practice. Each case was matched to 10 controls on calendar time and the general practice. In the second study, a subset of these cases defined as community-acquired, that is, not hospitalized in the prior year, were matched on practice and age with controls also not hospitalized in the prior year.

Main Outcome Measures.—The incidence of *C difficile* and risk associated with gastric acid–suppressive agent use.

Results.—The incidence of *C difficile* in patients diagnosed by their general practitioners in the General Practice Research Database increased from less than 1 case per 100,000 in 1994 to 22 per 100,000 in 2004. The adjusted rate ratio of *C difficile*–associated disease with current use of proton pump inhibitors was 2.9 (95% confidence interval [CI], 2.4-3.4) and with H_2-receptor antagonists the rate ratio was 2.0 (95% CI, 1.6-2.7). An elevated rate was also found with the use of nonsteroidal anti-inflammatory drugs (rate ratio, 1.3; 95% CI, 1.2-1.5).

Conclusions.—The use of acid-suppressive therapy, particularly proton pump inhibitors, is associated with an increased risk of community-acquired *C difficile*. The unexpected increase in risk with nonsteroidal anti-inflammatory drug use should be investigated further.

► Although the association with gastric acid–suppressive agents and the occurrence of *C difficile*–associated diarrhea is not surprising, and has been shown in hospitalized patients previously, this study is important for several reasons. One, it establishes very nicely the increase in the rate of community-acquired *C difficile*. The increase over a decade among the patients of British general practitioners has grown 22-fold! In this study, no patient with community-acquired disease was hospitalized within the previous year. Two, it demonstrates that more than half of the patients did not have exposure to antibiotics within the previous 90 days (the authors' definition of exposure). Three, it raises the possibility that nonsteroidal anti-inflammatory agents may be associated with an increased risk of *C difficile*. Physicians must consider *C difficile* disease in all patients, including those who have not received antibiotics, and this problem is increasing in importance in the general public in England and North America. With changes in virulence documented below (see Abstracts 16–7 and 16–8), and more severe disease, the changing epidemiology of this organism must be watched carefully.

D. R. Snydman, MD

12 Human Immunodeficiency Virus

An Improvement in Virologic Response to Highly Active Antiretroviral Therapy in Clinical Practice From 1996 Through 2002

Moore RD, Keruly JC, Gebo KA, et al (Johns Hopkins Univ, Baltimore, Md)

J Acquir Immune Defic Syndr 39:195-198, 2005 12–1

Introduction.—Early studies of highly active antiretroviral therapy (HAART) use in clinical practice suggested suboptimal rates of viral suppression. HAART regimens and expertise in the use of HAART have since evolved, and we sought to determine how virologic response to HAART has changed in clinical practice. We compared all patients who started a first HAART regimen from 1996 through 2002 in a longitudinal cohort of HIV-infected patients in care in Baltimore. There were significant improvements in suppressing HIV RNA to <400 copies/mL, ranging from 43.8% (1996) to 72.4% (2001–2002) by 6 months and from 60.1% (1996) to 79.9% (2001–2002) by 12 months (both $P < 0.01$ for trend). There were also significant improvements in CD4 cell response. Over time, there was a significant increase in the use of a nonnucleoside reverse transcriptase inhibitor (NNRTI) or boosted protease inhibitor (PI) regimen compared with a single PI as well as an increase in the number of patients who were antiretroviral (ARV) naive. There was also a significant temporal trend from 1996 through 2002 in achieving a suppressed HIV RNA level, adjusting for being ARV naive, specific HAART regimen, CD4 cell count, HIV-1 RNA level, and demographic factors. This suggests that improved virologic response may also be attributable to other factors such as a greater focus on medication adherence, improved ARV tolerability, and ease of dosing.

► This study certainly documents with precision the improvements in management of HIV-infected individuals. Efavirenz- or ritonavir-boosted protease inhibitors as the basis for HAART are now used with improved adherence, and to a better effect. Of note, in this cohort there was an increase in the number of infected African Americans, infected women, and those acquiring HIV infection through heterosexual contact. In concordance with the increase in adherence, there were increases in CD4 cells and fewer opportunistic infections.

D. R. Snydman, MD

Infection With Multidrug Resistant, Dual-Tropic HIV-1 and Rapid Progression to AIDS: A Case Report

Markowitz M, Mohri H, Mehandru S, et al (Rockefeller Univ, New York; ViroLogic, San Francisco; Cabrini Med Ctr, New York)

Lancet 365:1031-1038, 2005 12–2

Background.—Rapid progression to AIDS after acute HIV-1 infection, though uncommon, has been noted, as has the transmission of multidrug resistant viruses. Here, we describe a patient in whom these two factors arose concomitantly and assess the effects.

Methods.—We did a case study of a patient with HIV-1 seroconversion. We genotyped the virus and host genetic markers by PCR and nucleotide sequencing. To ascertain the drug susceptibility of our patient's HIV-1 we did phenotypic studies with the PhenoSense assay. We assessed viral coreceptor use via syncytium formation in vitro and with a modified PhenoSense assay.

Findings.—Our patient seems to have been recently infected by a viral variant of HIV-1 resistant to multiple classes of antiretroviral drugs. Furthermore, his virus population is dual tropic for cells that express CCR5 or CXCR4 coreceptor. The infection has resulted in progression to symptomatic AIDS in 4–20 months.

Interpretation.—The intersection of multidrug resistance and rapid development of AIDS in this patient is of concern, especially in view of his case history, which includes high-risk sexual contacts and use of metamfetamine. The public health ramifications of such a case are great.

► This is a very important case that was highlighted at last year's HIV conference. The documentation of superinfection with a virus that had dual tropism of CCR5 and CXCR4 coreceptor is notable and may be associated with accelerated rates of CD4 depletion and rapid progression to AIDS. While rapid progression to AIDS after acute HIV-1 infection and transmission of drug resistance have both been reported previously, the features of this case, namely the convergence of both multidrug resistance and rapid progression, make it unique. Fortunately, it is currently rare, but clinicians should be aware of such a possibility. The patient did have promiscuous sex with multiple partners and did use crystal methamphetamine, which may have a factor in disease progression. In animal models, methamphetamine does enhance feline immunodeficiency virus replication. Whether the use of this substance has such an effect or stimulates increased or prolonged sexual activity is not clear. This case illustrates both treatment and public health challenges to HIV management in a unique way.

D. R. Snydman, MD

Expanded Screening for HIV in the United States—An Analysis of Cost-Effectiveness

Paltiel AD, Weinstein MC, Kimmel AD, et al (Yale School of Medicine, New Haven, Conn; Harvard School of Public Health, Boston; Harvard Med School, Boston; et al)

N Engl J Med 352:586-595, 2005 12–3

Background.—Although the Centers for Disease Control and Prevention (CDC) recommend routine HIV counseling, testing, and referral (HIVCTR) in settings with at least a 1 percent prevalence of HIV, roughly 280,000 Americans are unaware of their human immunodeficiency virus (HIV) infection. The effect of expanded screening for HIV is unknown in the era of effective antiretroviral therapy.

Methods.—We developed a computer simulation model of HIV screening and treatment to compare routine, voluntary HIVCTR with current practice in three target populations: "high-risk" (3.0 percent prevalence of undiagnosed HIV infection; 1.2 percent annual incidence); "CDC threshold" (1.0 percent and 0.12 percent, respectively); and "U.S. general" (0.1 percent and 0.01 percent). Input data were derived from clinical trials and observational cohorts. Outcomes included quality-adjusted survival, cost, and cost-effectiveness.

Results.—In the high-risk population, the addition of one-time screening for HIV antibodies with an enzyme-linked immunosorbent assay (ELISA) to current practice was associated with earlier diagnosis of HIV (mean CD4 cell count at diagnosis, 210 vs. 154 per cubic millimeter). One-time screening also improved average survival time among HIV-infected patients (quality-adjusted survival, 220.7 months vs. 219.8 months). The incremental cost-effectiveness was $36,000 per quality-adjusted life-year gained. Testing every five years cost $50,000 per quality-adjusted life-year gained, and testing every three years cost $63,000 per quality-adjusted life-year gained. In the CDC threshold population, the cost-effectiveness ratio for one-time screening with ELISA was $38,000 per quality-adjusted life-year gained, whereas testing every five years cost $71,000 per quality-adjusted life-year gained, and testing every three years cost $85,000 per quality-adjusted life-year gained. In the U.S. general population, one-time screening cost $113,000 per quality-adjusted life-year gained.

Conclusions.—In all but the lowest-risk populations, routine, voluntary screening for HIV once every three to five years is justified on both clinical and cost-effectiveness grounds. One-time screening in the general population may also be cost-effective.

► Two studies, the one cited and another by Sanders et al,[1] came to the same conclusion about the cost effectiveness of screening for HIV. In high-risk populations, the cost effectiveness of screening is considerable given current financial assumptions about cost-effectiveness analyses; that is, any intervention at $50,000 or less per quality-adjusted year of life screened is quite cost effective. In the sensitivity analysis of the current study, there were 3 areas of uncertainty. First, the effect of HIV counseling, testing, and referral will be inversely related to the frequency of background testing already performed elsewhere in other clinics that often are involved with intravenous drug abuse treatment, family planning, insurance applications, and prisons. Second, acceptance of testing and treatment remains another area of imprecision. Third, the impact of testing on secondary transmission needs more study. In the model, testing could have a profound impact on this variable, with even minimal improvements in those receiving therapy.

D. R. Snydman, MD

Reference

1. Sanders GD, Bayoumi AM, Sundaram V, et al: Cost-effectiveness of screening for HIV in the era of highly active antiretroviral therapy. *N Engl J Med* 352:570-585, 2005.

Intermittent HIV-1 Viremia (Blips) and Drug Resistance in Patients Receiving HAART

Nettles RE, Kieffer TL, Kwon P, et al (Johns Hopkins Univ, Baltimore, Md; NIH, Bethesda, Md; Johns Hopkins Bloomberg School of Public Health, Baltimore, Md; et al)

JAMA 293:817-829, 2005 12–4

Context.—Many patients infected with human immunodeficiency virus type 1 (HIV-1) and receiving highly active antiretroviral therapy experience intermittent episodes of detectable viremia ("blips"), which may raise concerns about drug resistance, lead to costly repeat measurements of viral RNA, and sometimes trigger alterations in therapy.

Objective.—To test the hypothesis that blips represent random biological and statistical variation around mean steady-state HIV-1 RNA levels slightly below 50 copies/mL rather than biologically significant elevations in viremia.

Design, Setting, and Patients.—Between June 19, 2003, and February 9, 2004, patients receiving therapy underwent intensive sampling (every 2-3 days) over 3 to 4 months to define the frequency, magnitude, and duration of blips and their association with drug levels and other clinical variables. Blips were defined as HIV-1 RNA measurements greater than or equal to 50 copies/mL preceded and followed by measurements less than 50 copies/mL without a change in treatment. To determine whether blips result from or lead to drug resistance, an ultrasensitive genotyping assay was used to detect drug resistance mutations before, during, and after blips. Patients were 10 HIV-1–infected asymptomatic adults recruited by clinicians and followed up in the Moore Clinic at the Johns Hopkins Hospital. Patients had suppression of viremia to below 50 copies/mL while receiving a stable antiretroviral regimen for 6 months or longer.

Main Outcome Measures.—At each time point, plasma HIV-1 RNA levels were measured in 2 independent laboratories and drug resistance mutations were analyzed by clonal sequencing.

Results.—With the intensive sampling, blips were detected in 9 of 10 patients. Statistical analysis was consistent with random assay variation around a mean viral load below 50 copies/mL. Blips were not concordant on independent testing and had a short duration (median, <3 days) and low magnitude (median, 79 copies/mL). Blip frequency was not associated with demographic, clinical, or treatment variables. Blips did not occur in relation to illness, vaccination, or directly measured antiretroviral drug concentrations. Blips were marginally associated ($P = .08$) with reported episodes of nonadherence. Most importantly, in approximately 1000 independent clones sequenced for both protease and reverse transcriptase, no new resistance mutations were seen before, during, or shortly after blips.

Conclusion.—Most blips in this population appear to represent random biological and statistical variation around mean HIV-1 levels below 50 copies/mL rather than clinically significant elevations in viremia.

► This is a beautifully done study, albeit on only 10 patients. Sheldon Wolff, MD, one of my former mentors, former chair of Medicine at Tufts and former head of the National Institute of Allergy and Infectious Diseases, used to say that studying one patient really well can provide more information about biology than studying many patients in lesser detail. This study is such an example. It does provide some reassurance. Blips in HIV viral load detection have been thought to represent a number of different phenomena. They are thought to occur in the setting of reduced drug concentration in patients receiving highly active antiretroviral therapy, either because of a transient lack of adherence or reduced bioavailability, or to arise from heightened immune activation. There is concern in caring for patients with blips that this will lead to increased failure or drug resistance. The authors conclude that blips are normal variations around a low biologic threshold and are not associated with drug resistance mutations. In fact, the level of mutation analysis was such that at least for these 9 patients, the investigators could rule out blips caused by viral resistance.

D. R. Snydman, MD

Placebo-controlled Phase 3 Trial of a Recombinant Glycoprotein 120 Vaccine to Prevent HIV-1 Infection

Gurwith M, for the rgp120 HIV Vaccine Study Group (VaxGen, Brisbane, Calif; et al)

J Infect Dis 191:654-665, 2005 12–5

Background.—A vaccine is needed to prevent human immunodeficiency virus type 1 (HIV-1) infection.

Methods.—A double-blind, randomized trial of a recombinant HIV-1 envelope glycoprotein subunit (rgp120) vaccine was conducted among men who have sex with men and among women at high risk for heterosexual transmission of HIV-1. Volunteers received 7 injections of either vaccine or placebo (ratio, 2:1) over 30 months. The primary end point was HIV-1 seroconversion over 36 months.

Results.—A total of 5403 volunteers (5095 men and 308 women) were evaluated. The vaccine did not prevent HIV-1 acquisition: infection rates were 6.7% in 3598 vaccinees and 7.0% in 1805 placebo recipients; vaccine efficacy (VE) was estimated as 6% (95% confidence interval, −17% to 24%). There were no significant differences in viral loads, rates of antiretroviral-therapy initiation, or the genetic characteristics of the infecting HIV-1 strains between treatment arms. Exploratory subgroup analyses showed nonsignificant trends toward efficacy in preventing infection in the highest risk (VE, 43%; $n = 247$) and nonwhite (VE, 47%; $n = 914$) volunteers ($P = .10$, adjusted for multiple subgroup comparisons).

Conclusions.—There was no overall protective effect. The efficacy trends in subgroups may provide clues for the development of effective immunization approaches.

► The "holy grail" of HIV prevention is the development of a vaccine. After over 2 decades of study, we are yet to reach the point at which we have viable candidates. The one studied in this multi–million dollar effort was not successful. I chose this study as representative of the problems inherent in HIV vaccine development. The vaccine tested was a recombinant envelope vaccine utilizing a recombinant gp 120. It was previously shown to protect chimpanzees and was associated with an antibody response. However, the vaccine lacked a diverse T-cell response. The vaccine did produce neutralizing and CD4-blocking antibody in humans yet failed to prevent HIV infection, and also failed to alter any viral load levels or genetic characteristics of the virus that infected those who acquired HIV-1. This study will be useful as a benchmark for future vaccine studies, and the sera should prove useful for comparison, and it proves that vaccine trials aimed at preventing HIV infection can be performed. There were several interesting results from this trial. African Americans had a stronger antibody response to the rgp 120 vaccine than others. Also, persons with a relatively strong anti–gp 120 antibody response were a little less likely to become infected with HIV-1. But without any overall effectiveness, this subset analysis may be meaningless or imply that those with a lower response were more likely to become infected. In my view, one had to start somewhere, so despite some complaints about the cost and potential for success, this study is important as setting a baseline standard against which future efforts can be measured.

D. R. Snydman, MD

13 Fungal Infections

Efficacy and Safety of Caspofungin for Treatment of Invasive Aspergillosis in Patients Refractory to or Intolerant of Conventional Antifungal Therapy

Maertens J, for the Caspofungin Salvage Aspergillosis Study Group (Univ Hosp, Gasthuisberg, Leuven, Belgium; et al)

Clin Infect Dis 39:1563-1571, 2004 13–1

Background.—Invasive aspergillosis (IA) is an important cause of morbidity and mortality among immunocompromised patients. Echinocandins are novel antifungal molecules with in vitro and in vivo activity against Aspergillus species.

Methods.—We investigated the efficacy and safety of caspofungin in the treatment of IA. Ninety patients with IA who were refractory to or intolerant of amphotericin B, lipid formulations of amphotericin B, or triazoles were enrolled to receive caspofungin.

Results.—Efficacy was assessed for 83 patients who had infection consistent with definitions of IA and who received ≥1 dose of study drug. Common underlying conditions included hematologic malignancy (48% of patients), allogeneic blood and marrow transplantation (25% of patients), and solid-organ transplantation (11% of patients). Seventy-one patients (86%) were refractory to and 12 patients (14%) were intolerant of previous therapy. A favorable response to caspofungin therapy was observed in 37 (45%) of 83 patients, including 32 (50%) of 64 with pulmonary aspergillosis and 3 (23%) of 13 with disseminated aspergillosis. Two patients discontinued caspofungin therapy because of drug-related adverse events. Drug-related nephrotoxicity and hepatotoxicity occurred infrequently.

Conclusion.—Caspofungin demonstrated usefulness in the salvage treatment of IA.

► The echinocandins are a novel class of parenterally administered semisynthetic lipopeptides with a pathogen- specific mechanism for noncompetitive inhibition of the biosynthesis of 1,3 β glucans in the fungal cell wall. They have documented activity in vitro and in vivo against *Candida* and *Aspergillus* species. Caspofungin is the first in an emerging class of compounds (2 others are either licensed recently or close to licensure). The safety profile and effectiveness in comparative trials has made these drugs a drug of choice for invasive *Candida* infections,[1] especially because we are seeing more nonalbicans *Can-*

dida. Their use in aspergillosis is not as well accepted, and there is a suspicion that this class is not as good as voriconazole.

It is important to note that complete responses were rare, and partial responses were common. Of course, almost 40% of the patients enrolled were refractory to the therapy they had previously received. In addition, the requirements for a complete response were quite stringent in that complete resolution of signs and symptoms, including CT scan findings at the site of infection, were necessary. Partial responses might include a small residual infiltrate at the pulmonary site. This classification scheme is comparable to previously published data and compares favorably to voriconazole salvage therapy data. Toxicity was minimal, and assuming its tolerability, caspofungin can be considered to be appropriate for treatment of invasive aspergillosis. Because each agent has a different mechanism of action, trials or usage in combination with the azole compounds are being contemplated.

D. R. Snydman, MD

Reference

1. 2005 YEAR BOOK OF MEDICINE, pp 103-105.

Voriconazole Versus a Regimen of Amphotericin B Followed by Fluconazole for Candidaemia in Non-neutropenic Patients: A Randomised Non-inferiority Trial

Kullberg BJ, Sobel JD, Ruhnke M, et al (Nijmegen Univ, The Netherlands; Wayne State Univ, Detroit; Humboldt Univ, Berlin; et al)

Lancet 366:1435-1442, 2005 13–2

Background.—Voriconazole has proven efficacy against invasive aspergillosis and oesophageal candidiasis. This multicentre, randomised, non-inferiority study compared voriconazole with a regimen of amphotericin B followed by fluconazole for the treatment of candidaemia in non-neutropenic patients.

Methods.—Non-neutropenic patients with a positive blood culture for a species of candida and clinical evidence of infection were enrolled. Patients were randomly assigned, in a 2:1 ratio, either voriconazole (n=283) or amphotericin B followed by fluconazole (n=139). The primary efficacy analysis was based on clinical and mycological response 12 weeks after the end of treatment, assessed by an independent data-review committee unaware of treatment assignment.

Findings.—Of 422 patients randomised, 370 were included in the modified intention-to-treat population. Voriconazole was non-inferior to amphotericin B/fluconazole in the primary efficacy analysis, with successful outcomes in 41% of patients in both treatment groups (95% CI for difference −10.6% to 10.6%). At the last evaluable assessment, outcome was successful in 162 (65%) patients assigned voriconazole and 87 (71%) assigned amphotericin B/fluconazole (p=0.25). Voriconazole cleared blood cultures as quickly as amphotericin B/fluconazole (median time to negative blood culture, 2.0 days). Treatment discontinuations due to all-cause adverse events were more frequent in the voriconazole group, although most discontinuations were due to non-drug-related events and there were significantly fewer serious adverse events and cases of renal toxicity than in the amphotericin B/fluconazole group.

Interpretation.—Voriconazole was as effective as the regimen of amphotericin B followed by fluconazole in the treatment of candidaemia in non-neutropenic patients, and with fewer toxic effects.

Relevance to Practice.—There are several options for treatment of candidaemia in non-neutropenic patients, including amphotericin B, fluconazole, voriconazole, and echinocandins. Voriconazole can be given both as initial intravenous treatment and as an oral stepdown agent.

▶ The choice of the best first-line treatment for invasive candidiasis in the nonneutropenic population remains controversial. Fluconazole and caspofungin have been shown to be equivalent to amphotericin B. With increasing fluconazole-resistant species being isolated, attention is being paid to alternative agents. This large multicenter study demonstrates that voriconazole is as useful as amphotericin B for the treatment of invasive candidiasis in nonneutropenic patients. As the authors note, more than 50% of the cases of invasive candidiasis were caused by non-albicans species. My own practice at this juncture is to use caspofungin if we have documented invasive candidiasis until we know the species. The decision analysis in Abstract 13–3 does not detract from this stance since it uses a model of empiric use, not documented infections. With these data, we now have confidence that voriconazole may also be used for the treatment of invasive candidiasis.

D. R. Snydman, MD

Empirical Anti-*Candida* Therapy Among Selected Patients in the Intensive Care Unit: A Cost-Effectiveness Analysis

Golan Y, Wolf MP, Pauker SG, et al (Tufts-New England Med Ctr, Boston)

Ann Intern Med 143:857-869, 2005 13–3

Background.—Mortality from invasive candidiasis is high. Low culture sensitivity and treatment delay contribute to increased mortality, but nonselective early therapy may result in excess costs and drug resistance.

Objective.—To determine the cost-effectiveness of anti-*Candida* strategies for high-risk patients in the intensive care unit (ICU).

Design.—Cost-effectiveness decision model.

Data Sources.—Published data to 10 May 2005, identified from MEDLINE and Cochrane Library searches, ICU databases, expert estimates, and actual hospital costs.

Target Population.—Patients in the ICU with suspected infection who have not responded to antibacterial therapy.

Time Horizon.—Lifetime.

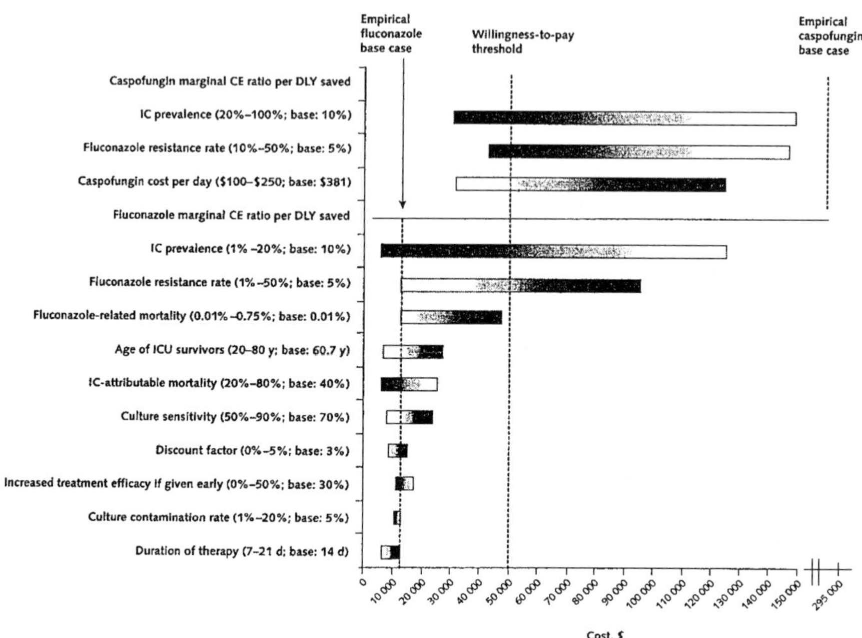

FIGURE 2.—The darker portion of each bar represents the higher values for the corresponding sensitivity range tested. For example, for fluconazole-related mortality, 0.75% is to the right of the bar. For invasive candidiasis (*IC*) prevalence, 20% is to the left of the bar. The upper 3 analyses and the lower 10 analyses examined the effect of varying the value of base-case estimates on the marginal CE ratio of empirical caspofungin and fluconazole, respectively. The horizontal axis represents the discounted incremental CE ratio for each value on the vertical axis. The width of the bar associated with each variable illustrates the range for the CE ratio. The upper and lower limits followed by the base-case value for each variable tested are in parentheses. The bars are ordered from least width at the bottom to the greatest width at the top. The comparator for analyses of fluconazole CE ratio, excluding the analysis of fluconazole resistance rates, is culture-based fluconazole, the next most effective treatment strategy. For the analysis of fluconazole resistance rates, culture-based fluconazole is replaced with culture-based caspofungin as the next most effective strategy at a fluconazole resistance rate of 17%. The comparator for analyses of caspofungin CE ratio, excluding the analysis of fluconazole resistance rates, is empirical fluconazole, the next most effective treatment strategy. For the analysis of fluconazole resistance rates, empirical fluconazole is replaced with culture-based caspofungin at a fluconazole resistance rate of 34%. Because the effectiveness and cost of both empirical and culture-based caspofungin are not affected by fluconazole resistance, any further increase in fluconazole resistance rates has no effect on the marginal CE ratio of empirical caspofungin. ICU = intensive care unit. (Courtesy of Golan Y, Wolf MP, Pauker SG, et al: Empirical anti-*Candida* therapy among selected patients in the intensive care unit: A cost-effectiveness analysis. *Ann Intern Med* 143:857-869, 2005.)

Perspective.—Societal.

Interventions.—Fluconazole, caspofungin, amphotericin B, or lipid formulation of amphotericin B given as either empirical or culture-based therapy and no anti-*Candida* therapy.

Outcome Measures.—Incremental life expectancy and incremental cost per discounted life-year (DLY) saved.

Results of Base-Case Analysis.—Ten percent of the target population will have invasive candidiasis. Empirical caspofungin therapy is the most effective strategy but is expensive ($295,115 per DLY saved). Empirical fluconazole therapy is the most reasonable strategy ($12,593 per DLY saved) and decreases mortality from 44.0% to 30.4% in patients with invasive candidiasis and from 22.4% to 21.0% in the overall target cohort (Fig 2).

Results of Sensitivity Analysis.—Empirical fluconazole therapy is reasonable for likelihoods of invasive candidiasis greater than 2.5% or fluconazole resistance less than 24.0%. For higher resistance levels, empirical caspofungin therapy is preferred. For low prevalences of invasive candidiasis, culture-based fluconazole is reasonable. For prevalences exceeding 60%, empirical caspofungin therapy is reasonable. For caspofungin to be reasonable at a prevalence of 10%, its cost must be reduced by 58%.

Limitations.—Less severe illness and limited use of broad-spectrum antimicrobial agents, typical of smaller hospitals, could result in a lower risk for invasive candidiasis.

Conclusions.—In patients in the ICU with suspected infection who have not responded to antibiotic treatment, empirical fluconazole should reduce mortality at an acceptable cost. The use of empirical strategies in low-risk patients is not justified.

▶ I have selected this study, which is a work done by some of my faculty, because it is an outstanding piece of work, formalizing, in a decision analysis, thresholds for the use of empiric antifungal therapy for patients in the ICU. The diagram I have chosen summarizes those thresholds. It illustrates the thresholds at which fluconazole is the preferred option and compares them with those thresholds at which caspofungin is the preferred option. In no model is lipid amphotericin the preferred option, and voriconazole was not modeled. What I particularly like about this analysis is that it takes into account likelihood of antifungal resistance, cost, attributable mortality, and likelihood of culture contamination as well as efficacy. It is important to recognize that the population on which this analysis is based comprises those patients with fever, hypothermia, and unexplained hypotension despite 3 days of antibacterial therapy. One might argue with the prevalence estimates of fluconazole-resistant candida, but the authors have performed a sensitivity analysis over a wide range of estimates. It is interesting to note that caspofungin is the most effective strategy in the base-case analysis, but the cost of this agent makes it not cost effective at present cost. The authors have limited the amount of exposure of empiric anti-*Candida* therapy to an estimate of 7% of patients, which should limit the likelihood of resistance. It should be noted, however, that the use of fluconazole as the strategy should be effective with resistance rates as high as 43%.

D. R. Snydman, MD

14 New Antibiotics

Ertapenem Versus Piperacillin/Tazobactam for Diabetic Foot Infections (SIDESTEP): Prospective, Randomized, Controlled, Double-blinded, Multicentre Trial

Lipsky BA, Armstrong DG, Citron DM, et al (Univ of Washington, Seattle; Rosalind Franklin Univ of Medicine and Science, Chicago; RM Alden Research Lab, Santa Monica, Calif; et al)

Lancet 366:1695-1703, 2005 14–1

Background.—Diabetic foot infections are a common and serious problem, yet few randomised trials of adequate quality have compared the efficacy of the various antibiotic regimens available for their treatment. Our aim was to assess the efficacy and safety of ertapenem versus piperacillin/tazobactam for foot infections.

Methods.—We did a randomised, double-blinded, multicentre trial in adults (n=586) with diabetes and a foot infection classified as moderate-to-severe and requiring intravenous antibiotics. We assigned patients intravenous ertapenem (1 g daily; n=295) or piperacillin/tazobactam (3.375 g every 6 h; n=291) given for a minimum of 5 days, after which oral amoxicillin/clavulanic acid (875/125 mg every 12 h) could be given for up to 23 days. Investigators retained the option to administer vancomycin to patients in either group to ensure adequate coverage for potentially antibiotic resistant Enterococcus spp and meticillin-resistant *Staphylococcus aureus* (MRSA). Our primary outcome was the proportion of patients with a favourable clinical response (cure or improvement) on the day that intravenous antibiotic was discontinued. Analyses were by an evaluable-patient only approach. This study is registered with ClinicalTrials.gov, number NCT00229112.

Findings.—Of the 576 patients treated, 445 were available for assessment at the end of intravenous therapy. Both baseline characteristics and favourable clinical response rates were similar for the 226 who received ertapenem and the 219 who received piperacillin/tazobactam (94%vs 92%, respectively; between treatment difference 1.9%, 95% CI −2.9 to 6.9). Rates of favourable microbiological responses (eradication rates and clinical outcomes, by pathogen) and adverse events did not differ between groups.

Interpretation.—Clinical and microbiological outcomes for patients treated with ertapenem were equivalent to those for patients treated with piperacillin/tazobactam, suggesting that this once-daily antibiotic should be

TABLE 5.—Favourable Clinical Response Rates, for Species With at Least 20 Isolates at FUA, by Baseline Pathogen

	Ertapenem (n=173)*	Piperacillin/Tazobactam (n=151)*	Observed Differences (95% CI)
Gram-positive aerobic cocci	149/176 (84·7%)	132/166 (79·5%)	5.1 (−3·1 to 13·6)
Enterococcus†	19/22 (86·4%)	8/9 (88·9%)	−2·5
Enterococcus faecalis	13/15 (86·7%)	12/16 (75·0%)	11·7 (−19·2 to 41·1)
Staphylococcus aureus	75/90 (83·3%)‡	62/79 (78·5%)	4·9 (−7·6 to 17·2)
Meticillin resistant	14/18 (77·8%)	10/15 (66·7%)	11.1 (−19·8 to 42·7)
Meticillin susceptible	60/71 (84·5%)	52/64 (81·3%)	3·3 (−9·9 to 17·1)
Streptococcus agalactiae	15/21 (71·4%)	22/26 (84·6%)	−13·2 (−38·3 to 10·9)
Gram-negative aerobic bacilli	64/73 (87·7%)	43/56 (76·8%)	10·9 (−2·3 to 25·2)
Enterobacteriaceae§	36/42 (85·7%)	26/33 (78·8%)	6·9 (−11·1 to 25·9)
Pseudomonas aeruginosa	15/18 (83·3%)	7/10 (70·0%)	13·3 (−18·2 to 48·7)
Gram-positive anaerobic cocci	66/74 (89·2%)	48/62 (77·4%)	11·8 (−0·8 to 25·2)
Peptostreptococcus magnus	34/38 (89·5%)	24/27 (88·9%)	0·6 (−15·4 to 20·6)
Peptostreptococcus asaccharolyticus	10/11 (90·9%)	7/11 (63·6%)	27·3 (−10·9 to 58·6)
Gram-positive anaerobic bacilli¶	23/26 (88·5%)	12/17 (70·6%)	17·9 (−6·9 to 45·1)
Gram-negative anaerobic bacilli‖	33/40 (82·5%)	28/40 (70·0%)	12·5 (−7·2 to 31·3)
Gram-negative anaerobic coccobacilli**	21/25 (84·0%)	11/16 (68·8%)	15·3 (−10·8 to 43·3)

Data are number of pathogens with associated favourable assessment/number of pathogens assessed (observed response) unless otherwise indicated.
*Number observed calculated by pooling across baseline severity.
†No species identifed.
‡Oxacillin susceptibility not provided for one isolate.
§Includes *Enterobacter* spp, *Escherichia* spp, *Klebsiella* spp, *Morganella* spp, *Proteus* spp, and *Providencia* spp.
¶Includes *Clostridium* spp, *Eubacterium* spp, and *Propionbacterium* spp.
‖Includes *Porphyomonas* spp and *Prevotella* spp.
**Includes *Bacteroides* spp.
Abbreviation: FUA, Follow-up assessment.
(Courtesy of Lipsky BA, Armstrong DG, Citron DM, et al: Ertapenem versus piperacillin/tazobactam for diabetic foot infections (SIDESTEP): Prospective, randomized, controlled, double-blinded, multicentre trial. *Lancet* 366:1695-1703, 2005. Reprinted with permission from Elsevier.)

considered for parenteral therapy of diabetic foot infections, when deemed appropriate (Table 5).

► There are very few studies that have prospectively evaluated the treatment of diabetic foot infections. This study was selected because it has a number of strengths and provides data for a relatively new antimicrobial agent to be used for this indication. Among the strengths, a large number of patients were included, which allowed the authors to better characterize the microbiology and outcomes of patients with diabetic foot infection. In addition, it used a multicenter double-blind study design and adopted the newly developed diabetic foot infection classification guidelines. The study clearly illustrates the equivalence of ertapenem, a carbapenem that can be given once a day to piperacillin/tazobactam and extended-spectrum penicillin and beta-lactamase inhibitor combination. The authors also emphasize the need for proper wound care and appropriate surgical debridement when necessary. Although they did track this latter procedure, the results are not reported, and some sites of enrollment did not track this modality closely. It will be of interest to see if a follow-up publication dissects risk factors for failure. Of note, even though *Pseudomonas* spp was occasionally isolated, bacteriologic eradication was equivalent in the ertapenem arm, despite the fact that ertapenem does not have significant activity against *Pseudomonas* spp.

D. R. Snydman, MD

Safety and Efficacy of Tigecycline in Treatment of Skin and Skin Structure Infections: Results of a Double-blind Phase 3 Comparison Study With Vancomycin-Aztreonam

Breedt J, for the Tigecycline 305 cSSSI Study Group (Eugene Marais Hosp, Les Marais, Pretoria, Republic of South Africa; et al)

Antimicrob Agents Chemother 49:4658-4666, 2005 14–2

Introduction.—In a randomized, double-blind, controlled trial, 546 patients with complicated skin and skin structure infections received tigecycline 100 mg/day (a 100-mg initial dose and then 50 mg intravenously twice daily) or the combination of vancomycin 2 g/day (1 g intravenously twice daily) and aztreonam 4 g/day (2 g intravenously twice daily) for up to 14 days. The primary end point was the clinical response in the clinical modified intent-to-treat (c-mITT) and clinically evaluable (CE) populations at the test-of-cure visit 12 to 92 days after the last dose. The microbiologic response at the test-of-cure visit was also assessed. Safety was assessed by physical examination, laboratory results, and adverse event reporting. Five hundred twenty patients were included in the c-mITT population (tigecycline group, $n = 261$; combination group, $n = 259$), and 436 were clinically evaluable (tigecycline group, $n = 223$; combination group, $n = 213$). The clinical responses in the tigecycline and the combination vancomycin and aztreonam groups were similar in the c-mITT population (84.3% versus 86.9%; difference, −2.6% [95% confidence interval, −9.0, 3.8]; $P =$

0.4755) and the CE population (89.7% versus 94.4%; difference, −4.7% [95% confidence interval, −10.2, 0.8]; $P = 0.1015$). Microbiologic eradication (documented or presumed) occurred in 84.8% of the patients receiving tigecycline and 93.2% of the patients receiving vancomycin and aztreonam (difference, −8.5 [95% confidence interval, −16.0, −1.0]; $P = 0.0243$). The numbers of patients reporting adverse events were similar in the two groups, with increased nausea and vomiting rates in the tigecycline group and an increased incidence of rash and increases in alanine aminotransferase and aspartate aminotransferase levels in the combination vancomycin and aztreonam group. Tigecycline was shown to be safe and effective for the treatment of complicated skin and skin structure infections.

► Tigecycline is the first glycylcycline drug, a derivative of tetracycline compounds. It has very interesting activity, including activity against methicillin-resistant *Staphylococcus aureus* (MRSA), vancomycin-resistant enterococci (VRE), many multidrug-resistant gram-negative organisms, including some nonfermenters, such as *Acinetobacter* species and *Stenotrophomonas maltophilia*. It is also active against anaerobic bacteria. The mechanism of action is binding to bacterial 30S ribosome, and blocking protein synthesis, and in contrast to the tetracycline compounds, it is designed to circumvent resistance mechanisms, such as efflux pumps, and ribosomal mechanisms of protection. The data suggest that tigecycline, given in a dose of 100 mg to load, then 50 mg IV, twice a day is equivalent to vancomycin and aztreonam for skin and skin structure infections. It will be of great interest to see how this agent develops, now that it is licensed in the United States, because it has broad activity, and I can see it being an option for *Acinetobacter* species and other difficult-to-treat organisms for which there are very few other choices.

D. R. Snydman, MD

15 Clinical Diagnostics

A Prospective, Randomized, and Comparative Study of 3 Different Methods for the Diagnosis of Intravascular Catheter Colonization

Bouza E, Alvarado N, Alcalá L, et al (Hospital General Universitario Gregorio Marañon, Madrid)

Clin Infect Dis 40:1096-1100, 2005 15–1

Background.—Demonstration of catheter tip colonization is usually performed by use of Maki's semiquantitative technique, although the superiority of quantitative techniques has been claimed on the basis of their purported ability to detect both endoluminal and exoluminal microorganisms.

Methods.—We prospectively compared Maki's semiquantitative technique and the quantitative methods of sonication and vortexing for the detection of colonization of intravascular catheter tips and catheter-related bloodstream infections. All 3 techniques were performed on the tip of each catheter, and the order in which each technique was performed was randomly assigned.

Results.—Of the 1000 catheter tips that were processed, 329 (32.9%) had positive results for at least 1 of the 3 techniques when a breakpoint of ≥100 colony-forming units (cfu)/catheter segment was used for the quantitative techniques and a breakpoint of ≥15 cfu was used for Maki's technique. Eighty-two of the catheter tips for which results were positive were from patients with catheter-related bloodstream infections. For each technique, the likelihood of detection decreased progressively depending on the order in which the technique was performed (i.e., second vs. first and third vs. second). The likelihood of detection of catheter colonization for each technique, when the technique was performed first and when 2 breakpoints (≥100 cfu/catheter segment [criterion B] and ≥1000 cfu/catheter segment [criterion A]) were used for the quantitative techniques and a breakpoint of ≥15 cfu was used for Maki's technique, was as follows: 99.1% and 100% for Maki's technique, 95.1% and 92.9% for sonication, and 93.1% and 72.8% for vortexing (for criteria B and A, respectively). No inferiority of Maki's technique could be demonstrated when results were compared according to whether catheter placement was short term (i.e., <7 days) or long term (i.e., ≥7 days), either for the detection of colonization or for the detection of catheter-related bloodstream infections.

Conclusions.—According to data from the present study, the quantitative techniques of sonication and vortexing were not superior to Maki's tech-

TABLE 3.—Diagnostic Yield of the Different Techniques Used for the Detection of Colonization in Patients With Catheter-related Bloodstream Infection (With Breakpoints of ≥15 cfu, for Maki's Technique, and ≥100 cfu/Catheter Segment, for Quantitative Techniques) by Duration of Catheterization

Procedure Order	Short-term Catheters (n = 142)			Long-term Catheters (n = 227)		
	Maki's Technique	Sonication	Vortexing	Maki's Technique	Sonication	Vortexing
Sensitivity[a]	90.0 (55.5-99.7)	90.0 (55.5-99.7)	90.0 (55.5-99.7)	87.5 (77.6-94.1)	91.7 (82.7-96.9)	83.3 (72.7-91.1)
Specificity[b]	81.8 (74.2-88.0)	81.8 (74.2-88.0)	87.1 (80.2-92.3)	77.4 (70.0-83.7)	78.7 (71.4-84.9)	80.0 (72.8-86.0)
Positive PV[c]	27.3 (13.3-45.5)	27.3 (13.3-45.5)	34.6 (17.2-55.7)	63.6 (53.4-73.1)	65.3 (55.2-74.5)	63.2 (52.6-72.8)
Negative PV[d]	99.1 (95.0-100)	99.1 (95.0-100)	99.1 (95.2-100)	93.8 (88.1-97.3)	96.8 (92.1-99.1)	93.9 (88.4-97.3)
Positive LR (95% CI)	5.0 (1.8-13.5)	5.0 (1.8-13.5)	7.0 (2.5-19.6)	3.9 (2.4-6.4)	4.3 (2.6-7.1)	4.2 (2.5-7.0)
Negative LR (95% CI)	0.12 (0.02-0.97)	0.12 (0.02-0.97)	0.11 (0.01-0.91)	0.16 (0.08-0.34)	0.11 (0.04-0.25)	0.21 (0.11-0.40)

NOTE. Data are % (95% CI) unless indicated otherwise. Long-term catheters, catheters that were in place for ≥7 days; LR, likelihood ratio; PV, predictive value; short-term catheters, catheters that were in place for <7 days.

[a] P values for the comparison of the sensitivity of the different methods for short-term and long-term catheters, respectively, were as follows: for Maki's technique vs. sonication, $P = 1$ and $P = .375$; for Maki's technique vs. vortexing, $P = 1$ and $P = .549$; and for sonication vs. vortexing, $P = 1$ and $P = .031$. $P < .017$ was considered to be statistically significant (for 3 comparisons with Bonferroni correction).

[b] P values for the comparison of the specificity of the different methods for short-term and long-term catheters, respectively, were as follows: for Maki's technique vs. sonication, $P = 1$ and $P = .791$; for Maki's technique vs. vortexing, $P = .039$ and $P = .424$; and for sonication vs. vortexing, $P = .039$ and $P = .687$. $P < 017$ was considered to be statistically significant (for 3 comparisons with Bonferroni correction).

[c] P values for the comparison of the positive predictive value of the different methods for short-term and long-term catheters, respectively, were as follows: for Maki's technique vs. sonication, $P = 1$ and $P = .883$; for Maki's technique vs. vortexing, $P = .565$ and $P = 1$; and for sonication vs. vortexing, $P = .565$ and $P = .767$. $P < 017$ was considered to be statistically significant (for 3 comparisons with Bonferroni correction).

[d] P values for the comparison of the negative predictive value of the different methods for short-term and long-term catheters, respectively, were as follows: for Maki's technique vs. sonication, $P = 1$ and $P = .376$; for Maki's technique vs. vortexing, $P = 1$ and $P = 1$; and for sonication vs. vortexing, $P = 1$ and $P = .378$. $P < .017$ was considered to be statistically significant (for 3 comparisons with Bonferroni correction).

(Courtesy of Bouza E, Alvarado N, Alcalá L, et al: A prospective, randomized, and comparative study of 3 different methods for the diagnosis of intravascular catheter colonization. *Clin Infect Dis* 40:1096-1100, 2005. Reproduced by permission of the University of Chicago, Publisher.)

nique under the test conditions used. The greater simplicity of Maki's semiquantitative technique makes it the procedure of choice for routine work in the microbiology laboratory (Table 3).

▶ The studies by Maki on catheter-associated bloodstream infections have defined the pathophysiologic mechanism, and have developed methodologies at prevention. The "roll plate" technique was the first in his series to develop his hypotheses and uses the concept that the intracutaneous segment can be sterilely remove, and rolled 4 times back and forth on a blood agar plate in the microbiology laboratory, and then the plate can be incubated and the colonies counted semiquantitatively. There have been a number of studies challenging the clinical utility of the Maki roll plate technique for diagnosing IV catheter infections and catheter-related bloodstream infections. The argument has been put forth that the roll plate technique will miss those infections that arise intraluminally; however, the use of sonication and flushing of catheters in the laboratory, with serial dilutions of the sonicate for culture, are too time-consuming for most busy clinical microbiology laboratories. The study cited here, with analysis of 1000 catheters, 82 catheter-related bloodstream infections, and 329 semiquantitative catheter cultures that were positive is the largest and most comprehensive to date. It is reassuring to note that the procedure we have in place has stood the test of time and has the best sensitivity and specificity.

D. R. Snydman, MD

Do Emergency Department Blood Cultures Change Practice in Patients With Pneumonia?

Kennedy M, Bates DW, Wright SB, et al (Harvard Med School; Brigham and Women's Hosp, Boston; Beth Israel Deaconess Med Ctr, Boston)
Ann Emerg Med 46:393-400, 2005 15–2

Study Objective.—Although it is considered standard of care to obtain blood cultures on patients hospitalized for pneumonia, several studies have questioned the utility and cost-effectiveness of this practice. The objective of this study is to determine the impact of emergency department (ED) blood cultures on antimicrobial therapy for patients with pneumonia.

Methods.—We performed a prospective, observational, cohort study of consecutive adult (age ≥18 years) patients treated at an urban university ED between February 1, 2000 and February 1, 2001. Inclusion criteria were radiographic evidence of pneumonia, clinical evidence of pneumonia, and blood culture obtained. Blood cultures were classified as positive, negative, or contaminant based on previously established criteria. Additionally, data were collected on antimicrobial sensitivities, empiric antibiotic therapy, antibiotic changes, and reasons for changes.

Results.—There were 3,926 ED visits with blood cultures obtained for any reason, of which 3,762 (96%) were available for review. Of these, 414 of 3,762 (11%) patients met pneumonia study inclusion criteria, and blood

TABLE 2.—Infections Resistant to Empiric Therapy

Subject Characteristics	Initial Antibiotic(s)	Organism Characteristics	Final Antibiotic
82-y-old man Nursing home resident Comorbidities: CHF, MI, dementia	Metronidazole, ceftriaxone	*S aureus* Resistant: oxacillin, levofloxacin, clindamycin; Intermediate resistance: gentamicin	Vancomycin
58-y-old man Comordities: alcoholism, CHF, CVD, mild DM, pancreatitis	Clindamycin, levofloxacin	*S aureus* Resistant: penicillin, erythromycin, clindamycin, levofloxacin	Gentamicin, cefazolin
76-y-old woman Nursing home resident Comorbidities: CHF, COPD	Amikacin	*S aureus* Resistant: oxacillin, levofloxacin, penicillin, tetracycline, erythromycin, clindamycin	Vancomycin, tobramycin
85-y-old woman Nursing home resident Comorbidities: COPD, MI	Levofloxacin	*E coli* Resistant: ampicillin, trimethoprim, ciprofloxacin, piperacillin, cefuroxime, levofloxacin	Ceftriaxone

Abbreviations: CHF, Congestive heart failure; *MI*, myocardial infarction; *CVD*, cardiovascular disease; *DM*, mild diabetes mellitus.
(Courtesy of Kennedy M, Bates DW, Wright SB, et al: Do emergency department blood cultures change practice in patients with pneumonia? *Ann Emerg Med* 46:393-400, 2005.)

TABLE 4.—Summary of Rates of Bacteremia, Resistant Infections, and Impact of Blood Cultures on Antibiotic Management in Studies of Patients With Pneumonia

Study/Study Design	Bacteremia (% of Total Enrolled)	Subjects With Change In Antibiotic Therapy Because of Blood Culture (% of Total Enrolled)	Subjects With Infection Resistant to Empiric Therapy (% of Total Enrolled)
This study/prospective study of 414 ED patients with pneumonia	7.0	3.6	1.0
Campbell et al, 2003/prospective study of 760 patients hospitalized for CAP	5.66	1.97	0.4
Waterer et al, 2001/prospective study of 209 patients with CAP	13.9	5.7	Not reported
Waterer et al, 1999/retrospective study of 74 patients with bacteremic pneumococcal pneumonia	N/A	Not comparable*	2.7
Chalasani et al, 1995/retrospective study of 517 patients hospitalized for CAP	6.6	1.4	Not reported
Woodhead et al, 1991/prospective study of 86 patients hospitalized for CAP	10.5	Not reported	Not reported

*This study included only subjects with bacteremia; 41.9% of bacteremic subjects had a change in antibiotic management because of blood cultures, but only 2.7% of infections in bacteremic subjects were resistant to empiric therapy.

(Courtesy of Kennedy M, Bates DW, Wright SB, et al: Do emergency department blood cultures change practice in patients with pneumonia? *Ann Emerg Med* 46:393-400, 2005.)

cultures identified 29 of 414 (7.0%) patients with true bacteremia. In the 414 patients, blood culture results altered therapy for 15 patients (3.6%) with suspected pneumonia, of which 11 (2.7%) patients had their coverage narrowed; only 4 (1.0%) patients had their coverage broadened because of resistance to empiric therapy. For the 11 patients with bacteremia whose therapy was not altered, culture results actually supported narrowing therapy in 8 (1.9%) cases, but this was not done.

Conclusion.—Blood cultures rarely altered therapy for patients presenting to the ED with pneumonia. More discriminatory blood culture use may potentially reduce resource utilization (Tables 2 and 4).

► The Joint Commission on Hospital Accreditation and large organizations that set standards for quality indicators have determined that blood cultures should be obtained before initiating therapy for community-acquired pneumonia. The authors have examined the clinical impact of such a practice and determined that rarely will cultures affect therapy. They determined that 100 patients would have to be cultured to find 1 isolate resistant to the empiric therapy chosen. And in 3 of the cases that were transfers from nursing homes, one can suggest that methicillin-resistant *Staphylococcus aureus* (MRSA) would be a consideration that should be covered. In addition, bacteremia was documented in only 7% of cases, and when documented, did not lead to a change in therapy most of the time. This is in accordance with studies of our own that we published more than a decade ago with respect to all hospitalized patients with bacteremia. Often no change takes place, even when indicated, and the usual response is to increase the number of antibiotics, not narrow the spectrum. The authors appropriately challenge the validity of the standards. Studies to develop predictors of when blood cultures would be useful are sorely needed, and a predictive instrument concerning such use for this indication might be warranted.

D. R. Snydman, MD

16 Health Care Associated Infections

Infections Associated With Tumor Necrosis Factor-α Antagonists
Crum NF, Lederman ER, Wallace MR (Naval Med Ctr San Diego, Calif; United States Naval Med Research Unit 2 (ERL), Jakarta, Indonesia)
Medicine 84:291-302, 2005 16–1

Introduction.—Tumor necrosis factor (TNF)-α antagonists are promising therapeutic agents for patients with severe autoimmune and rheumatologic conditions. Unfortunately, their use has been associated with an increased rate of tuberculosis, endemic mycoses, and intracellular bacterial infections. Infliximab, 1 of 3 available drugs in this novel class, appears to be associated with the greatest risk of infection, likely because of its long half-life and induction of monocyte apoptosis. Prospective trials are necessary to determine the exact risk associated with these agents, particularly the newer TNF-α antagonists. More specific TNF-α blockers, which reduce inflammation while maintaining adequate immunity, are needed. In the meantime, a thorough work-up is mandatory for all febrile illness occurring in TNF-α blocker recipients. We present 4 patients who developed severe infections during TNF-α antagonist therapy, review the literature, and discuss current guidelines for surveillance and prophylaxis.

► On the basis of current data, the overall risk of severe infections appears to be low with the use of TNF-α blockers. It is estimated that the risk is 0.02 to 0.05 cases per person year. The risk is also highest in the first 3 months of treatment. As these drugs become more commonly used for psoriasis, and Crohn's disease, one can expect to see more cases of infections. As the authors point out, most of the infections are due to pathogens with significant cell-mediated immunity as the host defense mechanism that keeps the agent in check. Although the authors imply that infliximab may be more likely associated with infections than other TNF-α antagonists, I think the jury is still out on the relative risks associated with each agent. The physician must be aware of the risk of severe infections, including *Staphylococcus aureus*, as well as the reactivation infections documented in this case series.

D. R. Snydman, MD

Progressive Multifocal Leukoencephalopathy in a Patient Treated With Natalizumab

Langer-Gould A, Atlas SW, Green AJ, et al (Stanford Univ, Calif; Univ of California, San Francisco)

N Engl J Med 353:375-381, 2005 16–2

Introduction.—We describe the clinical course of a patient with multiple sclerosis in whom progressive multifocal leukoencephalopathy (PML), an opportunistic viral infection of the central nervous system, developed during treatment with interferon beta-1a and a selective adhesion-molecule blocker, natalizumab. The first PML lesion apparent on magnetic resonance imaging was indistinguishable from a multiple sclerosis lesion. Despite treatment with corticosteroids, cidofovir, and intravenous immune globulin, PML progressed rapidly, rendering the patient quadriparetic, globally aphasic, and minimally responsive. Three months after natalizumab therapy was discontinued, changes consistent with an immune-reconstitution inflammatory syndrome developed. The patient was treated with systemic cytarabine, and two months later, his condition had improved.

► This case report is 1 of 3 reports of the development of progressive multifocal encephalopathy caused by papovavirus in patients receiving interferon–β-1a with natalizumab (Tysabri), a monoclonal antibody against α-4 integrins. At least 1 of the cases reported have been with the use of natalizumab alone. This alarming development has obviously put the use of this agent on hold by the Food and Drug Administration. JC virus, the cause of PML, is a ubiquitous virus, and evidence of infection can be found in about 80% of adults. The occurrence of PML typically takes place in other forms of immunosuppression, namely HIV infection, chemotherapy for lymphoma, or other diseases, such as transplant recipients who are on chronic immunosuppression.

There are several important points that can be noted in this case report as follows: (1) the lesions showed up on MRI before onset of symptoms; (2) the patient had a reconstitution syndrome with discontinuation of interferon and natalizumab therapy; and (3) the patient actually had some neurologic improvement, although in other cases reported to date, most patients have died with progressive neurologic disease. In the case reported here, the authors used cytarabine, and the patient improved, although the reasons for improvement are not clear. As the authors point out, cytarabine failed to show efficacy in patients with HIV who had PML, and the response in this patient should not be construed as a sign that this treatment is appropriate for this disease.

D. R. Snydman, MD

Risk Factors for Hematogenous Complications of Intravascular Catheter–Associated *Staphylococcus aureus* Bacteremia

Fowler VG Jr, Justice A, Moore C, et al (Duke Univ, Durham, NC; Univ of Oxford, England)

Clin Infect Dis 40:695-703, 2005 16–3

Background.—The role of both host and pathogen characteristics in hematogenous seeding following *Staphylococcus aureus* bacteremia is incompletely understood.

Methods.—Consecutive patients with intravascular catheter-associated *Staphylococcus aureus* bacteremia were prospectively recruited over a 91-month period. The corresponding bloodstream isolates were examined for the presence of 35 putative virulence determinants. Patient and bacterial characteristics associated with the development of hematogenous complications (HCs) (i.e., septic arthritis, vertebral osteomyelitis, or endocarditis) were defined.

Results.—HC occurred in 42 (13%) of 324 patients. Patient characteristics at diagnosis that were associated with HC included community onset (relative risk [RR], 2.25; 95% confidence interval [CI], 1.24-4.07; *P*=.007), increased symptom duration (odds ratio for each day, 1.14; 95% CI, 1.06-1.2; *P*<.001), presence of a long-term intravascular catheter or noncatheter prosthesis (RR, 4.02; 95% CI, 1.74-9.27; *P*<.001), hemodialysis dependence (RR, 3.84; 95% CI, 2.08-7.10; *P*<.001), and higher APACHE II score (*P*=.02). Bacterial characteristics included sea (RR, 2.03; 95% CI, 1.16-3.55; *P*=.011) and methicillin-resistant S. aureus (MRSA) (RR, 2.09; 95% CI, 1.19-3.67; *P*=.015). Subsequent failure to remove a catheter was also associated with HC (RR, 2.28; 95% CI, 1.22-4.27; *P*=.011). On multivariable analysis, symptom duration, hemodialysis dependence, presence of a long-term intravascular catheter or a noncatheter device, and infection with MRSA remained significantly associated with HC.

TABLE 3.—Final Multivariable Analysis of Patient and Bacterial Characteristics Associated With Hematogenous Complications of Intravascular Catheter-associated *Staphylococcus aureus* Bacteremia

Independent Variable	OR (95%) CI)	*P*
Hemodialysis dependence only[a]	72 (8.2-630)	<.001
Permanent foreign body only[b]	4.2 (1.1-17)	.04
Both hemodialysis dependence and permanent foreign body[c]	11 (3.2-38)	<.001
Duration of symptoms before diagnosis[d]	1.15 (1.06-1.24)	<.001
Methicillin-resistant bacterial isolate	2.3 (1.1-4.7)	.03

[a] Includes 2 patients with uncomplicated bacteremia and 3 patients with hematogenous complications.

[b] Includes 32 patients with uncomplicated bacteremia and 20 patients with hematogenous complications. To present a parsimonious model, both patients with long-term catheters and those with noncatheter prostheses were included.

[c] Includes 88 patients with uncomplicated bacteremia and 26 patients with hematogenous complications.

[d] OR is for each day of symptoms before diagnosis.

(Courtesy of Fowler VG Jr, Justice A, Moore C, et al: Risk factors for hematogenous complications of intravascular catheter—associated *Staphylococcus aureus* bacteremia. *Clin Infect Dis* 40:695-703, 2005. Reproduced by permission of the publisher, University of Chicago.)

Conclusions.—This investigation identifies 4 host- and pathogen-related risk factors for hematogenous bacterial seeding and reaffirms the importance of prompt catheter removal (Table 3).

► What differentiates this study from previous ones is the exhaustive molecular studies of *S aureus* isolates obtained from catheter-associated blood stream infections. Methicillin resistance and the failure to remove a foreign body as well as hemodialysis dependence were all independent risk factors for hematogenous complications. In addition, the duration of symptoms before a diagnosis was also significant. The data also suggest that failure to remove a catheter is independently associated with a risk of a hematogenous complication. Although this was a single center study and conducted during a long interval, the completeness of the data base and the rigor of the molecular studies make it a notable contribution. The increased risk for hematogenous seeding for MRSA also suggests some as yet unidentified molecular factors that can enhance virulence of this organism.

D. R. Snydman, MD

A Hospital Outbreak of *Clostridium difficile* Disease Associated With Isolates Carrying Binary Toxin Genes

McEllistrem MC, Carman RJ, Gerding DN, et al (Univ of Pittsburgh, Pa; TechLab, Blacksburg, Va; Hines Veterans Affairs Hosp, Ill)

Clin Infect Dis 40:265-272, 2005 16–4

Introduction.—The binary toxin genes *cdt* and *cdtB* have been detected in ~5% of *Clostridium difficile* strains. Severe *C. difficile* disease (CDD) may be associated with strains that carry the binary toxin genes.

Methods.—From April 2001 through March 2002, 8 severe and 41 nonsevere cases of nosocomial CDD were studied. Severe cases of CDD were defined by the presence of ≥2 of the following criteria: (1) abdominal pain, (2) a white blood cell count of >20,000 or <1500 cells/mm^3, and (3) ileus or bowel wall thickening with ascites. Underlying disease was assessed by 2 methods: a modified Horn score and the presence of comorbid conditions. The presence of *cdtA*, *cdtB*, and the toxin A and toxin B genes was determined, and molecular subtyping was performed.

Results.—All strains were positive for the toxin A and B genes, and 65.3% of the strains carried the *cdtA* and *cdtB* genes. Strains that carried the binary toxin genes accounted for 87.5% of the cases of severe CDD and 61.0% of the nonsevere cases (P = .23). Severity of CDD was not associated with either severe underlying disease or comorbid conditions. The strains that caused severe CDD belonged to 4 protein profile groups and ≥3 restriction endonuclease analysis (REA) groups. All (i.e., 5 of 5) strains in REA group BI, compared with none (i.e., 0 of 7) of the strains in REA group J carried the binary toxin genes (P = .001). Strains that belonged to REA groups BK and BR also carried the binary toxin genes.

Conclusions.—The binary toxin genes were present in nearly two-thirds of the *C. difficile* strains, and they were correlated with the REA group. Severity of CDD was not closely associated with a specific clone or underlying disease, but it may be associated with the presence of the binary toxin genes. Larger studies are needed to discern whether a true association exists and whether the binary toxin alters the pathogenicity of the *C. difficile* strain.

► The main virulence genes for *C difficile* are the toxin A and B genes. The binary toxin, an actin-specific adenosine diphosphate–ribosyltransferase, has been reported to be found in about 5% of isolates. And it has been thought to be associated with more severe forms of disease. What is clear currently is that many medical centers are seeing outbreaks of *C difficile*–associated disease that are much more severe. Toxic megacolon that requires surgery and may also result in death seems to be more common. It has been thought that these cases are due to the presence of binary toxin. However, other virulence factors or underlying diseases may contribute to severity. This limited study does not show a clear association of the presence of binary toxin with severe *C difficile*–associated disease, but a trend. This may be a power issue or the use of a retrospective analysis of cases. Nevertheless, this selection should underscore for the internist the changing clinical spectrum of *C difficile*– associated disease. Of interest is that binary toxin was found in a majority of all isolates of *C difficile*.

D. R. Snydman, MD

Toxin Production by an Emerging Strain of *Clostridium difficile* Associated With Outbreaks of Severe Disease in North America and Europe

Warny M, Pepin J, Fang A, et al (Acambis Inc, Cambridge, Mass; Univ of Sherbrooke, Quebec, Canada; Centers for Disease Control and Prevention, Atlanta, Ga; et al)

Lancet 366:1079-1084, 2005 16–5

Background.—Toxins A and B are the primary virulence factors of *Clostridium difficile*. Since 2002, an epidemic of *C difficile*-associated disease with increased morbidity and mortality has been present in Quebec province, Canada. We characterised the dominant strain of this epidemic to determine whether it produces higher amounts of toxins A and B than those produced by non-epidemic strains.

Methods.—We obtained isolates from 124 patients from Centre Hospitalier Universitaire de Sherbrooke in Quebec. Additional isolates from the USA, Canada, and the UK were included to increase the genetic diversity of the toxinotypes tested. Isolate characterisation included toxinotyping, pulsed-field gel electrophoresis (PFGE), PCR ribotyping, detection of a binary toxin gene, and detection of deletions in a putative negative regulator for toxins A and B (*tcd*C). By use of an enzyme-linked immunoassay, we measured the in-vitro production of toxins A and B by epidemic strain and non-dominant strain isolates.

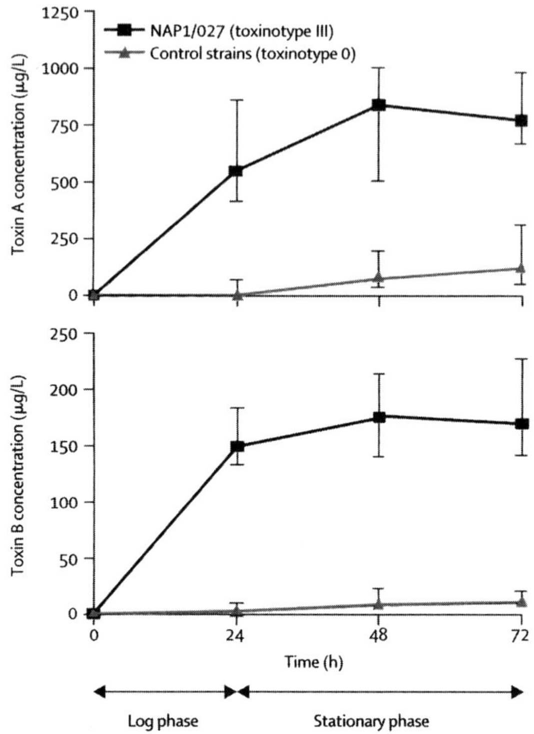

FIGURE 3.—In vitro production of toxins A and B by *C difficile* isolates. Median concentration and IQRs are shown. *C difficile* strains included 25 toxinotype 0 and 15 NAP1/027 strains (toxinotype III from various locations. (Courtesy of Warny M, Pepin J, Fang A, et al: Toxin production by an emerging strain of *Clostridium difficile* associated with outbreaks of severe disease in North America and Europe. *Lancet* 366:1079-1084, 2005. Reprinted with permission from Elsevier.)

Findings.—The epidemic strain was characterised as toxinotype III, North American PFGE type 1, and PCR-ribotype 027 (NAP1/027). This strain carried the binary toxin gene *cdt*B and an 18-bp deletion in *tcd*C. We isolated this strain from 72 patients with *C difficile*-associated disease (58 [67%] of 86 with health-care-associated disease; 14 [37%] of 38 with community-acquired disease). Peak median (IQR) toxin A and toxin B concentrations produced in vitro by NAP1/027 were 16 and 23 times higher, respectively, than those measured in isolates representing 12 different PFGE types, known as toxinotype 0 (toxin A, median 848 µg/L [IQR 504-1022] *vs* 54 µg/L [23-203]; toxin B, 180 µg/L [137-210] *vs* 8 µg/L [5-25]; $p<0.0001$ for both toxins).

Interpretation.—The severity of *C difficile*-associated disease caused by NAP1/027 could result from hyperproduction of toxins A and B. Dissemination of this strain in North America and Europe could lead to important changes in the epidemiology of *C difficile*-associated disease (Fig 3).

► This article underscores the changing epidemiology of *C difficile*-associated diarrhea with the production of binary toxin. These cases have become very common, and the number of reports is a direct indicator of the medical consequences and common disease we are seeing.

The next article (Abstract 16–6) best illustrates the increase in toxin production, and although it does not directly link toxin production to severity of illness, there is indirect evidence of this with the association of outbreaks with high mortality rates. The mechanism behind the high rates of transmission of this strain are not well understood but may be related to increased use of fluoroquinolones.

D. R. Snydman, MD

Mortality Attributable to Nosocomial *Clostridium difficile*-Associated Disease During an Epidemic Caused by a Hypervirulent Strain in Quebec

Pépin J, Valiquette L, Cossette B (Univ of Sherbrooke, Quebec, Canada; Centre hospitalier universitaire de Sherbrooke, Quebec, Canada)

CMAJ 173:1037-1041, 2005 16–6

Background.—Since 2002 an epidemic of *Clostridium difficile*-associated disease (CDAD) caused by a hypervirulent toxinotype III ribotype 027 strain has spread to many hospitals in Quebec. The strain has also been found in the United States, the United Kingdom and the Netherlands. The effects of this epidemic on mortality and duration of hospital stay remain unknown. We measured these effects among patients admitted to a hospital in Quebec during 2003 and 2004.

Methods.—We compared mortality and total length of hospital stay among inpatients in whom nosocomial CDAD developed and among control subjects without CDAD matched for sex, age, Charlson Comorbidity Index score and length of hospital stay up to the diagnosis of CDAD in the corresponding case.

Results.—Thirty days after diagnosis 23.0% (37/161) of the patients with CDAD had died, compared with 7.0% (46/656) of the matched control subjects ($p < 0.001$). Twelve months after diagnosis, mortality was 37.3% (60/161) among patients with CDAD and 20.6% (135/656) among the control subjects ($p < 0.001$), for a cumulative attributable mortality of 16.7% (95% confidence interval 8.6%-25.2%). Each case of nosocomial CDAD led, on average, to 10.7 additional days in hospital.

Interpretation.—This study documented a high attributable mortality among elderly patients with CDAD mostly caused by a hypervirulent strain, which represents a dramatic change in the severity of this infection (Table 2).

► This analysis attempts to determine the proportion of deaths attributable to *C difficile*-associated diarrhea (CDAD) in Quebec, Canada, a province with high nosocomial CDAD rates and high mortality rates. This analysis underscored the disproportionate impact on the elderly population, and the authors estimate between 1000 and 3000 elderly people in Quebec may have died as a result of nosocomial CDAD. The authors recognize that there are limitations to this analysis, and to be accurate, they should be pointed out. For example, they

TABLE 2.—Mortality at 30 Days and 1 Year Among Patients in Whom Nosocomial *Clostridium difficile*-associated Disease (CDAD) Developed and in Matched Control Subjects Without CDAD, by Age and Charlson Comorbidity Index Score

	Mortality at 30 D			Mortality at 1 Yr		
Variable	No. (%) of Case Subjects	No. (%) of Control Subjects	Attributable Mortality (95% CI), %	No. (%) of Case Subjects	No. (%) of Control Subjects	Attributable Mortality (95% CI), %
Age, yr						
18-64	1/16 (6.3)	2/64 (3.1)	3.2 (−7.4 to 29.3)	1/16 (6.3)	7/64 (10.9)	−4.7 (−22.0 to 17.1)
65-74	12/62 (19.4)	13/257 (5.1)	14.3 (5.0 to 26.9)	23/62 (37.1)	41/257 (16.0)	21.1 (8.4 to 35.0)
≥75	24/83 (28.9)	31/335 (9.3)	19.7 (9.8 to 31.2)	36/83 (43.4)	87/335 (26.0)	17.4 (5.6 to 29.6)
Charlson Comorbidity Index score						
0	0/11 (0)	1/55 (1.8)	−1.8 (−30.4 to 11.0)	0/11 (0)	1/55 (1.8)	−1.8 (−30.4 to 11.0)
1-3	16/69 (23.2)	16/305 (5.2)	17.9 (8.4 to 30.1)	20/69 (29.0)	48/305 (15.7)	13.3 (2.2 to 26.2)
4-6	15/59 (25.4)	23/225 (10.2)	15.2 (4.0 to 28.9)	28/59 (47.5)	59/225 (26.2)	21.2 (6.8 to 35.6)
≥7	6/22 (27.3)	6/71 (8.5)	18.8 (0.4 to 42.5)	12/22 (54.5)	27/71 (38.0)	16.5 (−8.6 to 39.7)

Note: CI = confidence interval.

(Courtesy of Pépin J, Valiquette L, Cossette B: Mortality attributable to nosocomial *Clostridium difficile*–associated disease during an epidemic caused by a hypervirulent strain in Quebec. *CMAJ* 173:1037-1041, 2005. Reprinted by permission of the publisher.

were unable to match completely cases to controls (in a 5:1 match), and the attributable mortality rate was being measured at a time when an outbreak of this new more virulent strain was circulating in the population. They also point out that a longer hospital stay might be a cause for acquisition of *C difficile*, but the authors did control for this variable by only taking the first hospital stay as the time of exposure. These data underscore the need to prevent and treat *C difficile* more effectively and this "old" disease becomes a newly emerging pathogen.

D. R. Snydman, MD

An Epidemic, Toxin Gene–Variant Strain of *Clostridium difficile*

McDonald LC, Killgore GE, Thompson A, et al (Centers for Disease Control and Prevention, Atlanta, Ga; Univ of Vermont, Burlington; Loyola Univ, Hines, Ill)
N Engl J Med 353:2433-2441, 2005 16–7

Background.—Recent reports suggest that the rate and severity of *Clostridium difficile*–associated disease in the United States are increasing and that the increase may be associated with the emergence of a new strain of *C. difficile* with increased virulence, resistance, or both.

Methods.—A total of 187 *C. difficile* isolates were collected from eight health care facilities in six states (Georgia, Illinois, Maine, New Jersey, Oregon, and Pennsylvania) in which outbreaks of *C. difficile*–associated disease had occurred between 2000 and 2003. The isolates were characterized by restriction-endonuclease analysis (REA), pulsed-field gel electrophoresis (PFGE), and toxinotyping, and the results were compared with those from a database of more than 6000 isolates obtained before 2001. The polymerase chain reaction was used to detect the recently described binary toxin CDT and a deletion in the pathogenicity locus gene, *tcdC*, that might result in increased production of toxins A and B.

Results.—Isolates that belonged to one REA group (BI) and had the same PFGE type (NAP1) were identified in specimens collected from patients at all eight facilities and accounted for at least half of the isolates from five facilities. REA group BI, which was first identified in 1984, was uncommon among isolates from the historic database (14 cases). Both historic and current (obtained since 2001) BI/NAP1 isolates were of toxinotype III, were positive for the binary toxin CDT, and contained an 18-bp *tcdC* deletion. Resistance to gatifloxacin and moxifloxacin was more common in current BI/NAP1 isolates than in non-BI/NAP1 isolates (100 percent vs. 42 percent, $P<0.001$), whereas the rate of resistance to clindamycin was the same in the two groups (79 percent). All of the current but none of the historic BI/NAP1 isolates were resistant to gatifloxacin and moxifloxacin ($P<0.001$).

Conclusions.—A previously uncommon strain of *C. difficile* with variations in toxin genes has become more resistant to fluoroquinolones and has emerged as a cause of geographically dispersed outbreaks of *C. difficile*–associated disease.

A Predominantly Clonal Multi-Institutional Outbreak of *Clostridium difficile*–Associated Diarrhea With High Morbidity and Mortality

Loo VG, Poirier L, Miller MA, et al (McGill Univ, Montreal; Université de Montréal; Hôpital Jean Talon, Montreal; et al)

N Engl J Med 353:2442-2449, 2005 16–8

Background.—In March 2003, several hospitals in Quebec, Canada, noted a marked increase in the incidence of *Clostridium difficile*–associated diarrhea.

Methods.—In 2004 we conducted a prospective study at 12 Quebec hospitals to determine the incidence of nosocomial *C. difficile*–associated diarrhea and its complications and a case–control study to identify risk factors for the disease. Isolates of *C. difficile* were typed by pulsed-field gel electrophoresis and analyzed for binary toxin genes and partial deletions in the toxin A and B repressor gene *tcdC*. Antimicrobial susceptibility was evaluated in a subgroup of isolates.

Results.—A total of 1703 patients with 1719 episodes of nosocomial *C. difficile*–associated diarrhea were identified. The incidence was 22.5 per 1000 admissions. The 30-day attributable mortality rate was 6.9 percent. Case patients were more likely than matched controls to have received fluoroquinolones (odds ratio, 3.9; 95 percent confidence interval, 2.3 to 6.6) or cephalosporins (odds ratio, 3.8; 95 percent confidence interval, 2.2 to 6.6). A predominant strain, resistant to fluoroquinolones, was found in 129 of 157 isolates (82.2 percent), and the binary toxin genes and partial deletions in the *tcdC* gene were present in 132 isolates (84.1 percent).

Conclusions.—A strain of *C. difficile* that was resistant to fluoroquinolones and had binary toxin and a partial deletion of the *tcdC* gene was responsible for this outbreak of *C. difficile*–associated diarrhea. Exposure to fluoroquinolones or cephalosporins was a risk factor.

► There is very little question that the epidemiology of *C difficile* is changing and that a new or many new strains are evolving. The disease is much more severe, toxic megacolon is not uncommon, mortality rate seems to be increasing among these patients, and even community-acquired disease with little or no antibiotic exposure is being reported. As these 2 reports (Abstracts 16–7 and 16–8) illustrate, what we know is that many of these strains make a variant toxin called the binary toxin; these strains have a genetic deletion of a regulatory gene that may confer increased virulence, and many of these strains are resistant to the newer-generation quinolones. It is not known if the use of these newer-generation fluoroquinolones is the major risk factor, although in some outbreaks this appears to be the case. Hospital and commercial laboratories do not have the capability to diagnose these isolates, which makes surveillance and recognition all the more problematic. We have no idea how to treat this severe disease, but recognition is obviously important and surgical intervention may be necessary, something that has rarely been necessary in the past 20 years with better diagnosis and treatment. Infection control and containment of the strains within institutions is critical to the elimination of this organism. However, with the widespread reporting in the United States and Canada as well as Europe, and molecular epidemiologic studies to demonstrate identity in all geographic locales, it may be too late to contain this worrisome strain.

D. R. Snydman, MD

17 Vaccines

A Vaccine to Prevent Herpes Zoster and Postherpetic Neuralgia in Older Adults

Oxman MN, for the Shingles Prevention Study Group (VA San Diego Healthcare System, Calif; et al)

N Engl J Med 352:2271-2284, 2005 17–1

Background.—The incidence and severity of herpes zoster and postherpetic neuralgia increase with age in association with a progressive decline in cell-mediated immunity to varicella–zoster virus (VZV). We tested the hypothesis that vaccination against VZV would decrease the incidence, severity, or both of herpes zoster and postherpetic neuralgia among older adults.

Methods.—We enrolled 38,546 adults 60 years of age or older in a randomized, double-blind, placebo-controlled trial of an investigational live attenuated Oka/Merck VZV vaccine ("zoster vaccine"). Herpes zoster was diagnosed according to clinical and laboratory criteria. The pain and discomfort associated with herpes zoster were measured repeatedly for six months. The primary end point was the burden of illness due to herpes zoster, a measure affected by the incidence, severity, and duration of the associated pain and discomfort. The secondary end point was the incidence of postherpetic neuralgia.

Results.—More than 95 percent of the subjects continued in the study to its completion, with a median of 3.12 years of surveillance for herpes zoster. A total of 957 confirmed cases of herpes zoster (315 among vaccine recipients and 642 among placebo recipients) and 107 cases of postherpetic neuralgia (27 among vaccine recipients and 80 among placebo recipients) were included in the efficacy analysis. The use of the zoster vaccine reduced the burden of illness due to herpes zoster by 61.1 percent ($P<0.001$), reduced the incidence of postherpetic neuralgia by 66.5 percent ($P<0.001$), and reduced the incidence of herpes zoster by 51.3 percent ($P<0.001$). Reactions at the injection site were more frequent among vaccine recipients but were generally mild.

Conclusions.—The zoster vaccine markedly reduced morbidity from herpes zoster and postherpetic neuralgia among older adults.

► This study was a prodigious undertaking and encompassed over 38,000 subjects enrolled over 3 years with another 3 years of follow-up! The VZV used in this study reduced dramatically the burden of illness caused by herpes zoster among those older than 60 years. Before clinicians adopt the practice of administering VZV to adults, it must be noted that the potency of the vaccine used in this study was 14 times greater than that in the currently licensed vaccine. This trial not only demonstrated a reduced likelihood of herpes zoster, but among those who did get herpes zoster, the burden of illness, that is, postherpetic neuralgia persistence and severity, were reduced as well. Ultimately, since the vaccine was safe, it will probably be produced for use among the growing population of baby-boomers, now at increasing risk for herpes zoster as immunity wanes. A superficial cost-effectiveness analysis would indicate that the vaccine should be cost effective, especially as older individuals live longer and more productive lives. Also to be added to the equation is the changing burden of illness, with most children receiving immunization, which confers a lower likelihood of herpes zoster. But for baby-boomers who developed chickenpox, the risk of herpes zoster is significant and this vaccine may well confer benefit.

D. R. Snydman, MD

Efficacy of an Acellular Pertussis Vaccine Among Adolescents and Adults

Ward JI, for the APERT Study Group (UCLA, Torrance, Calif; et al)

N Engl J Med 353:1555-1563, 2005 17–2

Background.—Pertussis immunization of adults may be necessary to improve the control of a rising burden of disease and infection. This trial of an acellular pertussis vaccine among adolescents and adults evaluated the incidence of pertussis, vaccine safety, immunogenicity, and protective efficacy.

Methods.—Bordetella pertussis infections and illnesses were prospectively assessed in 2781 healthy subjects between the ages of 15 and 65 years who were enrolled in a national multicenter, randomized, double-blind trial of an acellular pertussis vaccine. Subjects received either a dose of a tricomponent acellular pertussis vaccine or a hepatitis A vaccine (control) and were monitored for 2.5 years for illnesses with cough that lasted for more than 5 days. Each illness was evaluated with use of a nasopharyngeal aspirate for culture and polymerase-chain-reaction assay, and serum samples from patients in both acute and convalescent stages of illness were analyzed for changes in antibodies to nine B. pertussis antigens.

Results.—Of the 2781 subjects, 1391 received the acellular pertussis vaccine and 1390 received the control vaccine. The groups had similar ages and demographic characteristics, and the median duration of follow-up was 22 months. The acellular pertussis vaccine was safe and immunogenic. There were 2672 prolonged illnesses with cough, but the incidence of this nonspecific outcome did not vary between the groups, even when stratified according to age, season, and duration of cough. On the basis of the primary pertussis case definition, vaccine protection was 92 percent (95 percent confidence interval, 32 to 99 percent). Among unimmunized controls with illness, 0.7 percent to 5.7 percent had *B. pertussis* infection, and the percentage increased with the duration of cough. On the basis of other case definitions, the incidence of pertussis in the controls ranged from 370 to 450 cases per 100,000 person-years.

Conclusions.—The acellular pertussis vaccine was protective among adolescents and adults, and its routine use might reduce the overall disease burden and transmission to children.

► The other day I received a call from an internist asking about the use of pertussis vaccine in adults. He indicated to me that a patient of his had told him this was recommended by AARP! I was unaware of this recommendation but aware of these data, and as of this writing, the ACIP is deliberating the recommendations as is the CDC. These data indicate the effectiveness of the acellular pertussis vaccine in adolescents older than 15 years and adults younger than 65 years. Two vaccines have now been licensed, and they both have about one third the antigenic component used for children. A single dose is effective. Given the burden of pertussis in adolescents and adults, and increase in cases with attendant morbidity and cost as well as difficulty in making a diagnosis, it is anticipated that a booster dose of vaccine will be recommended for some patients, particularly health care workers and those working with children and adolescents. Another strategy might be the immunization with booster doses of all adolescents. Those physicians caring for such populations are cautioned to pay attention to recommendations that will be forthcoming in 2006.

D. R. Snydman, MD

18 Miscellaneous

Cytomegalovirus Infection in Critically Ill Patients

Jaber S, Chanques G, Borry J, et al (Univ Hosp of Montpellier, France)

Chest 127:233-241, 2005 18–1

Objective.—To determine the prevalence, associated findings, and consequences of cytomegalovirus (CMV) antigenemia in critically ill patients.

Design.—A retrospective, case-control clinical study.

Setting.—A 12-bed university hospital medical-surgical ICU.

Patients.—Two hundred thirty-seven patients with fever for > 72 h, without proven evidence of bacteriologic and/or fungal origin, and whose pp65 antigenemia assays were studied. Patients with HIV infection and transplant recipients were excluded.

Interventions.—None.

Measurements and Results.—CMV antigenemia was diagnosed within 20 ± 12 days (mean ± SD) after ICU admission in 17% patients in whom the pathology was suspected. The 40 patients in the CMV group were matched with 40 other patients in the control group. CMV infection was linked to renal failure (58% vs 33%, respectively; $p = 0.02$) and steroid use (55% vs 33%, respectively; $p = 0.04$). Patients with CMV had a significantly longer stay in the ICU (41 ± 28 days vs 31 ± 22 days, respectively; $p = 0.04$), a longer duration of mechanical ventilation (35 ± 27 days vs 24 ± 20 days, respectively; $p = 0.03$), a higher rate of nosocomial infection (75% vs 50%, respectively; $p = 0.04$), and a higher mortality (50% vs 28%, $p = 0.02$).

Conclusions.—CMV antigenemia is not an uncommon diagnosis in critically ill ICU patients with unexplained prolonged fever after 10 days of hospitalization, regardless of their immune system status. Although associated with a higher morbidity and mortality, the clinical significance of CMV is unknown. Further prospective studies should evaluate the impact on ICU outcome and whether CMV is truly a pathogen or simply another indicator of immunosuppression.

► A few days before writing this comment, I was asked about a patient in the surgical ICU with a very high CMV viral load, and pulmonary infiltrates. The question was whether CMV was contributing to the patient's illness. The study cited here raises more questions than answers, but the data illustrate the problem with CMV and its reactivation in the ICU setting. The authors cite the prospective studies, which show a high degree of variability, but the important take-home message is that CMV can reactivate in about 10% to 15% of patients in the ICU. We know that bacteremia can upregulate tumor necrosis factor alfa, which reactivates latent CMV infection. So the association with bacteremia is not surprising. Whether this is an "epi" phenomenon, that is, a manifestation of immunosuppression, and not a cause, or whether this is a cause of disease, will need to be put to the test of an intervention trial. The higher mortality rate is also quite striking, and the same issue can be raised; that is, is CMV reactivation an indicator of the severity of illness or the cause of illness? Additional studies should be done in the ICUs to sort out these relationships.

D. R. Snydman, MD

An Evaluation of *Echinacea angustifolia* in Experimental Rhinovirus Infections

Turner RB, Bauer R, Woelkart K, et al (Univ of Virginia, Charlottesville; Karl-Franzens-Universitaet, Graz, Austria; Med Univ of South Carolina, Charleston; et al)

N Engl J Med 353:341-348, 2005 18–2

Background.—Echinacea has been widely used as an herbal remedy for the common cold, but efficacy studies have produced conflicting results, and there are a variety of echinacea products on the market with different phytochemical compositions. We evaluated the effect of chemically defined extracts from *Echinacea angustifolia* roots on rhinovirus infection.

Methods.—Three preparations of echinacea, with distinct phytochemical profiles, were produced by extraction from *E. angustifolia* roots with supercritical carbon dioxide, 60 percent ethanol, or 20 percent ethanol. A total of 437 volunteers were randomly assigned to receive either prophylaxis (beginning seven days before the virus challenge) or treatment (beginning at the time of the challenge) either with one of these preparations or with placebo. The results for 399 volunteers who were challenged with rhinovirus type 39 and observed in a sequestered setting for five days were included in the data analysis.

Results.—There were no statistically significant effects of the three echinacea extracts on rates of infection or severity of symptoms. Similarly, there were no significant effects of treatment on the volume of nasal secretions, on polymorphonuclear leukocyte or interleukin-8 concentrations in nasal-lavage specimens, or on quantitative-virus titer.

Conclusions.—The results of this study indicate that extracts of *E. angustifolia* root, either alone or in combination, do not have clinically significant effects on infection with a rhinovirus or on the clinical illness that results from it.

► *E angustifolia* roots were used in the 1800s as a common cold remedy, and they have had a resurgence in popularity in the last decade, coincident with the passage of the Dietary Supplement Health and Education Act of 1994, which liberalized such dietary supplements and the use of herbal medications. The market for herbal medications is billions of dollars and the use of echinacea is rampant among college students and others who want to prevent or treat colds. The clinical data regarding the effectiveness is controversial, and the authors have undertaken a study, on the basis of their well-developed cold model, using volunteers infected with rhinovirus, to establish any effect, either with respect to symptom relief, or viral replication, for echinacea. Although experimental, the rhinovirus model used does appear to reflect the impact of an intervention on natural infection, but, as the authors conclude, they found no effect.

D. R. Snydman, MD

Effect of Multivitamin and Multimineral Supplements on Morbidity From Infections in Older People (MAVIS trial): Pragmatic, Randomised, Double Blind, Placebo Controlled Trial

Avenell A, Campbell MK, Cook JA, et al (Univ of Aberdeen, Foresterhill, Scotland)

BMJ 331:324-327, 2005 18–3

Objective.—To examine whether supplementation with multivitamins and multiminerals influences self reported days of infection, use of health services, and quality of life in people aged 65 or over.

Design.—Randomised, placebo controlled trial, with blinding of participants, outcome assessors, and investigators.

Setting.—Communities associated with six general practices in Grampian, Scotland.

Participants.—910 men and women aged 65 or over who did not take vitamins or minerals.

Interventions.—Daily multivitamin and multimineral supplementation or placebo for one year.

Main Outcome Measures.—Primary outcomes were contacts with primary care for infections, self reported days of infection, and quality of life. Secondary outcomes included antibiotic prescriptions, hospital admissions, adverse events, and compliance.

Results.—Supplementation did not significantly affect contacts with primary care and days of infection per person (incidence rate ratio 0.96, 95% confidence interval 0.78 to 1.19 and 1.07, 0.90 to 1.27). Quality of life was not affected by supplementation. No statistically significant findings were found for secondary outcomes or subgroups.

Conclusion.—Routine multivitamin and multimineral supplementation of older people living at home does not affect self reported infection related morbidity.

► This is the third study I have chosen[1,2] that explores the use of vitamin supplements to prevent infections. This has been a controversial topic, in part because of early trials that suggested benefit and a subsequent meta-analysis that suggested a need for more trials. In theory, there may be merit, because vitamin and mineral intake in people older than 65 years may be suboptimal and, therefore, influence immunity to infection. On the basis of this and 2 other trials, it would appear that, for purposes of infection prevention, one cannot recommend vitamins or mineral supplements.

D. R. Snydman, MD

References

1. 2004 Year Book of Medicine, pp 163-165.
2. 2005 Year Book of Medicine, pp 143-144.

A Pilot Randomized Double-blind Placebo-controlled Trial on the Use of Antibiotics on Urinary Catheter Removal to Reduce the Rate of Urinary Tract Infection: The Pitfalls of Ciprofloxacin

Wazait HD, Patel HR, Van Der Meulen J, et al (Royal Coll of Surgeons of England, London; Whittington Hosp NHS Trust, London; London School of Hygiene and Tropical Medicine)

BJU Internatl 94:1048-1050, 2004 18–4

Background.—Catheter-associated urinary tract infection (CAUTI) is the most prevalent form of nosocomial infection. The most important factor in the development of CAUTI is the duration of catheterization. Other important factors are age, female sex, and the presence of diabetes mellitus and elevated serum creatinine levels. Most patients with CAUTI are asymptomatic, and treatment is not recommended with the catheter in place. Systemic antibiotics can be used, but their use is complicated by the development of antimicrobial resistance. The purpose of the present study was to determine whether a short course of antibiotics initiated at the removal of a short-term urethral catheter might decrease the incidence of subsequent urinary tract infection (UTI).

Methods.—Patients were recruited over 4 months from a mixture of medical and surgical wards at one hospital. Patients included in the study had a urethral catheter in situ for 48 hours or more but no longer than 7 days. Patients who had undergone recent genitourinary surgery or who were on antibiotic therapy were excluded. The study patients were randomly assigned to receive a 48-hour course of either ciprofloxacin or placebo tablets beginning 2 hours before catheter removal. A catheter specimen of urine was obtained at the start of the trial medication. Follow-up examinations were performed at 7 and 14 days after removal of the catheter. Included in the follow up was a questionnaire for UTI symptoms. Midstream urine samples were also obtained at follow-up.

Results.—A total of 48 patients was enrolled (25 receiving ciprofloxacin and 23 receiving placebo). Of the ciprofloxacin group, 4 patients (16%) had a UTI at the follow-up after catheter removal, and 2 patients were symptomatic. The UTI in 2 patients, including 1 that was symptomatic, was newly developed after removal of the catheter. The other 2 UTIs resulted from failure to resolve a CAUTI. All of the UTIs in the ciprofloxacin group were resistant to ciprofloxacin. In the placebo group, 3 patients (13%) had a UTI on follow-up after removal, and one of these patients was symptomatic. The UTI in the symptomatic patient was also resistant to ciprofloxacin. The other 2 patients were asymptomatic, and their UTIs resulted from a failure to resolve a CAUTI; one of these infections was resistant to ciprofloxacin.

Conclusions.—There is a real risk of UTI after removal of a urethral catheter, even in patients with no evidence of CAUTI before removal. UTIs occurring after removal of a short-term urinary catheter had a high rate of resistance to ciprofloxacin. There was no discernible benefit from the use of prophylactic ciprofloxacin for reducing the UTI rate after catheter removal.

► Catheter-associated UTI is the most common cause of nosocomial infection, and the question of management or use of "prophylactic antibiotics" does come up from time to time. Although it is known that antibiotics should not be given during catheterization, there is no unanimity of opinion regarding what to do after catheter removal. This study attempts to answer the question, and the findings are very instructive. (1) Ciprofloxacin resistance is common when it is used prophylactically. (2) Symptomatic urinary tract infection occurs in about 7% to 8% of patients once the catheter is removed. (3) Asymptomatic bacteriuria also occurs in another 7% of patients. It would seem the lesson learned is to monitor patients carefully and treat symptomatically rather than give "prophylactic" antibiotics.

D. R. Snydman, MD

Amoxicillin-Clavulanate vs Ciprofloxacin for the Treatment of Uncomplicated Cystitis in Women: A Randomized Trial

Hooton TM, Scholes D, Gupta K, et al (Univ of Washington, Seattle; Group Health Cooperative, Seattle)

JAMA 293:949-955, 2005 18–5

Context.—The high prevalence of resistance to trimethoprim-sulfamethoxazole and other antimicrobials among *Escherichia coli* causing acute cystitis in women has led to increased use of alternative antibiotics. One such antibiotic, amoxicillin-clavulanate, has not been well studied.

Objective.—To compare the efficacy of a 3-day regimen of amoxicillin-clavulanate to that of a 3-day regimen of ciprofloxacin in the treatment of acute cystitis in women. The primary study hypothesis was that the amoxicillin-clavulanate and ciprofloxacin treatment groups would differ in clinical cure.

Design, Setting, and Patients.—Randomized, single-blind treatment trial of 370 women, aged 18 to 45 years, with symptoms of acute uncomplicated cystitis and a urine culture with at least 10^2 colony-forming units of uropathogens per milliliter from a university student health center or a health maintenance organization.

Interventions.—Women were randomly assigned to receive amoxicillin-clavulanate (500 mg/125 mg twice daily) or ciprofloxacin (250 mg twice daily) for 3 days and were followed up for 4 months.

Main Outcome Measures.—The main outcome measure was clinical cure. Secondary study outcomes of interest were microbiological cure and vaginal *E coli* colonization at the 2-week follow-up visit.

Results.—Clinical cure was observed in 93 (58%) of 160 women treated with amoxicillin-clavulanate compared with 124 (77%) of 162 women treated with ciprofloxacin (P<.001). Amoxicillin-clavulanate was not as effective as ciprofloxacin even among women infected with strains susceptible to amoxicillin-clavulanate (65 [60%] of 109 women in the amoxicillin-clavulanate group vs 114 [77%] of 149 women in the ciprofloxacin group; P=.004). The difference in clinical cure rates occurred almost entirely within the first 2 weeks after therapy. Microbiological cure at 2 weeks was observed in 118 (76%) of 156 women treated with amoxicillin-clavulanate compared with 153 (95%) of 161 women treated with ciprofloxacin (P<.001). At this visit, 45% of women in the amoxicillin-clavulanate group compared with 10% in the ciprofloxacin group had vaginal colonization with *E coli* (P<.001).

Conclusions.—A 3-day regimen of amoxicillin-clavulanate is not as effective as ciprofloxacin for the treatment of acute uncomplicated cystitis, even in women infected with susceptible strains. This difference may be due to the inferior ability of amoxicillin-clavulanate to eradicate vaginal *E coli*, facilitating early reinfection.

► Acute uncomplicated urinary tract infections are among the most common infections in women encountered by clinicians. The Seattle group has been the most influential group to define the pathogenesis and treatment of these infections in a multitude of elegantly designed studies. This study is another important one, which analyzes the comparative efficacy of amoxicillin-clavulanate versus ciprofloxacin for uncomplicated cystitis in women. The authors conclude that ciprofloxacin is clinically superior to amoxicillin-clavulanate for uncomplicated urinary tract infections in women—that is, those that require 3 days of therapy. Their investigations suggest that the reason relapse is common in the amoxicillin-clavulanate group is due to failure to eradicate *E coli* from the vaginal flora. Interestingly, the lack of susceptibility of *E coli* to amoxicillin-clavulanate, which was somewhat more common than for ciprofloxacin, did not, in itself, account for more frequent failures. As the authors point out, although β-lactam antibiotics have been used for years for urinary tract infections, they have not been as effective as either trimethoprim-sulfamethoxazole or the quinolones. Current recommendations still favor the use of trimethoprim-sulfamethoxazole in regions where resistance of *E coli* to this agent is less than 20%. But based on these data, ciprofloxacin, at a dosage of 250 mg orally twice a day, would be the recommended alternative.

D. R. Snydman, MD

PART THREE

HEMATOLOGY AND ONCOLOGY

PATRICK J. LOEHRER, SR, MD

Introduction

The field of oncology has been evolving during the past several decades. We now recognize that therapies have both short-term and long-term consequences. Several articles address these issues. The other areas of cancer prevention and screening have also grown. Advances continue in early staging and the molecular markers of solid tumors.

This YEAR BOOK section highlights the breadth and depth that oncology research presented this year.

Patrick J. Loehrer, Sr, MD

19 Lung Cancer

Vinorelbine Plus Cisplatin vs Observation in Resected Non–Small-Cell Lung Cancer

Winton T, for the National Cancer Institute of Canada Clinical Trials Group and the National Cancer Institute of the United States Intergroup JBR.10 Trial Investigators (Natl Cancer Inst of Canada, Kingston, Ont, Canada; et al)

N Engl J Med 352:2589-2597, 2005 19–1

Background.—We undertook to determine whether adjuvant vinorelbine plus cisplatin prolongs overall survival among patients with completely resected early-stage non–small-cell lung cancer.

Methods.—We randomly assigned patients with completely resected stage IB or stage II non–small-cell lung cancer to vinorelbine plus cisplatin or to observation. The primary end point was overall survival; principal secondary end points were recurrence-free survival and the toxicity and safety of the regimen.

Results.—A total of 482 patients underwent randomization to vinorelbine plus cisplatin (242 patients) or observation (240); 45 percent of the patients had pathological stage IB disease and 55 percent had stage II, and all had an Eastern Cooperative Oncology Group performance status score of 0 or 1. In both groups, the median age was 61 years, 65 percent were men, and 53 percent had adenocarcinomas. Chemotherapy caused neutropenia in 88 percent of patients (including grade 3 febrile neutropenia in 7 percent) and death from toxic effects in two patients (0.8 percent). Nonhematologic toxic effects of chemotherapy were fatigue (81 percent of patients), nausea (80 percent), anorexia (55 percent), vomiting (48 percent), neuropathy (48 percent), and constipation (47 percent), but severe (grade 3 or greater) toxic effects were uncommon (<10 percent). Overall survival was significantly prolonged in the chemotherapy group as compared with the observation group (94 vs. 73 months; hazard ratio for death, 0.69; P=0.04), as was relapse-free survival (not reached vs. 46.7 months; hazard ratio for recurrence, 0.60; P<0.001). Five-year survival rates were 69 percent and 54 percent, respectively (P=0.03).

Conclusions.—Adjuvant vinorelbine plus cisplatin has an acceptable level of toxicity and prolongs disease-free and overall survival among patients with completely resected early-stage non–small-cell lung cancer.

► The standard of care for resected stage IB and II non–small cell lung cancer now includes adjuvant chemotherapy. The trial reported by Winton et al supports this recommendation. In this Intergroup study, patients with completely resected stage IB or II non–small cell lung cancer were randomly assigned to either an observation arm or adjuvant chemotherapy consisting of cisplatin plus vinorelbine. Although 4 cycles of therapy were planned, the median number of cycles delivered was 3, and 77% of patients required dose modifications to their regimen. Overall, the regimen was generally well tolerated, and only 1 patient died of a chemotherapy-related cause. Those patients assigned chemotherapy had significantly longer median and overall survival rates compared with those followed up with observation alone. The treatment effect seemed most pronounced in those with stage II disease, but the number of patients with stage I disease and the number of events on both arms with stage I disease were small. No patients in this trial received adjuvant radiotherapy, which may have a detrimental effect on survival. Those patients with *ras* mutations did not seem to benefit from adjuvant chemotherapy, although this needs to be validated in a prospective study.

N. H. Hanna, MD

EGF Receptor Gene Mutations Are Common in Lung Cancers From "Never Smokers" and Are Associated With Sensitivity of Tumors to Gefitinib and Erlotinib

Pao W, Miller V, Zakowski M, et al (Mem Sloan-Kettering Cancer Ctr, New York; Washington Univ, St Louis)

Proc Natl Acad Sci U S A 101:13306-13311, 2004 19–2

Introduction.—Somatic mutations in the tyrosine kinase (TK) domain of the epidermal growth factor receptor (EGFR) gene are reportedly associated with sensitivity of lung cancers to gefitinib (Iressa), kinase inhibitor. In-frame deletions occur in exon 19, whereas point mutations occur frequently in codon 858 (exon 21). We found from sequencing the *EGFR* TK domain that 7 of 10 gefitinib-sensitive tumors had similar types of alterations; no mutations were found in eight gefitinib-refractory tumors ($P = 0.004$). Five of seven tumors sensitive to erlotinib (Tarceva), a related kinase inhibitor for which the clinically relevant target is undocumented, had analogous somatic mutations, as opposed to none of 10 erlotinib-refractory tumors ($P = 0.003$). Because most mutation-positive tumors were adenocarcinomas from patients who smoked <100 cigarettes in a lifetime ("never smokers"), we screened *EGFR* exons 2-28 in 15 adenocarcinomas resected from untreated never smokers. Seven tumors had TK domain mutations, in contrast to 4 of 81 non-small cell lung cancers resected from untreated former or current smokers ($P = 0.0001$). Immunoblotting of lysates from cells transiently transfected with various *EGFR* constructs demonstrated that, compared to wild-type protein, an exon 19 deletion mutant induced diminished levels of phosphotyrosine, whereas the phosphorylation at tyrosine 1092 of an exon 21 point mutant was inhibited at 10-fold lower concentrations of drug. Collectively, these data show that adenocarcinomas from never smokers comprise a distinct subset of lung cancers, frequently containing mutations within the TK domain of *EGFR* that are associated with gefitinib and erlotinib sensitivity.

Gefitinib-Sensitizing EGFR Mutations in Lung Cancer Activate Anti-Apoptotic Pathways

Sordella R, Bell DW, Haber DA, et al (Harvard Med School, Charleston, Mass)
Science 305:1163-1167, 2004 19–3

Background.—Studies have suggested that receptor tyrosine kinases of the epidermal growth factor receptor (EGFR) family regulate essential cellular functions, including proliferation, survival, migration, and differentiation, and may be a key factor in the etiology and progression of solid tumors. EGFR is frequently overexpressed in non–small cell lung cancers (NSCLCs) of the breast, lung, colon, ovaries, and brain. This observation spurred the development of specific pharmacological inhibitors, such as gefitinib, which disrupts EGFR kinase activity by binding the adenosine triphosphate (ATP) pocket within the catalytic domain. Nearly all gefitinib-responsive lung cancers contain somatic mutations within the EGFR kinase domain, while no mutations have been observed in nonresponsive cases. These heterozygous mutations include both small in-frame deletions and missense substitutions clustered within the ATP-binding pocket. Previous studies have shown that both of these mutations result in increased EGF-dependent receptor activation.

Methods.—Cell lines stably transfected with mutant EGFRs facilitated comparison of the phosphorylation status of the major downstream targets of EGFR in a shared cellular background, including EGF-induced activation of extracellular signal-regulated kinase (Erk 1) and Erk 2 via Ras, of Akt via phospholipase C γ and phosphatidylinositol 3-kinase (PI3K), and of activator of transcription status 3 (STAT3) and STAT5 via Janus kinase 2 (JAK2).

Results.—Ras-mediated activation of the Erk kinases was found to contribute significantly to the proliferative activity of EGFR, whereas activation of Akt and STATs is linked mainly to an anti-apoptotic function.

Conclusions.—The effectiveness of gefitinib in lung cancers harboring mutant EGFRs may be a reflection of both its inhibition of critical anti-apoptotic pathways on which these cells have become strictly dependent and altered biochemical properties of the mutant receptors.

► Erlotinib and gefitinib are EGFR tyrosine kinase inhibitors. Each agent has an approximate 10% response rate in US patients and a higher response rate (20%-30%) in an Asian patient population. In addition, response rates with these agents also seem to correlate with smoking status, tumor histology, and sex. Previously, Lynch et al[1] and Paez et al[2] reported that tumor sensitivity to gefitinib was dependent on the presence of EGFR mutations in exons 18 to 21. Pao et al (Abstract 19–2) are the first to report similar findings with erlotinib. Furthermore, the incidence of EGFR mutations is significantly higher in those patients who never smoked. There are two "hot spots" for mutations—

namely, in exon 19 and 21. In exon 19 there are in-frame deletions that eliminate 4 amino acids, and in exon 21 there are point mutations that result in amino acid substitution. Why certain tumors have mutant EGFR while others do not requires further investigation.

In a related article by Sordella et al (Abstract 19–3), activated mutations of EGFR are reported to activate Akt and signal transduction and activator of transcription (STAT) signaling pathways, which promote cell survival. Ras-mediated activation contributes to the proliferative activity of EGFR. Inhibition of Akt and STAT signaling may contribute to the efficacy of gefitinib or erlotinib.

N. H. Hanna, MD

References

1. Lynch T, Bell D, Sordella R, et al: Activating mutations in the epidermal growth factor receptor underlying responsiveness of non–small-cell lung cancer to gefitinib. *N Engl J Med* 350:2129-2139, 2004.
2. Paez J, Janne P, Lee J, et al: EGFR mutations in lung cancer: Correlation with clinical response to gefitinib therapy. *Science* 304:1497-1500, 2004.

[^{18}F]Fluorodeoxyglucose Uptake by Positron Emission Tomography Predicts Outcome of Non–Small-Cell Lung Cancer

Sasaki R, Komaki R, Macapinlac H, et al (Univ of Texas, Houston; Kobe Univ, Hyogo, Japan)

J Clin Oncol 23:1136-1143, 2005 19–4

Purpose.—To determine whether the standardized uptake value (SUV) of [^{18}F]fluorodeoxyglucose uptake by positron emission tomography could be a prognostic factor for non-small-cell lung cancer (NSCLC).

Patients and Methods.—One hundred sixty-two patients with stage I to IIIb NSCLC were analyzed. Overall survival (OS), disease-free survival (DFS), distant metastasis-free survival (DMFS), and local-regional control (LRC) were calculated by the Kaplan-Meier method and evaluated with the log-rank test. The prognostic significance was assessed by univariate and multivariate analyses.

Results.—There were 93 patients treated with surgery and 69 patients treated with radiotherapy. A cutoff of 5 for the SUV for the primary tumor showed the best discriminative value. The SUV for the primary tumor was a significant predictor of OS (P = .02) in both groups. Low SUVs (≤ 5.0) showed significantly better DFS rates than those with high SUVs (> 5.0; surgery group, P = .02; radiotherapy group, P = .0005). Low SUVs (≤ 5.0) indicated a significantly better DFS than those with high SUVs (> 5.0; stage I or II, P = .02; stage IIIa or IIIb, P = .004). However, using the same cutoff point of 5, the SUV for regional lymph nodes was not a significant indicator for DFS (P = .19), LRC (P = .97), or DMFS (P = .17). The multivariate analysis showed that the SUV for the primary tumor was a significant prognostic factor for OS (P = .03) and DFS (P = .001).

Conclusion.—The SUV of the primary tumor was the strongest prognostic factor among the patients treated by curative surgery or radiotherapy.

► Tumor stage is the most reliable prognostic variable when estimating outcomes in patients with NSCLC. [^{18}F]Fluorodeoxyglucose positron emission tomography (FDG-PET), especially in conjunction with CT imaging, is a useful modality to stage patients with lung cancer. As adjuvant therapy becomes more readily used in the setting of resected NSCLC, determining variables that will better predict for good versus poor outcomes becomes especially pertinent. The majority of patients undergoing surgical resection for stage I or II disease will be cured of their disease by surgery alone, and therefore, adjuvant chemotherapy will benefit only a small percentage of patients. Sasaki et al report the utility of assessing maximum uptake by PET imaging in lung cancer and its ability to predict for outcomes. In this analysis, patients with potentially curable stage I-III disease treated with either surgery or radiation therapy were analyzed. A cutoff SUV of 4 or 5 was determined to discriminate between good and poor risk groups. These data are consistent with other reports. Prospective trials are necessary to validate the use of PET in predicting outcomes. If validated, one could consider a randomized trial in only patients with tumors exhibiting high SUV uptake on PET and evaluating different postoperative strategies (even a no-treatment control arm).

N. H. Hanna, MD

20 Smoking

The Impact of Smoking Status on the Behavior and Survival Outcome of Patients With Advanced Non-small Cell Lung Cancer: A Retrospective Analysis

Toh C-K, Wong E-H, Lim W-T, et al (Natl Cancer Ctr, Singapore)

Chest 126:1750-1756, 2004 20–1

Study Objectives.—There are fundamental differences in characteristics between smokers and nonsmokers with non-small cell lung cancer (NSCLC). We aim to study the impact of smoking status on the behavior of the disease, and to identify differences in outcome between the two groups.

Design.—A retrospective analysis was done of patients with NSCLC seen during the period from January 1999 to August 2002. Clinical characteristics, survival outcome, and response to treatment were reviewed and compared between the smokers and nonsmokers.

Setting.—Department of Medical Oncology, National Cancer Center.

Results.—Of 317 patients analyzed, 117 patients (36.3%) were nonsmokers. Among the nonsmokers, 74.5% had adenocarcinoma and 73.9% were women. The smokers had poorer performance status, reported more weight loss, and had a higher mean age at diagnosis of almost 8 years than nonsmokers. One hundred eighty-seven patients (59%) had died as of December 31, 2002. The nonsmokers had a longer median survival, although this was not statistically significant. There were no statistically significant differences in survival and response to chemotherapy between the two groups after adjusting for known prognostic factors.

Conclusions.—Despite the known differences in mutational spectra and clinical characteristics between smokers and nonsmokers with NSCLC, no differences in terms of response to chemotherapy and survival outcome were observed. This could imply that this disease is equally aggressive in these two groups. More research is needed to further delineate and characterize the differences between these two etiologically different forms of NSCLC.

The Relationship Between Cigarette Smoking and Quality of Life After Lung Cancer Diagnosis

Garces YI, Yang P, Parkinson J, et al (Mayo Clinic College of Medicine, Rochester, Minn)

Chest 126:1733-1741, 2004 20–2

Study Objective.—To describe the relationship between cigarette smoking and quality of life (QOL) among lung cancer survivors as measured by the lung cancer symptom scale (LCSS).

Design and Setting.—The LCSS was mailed to eligible patients (1,506 patients) between 1999 and 2002. LCSS scores (total and individual QOL components) were compared among different groups of cigarette smokers via univariate independent group testing and multivariate linear models. The modeling process examined group differences adjusted for age, gender, stage, and time of LCSS assessment. LCSS scores were transformed onto a scale of 0 to 100 points in which higher LCSS scores corresponded to a lower QOL. A 10-point difference between groups was defined a priori as being clinically significant.

Results.—At the time of lung cancer diagnosis, 18% of the patients were never-smokers, 58% were former smokers, and 24% were current smokers. Among survey respondents completing the LCSS at follow-up assessment (1,028 respondents), the mean age was 65.2 years (SD, 10.8 years) and 45% were women. Thirty percent of baseline current smokers continued to smoke at the time of the follow-up assessment (ie, persistent smokers). The adjusted mean total LCSS scores for never-smokers and persistent smokers were 17.6 (SD, 4.02) and 28.7 (SD, 5.09), respectively ($p < 0.0001$). Seven of the individual LCSS QOL components (ie, appetite, fatigue, cough, shortness of breath, lung cancer symptoms, illness affecting normal activities, and overall QOL) were clinically and statistically ($p < 0.001$) different between never-smokers and persistent smokers. No clinically significant differences were noted for pain or hemoptysis. Former smokers had intermediate LCSS scores. No dose-response trends were observed between the number of packs of cigarettes smoked per day or the total number of pack-years smoked and the adjusted scores.

Conclusion.—The hypothesized relationship between smoking status and QOL was supported by this correlational study. Our findings suggest that persistent cigarette smoking after a lung cancer diagnosis negatively impacts QOL scores.

▶ Approximately 10% of patients who have lung cancer in the United States are never-smokers. The incidence is higher in other countries, particularly in Asia. The clinical behavior of lung cancer in smokers compared with never-smokers may differ because it is based on different mutations that result in lung cancer development. Toh et al (Abstract 20–1) report the clinical differences between never-smokers and smokers who had lung cancer and were seen at the National Cancer Center in Singapore over a 3-year period. While never-smokers were diagnosed with lung cancer at an earlier age, were predominantly female, and had adenocarcinoma, their clinical outcomes did not differ from smokers with lung cancer. That is, the response to chemotherapy, duration of response, and survival times were not significantly different. This may be explained by the nonspecific mechanisms for which chemotherapy causes cytotoxicity.

Garces et al (Abstract 20–2) from the Mayo Clinic evaluated the quality-of-life differences in patients diagnosed with lung cancer according to smoking status. Their findings suggest that persistent cigarette smoking after a lung cancer diagnosis negatively impacts on quality of life. Namely, persistent smokers were found to have worse appetite, fatigue, coughing, dyspnea, symptomatic distress effect on activities, and worse overall quality of life compared with never-smokers. Former smokers had intermediate scores. While significant advances have been made in understanding the molecular defects in lung cancer, which have translated into improved therapeutic outcomes, continued efforts to discourage smoking will ultimately result in making lung cancer an uncommon disease once again.

N. H. Hanna, MD

21 Breast Cancer

Tamoxifen Treatment for Breast Cancer and Risk of Endometrial Cancer: A Case–Control Study

Swerdlow AJ, for the British Tamoxifen Second Cancer Study Group (Inst of Cancer Research, Sutton, Surrey, England)

J Natl Cancer Inst 97:375-384, 2005 21–1

Background.—Tamoxifen treatment of breast cancer is associated with an increased risk of endometrial cancer, but tamoxifen-related risks of endometrial cancer are unclear in premenopausal women, in long-term users of tamoxifen, and in women for whom several years have passed since ending treatment. We conducted a case-control study in Britain to investigate these risks.

Methods.—We compared treatment information on 813 case patients who had endometrial cancer after their diagnosis for breast cancer and 1067 control patients who had breast cancer but not subsequent endometrial cancer. We assessed risk by conditional logistic regression analysis. All statistical tests were two-sided.

Results.—Overall, tamoxifen treatment, compared with no treatment, was associated with an increased risk of endometrial cancer (odds ratio [OR] = 2.4; 95% confidence interval [CI] = 1.8 to 3.0). Risk increased statistically significantly (P_{trend}<.001) with duration of treatment (for ≥ 5 years of treatment compared with no treatment, OR = 3.6, 95% CI = 2.6 to 4.8). As an indication of background levels of treatment, 16% of control patients received 5 years or more of treatment. Risk of endometrial cancer adjusted for treatment duration did not diminish in follow-up to at least 5 years after the last treatment ended. Risk of endometrial cancer was not associated with the daily dose of tamoxifen and was comparable in pre- and postmenopausal women. Ever treatment with tamoxifen was associated with a much greater risk of Mullerian and mesodermal mixed endometrial tumors (OR = 13.5, 95% CI = 4.1 to 44.5) than of adenocarcinoma (OR = 2.1, 95% CI = 1.6 to 2.7) or clear cell and papillary serous tumors (OR = 3.1, 95% CI = 0.8 to 17.9).

Conclusions.—There is an increasing risk of endometrial cancer associated with longer tamoxifen treatment, extending well beyond 5 years. The increased risk of endometrial cancer associated with tamoxifen treatment should be considered clinically for both premenopausal and postmenopausal women during treatment and for at least 5 years after the last treatment.

► This study provides 2 observations that are particularly noteworthy. First, risk of endometrial cancer continues to increase out to 10 years of treatment, whereas evidence to date does not support increased efficacy for treatment that extends beyond 5 years. This would suggest that, at least at the current time, treatment should be limited to 5 years of therapy. Secondly, the increase in risk of mixed mesodermal sarcoma (13.5-fold increase) of the uterus increases to a much greater extent than the risk for endometrial carcinoma (2.1-fold increase). Because these lesions have a much worse prognosis than endometrial carcinoma stage for stage, this adds further caution to the use of extended duration tamoxifen. To put these 2 considerations into context, the benefits of tamoxifen far outweigh the risks. Further, the largest study of tamoxifen as a preventive for breast cancer[1] did not show the marked increase in risk of mixed mesodermal sarcomas. The bottom line is that the risk of endometrial cancer must be taken into account when recommending tamoxifen therapy but should not limit its appropriate use.

J. T. Thigpen, MD

Reference

1. Bernstein L, Deapen D, Cerhan JR, et al: Tamoxifen therapy for breast cancer and endometrial cancer risk. *J Natl Cancer Inst* 91:1654-1662, 1999.

The Results of Frozen Section, Touch Preparation, and Cytological Smear Are Comparable for Intraoperative Examination of Sentinel Lymph Nodes: A Study in 133 Breast Cancer Patients

Brogi E, Torres-Matundan E, Tan LK, et al (Memorial Sloan-Kettering Cancer Ctr, New York)

Ann Surg Oncol 12:173-180, 2005 21–2

Background.—The goal of intraoperative sentinel lymph node (SLN) examination is to avoid reoperation for a positive SLN, but the ideal method of intraoperative SLN examination remains unclear, and published results vary widely.

Methods.—We evaluated the sensitivity of intraoperative frozen section (FS), touch preparation (TP), and cytological smear (CS) in 305 SLNs from 133 breast cancer patients. Each SLN was received fresh and cut into 2- to 3-mm slices; TP and CS from each cut surface and an FS of the entire SLN were obtained. Postoperative evaluation of the SLN consisted of 1 hematoxylin and eosin-stained section and of one hematoxylin and eosin-stained and one immunohistochemically stained section for cytokeratin from each of two levels 50 µm apart. Tumor cells found by any method, including immunohistochemistry, identified a positive SLN. Three pathologists blinded to the final SLN diagnosis reviewed all TP, CS, and FS; the consensus diagnosis (concordance of two or more) was used for the study.

Results.—FS, TP, and CS had comparable sensitivities (59%, 57%, and 59%, respectively). Each method was more sensitive in detecting macrometastases (>2 mm; 96%, 93%, and 93%, respectively) than micrometastases (≤2 mm; 27%, 27%, and 30%, respectively). The combination of methods only marginally improved the intraoperative sensitivity. TP and CS were each responsible for a single false-positive result.

Conclusions.—FS, TP, and CS are comparable for the intraoperative detection of SLN metastases, and each method is substantially better at detecting macrometastases than micrometastases. The combination of two or more techniques only marginally improves the sensitivity over that achieved by a single method.

► Ideally, the surgical management of breast cancer is accomplished with a single operation. This was not difficult in the era of modified radical mastectomy but has become more challenging with the need to obtain negative margins as part of lumpectomy and the intraoperative evaluation of the SLN for metastases. As illustrated in this report, FS, TP, and CS are equally sensitive in detecting SLN metastases. All 3 techniques perform well when metastases larger than 2 mm are present, and none are particularly effective for detecting micrometastases. Whether the detection of micrometastases intraoperatively is important is uncertain, since their impact on both local recurrence in the axilla and prognosis is a matter of debate. The results of 2 prospective trials, the NSABP B32 study and the American College of Surgeons Oncology Group Z10 trial, both of which are closed to accrual, should help to resolve this issue. At present, the choice of FS, TP, or CS appears to be one of institutional preference.

M. Morrow, MD

Significantly Higher Pathologic Complete Remission Rate After Neoadjuvant Therapy With Trastuzumab, Paclitaxel, and Epirubicin Chemotherapy: Results of a Randomized Trial in Human Epidermal Growth Factor Receptor 2–Positive Operable Breast Cancer

Buzdar AU, Ibrahim NK, Francis D, et al (Univ of Texas, Houston)

J Clin Oncol 23:3676-3685, 2005 21–3

Purpose.—The objective of this study was to determine whether the addition of trastuzumab to chemotherapy in the neoadjuvant setting could increase pathologic complete response (pCR) rate in patients with human epidermal growth factor receptor 2 (HER2)–positive disease.

Patients and Methods.—Forty-two patients with HER2-positive disease with operable breast cancer were randomly assigned to either four cycles of paclitaxel followed by four cycles of fluorouracil, epirubicin, and cyclophosphamide or to the same chemotherapy with simultaneous weekly trastuzumab for 24 weeks. The primary objective was to demonstrate a 20% improvement in pCR (assumed 21% to 41%) with the addition of trastuzumab to chemotherapy. The planned sample size was 164 patients.

Results.—Prognostic factors were similar in the two groups. After 34 patients had completed therapy, the trial's Data Monitoring Committee stopped the trial because of superiority of trastuzumab plus chemotherapy. pCR rates were 25% and 66.7% for chemotherapy (n = 16) and trastuzumab plus chemotherapy (n = 18), respectively (P = .02). The decision was based on the calculation that, if study continued to 164 patients, there was a 95% probability that trastuzumab plus chemotherapy would be superior. Of the 42 randomized patients, 26% in the chemotherapy arm achieved pCR compared with 65.2% in the trastuzumab plus chemotherapy arm (P = .016). The safety of this approach is not established, although no clinical congestive heart failure was observed. A more than 10% decrease in the cardiac ejection fraction was observed in five and seven patients in the chemotherapy and trastuzumab plus chemotherapy arms, respectively.

Conclusion.—Despite the small sample size, these data indicate that adding trastuzumab to chemotherapy, as used in this trial, significantly increased pCR without clinical congestive heart failure.

► Although the concept that preoperative chemotherapy would be superior to postoperative chemotherapy by allowing more prompt treatment of subclinical micrometastases is an attractive one, a meta-analysis of randomized trials of preoperative versus postoperative chemotherapy reveals no difference in survival based on the timing of administration of chemotherapy.[1] At present, in operable breast cancer, the only proven benefit of preoperative chemotherapy is to increase the rate of breast-conserving surgery. However, pCR occurs in only about 26% of patients.[2] In the small study of neoadjuvant chemotherapy plus trastuzumab reported by Buzdar et al, a dramatic 65% pathologic complete remission rate was observed in the 18 patients treated with the combination treatment, compared with 26% for patients treated with chemotherapy alone. This dramatic result was initially viewed with some skepticism based on both the very small sample size and concerns about cardiotoxicity in patients receiving the combination therapy. However, these findings are consistent with the clear benefits of postoperative trastuzumab presented at the 2005 American Society of Clinical Oncology meeting. While careful monitoring of cardiac toxicity is essential, preoperative trastuzumab is a viable option for the women with a HER2 overexpressing tumor too large to allow primary breast-conserving therapy. As responses to drug therapy improve, the inability to reliably determine the extent of viable residual tumor remains a major deterrent to the maximum use of breast-conserving therapy.

M. Morrow, MD

References

1. Mauri D, Pavlidis N, Ioannidis JP: Neoadjuvant versus adjuvant systemic treatment in breast cancer: A meta-analysis. *J Natl Cancer Inst* 97:188-194, 2005.
2. Bear HD, Anderson S, Brown A, et al: The effect on tumor response of adding sequential preoperative docetaxel to preoperative doxorubicin and cyclophosphamide: Preliminary results from National Surgical Adjuvant Breast and Bowel Project Protocol B-27. *J Clin Oncol* 21:4165-4174, 2003.

Sentinel Node Biopsy After Neoadjuvant Chemotherapy in Breast Cancer: Results From National Surgical Adjuvant Breast and Bowel Project Protocol B-27

Mamounas EP, Brown A, Anderson S, et al (Natl Surgical Adjuvant Breast and Bowel Project; Univ of Pittsburgh, Pa; Allegheny Gen Hosp, Pittsburgh, Pa; et al)

J Clin Oncol 23:2694-2702, 2005 21–4

Purpose.—Experience with sentinel node biopsy (SNB) after neoadjuvant chemotherapy is limited. We examined the feasibility and accuracy of this procedure within a randomized trial in patients treated with neoadjuvant chemotherapy.

Patients and Methods.—During the conduct of National Surgical Adjuvant Breast and Bowel Project trial B-27, several participating surgeons attempted SNB before the required axillary dissection in 428 patients. All underwent lymphatic mapping and an attempt to identify and remove a sentinel node. Lymphatic mapping was performed with radioactive colloid (14.7%), with lymphazurin blue dye alone (29.9%), or with both (54.7%).

Results.—Success rate for the identification and removal of a sentinel node was 84.8%. Success rate increased significantly with the use of radioisotope (87.6% to 88.9%) versus with the use of lymphazurin alone (78.1%, $P = .03$). There were no significant differences in success rate according to clinical tumor size, clinical nodal status, age, or calendar year of random assignment. Of 343 patients who had SNB and axillary dissection, the sentinel nodes were positive in 125 patients and were the only positive nodes in 70 patients (56.0%). Of the 218 patients with negative sentinel nodes, nonsentinel nodes were positive in 15 (false-negative rate, 10.7%; 15 of 140 patients). There were no significant differences in false-negative rate according to clinical patient and tumor characteristics, method of lymphatic mapping, or breast tumor response to chemotherapy.

Conclusion.—These results are comparable to those obtained from multicenter studies evaluating SNB before systemic therapy and suggest that the sentinel node concept is applicable following neoadjuvant chemotherapy.

► The accuracy of SNB after neoadjuvant chemotherapy has been unclear after a number of small single-institution studies reported wide variations in false-negative rates.[1-3] The report from the National Surgical Adjuvant Breast and Bowel Project, although not part of the protocol design of B-27, is the largest experience with SNB after neoadjuvant therapy and provides reassurance that the procedure is appropriate in this circumstance. The identification rate of 84.8% and the false-negative rate of 10.7% are consistent with multi-institutional studies of primary SNB reported during the same period (1996-2000). No relationship between tumor size, clinical nodal status at presentation, and extent of clinical or pathologic response to chemotherapy and the accuracy of SNB was observed. This study indicates that SNB is an accurate method of axillary staging in patients with operable breast cancer who receive preoperative chemotherapy.

M. Morrow, MD

References

1. Breslin TM, Cohen L, Sahin A, et al: Sentinel lymph node biopsy is accurate after neoadjuvant chemotherapy for breast cancer. *J Clin Oncol* 18:3480-3486, 2000.
2. Nason KS, Anderson BO, Byrd DR, et al: Increased false negative SNB rates after preoperative chemotherapy for invasive breast carcinoma. *Cancer* 89:2187-2194, 2000.
3. Haid A, Tausch C, Lang A, et al: Is sentinel lymph node biopsy reliable and indicated after preoperative chemotherapy in patients with breast carcinoma? *Cancer* 92:1080-1084, 2001.

22 Colorectal Cancer

Screening for the Lynch Syndrome (Hereditary Nonpolyposis Colorectal Cancer)

Hampel H, Frankel WL, Martin E, et al (Ohio State Univ, Columbus; Mount Carmel Health System, Columbus, Ohio; Riverside Methodist Hosp, Columbus, Ohio)

N Engl J Med 352:1851-1860, 2005 22–1

Background.—Germ-line mutations in the mismatch-repair genes *MLH1*, *MSH2*, *MSH6*, and *PMS2* lead to the development of the Lynch syndrome (hereditary nonpolyposis colorectal cancer), conferring a strong susceptibility to cancer. We assessed the frequency of such mutations in patients with colorectal cancer and examined strategies for molecular screening to identify patients with the syndrome.

Methods.—Patients with a new diagnosis of colorectal adenocarcinoma at the major hospitals in metropolitan Columbus, Ohio, were eligible for the study. Genotyping of the tumor for microsatellite instability was the primary screening method. Among patients whose screening results were positive for microsatellite instability, we searched for germ-line mutations in the *MLH1*, *MSH2*, *MSH6*, and *PMS2* genes with the use of immunohistochemical staining for mismatch-repair proteins, genomic sequencing, and deletion studies. Family members of carriers of the mutations were counseled, and those found to be at risk were offered mutation testing.

Results.—Of 1066 patients enrolled in the study, 208 (19.5 percent) had microsatellite instability, and 23 of these patients had a mutation causing the Lynch syndrome (2.2 percent). Among the 23 probands with the Lynch syndrome, 10 were more than 50 years of age and 5 did not meet the Amsterdam criteria or the Bethesda guidelines for the diagnosis of hereditary nonpolyposis colorectal cancer (including the use of age and family history to identify patients at high risk for the Lynch syndrome). Genotyping for microsatellite instability alone and immunohistochemical analysis alone each failed to identify two probands. In the families of 21 of the probands, 117 persons at risk were tested, and of these, 52 had Lynch syndrome mutations and 65 did not.

Conclusions.—Routine molecular screening of patients with colorectal adenocarcinoma for the Lynch syndrome identified mutations in patients and their family members that otherwise would not have been detected. These data suggest that the effectiveness of screening with immunohistochemical analysis of the mismatch-repair proteins would be similar to that of the more complex strategy of genotyping for microsatellite instability.

► This article demonstrates the feasibility of broad-scale screening for germline mutations. In addition, this trial demonstrates the limitations of known genetic mutations and screening.

P. J. Loehrer, Sr, MD

Use of Colonoscopy for Colorectal Cancer Screening: Evidence From the 2000 National Health Interview Survey

Subramanian S, Amonkar MM, Hunt TL (Research Triangle Inst Internatl, Waltham, Mass; Pfizer Corp, Peapack, NJ)
Cancer Epidemiol Biomarkers Prev 14:409-416, 2005 22–2

Background.—The use of colonoscopy as a primary screening tool for colorectal cancer is gaining momentum owing to several studies suggesting superior effectiveness and the recent, favorable decision by Medicare to cover all routine screening colonoscopies. This study documents the use of colonoscopy versus other tests to screen for colorectal cancer.

Materials and Methods.—Data from the 2000 National Health Interview Survey were analyzed. Fecal occult blood test (FOBT), sigmoidoscopy, and colonoscopy done for any reason and for routine screening only were analyzed for those ≥50 years without previously diagnosed colorectal cancer (n = 12,505).

Results.—The proportion of the total eligible population receiving any of the recommended tests for all possible reasons and for screening purposes only is 34.6% and 25.1%, respectively. For routine screening purposes, the test most commonly utilized was FOBT (55.6%) followed by colonoscopy (29.1%) and sigmoidoscopy (15.3%). When usage was assessed for all reasons, FOBT was still most commonly utilized (45.8%) followed by colonoscopy (38.7%) and sigmoidoscopy (15.5%). The elderly, non-White males and those with private insurance have a higher probability of receiving colonoscopy than FOBT. Several regional differences exist, including higher probability of undergoing sigmoidoscopy versus colonoscopy in the West.

Conclusions.—Only one fourth (upper limit one third) of the study population complied with colorectal cancer screening recommendations. Nearly one third of the routine screening tests done in 2000 were colonoscopies. This study provides baseline values that can be used to project future colonoscopy demand and identify potential supply barriers.

► Who undergoes colonoscopy in the United States? This article addresses this question and provides important baseline data. A major impact in the performance of colonoscopy has been changes in Medicare coverage in 2001. Despite its obvious limitations, fecal occult blood tests (OBT) is the most common screening tool, but the highest proportion of screening colonoscopies were those 80 years or older (37.7%), black (36.4%), and geographic location in South (33.8%). Overall, only 25% of those surveyed received any of the recommended screening tests. This article tells us how low the bar is currently set.

P. J. Loehrer, Sr, MD

Preoperative Versus Postoperative Chemoradiotherapy for Rectal Cancer

Sauer R, for the German Rectal Cancer Study Group (Univ of Erlangen, Germany; et al)

N Engl J Med 351:1731-1740, 2004 22–3

Background.—Postoperative chemoradiotherapy is the recommended standard therapy for patients with locally advanced rectal cancer. In recent years, encouraging results with preoperative radiotherapy have been reported. We compared preoperative chemoradiotherapy with postoperative chemoradiotherapy for locally advanced rectal cancer.

Methods.—We randomly assigned patients with clinical stage T3 or T4 or node-positive disease to receive either preoperative or postoperative chemoradiotherapy. The preoperative treatment consisted of 5040 cGy delivered in fractions of 180 cGy per day, five days per week, and fluorouracil, given in a 120-hour continuous intravenous infusion at a dose of 1000 mg per square meter of body-surface area per day during the first and fifth weeks of radiotherapy. Surgery was performed six weeks after the completion of chemoradiotherapy. One month after surgery, four five-day cycles of fluorouracil (500 mg per square meter per day) were given. Chemoradiotherapy was identical in the postoperative-treatment group, except for the delivery of a boost of 540 cGy. The primary end point was overall survival.

Results.—Four hundred twenty-one patients were randomly assigned to receive preoperative chemoradiotherapy and 402 patients to receive postoperative chemoradiotherapy. The overall five-year survival rates were 76 percent and 74 percent, respectively ($P=0.80$). The five-year cumulative incidence of local relapse was 6 percent for patients assigned to preoperative chemoradiotherapy and 13 percent in the postoperative-treatment group ($P=0.006$). Grade 3 or 4 acute toxic effects occurred in 27 percent of the patients in the preoperative-treatment group, as compared with 40 percent of the patients in the postoperative-treatment group ($P=0.001$); the corresponding rates of long-term toxic effects were 14 percent and 24 percent, respectively ($P=0.01$).

Conclusions.—Preoperative chemoradiotherapy, as compared with postoperative chemoradiotherapy, improved local control and was associated with reduced toxicity but did not improve overall survival.

▶ These investigators from Germany and Austria looked at locally advanced rectal cancer and compared preoperative chemoradiation therapy to postoperative chemoradiation therapy. The doses were reasonable, and more than 800 patients were on the study. Preoperative chemoradiotherapy had approximately half of the local recurrence rate that was seen in the postoperative part. The overall survival rates were approximately 75% in both arms, so there was no significant difference. This is a good figure, considering that approximately two thirds of the patients were T3 and more than half the patients were node positive.

There are some who would probably argue that improving local control does not make any difference if there is no improvement in survival rate. Most of such individuals have probably never cared for patients with recurrent rectal carcinoma and probably never dealt with the problem of local recurrence, which, in this particular disease, is a particularly miserable problem to manage, frequently because of the intractable pelvic pain that is extremely difficult to control.

I think this study has been well done, and I believe the questions have been answered. The problem will still be getting surgeons to agree to preoperative treatment, which is not always easy to achieve in the United States.

E. Glatstein, MD

American Society of Clinical Oncology Recommendations on Adjuvant Chemotherapy for Stage II Colon Cancer

Benson AB III, Schrag D, Somerfield MR, et al (American Society of Clinical Oncology, Alexandria, Va)

J Clin Oncol 22:3408-3419, 2004 22–4

Purpose.—To address whether all medically fit patients with curatively resected stage II colon cancer should be offered adjuvant chemotherapy as part of routine clinical practice, to identify patients with poor prognosis characteristics, and to describe strategies for oncologists to use to discuss adjuvant chemotherapy in practice.

Methods.—An American Society of Clinical Oncology Panel, in collaboration with the Cancer Care Ontario Practice Guideline Initiative, reviewed pertinent information from the literature through May 2003.

Results.—A literature-based meta-analysis found no evidence of a statistically significant survival benefit of adjuvant chemotherapy for stage II patients.

Recommendations.—The routine use of adjuvant chemotherapy for medically fit patients with stage II colon cancer is not recommended. However, there are populations of patients with stage II disease that could be considered for adjuvant therapy, including patients with inadequately sampled nodes, T4 lesions, perforation, or poorly differentiated histology.

Conclusion.—Direct evidence from randomized controlled trials does not support the routine use of adjuvant chemotherapy for patients with stage II colon cancer. Patients and oncologists who accept the relative benefit in stage III disease as adequate indirect evidence of benefit for stage II disease are justified in considering the use of adjuvant chemotherapy, particularly for those patients with high-risk stage II disease. The ultimate clinical decision should be based on discussions with the patient about the nature of the evidence supporting treatment, the anticipated morbidity of treatment, the presence of high-risk prognostic features on individual prognosis, and patient preferences. Patients with stage II disease should be encouraged to participate in randomized trials.

► As there has been no trial conducted of sufficient power to clarify the role of adjuvant therapy for stage II colon cancer patients, this meta-analysis is of importance. Whereas fluoropyrimidine-based adjuvant therapy has a clear impact on stage III disease, this has not been clearly demonstrated in stage II disease. However, some subgroups deserve special consideration. This includes those patients with inadequate lymph node sampling. Other high-risk features, such as T4 lesions, perforation, aneuploidy may be associated with a poorer prognosis, but it remains unclear whether adjuvant therapy benefits this patient population. To truly detect clear benefit in a good-risk population would take more patients than has ever been attempted to be accrued. Talking points for health care providers to patients are well outlined in this article.

P. J. Loehrer, Sr, MD

Lymph Node Evaluation in Colorectal Cancer Patients: A Population-Based Study

Baxter NN, Virnig DJ, Rothenberger DA, et al (Univ of Minnesota, Minneapolis; Univ of Michigan, Ann Arbor)

J Natl Cancer Inst 97:219-225, 2005 22–5

Background.—Adequate lymph node evaluation is required for proper staging of colorectal cancer, and the number of lymph nodes examined is associated with survival. According to current guidelines, the recommended minimum number of lymph nodes examined to ensure adequate sampling is 12. We used data from the National Cancer Institute's Surveillance, Epidemiology, and End Results program to determine the proportion of colorectal cancer patients in the United States who receive adequate lymph node evaluation.

Methods.—For 116,995 adults with colorectal adenocarcinoma, diagnosed from 1988 through 2001, who underwent radical surgery and did not receive neoadjuvant radiation, we evaluated the number of lymph nodes, the likelihood of receiving adequate lymph node evaluation (i.e., at least 12 lymph nodes examined), and the influence of tumor and patient factors on lymph node evaluation. All statistical tests were two-sided.

Results.—Among all patients, the median number of lymph nodes examined was nine. Only 37% of all patients received adequate lymph node evaluation. The proportion of patients receiving adequate lymph node evaluation increased from 32% in 1988 to 44% in 2001 (P(trend)<.001, Cochran-Armitage test) (Fig 2). Advanced tumor stage was statistically significantly associated with adequate lymph node evaluation (odds ratio [OR] of receiving adequate lymph node evaluation=2.27, 95% confidence interval [CI] = 2.18 to 2.35). Older patients (≥71 years, OR = 0.45, 95% CI =

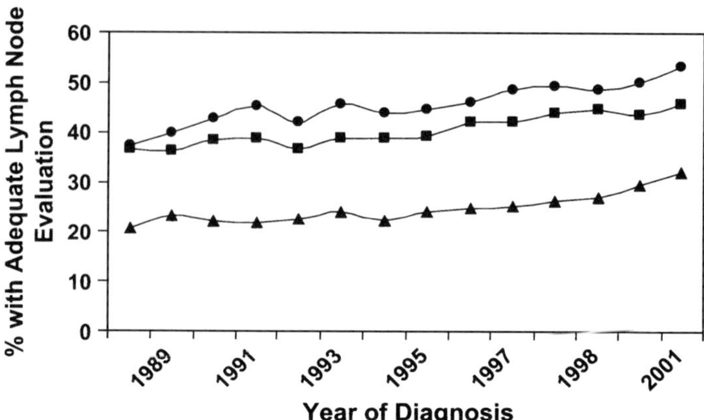

FIGURE 2.—Percentage of patients with adequate lymph node evaluation (ie, at least 12 lymph nodes evaluated) by stage of colorectal cancer disease over time. *Solid triangles* = percentage of patients with stage I disease who had adequate lymph node evaluation; *solid squares* = percentage of patients with stage II disease who had adequate lymph node evaluation; *solid circles* = percentage of patients with stage III disease who had adequate lymph node evaluation. (Courtesy of Baxter NN, Virnig DJ, Rothenberger DA, et al: Lymph node evaluation in colorectal cancer patients: A population-based study. *J Natl Cancer Inst* 97:219-225, 2005. By permission of Oxford University Press.)

0.44 to 0.47) were less likely to receive adequate lymph node evaluation than younger patients, and those with left-sided (OR = 0.45, 95% CI = 0.44 to 0.47) or rectal (OR = 0.52, 95% CI = 0.50 to 0.54) cancers were less likely to receive adequate lymph node evaluation than patients with right-sided cancers. In all analyses, geographic location was an important predictor of adequate lymph node evaluation, which ranged from 33% to 53%, depending on geographic location.

Conclusions.—In 2001, the majority of patients with colorectal cancer still received inadequate lymph node evaluation. The association of demographic variables, particularly patient age and geographic location, with adequate lymph node evaluation indicates that local surgical and pathology practice patterns may affect adequacy of lymph node evaluation.

► The progression-free and overall survival of colorectal cancer (CRC) patients with lymph node–negative (stage II) disease is significantly better than that of patients with lymph node–positive (stage III) disease. Yet, those patients with fewer lymph nodes sampled fare less well in both stage II and III disease based on both the International Union Against Cancer and the American Joint Committee on Cancer. The recommended minimum number of lymph nodes to ensure adequate staging is 12.[1,2] An example of the impact of the sample has been made by Swanson et al,[3] who found the 5-year survival of stage II CRC was 64% with samples of 1 or 2 lymph nodes, whereas it jumped to 86% when 24 or more lymph nodes were examined. This article by Baxter et al outlines the difference in lymph node sampling from the Surveillance, Epidemiology, and End Results (SEER) Database. In large part, the number of lymph nodes sampled falls into the laps of the pathologists and the technicians who initially prepare the surgical specimens. Sometimes, dissections take a bit more time, but as shown in Fig 2, some trends for improvement are seen, but still more than half of patients with CRC are inadequately staged.

P. J. Loehrer, Sr, MD

References

1. Sobin LH, Green FL: TNM classification: Clarification of number of regional lymph nodes for pNo. *Cancer* 92:452, 2001.
2. Wittekind CH, Wagner G: Colon and rectum, in Wittekind CH, Wagner G (eds): *TNM-Classification of Malignant Tumors*. New York, Springer, 1997, pp 64-67.
3. Swanson RS, Compton CC, Stewart AK, et al: The prognosis of T3N0 colon cancer is dependent on the number of lymph nodes examined. *Ann Surg Oncol* 10:65-71, 2003.

23 Prostate Cancer

Immediate Versus Deferred Hormonal Treatment for Patients With Prostate Cancer Who Are Not Suitable for Curative Local Treatment: Results of the Randomized Trial SAKK 08/88

Studer UE, Hauri D, Hanselmann S, et al (Swiss Group for Clinical Cancer Research, Bern, Switzerland; Univ of Bern, Switzerland)

J Clin Oncol 22:4109-4118, 2004 23–1

Purpose.—To determine if immediate hormonal therapy is advantageous compared with deferred treatment in newly diagnosed asymptomatic prostate cancer patients who, for any reason, were not candidates for curative local treatment.

Patients and Methods.—Between February 1988 and February 1992, 197 patients with a median age of 76 years (range, 56 to 86 years) were randomly assigned to receive either immediate or deferred orchiectomy on symptomatic progression. The two groups did not differ significantly in clinical or laboratory parameters; 67% had T3-4 tumors and 20% had lymph node metastases. Patient accrual was stopped prematurely because of a similar competing trial. Therefore, observation time was prolonged to achieve the desired number of events and statistical power.

Results.—Deferred orchiectomy was necessary in 58% of the patients. Median time to disease progression was 2.8 years less than for patients with immediate orchiectomy. However, overall pain-free time from random assignment to symptomatic progression after immediate or deferred orchiectomy, and performance status, were identical in both groups. Cancer-specific survival tended to be longer in the immediate group ($P = .09$) but there was no difference in overall survival between the two groups ($P = .96$). The median hemoglobin value decreased significantly after immediate orchiectomy ($P < .001$).

Conclusion.—For elderly, asymptomatic patients not undergoing curative local treatment, we were unable to show any major advantage of immediate compared with deferred hormonal treatment regarding quality of life or overall survival in our limited number of patients. Disabling complications were prevented in the deferred-treatment arm by careful follow-up; 42% of these patients never required any tumor-specific treatment.

► Prostate cancer may be an incidental finding, especially in elderly patients. Most data on timing of hormonal therapy for patients diagnosed with prostate cancer have been retrospective. Indeed, in the articles, 42% of patients selected randomly to the different treatment arms never received therapy for prostate cancer. This trial by Studer et al was stopped before the planned total accrual, but the follow-up and number of events still allowed a detection of a 15% difference in the 5-year survival with 88% power in which no obvious disease was noted. A trend for cancer specific survival ($P = .09$) was seen, but was of uncertain significance. This is another trial that supports the observation that the biology of the tumor has the biggest impact on survival.

P. J. Loehrer, Sr, MD

Operating Characteristics of Prostate-Specific Antigen in Men With an Initial PSA Level of 3.0 ng/mL or Lower

Thompson IM, Ankerst DP, Chi C, et al (Univ of Texas, San Antonio; Fred Hutchinson Cancer Research Ctr, Seattle; Univ of Colorado, Denver; et al)

JAMA 294:66-70, 2005 23–2

Context.—Three fourths of US men older than 50 years have been screened with prostate-specific antigen (PSA) for prostate cancer.

Objective.—To estimate the receiver operating characteristic (ROC) curve for PSA.

Design, Setting, and Participants.—Calculation of PSA ROC curves in the placebo group of the Prostate Cancer Prevention Trial, a randomized, prospective study conducted from 1993 to 2003 at 221 US centers. Participants were 18 882 healthy men aged 55 years or older without prostate cancer and with PSA levels less than or equal to 3.0 ng/mL and normal digital rectal examination results, followed up for 7 years with annual PSA measurement and digital rectal examination. If PSA level exceeded 4.0 ng/mL or rectal examination result was abnormal, a prostate biopsy was recommended. After 7 years of study participation, an end-of-study prostate biopsy was recommended in all cancer-free men.

Main Outcome Measures.—Operating characteristics of PSA for prostate cancer detection, including sensitivity, specificity, and ROC curve.

Results.—Of 8575 men in the placebo group with at least 1 PSA measurement and digital rectal examination in the same year, 5587 (65.2%) had had at least 1 biopsy; of these, 1225 (21.9%) were diagnosed with prostate cancer. Of 1213 cancers with Gleason grade recorded, 250 (20.6%) were Gleason grade 7 or greater and 57 (4.7%) were Gleason grade 8 or greater. The areas under the ROC curve (AUC) for PSA to discriminate any prostate cancer vs no cancer, Gleason grade 7 or greater cancer vs no or lower-grade cancer, and Gleason grade 8 or greater cancer vs no or lower-grade cancer were 0.678 (95% confidence interval [CI], 0.666-0.689), 0.782 (95% CI, 0.748-0.816), and 0.827 (95% CI, 0.761-0.893), respectively (all P values <.001 for AUC vs 50%). For detecting any prostate cancer, PSA cutoff values of 1.1, 2.1, 3.1, and 4.1 ng/mL yielded sensitivities of 83.4%, 52.6%, 32.2%, and 20.5%, and specificities of 38.9%, 72.5%, 86.7%, and 93.8%, respectively. Age-stratified analyses showed slightly better performance of PSA in men younger than 70 years vs those 70 years or older with AUC values of 0.699 (SD, 0.013) vs 0.663 (SD, 0.013) (P=.03).

Conclusion.—There is no cutpoint of PSA with simultaneous high sensitivity and high specificity for monitoring healthy men for prostate cancer, but rather a continuum of prostate cancer risk at all values of PSA.

► Prostate cancer remains 1 of the most common causes of malignancies in men. One of the unique aspects of this disease is that many men known to harbor prostate cancer will not die of the disease but rather of comorbid illnesses. This has clouded the impact of prostate cancer screening upon mortality end points. Having said this, PSA has been embraced by many as a serologic screening tool. Prostate biopsy (the definitive diagnostic tool) has not been routinely recommended in patients with PSA levels less than 4.0 ng/mL. This large prospective trial demonstrates that a specific PSA level that predicted low risk of disease could not be defined. Unfortunately, few African Americans were included in this trial. This article should shake the urology foundation. Does this mean that we should lower the threshold for biopsy? The answer in the words of the authors is: "While lowering the PSA threshold is likely to increase the detection of such aggressive cancers at an earlier stage, the unavoidable tradeoff is the increased detection of biologically inconsequential cancers." The history of prostate cancer varies from an indolent to an aggressive course. This should represent a call to arms that a better marker for disease is clearly needed.

P. J. Loehrer, Sr, MD

Radical Prostatectomy Versus Watchful Waiting in Early Prostate Cancer

Bill-Axelson A, for the Scandinavian Prostate Cancer Group Study No. 4 (Univ Hosp, Uppsala, Sweden; Univ of Helsinki; Örebro Univ, Sweden; et al)

N Engl J Med 352:1977-1984, 2005 23–3

Background.—In 2002, we reported the initial results of a trial comparing radical prostatectomy with watchful waiting in the management of early prostate cancer. After three more years of follow-up, we report estimated 10-year results.

Methods.—From October 1989 through February 1999, 695 men with early prostate cancer (mean age, 64.7 years) were randomly assigned to radical prostatectomy (347 men) or watchful waiting (348 men). The follow-up was complete through 2003, with blinded evaluation of the causes of death. The primary end point was death due to prostate cancer; the secondary end points were death from any cause, metastasis, and local progression.

Results.—During a median of 8.2 years of follow-up, 83 men in the surgery group and 106 men in the watchful-waiting group died (P=0.04). In 30 of the 347 men assigned to surgery (8.6 percent) and 50 of the 348 men assigned to watchful waiting (14.4 percent), death was due to prostate cancer. The difference in the cumulative incidence of death due to prostate cancer increased from 2.0 percentage points after 5 years to 5.3 percentage points after 10 years, for a relative risk of 0.56 (95 percent confidence interval, 0.36 to 0.88; P=0.01 by Gray's test). For distant metastasis, the corresponding increase was from 1.7 to 10.2 percentage points, for a relative risk in the surgery group of 0.60 (95 percent confidence interval, 0.42 to 0.86; P=0.004 by Gray's test), and for local progression, the increase was from 19.1 to 25.1 percentage points, for a relative risk of 0.33 (95 percent confidence interval, 0.25 to 0.44; P<0.001 by Gray's test).

Conclusions.—Radical prostatectomy reduces disease-specific mortality, overall mortality, and the risks of metastasis and local progression. The absolute reduction in the risk of death after 10 years is small, but the reductions in the risks of metastasis and local tumor progression are substantial.

► The frequent identification of asymptomatic prostate carcinoma at autopsy has led to debate regarding the merits of the routine use of radical prostatectomy. This prospective randomized trial directly compared the outcomes of radical prostatectomy and watchful waiting. The trial was initially reported after a mean follow-up of 6.2 years and demonstrated a 2% reduction in the risk of death due to prostate cancer and a 1.7% reduction in distant metastases with surgery. With additional follow-up, the absolute benefit in disease-specific mortality has increased from 2% to 5.3%, and the reduction in distant metastases is now 10.2%. A significant reduction in death from all causes is now observed in the surgery group. In addition, laminectomy and the use of hormone treatment were significantly less common ($P < .01$ and $P = .04$, respectively) in the surgery groups as was local disease progression. In exploratory analyses, these benefits did not vary according to prostate-specific antigen level at diagnosis or Gleason score, but the benefit of surgery appeared to be most evident in men younger than 65 years at diagnosis. Since the reduction in distant metastases has increased over time, it is likely that the survival benefits of surgery will increase further. Although surgery is associated with well-recognized side effects such as impotence and incontinence, the study indicates clear benefits for surgery over observation.

M. Morrow, MD

Five-Year Outcomes After Prostatectomy or Radiotherapy for Prostate Cancer: The Prostate Cancer Outcomes Study

Potosky AL, Davis WW, Hoffman RM, et al (Natl Cancer Inst, Bethesda, Md; New Mexico VA Health Care System, Albuquerque, NM; Fred Hutchinson Cancer Research Ctr, Seattle; et al)

J Natl Cancer Inst 96:1358-1367, 2004 23–4

Background.—Men treated for clinically localized prostate cancer with either radical prostatectomy or external beam radiotherapy usually survive many years with the side effects of these treatments. We present treatment-specific quality-of-life outcomes for prostate cancer patients 5 years after initial diagnosis.

TABLE 1.—Comparison of 5-year PCOS Survey Responders on Individual Urinary, Bowel, and Sexual Domain Items*

Domain	RP† (n = 901)	EBRT† (n = 286)	OR (95% CI)
Urinary			
No control or frequent leaks vs. total control or occasional leaks	14.4 (15.3)	4.9 (4.1)	4.4 (2.2 to 8.6)
Leaks ≥2 times per day‡	15.6 (16.1)	4.1 (3.6)	5.3 (2.6 to 10.8)
Wears any pads to stay dry‡	28.6 (28.6)	4.2 (4.2)	9.4 (4.7 to 18.9)
Frequent urination more than half the time‡	10.6 (10.1)	8.9 (9.3)	1.1 (0.6 to 1.9)
Bothered by dripping or leaking urine§	13.9 (14.3)	3.0 (2.6)	6.5 (2.7 to 15.6)
Bowel‖			
Diarrhea‡	23.3 (23.9)	28.8 (26.7)	0.84 (0.55 to 1.26)
Painful bowel movements‡	10.4 (11.5)	12.2 (9.4)	1.31 (0.73 to 2.35)
Bowel urgency‡	17.7 (19.3)	33.4 (28.5)	0.56 (0.36 to 0.87)
Wetness in rectal area‡	13.8 (14.8)	20.6 (18.3)	0.75 (0.47 to 1.20)
Painful hemorrhoids‡	11.0 (10.2)	15.7 (19.6)	0.43 (0.25 to 0.74)
Bothered by frequent bowel movement to pain, or urgency§	4.3 (4.8)	5.0 (4.0)	1.23 (0.52 to 2.89)
Sexual			
No/little vs. some/a lot of interest in sexual activity	46.5 (48.9)	55.2 (47.4)	1.1 (0.73 to 1.6)
No sexual activity vs. any sexual activity	48.9 (50.7)	51.3 (43.9)	1.4 (0.93 to 2.0)
Erection insufficient for intercourse‡	76.9 (79.3)	73.1 (63.5)	2.5 (1.6 to 3.8)
Bothered by sexual dysfunction§	47.4 (46.7)	42.0 (44.6)	1.1 (0.75 to 1.6)

*Model-based odds ratios (with external beam radiotherapy patients as referent group) and adjusted percentages are from separate logistic regression models (for each row) each adjusting for treatment propensity score, age at diagnosis, baseline function, race/ethnicity, comorbidity, and educational level. All estimates were weighted to total eligible cases.

†Values in columns are unadjusted percentages (adjusted percentages).

‡Percentages and odds ratio for yes versus no/none.

§For bother items, percentages refer to patients reporting a large or moderate problem versus a small or no problem.

‖For the five bowel function items, percentages refer to patients reporting having the problem every day or some days versus rarely or never.

Abbreviations: PCOS, Prostate Cancer Outcomes Study; *RP*, radical prostatectomy; *EBRT*, external beam radiotherapy; *OR*, odds ratio; *CI*, confidence interval.

(Courtesy of Potosky AL, Davis WW, Hoffman RM, et al: Five-year outcomes after prostatectomy or radiotherapy for prostate cancer: The prostate cancer outcomes study. *J Natl Cancer Inst* 96:1358-1367, 2004, by permission of Oxford University Press.)

Methods.—The cohort consisted of men aged 55-74 years who were newly diagnosed with clinically localized prostate cancer in 1994-1995 and were treated with radical prostatectomy (n = 901) or external beam radiotherapy (n = 286). We used clinical and quality-of-life data previously collected at the time of diagnosis (i.e., baseline) and at the 2-year follow-up and data newly collected at 5 years after diagnosis to compare urinary, bowel, and sexual function and to examine temporal changes in those functions. Odds ratios (ORs) and adjusted percentages were calculated by logistic regression. All statistical tests were two-sided.

Results.—At 5 years after diagnosis, overall sexual function declined in both groups to approximately the same level. However, at 5 years after diagnosis, erectile dysfunction was more prevalent in the radical prostatectomy group than in the external beam radiotherapy group (79.3% versus 63.5%; OR = 2.5, 95% confidence interval [CI] = 1.6 to 3.8). Approximately 14%-16% of radical prostatectomy and 4% of external beam radiotherapy patients were incontinent at 5 years (OR = 4.4, 95% CI = 2.2 to

8.6). Bowel urgency and painful hemorrhoids were more common in the external beam radiotherapy group than in the radical prostatectomy group. All of these differences remained statistically significant after adjustment for confounders and for differences between treatment groups in some baseline characteristics.

Conclusions.—At 5 years after diagnosis, men treated with radical prostatectomy for localized prostate cancer continue to experience worse urinary incontinence than men treated with external beam radiotherapy. However, the two treatment groups were more similar to each other with respect to overall sexual function, mostly because of a continuing decline in erectile function among the external beam radiotherapy patients between years 2 and 5 (Table 1).

▶ The controversy over the management of clinically localized prostate cancer continues. This study represents what is called the Prostate Cancer Outcomes Study, which tried to assess the long-term health-related quality of life outcomes for patients diagnosed and treated with prostate cancer in the community-based setting in 1994 and 1995. The patients were not randomized to their respective treatments, and for the early stage patients, over 900 received radical prostatectomy versus 286 who received external-beam radiation therapy. As evidence of the lack of comparability, Table 4 in the original article shows a statistically significant younger age group for the prostatectomy patients, a more favorable PSA, and a trend toward more favorable Gleason scores. In terms of quality of life, the men treated with radical prostatectomy had worse problems with urinary incontinence than men treated with external beam. The potency issues were quite comparable between the 2 groups.

The controversy over treatment for early stage prostate cancer will continue until someone really is able to carry out a well-designed clinical study in which the treatment itself is the variable that is randomized. The only other possibility to resolve this controversy would be the development of a third form of effective, curative treatment that did not have the problems associated with either of these other 2 modalities.

E. Glatstein, MD

▶ This article emphasizes the significant long-term side effects associated with both radical prostatectomy and external beam radiotherapy for the treatment of localized prostate cancer. Differences in urinary and sexual dysfunction are present between treatments, and this information may be useful to men attempting to make a treatment choice. The 5-year follow-up in this study also documents a significant decline in sexual functioning between years 2 and 5 after treatment in men receiving external beam radiotherapy. Although techniques of surgery and radiotherapy have improved since the treatment of this patient sample in 1994-1995, this study still provides valuable information on the incidence and duration of side effects of local therapy for prostate cancer.

M. Morrow, MD

24 Myeloid Suppressor Cell Tumors

Secondary Surgical Cytoreduction for Advanced Ovarian Carcinoma
Rose PG, for the Gynecologic Oncology Group (Case Western Reserve Univ, Cleveland, Ohio; et al)
N Engl J Med 351:2489-2497, 2004 24–1

Background.—We evaluated the effect of adding secondary cytoreductive surgery to postoperative chemotherapy on progression-free survival and overall survival among patients who had advanced ovarian cancer and residual tumor exceeding 1 cm in diameter after primary surgery.

Methods.—Women were enrolled within six weeks after primary surgery. If, after three cycles of postoperative paclitaxel plus cisplatin, a patient had no evidence of progressive disease, she was randomly assigned to undergo secondary cytoreductive surgery followed by three more cycles of chemotherapy or three more cycles of chemotherapy alone.

Results.—We enrolled 550 women. After completing three cycles of postoperative chemotherapy, 216 eligible patients were randomly assigned to receive secondary surgical cytoreduction followed by chemotherapy and 208 to receive chemotherapy alone. Surgery was declined by or medically contraindicated in 15 patients who were assigned to secondary surgery (7 percent). As of March 2003, 296 patients had died and 82 had progressive disease. The likelihood of progression-free survival in the group assigned to secondary surgery plus chemotherapy, as compared with the chemotherapy-alone group, was 1.07 (95 percent confidence interval, 0.87 to 1.31; P=054), and the relative risk of death was 0.99 (95 percent confidence interval, 0.79 to 1.24; P=0.92).

Conclusions.—For patients with advanced ovarian carcinoma in whom primary cytoreductive surgery was considered to be maximal, the addition of secondary cytoreductive surgery to postoperative chemotherapy with paclitaxel plus cisplatin does not improve progression-free survival or overall survival.

► The typical patient with ovarian cancer is diagnosed at the time of laparotomy and undergoes a maximum debulking of primary and metastatic tumor throughout the abdomen followed by postoperative chemotherapy. However, efforts to improve survival among patients with stage III ovarian cancer have had very limited success. These investigators from the Gynecologic Oncology Group randomized patients to receive a second surgical debulking after chemotherapy in an effort to minimize residual tumor burden a second time. After 3 cycles of Taxol, then Cisplatin, patients were randomized and assigned to undergo a second debulking surgery followed by 3 more cycles of chemotherapy versus continuation of chemotherapy alone. Obviously, the patients could not have had progressive disease in between their surgeries. With 550 patients, 216 were randomly assigned to receive a second surgical debulking followed by more chemotherapy and another 218 were randomized to receive continuing Taxol and Cisplatin. The authors conclude that the second surgical procedure showed no advantage over the continuation of chemotherapy.

This is an important study because it sheds some light on the importance of debulking surgery. The point is that once the surgical debulking has been done, it is up to the drugs at that point. More surgery is not better.

E. Glatstein, MD

Mortality in Overweight and Underweight Children With Acute Myeloid Leukemia

Lange BJ, Gerbing RB, Feusner J, et al (Children's Hosp of Philadelphia; Children's Oncology Group, Arcadia, Calif; Children's Hosp of Oakland, Calif; et al)

JAMA 293:203-211, 2005 24–2

Context.—Current treatment for acute myeloid leukemia (AML) in children cures about half the patients. Of the other half, most succumb to leukemia, but 5% to 15% die of treatment-related complications. Overweight children with AML seem to experience excess life-threatening and fatal toxicity. Nothing is known about how weight affects outcomes in pediatric AML.

Objective.—To compare survival rates in children with AML who at diagnosis are underweight (body mass index [BMI] ≤10th percentile), overweight (BMI ≥95th percentile), or middleweight (BMI = 11th-94th percentiles).

Design, Setting, and Participants.—Retrospective review of BMI and survival in 768 children and young adults aged 1 to 20 years enrolled in Children's Cancer Group-2961, an international cooperative group phase 3 trial for previously untreated AML conducted August 30, 1996, through December 4, 2002. Data were collected through January 9, 2004, with a median follow-up of 31 months (range, 0-78 months).

Main Outcome Measures.—Hazard ratios (HRs) for survival and treatment-related mortality.

Results.—Eighty-four of 768 patients (10.9%) were underweight and 114 (14.8%) were overweight. After adjustment for potentially confounding variables of age, race, leukocyte count, cytogenetics, and bone marrow transplantation, compared with middleweight patients, underweight patients were less likely to survive (HR, 1.85; 95% confidence interval [CI],

1.19-2.87; $P = .006$) and more likely to experience treatment-related mortality (HR, 2.66; 95% CI, 1.38-5.11; $P = .003$). Similarly, overweight patients were less likely to survive (HR, 1.88; 95% CI, 1.25-2.83; $P = .002$) and more likely to have treatment-related mortality (HR, 3.49; 95% CI, 1.99-6.10; $P<.001$) than middleweight patients. Infections incurred during the first 2 courses of chemotherapy caused most treatment-related deaths.

Conclusion.—Treatment-related complications significantly reduce survival in overweight and underweight children with AML.

► This is an interesting study that looks at the impact of body mass index upon survival and toxicity in children treated for AML. Little information exists regarding the pharmacology of chemotherapy in underweight patients, but malnutrition can impair the immune system and may also affect drug absorption. One might expect a decreased cure rate and less toxicity for overweight patients, but surprisingly the opposite was found. These differences in outcome are at least as good as what prospective treatment trials have demonstrated with novel treatments. Additional studies looking at pharmacokinetic, pharmacodynamics, and pharmacogenomics are clearly needed.

P. J. Loehrer, Sr, MD

► Treatment-related toxicity remains a significant problem in the treatment of patients with AML. Several previous reports have suggested that such toxicity may be greater in both malnourished and in overweight individuals. The report by Lange et al examines the outcome for underweight and overweight pediatric patients with newly diagnosed AML treated in the CCG-2961 study. Their findings show in a multivariate analysis that both underweight and overweight patients have a significantly worse outcome that is associated with increased treatment-related mortality. Both groups of patients were more likely to die before or during their first remission, with infections being the most common event. Of note is that overweight patients experienced more abdominal pain, hypertension, pulmonary problems, and coagulopathy. These are important findings but beg the question as to what can be done to prevent these complications. The risk of underdosing patients is a significant concern when curing AML remains a major challenge. In addition, improving the nutritional status or the obesity in newly diagnosed patients before initiating treatment is unlikely to be practical. Certainly, more knowledge concerning the pharmacokinetics of the critical induction chemotherapeutic agents in these different groups of patients is needed and provides the most rational solution to correcting the reported increased, treatment-related mortality. Such data are, unfortunately, nearly nonexistent, highlighting the timeliness of this challenge.

R. J. Arceci, MD, PhD

Molecular Responses in Patients With Chronic Myelogenous Leukemia in Chronic Phase Treated With Imatinib Mesylate

Cortes J, Talpaz M, O'Brien S, et al (Univ of Texas MD Anderson Cancer Ctr, Houston)

Clin Cancer Res 11:3425-3432, 2005 24–3

Purpose.—To determine the clinical significance of molecular response and relapse among patients with chronic myelogenous leukemia (CML) treated with imatinib.

Experimental Design.—We analyzed the results of quantitative PCR in 280 patients with CML in chronic phase who achieved complete cytogenetic remission with imatinib (117 after IFN-α failure and 163 previously untreated). Median follow-up was 31 months (range, 3-52 months).

Results.—Median BCR-ABL/ABL ratio before the start of therapy was 3944 (range, 0.252-170.53). A major molecular response (BCR-ABL/ABL ratio <0.05%) was achieved in 174 (62%), and transcripts became undetectable (complete molecular response) in 95 (34%). By multivariate analysis, only treatment with high-dose imatinib ($P = 0.02$) was associated with achievement of a major molecular response. Nine of 166 (5%) patients who achieved a major molecular response lost their cytogenetic remission, compared with 25 of 68 (37%) among those who did not achieve this response ($P < 0.0001$). Patients achieving a major molecular response 12 months after the start of therapy had significantly better complete cytogenetic remission duration than others. A >1-log reduction in transcript levels after 3 months of therapy predicted for an improved probability of achieving a major molecular response at 24 months. Increasing levels of BCR-ABL transcripts predicted for a loss of cytogenetic remission only among patients who did not achieve a major molecular response.

Conclusions.—Achieving a major molecular response, particularly within the first year of therapy, is predictive of a durable cytogenetic remission and may be the future goal of therapy in CML.

► The use of new standard therapies is constantly undergoing further revision and modification. The use of imatinib for the targeted treatment of CML is one such relatively new therapy whose use is being refined. In CML, the gold standard for clinical benefit is the development of molecular complete responses based on the PCR analysis for the BCR-ABL transcript. While greater than 90% of patients achieve a complete hematologic response and approximately 50% achieve a complete or major cytogenetic response, the achievement of molecular responses and the predictive role these responses play in long-term outcome have not previously been defined. These authors followed 280 patients with chronic-phase CML who achieved a complete cytogenetic response (CCR) with imatinib with quantitative PCR analysis for the BCR-ABL transcript. A major molecular response was achieved in 62% of the CCR patients studied. This compared to only about a third of patients who reach this goal without achieving CCR. Overall, 95% of the patients who achieved major molecular responses maintained their cytogenetic responses compared with only 63% of those who did not reach the level of a major molecular response. Based on multivariate analysis, the only variable associated with this outcome was the use of high-dose imatinib, suggesting that more intensive therapy, especially in the first year, may be critical to inducing these types of long-term benefits. This study provides some interesting insight into the ability to define the optimal status that one wishes to achieve with CML targeted therapy. The ability to induce a major molecular response within the first year is clearly critical for long-term benefit and for all patients may be the standard that needs to be achieved with combinations of targeted and other CML therapy (whether combinations with chemotherapy such as low-dose cytosine arabinoside or with interferon-α).

M. S. Gordon, MD

25 Cancer Prevention

Vitamin E in the Primary Prevention of Cardiovascular Disease and Cancer: The Women's Health Study: A Randomized Controlled Trial

Lee I-M, Cook NR, Gaziano JM, et al (Harvard Med School, Boston; Univ of Miami, Fla)

JAMA 294:56-65, 2005 25–1

Context.—Basic research provides plausible mechanisms and observational studies suggest that apparently healthy persons, who self-select for high intakes of vitamin E through diet or supplements, have decreased risks of cardiovascular disease and cancer. Randomized trials do not generally support benefits of vitamin E, but there are few trials of long duration among initially healthy persons.

Objective.—To test whether vitamin E supplementation decreases risks of cardiovascular disease and cancer among healthy women.

Design, Setting, and Participants.—In the Women's Health Study conducted between 1992 and 2004, 39 876 apparently healthy US women aged at least 45 years were randomly assigned to receive vitamin E or placebo and aspirin or placebo, using a 2 × 2 factorial design, and were followed up for an average of 10.1 years.

Intervention.—Administration of 600 IU of natural-source vitamin E on alternate days.

Main Outcome Measures.—Primary outcomes were a composite end point of first major cardiovascular event (nonfatal myocardial infarction, nonfatal stroke, or cardiovascular death) and total invasive cancer.

Results.—During follow-up, there were 482 major cardiovascular events in the vitamin E group and 517 in the placebo group, a nonsignificant 7% risk reduction (relative risk [RR], 0.93; 95% confidence interval [CI], 0.82-1.05; $P = .26$). There were no significant effects on the incidences of myocardial infarction (RR, 1.01; 95% CI, 0.82-1.23; $P = .96$) or stroke (RR, 0.98; 95% CI, 0.82-1.17; $P = .82$), as well as ischemic or hemorrhagic stroke. For cardiovascular death, there was a significant 24% reduction (RR, 0.76; 95% CI, 0.59-0.98; $P = .03$). There was no significant effect on the incidences of total cancer (1437 cases in the vitamin E group and 1428 in the placebo group; RR, 1.01; 95% CI, 0.94-1.08; $P = .87$) or breast (RR, 1.00; 95% CI, 0.90-1.12; $P = .95$), lung (RR, 1.09; 95% CI, 0.83-1.44; $P = .52$), or colon cancers (RR, 1.00; 95% CI, 0.77-1.31; $P = .99$). Cancer deaths also did not differ significantly between groups. There was no significant effect of vitamin E on total mortality (636 in the vitamin E group and 615 in the placebo group; RR, 1.04; 95% CI, 0.93-1.16; $P = .53$).

Conclusions.—The data from this large trial indicated that 600 IU of natural-source vitamin E taken every other day provided no overall benefit for major cardiovascular events or cancer, did not affect total mortality, and decreased cardiovascular mortality in healthy women. These data do not support recommending vitamin E supplementation for cardiovascular disease or cancer prevention among healthy women.

Low-Dose Aspirin and Vitamin E: Challenges and Opportunities in Cancer Prevention

Jacobs EJ, Thun MJ (American Cancer Society, Atlanta, Ga)
JAMA 294:105-106, 2005 25–2

Background.—Two recent articles from the Women's Health Study (WHS) have reported findings from a 10-year placebo-controlled randomized trial of low-dose aspirin and vitamin E in predominantly middle-aged women with no history of cancer or cardiovascular disease. The WHS showed that, in terms of noncancer outcomes, low-dose aspirin provided a reduction in stroke risk but had no apparent effect on myocardial infarction. There was an increased risk of gastrointestinal bleeding requiring transfusion. However, neither alternate-day, low-dose aspirin nor vitamin E showed any evidence of efficacy in reduction of overall cancer risk. The implications of these findings on cancer prevention in women were discussed.

Overview.—The null results from the WHS in terms of cancer prevention and low-dose aspirin do not contradict evidence from previous studies that moderate or high doses of aspirin may reduce the risk of certain cancers. The null results for vitamin E and cancer from the WHS are consistent with evidence from previous trials, which found that even relatively long-term α-tocopherol supplementation is unlikely to have any significant effect on cancer risk in women. Another trial of α-tocopherol in men (the Alpha-Tocopherol Beta Carotene [ATBC] trial) found an unexpected reduction in prostate cancer incidence among men. The ATBC trial included only male smokers though, and this association was not observed in the Heart Outcomes Prevention Evaluation—The Ongoing Outcomes (HOPE-TOO) trial or in 2 other observational studies.

Conclusions.—There have been some successes in cancer chemoprevention, such as the use of tamoxifen in breast cancer prevention, but no agent has been shown to be as effective in cancer prevention as statins are in the prevention of cardiovascular disease. However, it must be remembered that there are effective methods for reducing cancer incidence and mortality, although they have been underapplied. Included in these methods are reduction in tobacco use, colorectal cancer screening, and questioning patients about tobacco use and ensuring that patients who use tobacco are treated and counseled appropriately.

Low-dose Aspirin in the Primary Prevention of Cancer: The Women's Health Study: A Randomized Controlled Trial

Cook NR, Lee IM, Gaziano JM, et al (Harvard Med School, Boston; Harvard School of Public Health, Boston; Univ of Miami, Fla; et al)

JAMA 294:47-55, 2005 25–3

Context.—Basic research and observational evidence as well as results from trials of colon polyp recurrence suggest a role for aspirin in the chemoprevention of cancer.

Objective.—To examine the effect of aspirin on the risk of cancer among healthy women.

Design, Setting, and Participants.—In the Women's Health Study, a randomized 2 × 2 factorial trial of aspirin and vitamin E conducted between September 1992 and March 2004, 39 876 US women aged at least 45 years and initially without previous history of cancer, cardiovascular disease, or other major chronic illness were randomly assigned to receive either aspirin or aspirin placebo and followed up for an average of 10.1 years.

Intervention.—A dose of 100 mg of aspirin (n=19 934) or aspirin placebo (n=19 942) administered every other day.

Main Outcome Measures.—Confirmed newly diagnosed invasive cancer at any site, except for nonmelanoma skin cancer. Incidence of breast, colorectal, and lung cancer were secondary end points.

Results.—No effect of aspirin was observed on total cancer (n = 2865; relative risk [RR], 1.01; 95% confidence interval [CI], 0.94-1.08; *P* = .87), breast cancer (n = 1230; RR, 0.98; 95% CI, 0.87-1.09; *P* = .68), colorectal cancer (n = 269; RR, 0.97; 95% CI, 0.77-1.24; *P* = .83), or cancer of any other site, with the exception of lung cancer for which there was a trend toward reduction in risk (n = 205; RR, 0.78; 95% CI, 0.59-1.03; *P* = .08). There was also no reduction in cancer mortality either overall (n = 583; RR, 0.95; 95% CI, 0.81-1.11; *P* = .51) or by site, except for lung cancer mortality (n = 140; RR, 0.70; 95% CI, 0.50-0.99; *P* = .04). No evidence of differential effects of aspirin by follow-up time or interaction with vitamin E was found.

Conclusions.—Results from this large-scale, long-term trial suggest that alternate day use of low-dose aspirin (100 mg) for an average 10 years of treatment does not lower risk of total, breast, colorectal, or other site-specific cancers. A protective effect on lung cancer or a benefit of higher doses of aspirin cannot be ruled out.

► These articles (Abstracts 25–1 to 25–3) report the findings of the Women's Health Study, a prospective randomized trial evaluating the potential role of Vitamin E and aspirin on an every other day administration schedule. To their credit, these are large trials in a single sex with reasonable follow-up. Vitamin E had no impact on the prevention of cancer. It is somewhat more surprising that even aspirin did not appear to benefit patients, given that other trials have demonstrated a decreased incidence in the development of colorectal adenomas.[1-3] The impact of aspirin in other trials upon colorectal cancer has been unclear.[3,4] The reasons for the latter may be the use of alternate day aspirin or relatively short follow-up (as many cancers occur with longer follow-up). This does not negate the impact of aspirin in prevention of cardiovascular disease, or further exploring the roles of daily aspirin for chemoprevention. Until then, limiting the exposure to known carcinogens (eg, tobacco) still remains the best bet.

P. J. Loehrer, Sr, MD

References

1. Baron JA, Cole BF, Sandler RS, et al: A randomized trial to prevent colorectal adenomas. *N Engl J Med* 348:891-899, 2003.
2. Benamouzig R, Deyra J, Martin A, et al: Daily soluble aspirin and prevention of colorectal adenoma recurrence: One-year results of the APACC trial. *Gastroenterology* 125:328-336, 2003.
3. Sandler RS, Halabie S, Baron JA, et al: A randomized trial of aspirin to prevent colorectal adenomas in patients with previous colorectal cancer. *N Engl J Med* 348:883-890, 2003.
4. Gann PH, Manson JAE, Glynn RJ, et al: Low-dose aspirin and incidence of colorectal tumors in a randomized trial. *J Natl Cancer Inst* 85:1220-1224, 1993.

The Beta-Carotene and Retinol Efficacy Trial: Incidence of Lung Cancer and Cardiovascular Disease Mortality During 6-Year Follow-up After Stopping β-Carotene and Retinol Supplements

Goodman GE, Thornquist MD, Balmes J, et al (Fred Hutchinson Cancer Research Ctr, Seattle; Swedish Cancer Inst, Seattle; Univ of California, San Francisco; et al)

J Natl Cancer Inst 96:1743-1750, 2004 25–4

Background.—The Beta-Carotene and Retinol Efficacy Trial (CARET) tested the effect of daily beta-carotene (30 mg) and retinyl palmitate (25,000 IU) on the incidence of lung cancer, other cancers, and death in 18,314 participants who were at high risk for lung cancer because of a history of smoking or asbestos exposure. CARET was stopped ahead of schedule in January 1996 because participants who were randomly assigned to receive the active intervention were found to have a 28% increase in incidence of lung cancer, a 17% increase in incidence of death and a higher rate of cardiovascular disease mortality compared with participants in the placebo group.

Methods.—After the intervention ended, CARET participants returned the study vitamins to their study center and provided a final blood sample. They continue to be followed annually by telephone and mail self-report. Self-reported cancer endpoints were confirmed by review of pathology reports, and death endpoints were confirmed by review of death certificates. All statistical tests were two-sided.

Results.—With follow-up through December 31, 2001, the post-intervention relative risks of lung cancer and all-cause mortality for the active intervention group compared with the placebo group were 1.12 (95% confidence interval [CI] = 0.97 to 1.31) and 1.08 (95% CI = 0.99 to 1.17), respectively. Smoothed relative risk curves for lung cancer incidence and all-cause mortality indicated that relative risks remained above 1.0 throughout the post-intervention follow-up. By contrast, the relative risk of cardiovascular disease mortality decreased rapidly to 1.0 after the intervention was stopped. During the post-intervention phase, females had larger relative risks of lung cancer mortality (1.33 versus 1.14; $P = .36$), cardiovascular disease mortality (1.44 versus 0.93; $P = .03$), and all-cause mortality (1.37 versus 0.98; $P = .001$) than males.

Conclusions.—The previously reported adverse effects of beta-carotene and retinyl palmitate on lung cancer incidence and all-cause mortality in cigarette smokers and individuals with occupational exposure to asbestos persisted after drug administration was stopped although they are no longer statistically significant. Planned subgroup analyses suggest that the excess risks of lung cancer were restricted primarily to females, and cardiovascular disease mortality primarily to females and to former smokers.

► The incidence of lung cancer in the United States increased sharply in the 1940s and 1950s with increasing use of tobacco products decades earlier. The increased rates continued until the last decade, when a plateau of new cases was observed. More aggressive interventions to discourage smoking have been modestly successful. Despite this success, smoking rates and the incidence of lung cancer remains high in the United States. Observation data in the 1980s supported the use of beta-carotene and retinol as protective agents against cancer. CARET tested the effect of beta-carotene and retinol on the incidence of lung cancer and other cancers.

The study was closed prematurely in 1996 because of the observation that the incidence of lung cancer was significantly higher in the treated group. In addition, the incidence of cardiovascular disease mortality was also higher in the intervention group. Study participants discontinued their medication and were followed up. The incidence of cardiovascular mortality decreased precipitously in the intervention group once vitamin supplementation was discontinued; the incidence of lung cancer also decreased, although it still remained higher than the placebo group. This and other studies underscore the need to test chemoprevention strategies in a prospective manner before these interventions are widely adopted. One can not assume that an intervention is harmless and without risk. Indeed, an intervention that is hoped to prevent a molecularly complex disease, such as lung cancer, must be assumed to have profound biological effects on the host. This point has been further underscored with recent evidence that high-dose vitamin E supplementation and high-dose cyclo-oxygenase inhibitors may also have detrimental effects.

N. H. Hanna, MD

A Randomized Trial of Antioxidant Vitamins to Prevent Second Primary Cancers in Head and Neck Cancer Patients

Bairati I, Meyer F, Gélinas M, et al (L'Université Laval, Québec City; Centre Hospitalier de l'Université de Montréal; Universitaire de Sherbrooke, Québec; et al)

J Natl Cancer Inst 97:481-488, 2005 25–5

Background.—Although low dietary intakes of antioxidant vitamins and minerals have been associated with higher risks of cancer, results of trials testing antioxidant supplementation for cancer chemoprevention have been equivocal. We assessed whether supplementation with antioxidant vitamins could reduce the incidence of second primary cancers among patients with head and neck cancer.

Methods.—We conducted a multicenter, double-blind, placebo-controlled, randomized chemoprevention trial among 540 patients with stage I or II head and neck cancer treated by radiation therapy between October 1, 1994, and June 6, 2000. Supplementation with α-tocopherol (400 IU/day) and β-carotene (30 mg/day) or placebo began on the first day of radiation therapy and continued for 3 years after the end of radiation therapy. In the course of the trial, β-carotene supplementation was discontinued after 156 patients had enrolled because of ethical concerns. The remaining patients received α-tocopherol or placebo only. Survival was evaluated by Kaplan-Meier analysis. Cox proportional hazards models were used to estimate hazard ratios (HRs) and 95% confidence intervals (CIs). All statistical tests were two-sided.

Results.—After a median follow-up of 52 months, second primary cancers and recurrences of the first tumor were diagnosed in 113 and 119 participants, respectively. The effect of supplementation on the incidence of second primary cancers varied over time. Compared with patients receiving placebo, patients receiving α-tocopherol supplements had a higher rate of second primary cancers during the supplementation period (HR = 2.88, 95% CI = 1.56 to 5.31) but a lower rate after supplementation was discontinued (HR = 0.41, 95% CI = 0.16 to 1.03). Similarly, the rate of having a recurrence or second primary cancer was higher during (HR = 1.86, 95% CI = 1.27 to 2.72) but lower after (HR = 0.71, 95% CI = 0.33 to 1.53) supplementation with α-tocopherol. The proportion of participants free of second primary cancer overall after 8 years of follow-up was similar in both arms.

FIGURE 2.—Kaplan-Meier curves of survival until occurrence of a second primary cancer among participants randomly assigned to the supplement arm (*solid line*) or to the placebo arm (*dotted line*) for the entire follow-up period (**A**), during the first 3.5 years after randomization (**B**), and beyond 3.5 years after randomization (**C**). Data are shown only up to 8 years of follow-up because of the small numbers of participants beyond that time. (Courtesy of Bairati I, Meyer F, Gélinas M, et al: A randomized trial of antioxidant vitamins to prevent second primary cancers in head and neck cancer patients. *J Natl Cancer Inst* 97:481-488, 2005 by permission of Oxford University Press.)

FIGURE 2.

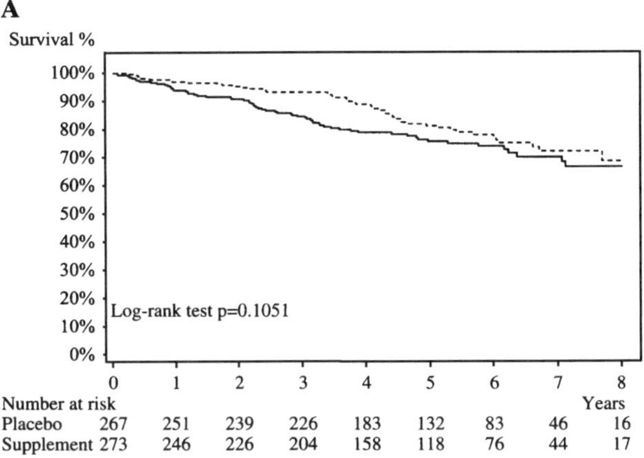

Number at risk									
Placebo	267	251	239	226	183	132	83	46	16
Supplement	273	246	226	204	158	118	76	44	17

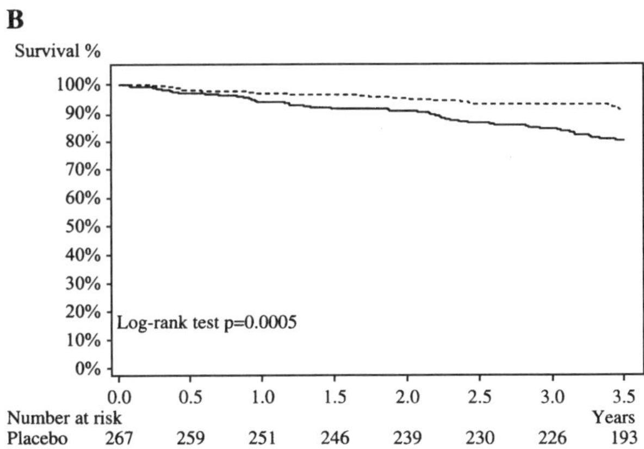

Number at risk								
Placebo	267	259	251	246	239	230	226	193
Supplement	273	261	246	234	226	213	204	162

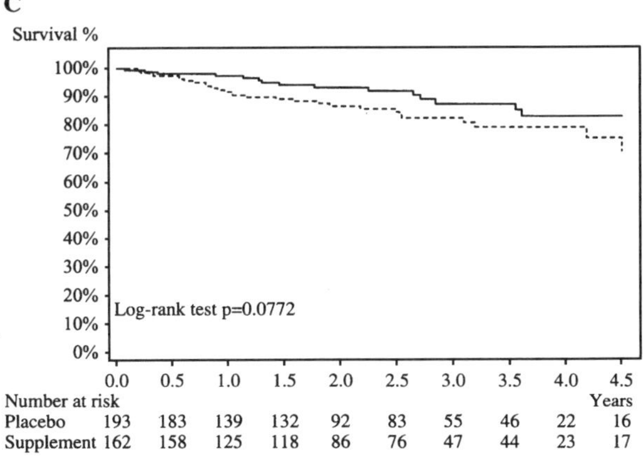

Number at risk										
Placebo	193	183	139	132	92	83	55	46	22	16
Supplement	162	158	125	118	86	76	47	44	23	17

Conclusions.—α-Tocopherol supplementation produced unexpected adverse effects on the occurrence of second primary cancers and on cancer-free survival (Fig 2).

► Patients with cancers of the head and neck are generally smokers who are at high risk of developing secondary cancers. Antioxidant interventions have been proposed as a means of reducing secondary cancers. This large, phase 3, multicenter study reported by Bairati et al evaluated placebo versus α-tocopherol (plus β-carotene initially) in patients undergoing treatment for stage I or II head and neck cancer who were also receiving radiotherapy. Treatment with β-carotene was discontinued after 156 patients because of ethical concerns regarding its effectiveness. Patients receiving the vitamin supplementation had a higher incidence of secondary cancers compared with the placebo group during the intervention. This effect was reversed in the period after the intervention was discontinued. Of note, more patients receiving vitamin supplementation reported side effects (generally mild); however, 16% of those receiving placebo also reported side effects. Importantly, those who continued to smoke had a significantly higher incidence of secondary cancers than did those who were nonsmokers (HR, 2.37). These study results should caution patients and physicians that the use of vitamin supplementation with α-tocopherol may be harmful with respect to the development of secondary cancers and accelerated cancer growth. Similarly, the Alpha-Tocopherol, Beta-Carotene Lung Cancer Prevention Study reported an adverse effect of β-carotene on lung cancer development during the intervention stage.[1]

N. H. Hanna, MD

Reference

1. The Alpha-Tocopherol, Beta-Carotene Cancer Prevention Study Group: The effect of vitamin E and beta carotene on the incidence of lung cancer and other cancers in male smokers. *N Engl J Med* 330:1029-1035, 1994.

26 Cancer Screening

Lessons From Controversy: Ovarian Cancer Screening and Serum Proteomics
Ransohoff DF (Univ of North Carolina, Chapel Hill)
J Natl Cancer Inst 97:315-319, 2005 26–1

Introduction.—In 2002 a study reported that a blood test, based on pattern-recognition proteomics mass spectroscopy analysis of serum, was nearly 100% sensitive and specific to detect ovarian cancer. Plans to introduce a commercial screening test by early 2004 were delayed amid concerns about whether the approach was reproducible and reliable. In this issue of JNCI, two commentaries discuss whether the initial results are reproducible and whether bias may account for results. This essay describes how threats to validity from chance and bias may cause erroneous results and inflated expectations in the kind of observational research being conducted in several "-omics" fields to assess molecular markers for diagnosis and prognosis of cancer. To address such threats and to realize the potential of new -omics technology will require application of appropriate rules of evidence in the design, conduct, and interpretation of clinical research about molecular markers.

Importance of Communication Between Producers and Consumers of Publicly Available Experimental Data
Liotta LA, Lowenthal M, Mehta A, et al (Natl Cancer Inst, Bethesda, Md)
J Natl Cancer Inst 97:310-314, 2005 26–2

Introduction.—The application of mass spectrometry to discover new cancer biomarkers is in its infancy. Many of these new markers are low-abundance proteins that exist as fragments associated with carrier proteins. Although reproducibility is key to the use of mass spectrometry for ion fingerprint analysis, the scientific community has yet to establish a common platform or standardized operating procedures that are necessary for intra- and inter-laboratory comparison. In an effort to assist others who are perfecting mass spectrometry platforms for profiling, ongoing experimental data were posted for public consumption. An unintended consequence of unrestricted access to experimental data is the risk of inappropriate conclusions drawn and publicly disseminated that could have been avoided by communication between the producers and consumers of the data. Such disputes, however, should not divert us from the validation of this promising new approach.

Signal in Noise: Evaluating Reported Reproducibility of Serum Proteomic Tests for Ovarian Cancer

Baggerly KA, Morris JS, Edmonson SR, et al (MD Anderson Cancer Ctr, Houston; Baylor College of Medicine, Houston)

J Natl Cancer Inst 97:307-309, 2005 26–3

Introduction.—Proteomic profiling of serum initially appeared to be dramatically effective for diagnosis of early-stage ovarian cancer, but these results have proven difficult to reproduce. A recent publication reported good classification in one dataset using results from training on a much earlier dataset, but the authors have since reported that they did not perform the analysis as described. We examined the reproducibility of the proteomic patterns across datasets in more detail. Our analysis reveals that the pattern that enabled successful classification is biologically implausible and that the method, properly applied, does not classify the data accurately. We show that the method used in previously published studies does not establish reproducibility and performs no better than chance for classifying the second dataset, in part because the second dataset is easy to classify correctly. We conclude that the reproducibility of the proteomic profiling approach has yet to be established.

► A report in 2002 in *The Lancet* of the use of proteomic profiling as a screening test for ovarian carcinoma suggested that this approach had a very high sensitivity and positive predictive value. Issues of reproducibility and reliability of the reported results have raised concerns about the validity of the initial report. Three articles (Abstracts 26–1 to 26–3) addressing these issues were published in the *Journal of the National Cancer Institute.* Baggerly et al (Abstract 26–3) report on an examination of the reproducibility of the proteomic patterns that enabled successful classification of patients as having ovarian carcinoma or not and note that the method reported in prior publications behaves no better than chance. Liotta et al raise a number of problems with the approach taken by Baggerly et al. Ransohoff (Abstract 26–1) discusses why appropriate study design and conduct are crucial in proper interpretation of data from studies of molecular markers. The discussions highlight important challenges in the promising field of proteomics involving study design and analysis, challenges that will have to be overcome if the promise of proteomics is to be realized. The immediate impact on the management of ovarian carcinoma is that there is still no validated screening test for the disease and that proteomic profiling cannot be regarded as having any current role in ovarian cancer screening.

J. T. Thigpen, MD

Lung Cancer Screening

Mulshine JL, Sullivan DC (Natl Cancer Inst, Bethesda, Md; Natl Cancer Inst, Rockville, Md)

N Engl J Med 352:2714-2720, 2005 26–4

Background.—Lung cancer is reported to account for 30% of all deaths from cancer in the United States and has now surpassed coronary artery disease as the leading cause of death among current and former smokers. Previous randomized trials showed no significant reduction in deaths from lung cancer with the use of screening that included a combination of chest radiography and cytologic analysis of sputum. A case vignette was used to explore the potential benefits of CT screening for the detection of lung cancer.

Methods.—A 60-year-old woman who had quit smoking 20 years earlier presents for a routine visit. She smoked 1 pack of cigarettes per day for 10 years before quitting smoking. Her medical history is unremarkable except for her smoking history, she feels well, and she reports engaging in regular physical exercise. Her husband was also a 1-pack-per-day smoker for at least 30 years but stopped smoking 10 years before the patient's presentation. The woman has asked her physician whether she and her husband should undergo CT scanning to screen for lung cancer. Evidence in support of various strategies is presented, along with a review of formal guidelines and clinical recommendations.

Results.—Overall, 55% to 85% of cancers detected in baseline scans and 60% to 100% of cancers detected in annual follow-up scans are stage 1 tumors. In contrast, only 16% of cancers diagnosed in the setting of routine clinical care in the United States are stage 1 cancers. An observational study from Japan reported a reduction in mortality for patients with lung cancers detected by CT screening. There was also an improvement in the overall 5-year survival rate, from 49% for cases detected by chest radiography to 84% for those detected by CT. One important concern about widespread CT screening is cost. At the present time, there is significant disparity in cost estimates for screening studies, and additional research is needed in this area.

Conclusions.—CT screening for detection of lung cancer has appeared to significantly increase the percentage of cases diagnosed in stage 1 among persons with a history of heavy smoking; however, the results of randomized trials are not yet available to assess whether such screening is effective in reducing mortality. In addition, false-positive test results are reportedly common, leading to undue worry, testing, and surgery in some patients. Thus, many persons who are interested in screening for lung cancer—such as the patient described in this vignette, who had a low risk for lung cancer—may be at greater risk of iatrogenic harm from such screening. These patients should be encouraged to participate in screening-management trials designed to define the best practice in this area.

Incidental Lung Cancers Identified at Coronial Autopsy: Implications for Overdiagnosis of Lung Cancer by Screening

Manser RL, Dodd M, Byrnes G, et al (Royal Melbourne Hosp, Victoria, Australia; Victorian Inst of Forensic Medicine, Southbank, Australia; Univ of Melbourne, Victoria, Australia; et al)

Respir Med 99:501-507, 2005 26–5

Background.—The extent to which overdiagnosis occurs in lung cancer screening programmes has been debated. Overdiagnosis refers to the detection by screening of cancers that would not have become clinically apparent or symptomatic before that individual died of other causes.

Methods.—A retrospective review of coronial autopsies performed in Victoria between April 1991 and February 2002 was conducted to determine the rate of incidental lung cancer in individuals who died of natural causes.

Results.—A total of 24,708 autopsy reports were searched electronically. We estimated that in 56% of these death was from natural causes. Amongst individuals who died naturally there were 167 cases of lung cancer, 47 of these were incidental including five carcinoid tumours, three small cell tumours, 11 cases of carcinoma in situ and 28 invasive nonsmall cell lung cancers. Of the incidental invasive nonsmall cell lung cancers, 86% were stage I.

Conclusions.—Although incidental lung cancer is uncommon, there are some lung cancers that remain undetected during life and do not contribute to death. These findings support the hypothesis that some lung cancers detected by screening may never progress to cause symptoms or death in that individual's lifetime and therefore may be overdiagnosed by screening.

► Lung cancer is the leading cause of cancer-related death in the United States. The majority of lung cancers are of non–small cell histologic type and are diagnosed as stage III or IV. The stage of disease is highly correlated with outcomes; therefore, detection of cancers at an early stage may lead to improved lung cancer mortality rates. Prior screening studies detected earlier stage lung cancers; however, lung cancer-specific mortality rates were not affected. These studies contained design flaws such as the use of screening in the control arm and poor compliance with the intervention arm. New technologies, including high-resolution CT scans, hold the promise of detecting earlier stage lung cancers. Thus, randomized trials comparing chest radiographs with CT have been conducted, and results are expected in the next 5 years. Mulshine and Sullivan (Abstract 26–4) outline an overview of lung cancer screening in the era of CT imaging. Studies evaluating CT imaging report a high detection rate of stage I tumors, usually adenocarcinomas. The 5-year survival rates for patients with these screened lung cancers appear better than the rates for historical controls. However, confirmation of the reduction in lung cancer mortality rates can only come with the results of randomized phase 3 studies. Mulshine and Sullivan describe the potential pitfalls of lung cancer screening, including overdiagnosis and length time bias. In support of this shortcoming, Manser and colleagues (Abstract 26–5) report the results of an autopsy series performed in Victoria, Australia, from 1991 to 2002. A total of 24,708 autopsies were conducted, and 167 cases of lung cancer were detected. These subjects had died of causes other than lung cancer. Their tumors consisted of all histologic subtypes, including carcinoid tumors and carcinomas in situ without an invasive component. The median tumor size was 3 cm. These findings support the hypothesis that some lung cancers are indolent and are not destined to affect a patient's health or life expectancy. These numbers are small, but this finding must be taken into account when considering future screening of lung cancer, particularly in those patients with a shortened life expectancy because of other comorbidities.

N. H. Hanna, MD

27 Supportive Care

Pain Education for Underserved Minority Cancer Patients: A Randomized Controlled Trial

Anderson KO, Mendoza TR, Payne R, et al (Univ of Texas, Houston; Baylor College of Medicine, Houston; Duke Univ, Durham, NC; et al)

J Clin Oncol 22:4918-4925, 2004 27–1

Purpose.—Previous studies found that African American and Hispanic cancer patients are at risk for undertreatment of pain. We evaluated the efficacy of a pain education intervention for underserved minority patients.

Patients and Methods.—Ninety-seven underserved African American and Hispanic outpatients with cancer-related pain were enrolled onto a randomized clinical trial of pain management education. The patients in the education group received a culture-specific video and booklet on pain management. The control group received a video and booklet on nutrition. A research nurse met with each patient to review the materials. We measured changes in pain intensity and pain-related interference 2 to 10 weeks after the intervention, as well as changes in quality of life, perceived pain control, functional status, analgesics, and physician pain assessments.

Results.—Physicians underestimated baseline pain intensity and provided inadequate analgesics for more than 50% of the sample. Although the ratings for pain intensity and pain interference decreased over time for both groups, there was no statistically significant difference between groups. Pain education did not affect quality of life, perceived pain control, or functional status. African American patients in the education but not the control group reported a significant decrease in pain worst ratings from baseline to first follow-up ($P < .01$), although this decrease was not maintained at subsequent assessments.

Conclusion.—Brief education had limited impact on pain outcomes for underserved minority patients, suggesting that more intensive education for patients and interventions for physicians are needed.

► Undertreatment of cancer-related pain is well documented. This is even more of a problem for the underserved population where education and resources are, at best, inconsistent. This was an attempt to cover the chasm. Unfortunately, the impact of this educational intervention was modest at best. However, it does represent an honest effort to make a difference.

P. J. Loehrer, Sr, MD

Inpatient Versus Outpatient Management of Low-Risk Pediatric Febrile Neutropenia: Measuring Parents' and Healthcare Professionals' Preferences

Sung L, Feldman BM, Schwamborn G, et al (Univ of Toronto; Hosp for Sick Children, Toronto; Dartmouth Med School, Hanover, NH)

J Clin Oncol 22:3922-3929, 2004 27–2

Purpose.—Our primary objective was to describe and compare parents' and healthcare professionals' strength of preference scores for outpatient oral antibiotic relative to inpatient parenteral antibiotic treatment for low-risk febrile neutropenic children. Our secondary objective was to identify predictors of strength of preference for oral outpatient treatment.

Methods.—Respondents were parents of children receiving cancer chemotherapy, and pediatric oncology healthcare professionals. First, the inpatient and outpatient options were described, and the respondent indicated their initially preferred option. The respondent next ranked how important seven factors (including "fear/anxiety" and "comfort") were in making their initial choice. The threshold technique was then used to elicit the respondent's strength of preference score for oral outpatient, relative to parenteral inpatient management.

Results.—There were 75 parent and 42 healthcare-professional respondents. There was no significant difference ($P = .08$) in the proportions of parents (40 of 75; 53%) and healthcare professionals (30 of 42; 71%) who initially would choose outpatient management. For parents, stronger preference for oral outpatient therapy was associated with higher anticipated quality of life for the parent and child at home relative to hospital, lower importance rank for "fear/anxiety," and higher importance rank for "comfort." Conversely, for professionals, only lower importance rank for "fear/anxiety" was associated with higher strength of preference scores for outpatient oral antibiotic management.

Conclusion.—Only 53% of parents would choose outpatient oral antibiotic management for low-risk febrile neutropenia. Predictors of strength of preference scores for outpatient oral antibiotic relative to inpatient parenteral antibiotic treatment differed between parent and professional respondents.

► This article by Sung et al represents an interesting vision of the present and future in clinical investigation and publishing. It says something about preferences of parents and health care professionals in comparing outpatient oral antibiotic versus inpatient IV antibiotic treatment for pediatric patients with cancer associated, low-risk, fever and neutropenia. The manuscript does not actually test outcomes in a real life experiment of 2 different approaches to managing fever and neutropenia, but examines hypothetical preferences on the basis of a script of questions of what might be. The study is what might be considered a "prequel" to a more definitive trial. The utility of the results from such studies could be important in planning such definitive trials. Of interest, only 53% of parents chose outpatient therapy while 71% of health care workers chose this option as preferable. The stated reasons for their choices were not surprisingly different. This type of information might be particularly informative in designing a trial testing the 2 possible treatment intervention strategies, but the ability to generalize from this set of parents and health care workers to others would have to be validated to be useful. Had this "preference" study been linked to an actual randomized clinical trial that tested the outcomes responses from participants in comparison with their prestudy preferences, a significant contribution to this field could have been made. As such, the presented study leaves one wondering about what might actually be true as compared to what people think reality is. While such methodologies are clearly useful in helping to plan needed accruals to clinical trials and the prediction of elections, one must question the need to publish such studies beyond knowing the methodology and including the results as part of the methods section of the actual clinical trials. Ironically, one of the stated limitations of the current study was "small sample sizes."

R. J. Arceci, MD, PhD

28 Long-term

Risk of Fracture After Androgen Deprivation for Prostate Cancer
Shahinian VB, Kuo Y-F, Freeman JL, et al (Univ of Texas, Galveston)
N Engl J Med 352:154-164, 2005 28–1

Background.—The use of androgen-deprivation therapy for prostate cancer has increased substantially over the past 15 years. This treatment is associated with a loss of bone-mineral density, but the risk of fracture after androgen-deprivation therapy has not been well studied.

Methods.—We studied the records of 50,613 men who were listed in the linked database of the Surveillance, Epidemiology, and End Results program and Medicare as having received a diagnosis of prostate cancer in the period from 1992 through 1997. The primary outcomes were the occurrence of any fracture and the occurrence of a fracture resulting in hospitalization. Cox proportional-hazards analyses were adjusted for characteristics of the patients and the cancer, other cancer treatment received, and the occurrence of a fracture or the diagnosis of osteoporosis during the 12 months preceding the diagnosis of cancer.

Results.—Of men surviving at least five years after diagnosis, 19.4 percent of those who received androgen-deprivation therapy had a fracture, as compared with 12.6 percent of those not receiving androgen-deprivation therapy ($P<0.001$). In the Cox proportional-hazards analyses, adjusted for characteristics of the patient and the tumor, there was a statistically significant relation between the number of doses of gonadotropin-releasing hormone received during the 12 months after diagnosis and the subsequent risk of fracture.

Conclusions.—Androgen-deprivation therapy for prostate cancer increases the risk of fracture.

► This represents an important observation to remember in patients treated with androgen deprivation. Earlier use of hormonal therapy will make this more relevant and defining the role of bisphosphonate therapy even more important.

P. J. Loehrer, Sr, MD

Risk of Cardiac Death After Adjuvant Radiotherapy for Breast Cancer

Giordano SH, Kuo Y-F, Freeman JL, et al (Univ of Texas MD Anderson Cancer Ctr, Houston; Univ of Texas Med Branch, Galveston)

J Natl Cancer Inst 97:419-424, 2005 28–2

Background.—Women with breast cancer who are treated with adjuvant radiation have a decreased risk of local recurrence but an increased risk of mortality from ischemic heart disease. Patients with left-sided breast tumors receive a higher dose of radiation to the heart than patients with right-sided tumors. Because radiation techniques have improved over time, we investigated whether the risk of death from ischemic heart disease after adjuvant breast radiotherapy decreased over time.

Methods.—We used the 12-registry 1973-2000 dataset from the National Cancer Institute's Surveillance, Epidemiology, and End Results (SEER) program. Women (n = 27,283) treated with adjuvant radiation for breast cancer diagnosed in 1973-1989 were included in the study. Ischemic heart disease mortality was calculated at 15 years and compared for women diagnosed during 1973-1979, 1980-1984, and 1985-1989. Cox proportional hazards models were used to calculate the hazard of death from ischemic heart disease for women diagnosed 1973-1988 and censored at 12 years. All statistical tests were two-sided.

Results.—There were no differences in age, race/ethnicity, disease stage, or follow-up time between the 13 998 women with left-sided and 13 285 with right-sided cancer. For women diagnosed in 1973-1979, there was a statistically significant difference in 15-year mortality from ischemic heart disease between patients with left-sided (13.1%, 95% confidence interval [CI] = 11.6 to 14.6) and those with right-sided (10.2%, 95% CI = 8.9 to 11.5) breast cancer (P = .02); no such difference was found for women diagnosed in 1980-1984 (9.4%, [95% CI = 8.1 to 10.6] versus 8.7% [95% CI = 7.4 to 10.0], respectively, P = .64) or 1985-1989 (5.8% [95% CI = 4.8 to 6.8] versus 5.2% [95% CI = 4.4 to 5.9], respectively, P = .98). In the Cox model, the hazard ratio [HR] for ischemic heart disease mortality for women with left-sided versus women with right-sided disease was 1.50 (95% CI = 1.19 to 1.87) in 1979. With each succeeding year after 1979, the hazard of death from ischemic heart disease for women with left-sided versus those with right-sided disease declined by 6% (HR = 0.94, 95% CI = 0.91 to 0.98).

Conclusions.—Risk of death from ischemic heart disease associated with radiation for breast cancer has substantially decreased over time (Table 2).

► This is, I believe, a very important article from investigators with the M. D. Anderson Hospital and the University of Texas Medical Branch at Galveston. There has been an increase in awareness over the last 20 years or so about potential complications of radiation therapy and management of breast cancer reflecting predominantly cardiac problems related to left-sided lesions. These investigators have looked at the Seer Program and looked at different 5-year cohorts with at least 15 years of follow-up in each of the cohorts. A total of over

TABLE 2.—Comparison of Percent Ischemic Heart Disease Mortality (With 95% Confidence Intervals) at 15 Years of Follow-Up Between Women With Left-Sided and Right-Sided Breast Cancers, Stratified by Stage of Disease at Time of Diagnosis

Cohort by Year of Diagnosis	All Patients			Patients With in situ/Localized Disease			Patients With Regional Disease		
	Left-Sided, %	Right-Sided, %	*P*	Left-Sided, %	Right-Sided, %	*P*	Left-Sided, %	Right-Sided, %	*P*
Overall	8.7 (8.0 to 9.3)	7.5 (6.9 to 8.2)	.07	7.6 (6.7 to 8.4)	6.7 (5.9 to 7.5)	.40	10.2 (9.1 to 11.3)	8.6 (7.6 to 9.6)	.09
1973-1979	13.1 (11.6 to 14.6)	10.2 (8.9 to 11.5)	.02	12.7 (10.3 to 15.2)	9.6 (7.5 to 11.8)	.14	13.3 (11.5 to 15.1)	10.6 (8.9 to 12.3)	.06
1980-1984	9.4 (8.1 to 10.6)	8.7 (7.4 to 10.0)	.64	8.9 (7.2 to 10.4)	8.7 (7.1 to 10.4)	.87	10.0 (7.9 to 12.1)	8.8 (6.8 to 10.9)	.38
1985-1989	5.8 (4.8 to 6.7)	5.2 (4.4 to 5.9)	.98	5.7 (4.5 to 6.8)	4.9 (4.0 to 5.8)	.79	6.0 (4.4 to 7.6)	5.7 (4.1 to 7.2)	.76

(Courtesy of Giordano SH, Kuo Y-F, Freeman JL, et al: Risk of cardiac death after adjuvant radiotherapy for breast cancer. *J Natl Cancer Inst* 97:419-424, 2005, by permission of Oxford University Press.)

27,000 patients have received adjuvant radiation therapy as part of their management. They looked at the ratio of ischemic heart injury for patients with left-sided versus right-sided disease. What their data show is that there has been a substantial decrease in the risk of death from ischemic heart disease associated with radiation therapy for the treatment of breast cancer. It would appear as though the radiation oncology community accepted the fact that there was a problem and tried to make modifications in their technique to reduce the risk. Fifteen years is probably a pretty good estimate that this is a real reduction, but the data can still be reviewed at a later point in time to account for a more complete follow-up.

What makes this really important, I believe, is that it does come from the Seer data, which are essentially a cross-section of community hospital practice. I think this is a very good study, and one that will be even further improved with 3-D treatment planning and more conformal radiation approaches. The intensity-modulated radiation therapy may further improve the cardiac injury problem secondary to radiation, but that one is more likely to have an expensive price, precisely because these patients, too, live, on the whole, for a long period of time. The spreading of dose around larger amounts of normal tissue will, in the long run, make for a higher proportion of radiation-induced cancer than what we have seen in the past. Although there are no data at this point to confirm that, I believe it is a predictable result.

E. Glatstein, MD

Development of Risk-Based Guidelines for Pediatric Cancer Survivors: The Children's Oncology Group Long-term Follow-up Guidelines From the Children's Oncology Group Late Effects Committee and Nursing Discipline

Landier W, Bhatia S, Eshelman DA, et al (Stanford Univ, Calif; USC Keck School of Medicine, Los Angeles; Univ of Texas, Dallas; et al)

J Clin Oncol 22:4979-4990, 2004 28–3

Introduction.—The Children's Oncology Group Long-Term Follow-Up Guidelines for Survivors of Childhood, Adolescent, and Young Adult Cancers are risk-based, exposure-related clinical practice guidelines intended to promote earlier detection of and intervention for complications that may potentially arise as a result of treatment for pediatric malignancies. Developed through the collaborative efforts of the Children's Oncology Group Late Effects Committee, Nursing Discipline, and Patient Advocacy Committee, these guidelines represent a statement of consensus from a multidisciplinary panel of experts in the late effects of pediatric cancer treatment. The guidelines are both evidence-based (utilizing established associations between therapeutic exposures and late effects to identify high-risk categories) and grounded in the collective clinical experience of experts (matching the magnitude of risk with the intensity of screening recommendations). They are intended for use beginning 2 or more years following the completion of cancer therapy; however, they are not intended to provide guidance for follow-up of the survivor's primary disease. A complementary set of patient education materials ("Health Links") was developed to enhance follow-up care and broaden the application of the guidelines. The information provided in these guidelines is important for health care providers in the fields of pediatrics, oncology, internal medicine, family practice, and gynecology, as well as subspecialists in many fields. Implementation of these guidelines is intended to increase awareness of potential late effects and to standardize and enhance follow-up care provided to survivors of pediatric cancer throughout the lifespan. The Guidelines, and related Health Links, can be downloaded in their entirety at *www.survivorshipguidelines.org*.

► The obvious consequence of improved treatment and outcomes for children with cancer is that there are an increasing number of survivors to monitor. And while more long-term survivors die of their initial or secondary cancers, other adverse late sequelae are important to understand not only for directing future therapeutic studies but also for anticipating and helping with future health needs of these surviving patients. And because these children are aging into adulthood, the need to engage not just pediatric specialists but also specialists in internal medicine and other adult disciplines is critical. The pediatric cooperative clinical trials groups have always been at the forefront of survivorship issues. The report by Landier et al carries on this tradition and significantly advances the field by developing evidence-based and risk-oriented guidelines for follow-up of survivors of childhood cancer. As noted in the report, these guidelines are designed to begin 2 to 3 years after stopping therapy for the primary malignancy. The guidelines are not designed to monitor the primary malignancy for relapse. However, in identifying in a preemptive fashion the adverse sequelae resulting from the primary disease and/or treatment, these guidelines should prove to be incredibly useful to all health care providers managing this group of patients. In addition, the development of patient education materials on long-term follow-up issues is a superb idea and should help both patients, their families, and health care providers to have a more common ground for follow-up discussion and testing.

R. J. Arceci, MD, PhD

29 Miscellaneous Topics

Differences Between Urologists in United States and Canada in Approach to Bladder Cancer
Chung D, Hersey K, Fleshner N (Univ of Toronto)
Urology 65:919-925, 2005 29–1

Objectives.—To determine the Canada-United States differences with respect to the detection, diagnosis, surveillance, and treatment of bladder cancer.

Methods.—A multiple-choice questionnaire was developed and mailed to 760 American and 516 Canadian urologists between November and December 2002. The areas assessed by the questionnaire included demographics, screening, superficial disease and recurrence, surveillance, muscle-invasive disease, advanced disease, and adjuvant systemic chemotherapy.

Results.—The survey was adequately completed by 32.3% of American urologists and 40.0% of Canadian urologists (overall response rate 36.2%). Canadian urologists tended to be older and had larger practices than U.S. urologists (P <0.05). With respect to bladder cancer detection, U.S. urologists were more likely to use intravenous urography and cystoscopy than were Canadian urologists (P <0.0001). For patients with superficial disease, a significant proportion of urologists in both countries did not routinely use adjuvant chemotherapy. For surveillance, Canadian urologists performed cystoscopy (P <0.0001) and upper tract imaging (P <0.0001) less frequently than U.S. urologists. Striking differences were noted in the approach to Stage T2a disease, with U.S. urologists advocating radical cystectomy more frequently (P <0.0001). With respect to the type of urinary diversion, Canadian urologists tended to favor conduits (P <0.0001, male and P = 0.002, female). Canadian urologists were also less likely to use adjuvant chemotherapy among patients with advanced disease.

Conclusions.—The results of our study have shown that the trend of urologists in the United States is toward more aggressive screening, closer surveillance, an earlier trigger for cystectomy, and more common indications for intravenous chemotherapy (Table 1 and Table 2).

► I find this article interesting. Although I am skeptical that the biology of bladder cancer is significantly different in the United States and Canada, the management of patients remains so. This is no doubt dependent upon training, biases, perceptions, and (dare I say) compensation. The differences in health

TABLE 1.—Baseline Demographics and Bladder Cancer Detection

Demographic	Canada (n)	United States (n)	*P* Value
Practice			<0.0001
Private	121 (72.5)	168 (71.8)	
Multisubspecialty		34 (14.5)	
HMO full-time		9 (3.8)	
Medical school full-time	46 (27.1)	23 (9.8)	
Decade residency completed			<0.0001
Before 1960	3 (1.8)		
1960s	21 (12.4)	1 (0.4)	
1970s	33 (19.5)	11 (4.7)	
1980s	58 (34.3)	31 (13.2)	
1990s and later	54 (32)	192 (81.7)	
Patients seen/month with bladder cancer (n)			<0.0001
0	3 (1.8)	2 (0.9)	
1-10	35 (20.7)	109 (46.6)	
11-20	63 (37.3)	87 (37.2)	
>20	68 (40.2)	36 (15.4)	
Radical cystectomies/yr			<0.0001
None	49 (29.0)	25 (10.7)	
1-5	65 (38.5)	173 (73.9)	
6-10	35 (20.7)	26 (11.1)	
11-25	17 (10.1)	6 (2.6)	
>25	3 (1.8)	4 (1.7)	
40-year-old nonsmoking woman with microscopic hematuria			
Urine cytology	95 (55.9)	146 (62.1)	0.232
Intravenous urography	21 (12.4)	156 (66.4)	<0.0001
Abdominal/pelvic ultrasonography	116 (68.2)	54 (23.0)	<0.0001
Abdominal/pelvic computed tomography	5 (2.9)	22 (9.4)	0.011
Cystoscopy	112 (65.9)	195 (83.0)	<0.0001
No investigations	9 (5.3)	3 (1.3)	0.018
Age for cystoscopy in nonsmoking woman with microscopic hematuria (yr)			<0.0001 (overall)
<30	27 (15.9)	89 (37.9)	
30-40	39 (22.9)	85 (36.2)	
41-50	76 (44.7)	53 (22.6)	
51-60	21 (12.4)	7 (3.0)	
61-65	3 (1.8)	0	
>65	4 (2.4)	1 (0.4)	
Age for cystoscopy in smoking woman with microscopic hematuria (yr)			<0.0001 (overall)
<30	70 (41.2)	157 (66.8)	
30-40	66 (38.8)	67 (28.5)	
41-50	32 (18.8)	10 (4.3)	
51-60	1 (0.6)		
61-65			
>65			

Note: Data in parentheses are percentages.

(Reprinted from Chung D, Hersey K, Fleshner N: Differences between urologists in United States and Canada in approach to bladder cancer. *Urology* 65:919-925, 2005.)

care systems are widely known. In addition, the number of trained urologists per capita is nearly twice as great as in the United States. This article raises questions about the standard of care and procedures that are based on evidence-based medicine. It remains bothersome to me about inappropriate use (and misuse) of intravesicular and systemic therapy in both countries. Bet-

TABLE 2.—Superficial Disease and Surveillance

Variable	Canada (n)	United States (n)	*P* Value
62-year-old with Ta G1-G2 resected			0.705 (overall)
Adjuvant intravesical chemotherapy	107 (62.9)	139 (59.1)	
No adjuvant intravesical chemotherapy	62 (36.5)	95 (40.4)	
Reasons			
Yes. All should have	17 (10)	17 (7.3)	
Yes. Only high risk	87 (51.2)	119 (50.9)	
No. No reduction recurrence	43 (25.3)	60 (25.6)	
No. Therapy too expensive	9 (5.3)	4 (1.7)	
No. Side effects too great	12 (7.1)	33 (14.1)	
62-year-old with Ta G1-G2 solitary recurrence			0.004 (overall)
Repeat TURBT	70 (41.2)	65 (27.8)	
Repeat TURBT and intravesical BCG	71 (41.8)	140 (59.6)	
Repeat TURBT and intravesical chemotherapy	27 (15.9)	30 (12.8)	
Repeat TURBT and systemic chemotherapy			
Radical cystectomy			
Radiotherapy			
Follow-up cystoscopy			<0.0001 (overall)
Every 3-5 mo	119 (70.4)	220 (93.6)	
Every 6-9 mo	46 (27.2)	15 (6.4)	
Every 10-12 mo	3 (1.8)	0 (0.0)	
Less than every 12 mo	0 (0.0)	0 (0.0)	
Image upper tracts			<0.0001 (overall)
Every 6-9 mo	4 (2.4)	4 (1.7)	
Every year	23 (13.7)	57 (24.3)	
Every 2-3 yr	79 (47.0)	129 (54.9)	
Never	62 (36.9)	45 (19.1)	
Why perform surveillance cystoscopy?			
To pick up more aggressive lesion at earlier stage	66 (39.3)	92 (39.1)	0.978
To prevent hematuria	1 (0.6)	2 (0.9)	0.768
Pays well	3 (1.8)	4 (1.7)	0.950
To pick up superficial lesion when smaller and easier to manage	118 (70.2)	159 (67.7)	0.582

Note: Data in parentheses are percentages.
Abbreviations: TURBT, Transurethral resection of bladder tumor; *BCG*, bacille Calmette-Guérin.
(Reprinted from Chung D, Hersey K, Fleshner N: Differences between urologists in United States and Canada in approach to bladder cancer. *Urology* 65:919-925, 2005. Copyright 2005, with permission from Elsevier Science.)

ter education and treatment guidelines might assist in minimizing some of these problem areas.

P. J. Loehrer, Sr, MD

Enrollment of Elderly Patients in Clinical Trials for Cancer Drug Registration: A 7-Year Experience by the US Food and Drug Administration

Talarico L, Chen G, Pazdur R (Food and Drug Administration, Rockville, Md)

J Clin Oncol 22:4626-4631, 2004 29–2

Purpose.—To analyze the age-related enrollment of cancer patients onto registration trials of new drugs or new indications approved by the US Food and Drug Administration from 1995 to 2002.

Patients and Methods.—This study involved retrospective analyses of demographic data of cancer patients enrolled onto registration trials. The data on 28,766 cancer patients from 55 registration trials were analyzed according to age distributions of ≥ 65, ≥ 70, and ≥ 75 years. The rates of enrollment in each age group for each cancer were compared with the corresponding rates in the US cancer population. The age distributions of the US cancer population were derived from the Surveillance, Epidemiology, and End Results Program of the National Cancer Institute for the period 1995 to 1999 based on the 2000 US Census.

Results.—The proportions of the overall patient populations aged ≥ 65, ≥ 70, and ≥ 75 years were 36%, 20%, and 9% compared with 60%, 46%, and 31%, respectively, in the US cancer population. Statistically significant under-representation of the elderly ($P < .001$) was noted in registration trials for all cancer treatment except for breast cancer hormonal therapies. Patients aged ≥ 70 years accounted for most of the under-representation.

Conclusion.—Elderly were under-represented in the registration trials of new cancer therapies. Various strategies may be needed to evaluate cancer therapies for the elderly in prospective clinical trials and to improve cancer care in the elderly population.

► As there has been no trial conducted of sufficient power to clarify the role of adjuvant therapy for stage II colon cancer patients, this meta-analysis is of importance. Whereas fluoropyrimidine-based adjuvant therapy has a clear impact on stage III disease, this has not been clearly demonstrated in stage II disease. However, some subgroups deserve special consideration. This includes those patients with inadequate lymph node sampling. Other high-risk features, such as T4 lesions, perforation, aneuploidy may be associated with a poorer prognosis, but it remains unclear whether adjuvant therapy benefits this patient population. To truly detect clear benefit in a good-risk population would take more patients than has ever been attempted to be accrued. Talking points for health care providers to patients are well outlined in this article.

P. J. Loehrer, Sr, MD

Suicide Risk in Cancer Patients From 1960 to 1999

Hem E, Loge JH, Haldorsen T, et al (Ullevål Univ, Norway; Univ of Oslo, Norway)

J Clin Oncol 22:4209-4216, 2004 29–3

Purpose.—Suicide risk is reportedly higher for cancer patients than for the general population, but estimates vary and analyses of trends are few. The aim of the present study was to determine whether cancer patients had a higher suicide risk between 1960 and 1999.

Patients and Methods.—A cohort comprising patients from the Cancer Registry of Norway 1960 to 1997 was linked to suicide diagnosis in the Register of Deaths at Statistics Norway and observed during 1960 to 1999. The cohort consisted of all cancer patients registered in the Cancer Registry of Norway 1960 to 1997 (N = 490,245 patients with 520,823 cancer diagnoses). Suicide was defined according to death certificates based on the International Classification of Diseases (versions 7, 8, 9, and 10).

Results.—During the period, 589 cancer patients (407 males and 182 females) committed suicide. The relative risk was elevated for males and females, with standardized mortality ratios (SMRs) of 1.55 (95% CI, 1.41 to 1.71) and 1.35 (95% CI, 1.17 to 1.56), respectively. Risk was highest in the first months after diagnosis. For both sexes, there was a significant decrease in the relative suicide risk over decades. The risk was markedly increased among male patients with cancer of respiratory organs (SMR, 4.08; 95% CI, 2.96 to 5.47). Otherwise, the SMRs varied from 0.76 to 3.67 across cancer types.

Conclusion.—Cancer may be a risk factor for suicide, particularly shortly after diagnosis. However, the relative risk gradually decreased during the period 1960 to 1999.

► Suicide in cancer patients is uncommon, but it remains a preventable cause of death. The risk factors for suicide (with or without cancer) are multifaceted including depression, as well as numerous other (eg, age, socioeconomic, education) factors. This article is a thorough review of an important topic, and places a special emphasis on the importance of physician-patient communication.

P. J. Loehrer, Sr, MD

Malignancies, Prothrombotic Mutations, and the Risk of Venous Thrombosis

Blom JW, Doggen CJM, Osanto S, et al (Leiden Univ, The Netherlands)

JAMA 293:715-722, 2005 29–4

Context.—Venous thrombosis is a common complication in patients with cancer, leading to additional morbidity and compromising quality of life.

Objective.—To identify individuals with cancer with an increased thrombotic risk, evaluating different tumor sites, the presence of distant metastases, and carrier status of prothrombotic mutations.

Design, Setting, and Patients.—A large population-based, case-control (Multiple Environmental and Genetic Assessment [MEGA] of risk factors for venous thrombosis) study of 3220 consecutive patients aged 18 to 70 years, with a first deep venous thrombosis of the leg or pulmonary embolism, between March 1, 1999, and May 31, 2002, at 6 anticoagulation clinics in the Netherlands, and separate 2131 control participants (partners of the patients) reported via a questionnaire on acquired risk factors for venous thrombosis. Three months after discontinuation of the anticoagulant therapy, all patients and controls were interviewed, a blood sample was taken, and DNA was isolated to ascertain the factor V Leiden and prothrombin 20210A mutations.

Main Outcome Measure.—Risk of venous thrombosis.

Results.—The overall risk of venous thrombosis was increased 7-fold in patients with a malignancy (odds ratio [OR], 6.7; 95% confidence interval [CI], 5.2-8.6) vs persons without malignancy. Patients with hematological malignancies had the highest risk of venous thrombosis, adjusted for age and sex (adjusted OR, 28.0; 95% CI, 4.0-199.7), followed by lung cancer and gastrointestinal cancer. The risk of venous thrombosis was highest in the first few months after the diagnosis of malignancy (adjusted OR, 53.5; 95% CI, 8.6-334.3). Patients with cancer with distant metastases had a higher risk vs patients without distant metastases (adjusted OR, 19.8; 95% CI, 2.6-149.1). Carriers of the factor V Leiden mutation who also had cancer had a 12-fold increased risk vs individuals without cancer and factor V Leiden (adjusted OR, 12.1; 95% CI, 1.6-88.1). Similar results were indirectly calculated for the prothrombin 20210A mutation in patients with cancer.

Conclusions.—Patients with cancer have a highly increased risk of venous thrombosis especially in the first few months after diagnosis and in the presence of distant metastases. Carriers of the factor V Leiden and prothrombin 20210A mutations appear to have an even higher risk.

► Trousseau's syndrome, which described an association between cancer and venous thrombosis was first discovered nearly 150 years ago. Although many studies have substantiated this association, they have suffered from a lack of power to determine the impact of various malignancies and known prothrombotic mutations. This article reinforces the relationship of cancer and clotting, and it also provides insight into those at highest risk.

P. J. Loehrer, Sr, MD

Estimated Radiation Risks Potentially Associated With Full-Body CT Screening

Brenner DJ, Elliston CD (Columbia Univ, New York)

Radiology 232:735-738, 2004 29–5

Purpose.—To estimate the radiation-related cancer mortality risks associated with single or repeated full-body computed tomographic (CT) examinations by using standard radiation risk estimation methods.

Materials and Methods.—The estimated dose to the lung or stomach from a single full-body CT examination is 14-21 mGy, which corresponds to a dose region for which there is direct evidence of increased cancer mortality in atomic bomb survivors. Total doses for repeated examinations are correspondingly higher. The authors used estimated cancer risks in a U.S. population derived from atomic bomb-associated cancer mortality data, together with calculated organ doses from a full-body CT examination, to estimate the radiation risks associated with single and multiple full-body CT examinations (Fig 1).

Results.—A single full-body CT examination in a 45-year-old adult would result in an estimated lifetime attributable cancer mortality risk of

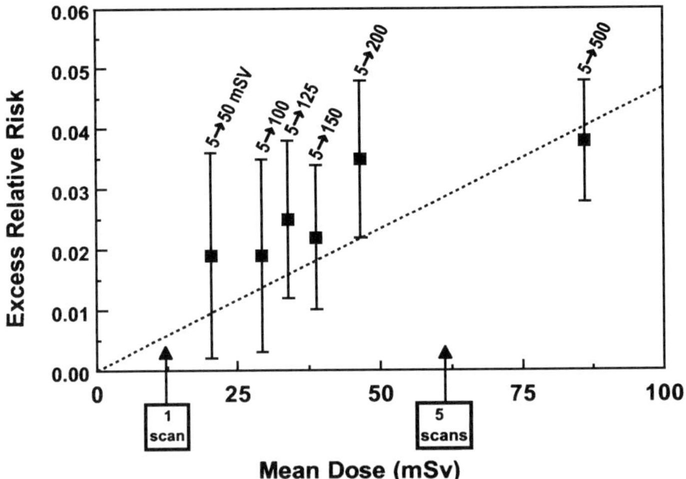

FIGURE 1.—Graph shows estimated excess relative risk (*black squares*) (±1 standard error [*error bars*]) of mortality (1950-1997) from solid cancer among groups of survivors in the life-span study cohort of atomic bomb survivors who were exposed to low doses (<500 mSv) of radiation. Dose limits for each group are shown above each data point. *Dashed line* represents result of zero-intercept linear fit to all life-span study data from 5 to 4,000 mSv (higher dose points not shown). *Arrows* refer to estimated doses from one and five full-body CT examinations. (Courtesy of Brenner DJ, Elliston CD: Estimated radiation risks potentially associated with full-body CT screening. *Radiology* 232:735-738, 2004. Reproduced with permission. Radiological Society of North America.)

around 0.08%, with the 95% credibility limits being a factor of 3.2 in either direction (Table 1). A 45-year-old adult who plans to undergo annual full-body CT examinations up to age 75 (30 examinations) would accrue an overall estimated lifetime attributable risk of cancer mortality of about

TABLE 1.—Estimated Organ Doses for a Typical Full-body CT Examination

Organ	Radiation Dose (mGy)
Thyroid	24.7
Bone surface	15.7
Esophagus	16.2
Lung	15.5
Stomach	14.4
Liver	14.0
Bladder	13.9
Breast (female)	12.3
Gonads (female)	12.2
Colon	11.6
Red bone marrow	9.9
Skin	7.5
Gonads (male)	2.6

Note: Doses were estimated for a full-body CT examination with a Volume Zoom scanner (Siemens) operated at 120 kV and 230 true mAs with a pitch of 1.75. The examination was from the C3 vertebra through the symphysis pubis. Dose estimation was performed with the ImPACT CT patient dosimetry calculator. Note if a lower amperage setting is used, the doses would be proportionally lower. The total effective dose (weighted average of organ doses) is 13.5 mSv for females and 11.6 mSv for males.

(Courtesy of Brenner DJ, Elliston CD: Estimated radiation risks potentially associated with full-body CT screening. *Radiology* 232:735-738, 2004. Reproduced with permission. Radiological Society of North America.)

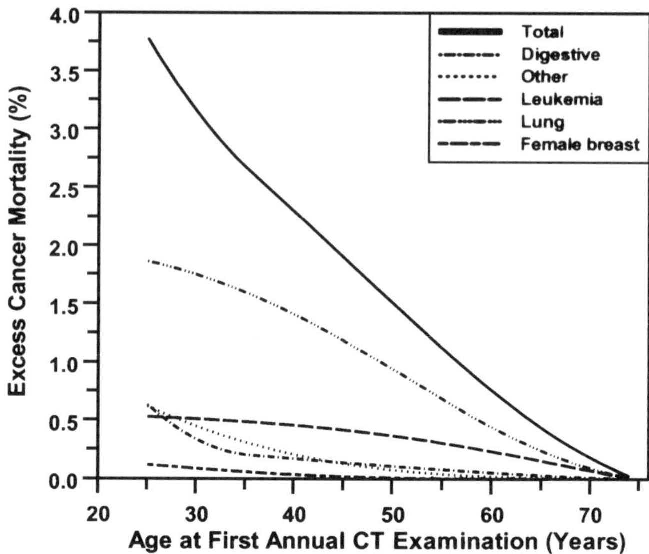

FIGURE 4.—Graph shows excess cancer mortality risks estimated to be associated with radiation from annual full-body CT examinations. Annual examinations are assumed to commence at the specified age and continue until age 75. (Courtesy of Brenner DJ, Elliston CD: Estimated radiation risks potentially associated with full-body CT screening. *Radiology* 232:735-738, 2004. Reproduced with permission. Radiological Society of North America.)

1.9%, with the 95% credibility limits being a factor of 2 in either direction (Fig 4).

Conclusion.—The authors provide estimates of lifetime cancer mortality risks from both single and annual full-body CT examinations. These risk estimates are needed to assess the utility of full-body CT examinations from both an individual and a public health perspective.

▶ These investigators from Columbia and New York do an important service in calling to our attention the dose of radiation that a patient would receive in a single full-body CT scan. They further go on to estimate the radiation-related cancer mortality risk associated with such examinations on an annual basis. This is an important article because it points out that the dose for whole-body scan is about 1 to 2 rad or cGy per peripheral body CT scan. These are not insignificant doses, and all too often the physicians who order these scans do not appreciate the dose that is being delivered. Nonetheless, for someone who has actually had a cancer, the information to be derived for that patient for his follow-up, at least for the first several years, easily justifies such intervention. Scanning people on an annual basis if they do not have cancer is a far more unjustifiable action.

E. Glatstein, MD

PART FOUR

KIDNEY, WATER, AND ELECTROLYTES

RENEE GARRICK, MD

Introduction

The majority of the articles selected for review this year were chosen by Saulo Klahr, MD, the longtime editor of the renal section of the YEAR BOOK OF MEDICINE. The editorial comments after each article were written by my colleagues and me. The articles selected have been divided into several sections. Each section focuses on a subsection of nephrology.

The first section focuses on articles that review the influence of blood pressure and metabolic disorders on the incidence, prevalence, and rate of progression of chronic kidney disease. These articles include an important subgroup analysis of the ALLHAT trial, which focused on hypertensive patients with reduced glomerular filtration rate (GFR). This post-hoc analysis suggested that in patients with a reduced GFR, the renal protective effect of lisinopril and amlodipine are not superior to those of chlorthalidone. As discussed in the commentary, the original design of ALLHAT, which was not stratified for proteinuria, and the degree of blood pressure control achieved during the early phases of the trial, may have influenced this analysis.

It is well-known that hypertension is a risk factor for the progression of chronic kidney disease (CKD), and many articles have suggested that optimal blood pressure control can help slow disease progression. Several articles published during the last year have sought to define the appropriate range of blood pressure control for patients with renal disease, and the findings suggest that, especially those with diabetes and/or proteinuria, systolic blood pressures below target range can worsen the rate of progression of renal disease.

Studies have continued to focus on the role of apolipoprotein E (APOE) and obesity in the progression of chronic renal disease. New data presented this year suggest that certain APOE alleles are associated with renal disease, and other APOE alleles are associated with cardiac disease. If these findings are confirmed, further studies may ultimately lead to the development of unique risk-screening panels.

The impending obesity epidemic heightens the potential impact of obesity on the prevalence and incidence of chronic kidney disease. Data from the Hypertension Detection and Follow-up Program (HD FP) suggest that the incidence of CKD varies with body mass index, a finding that further supports the need for obesity counseling as part of general medical care. The PAMELA study from Italy suggests that blood pressure elevation is separately related to changes in the lipids and glucose, a finding that offers interesting insight into the metabolic syndrome.

A possible role for uric acid in the pathogenesis of renal and cardiovascular disease has been suggested for many years. There is renewed interest in the potential link between essential hypertension, uric acid, and progressive renal disease. The role of uric acid is of particular interest, given the prevalence of diuretic-induced hyperuricemia.

The importance of accurate determination of renal function is self-evident; however, serum creatinine itself is a relatively insensitive marker of renal function. New determinations such as the serum concentration of cystatin-C may prove to be a better determinant of GFR.

The measurement of B-type natriuretic peptide (BNP) can be used to identify and monitor heart failure. Given the coexistence of heart disease and CKD, it is important to understand what, if any, impact CKD has on the clinical application of BNP measurements.

The second section focuses on the role of statin therapy in patients who have received a transplant, patients with chronic kidney disease, and patients on hemodialysis. The ALERT study was the first trial to demonstrate that statin therapy reduces the risk of major cardiac events in renal transplant patients. The advantage of treatment was not apparent until after more than 5 years of follow-up. The Four D trial studied hemodialysis patients with type 2 diabetes on statins for a median of 4 years and demonstrated no benefit from statin therapy on the primary end point of death due to cardiac disease. Pravastatin was studied on patients with chronic renal insufficiency, and the results suggested it may slow the progression of renal disease, especially in patients with proteinuria. As a group, these studies alert us to the risk of generalizing the results of studies in one patient population to different populations of patients and stress the need for careful study design and appropriate length of follow-up.

The third section focuses on glomerular disease and renal injury. The glomerular epithelial podocyte plays a pivotal role in glomerular injury. Several key articles this past year studied the effect of glomerular injury on podocyte migration and proliferation, and this avenue of investigation may provide key insights into the progression of glomerular injury. Another avenue of investigation has focused on the pathogenesis of hereditary focal segmental glomerular sclerosis (FSGS). Unlike the previously described podocyte mutations in hereditary FSGS, these studies suggest that an ion-channel (perhaps linked to angiotensin II and therefore amenable to pharmacologic therapy) may be involved.

After an injury, the kidney undergoes morphologic restoration of tubule damage and recovery of function. Recent studies suggest that bone marrow–derived cells do not significantly contribute to renal tubule restoration after an ischemic insult. This could influence the applicability of stem cell therapy in renal injury.

Several articles have focused on new immunosuppressive therapies, including the use of mycophenolate mofetil as compared to cytoxan for lupus nephritis, caspase inhibition to slow renal disease progression and polycystic kidney disease, and rapamycin therapy for the proteinuria and interstitial damage that accompanies membranous glomerular nephropathy.

Finally, the critical importance of careful control of hyperphosphatemia in the management of patients with renal insufficiency has been established; it is important that practicing internists understand and know how to apply the available dietary and pharmacologic agents.

The next section focuses on selected issues in acute renal failure. HIV-AIDS is now best addressed as a chronic disease. The existence of comorbid conditions and the occurrence of acute renal failure in patients on highly active antiretroviral therapy have been stressed during the past year.

An important finding is that phosphate-containing bowel preparations such as those used for colonoscopy and sigmoidoscopy can cause potentially irreversible renal failure in patients with normal renal function. They should be avoided.

The lack of utility of so-called renal dose dopamine has again been demonstrated. Importantly, the study included here demonstrated no effect of dopamine across a wide range of medical and surgical settings, including cardiac surgery, contrast-induced nephropathy, and nephrotoxin-induced acute renal failure.

The fifth section focuses on selected issues in chronic renal failure and transplantation. The number of patients with CKD has continued to increase. As such, it is important for practitioners to be familiar with the general medical needs of patients with CKD. In addition, the importance of a family history of kidney disease must be stressed, and internists must know how to measure kidney function and when to send patients to a kidney specialist.

There are several types of renal replacement therapy, including peritoneal dialysis, hemodialysis, and renal transplantation. New studies suggest that the long-term survival of patients may be influenced by the modality selected. Given the scarcity of organs, physicians and patients should become familiar with the availability of a paired kidney donation and with the availability of potentially less toxic immunosuppressive agents that may selectively block T-cell activation.

Renee Garrick, MD

30 Metabolic Factors and Renal Disease Progression

Renal Outcomes in High-Risk Hypertensive Patients Treated With an Angiotensin-Converting Enzyme Inhibitor or a Calcium Channel Blocker vs a Diuretic: A Report From the Antihypertensive and Lipid-Lowering Treatment to Prevent Heart Attack Trial (ALLHAT)

Rahman M, for the ALLHAT Collaborative Research Group (Case Western Reserve Univ, Cleveland, Ohio; et al)

Arch Intern Med 165:936-946, 2005 30–1

Background.—This study was performed to determine whether, in high-risk hypertensive patients with a reduced glomerular filtration rate (GFR), treatment with a calcium channel blocker or an angiotensin-converting enzyme inhibitor lowers the incidence of renal disease outcomes compared with treatment with a diuretic.

Methods.—We conducted post hoc analyses of the Antihypertensive and Lipid-Lowering Treatment to Prevent Heart Attack Trial (ALLHAT). Hypertensive participants 55 years or older with at least 1 other coronary heart disease risk factor were randomized to receive chlorthalidone, amlodipine, or lisinopril for a mean of 4.9 years. Renal outcomes were incidence of end-stage renal disease (ESRD) and/or a decrement in GFR of 50% or more from baseline. Baseline GFR, estimated by the simplified Modification of Diet in Renal Disease equation, was stratified into normal or increased (≥90 mL/min per 1.73 m^2, n = 8126), mild reduction (60-89 mL/min per 1.73 m^2, n = 18 109), or moderate-severe reduction (<60 mL/min per 1.73 m^2, n = 5662) in GFR. Each stratum was analyzed for effects of the treatments on outcomes.

Results.—In 448 participants, ESRD developed. Compared with patients taking chlorthalidone, no significant differences occurred in the incidence of ESRD in patients taking amlodipine in the mild (relative risk [RR], 1.47; 95% confidence interval [CI], 0.97-2.23) or moderate-severe (RR, 0.92; 95% CI, 0.68-1.24) reduction in GFR groups. Compared with patients taking chlorthalidone, no significant differences occurred in the incidence of

ESRD in patients taking lisinopril in the mild (RR, 1.34; 95% CI, 0.87-2.06) or moderate-severe (RR, 0.98; 95% CI, 0.73-1.31) reduction in GFR groups. In patients with mild and moderate-severe reduction in GFR, the incidence of ESRD or 50% or greater decrement in GFR was not significantly different in patients treated with chlorthalidone compared with those treated with amlodipine (odds ratios, 0.96 [$P = .74$] and 0.85 [$P = .23$], respectively) and lisinopril (odds ratios, 1.13 [$P = .31$] and 1.00 [$P = .98$], respectively). No difference in treatment effects occurred for either end point for patients taking amlodipine or lisinopril compared with those taking chlorthalidone across the 3 GFR subgroups, either for the total group or for participants with diabetes at baseline. At 4 years of follow-up, estimated GFR was 3 to 6 mL/min per 1.73 m^2 higher in patients assigned to receive amlodipine compared with chlorthalidone, depending on baseline GFR stratum.

Conclusions.—In hypertensive patients with reduced GFR, neither amlodipine nor lisinopril was superior to chlorthalidone in reducing the rate of development of ESRD or a 50% or greater decrement in GFR. Participants assigned to receive amlodipine had a higher GFR than those assigned to receive chlorthalidone, but rates of development of ESRD were not different between the groups.

► This subgroup analysis of the ALLHAT trial suggests that, across the range of GFR from 90 mL/min to 30 ML/min, in hypertensive patients with or without diabetes, amlodipine and lisinopril were not superior to chlorthalidone in slowing the progression of chronic kidney disease.

The design of ALLHAT may explain the differences reported between this and other studies that have suggested that ACEI/ARB are renal-protective, and a first-line therapy in hypertensive patients with proteinuria (over 200 mg/g creatinine), or diabetes.[1-3] Patients in ALLHAT were not stratified for proteinuria. Additionally, chlorthalidone achieved superior blood pressure control during the first 2 years of ALLHAT compared to that achieved with lisinopril, and in African American patients β-blockers were used as second-line therapy, which may have influenced the outcome. As such, this study alone should not alter current practice in proteinuric patients (over 200 mg/g creatinine) with hypertension and/or diabetes. Rather, in these patients best practice may be to add a thiazide-type diuretic (for cardiovascular protection) to ACEI/ARB therapy (for proteinuria protection).

R. Garrick, MD

References

1. Parving HH, Hommel E, Jensen BR, et al: Long-term beneficial effect of ACE inhibition on diabetic nephropathy in normotensive type 1 diabetic patients. *Kidney Int* 60:228-234, 2001.
2. K/DOQI clinical practice guidelines on hypertension and antihypertensive agents in chronic kidney disease. *Am J Kidney Dis* 43:S1-290, 2004.
3. Lewis EJ, Hunsicker LG, Clarke WR, et al: Renoprotective effect of the angiotensin-receptor antagonist irbesartan in patients with nephropathy due to type 2 diabetes. *N Engl J Med* 345:851-860, 2001.

The Effect of a Lower Target Blood Pressure on the Progression of Kidney Disease: Long-term Follow-up of the Modification of Diet in Renal Disease Study

Sarnak MJ, Greene T, Wang X, et al (Tufts-New England Med Ctr, Boston; Cleveland Clinic Found, Ohio; NIH, Bethesda, Md; et al)

Ann Intern Med 142:342-351, 2005 30–2

Background.—Hypertension is a risk factor for progression of chronic kidney disease. The optimal blood pressure to slow progression is unknown.

Objective.—To evaluate the effects of a low target blood pressure on kidney failure and all-cause mortality.

Design.—Long-term follow-up of the Modification of Diet in Renal Disease Study, a randomized, controlled trial conducted from 1989 to 1993.

Setting.—15 outpatient nephrology practices.

Participants.—840 persons with predominantly nondiabetic kidney disease and a glomerular filtration rate of 13 to 55 mL/min per 1.73 m^2.

Intervention.—A low target blood pressure (mean arterial pressure < 92 mm Hg) or a usual target blood pressure (mean arterial pressure < 107 mm Hg).

Measurements.—After the randomized trial was completed, kidney failure (defined as initiation of dialysis or kidney transplantation) and a composite outcome of kidney failure or all-cause mortality were ascertained through 31 December 2000.

Results.—Kidney failure occurred in 554 participants (66%), and the composite outcome occurred in 624 participants (74%). After Cox proportional hazards modeling and intention-to-treat analysis, the adjusted hazard ratios were 0.68 (95% CI, 0.57 to 0.82; $P < 0.001$) for kidney failure and 0.77 (CI, 0.65 to 0.91; $P = 0.0024$) for the composite outcome in the low target blood pressure group compared with the usual target blood pressure group. Evidence was insufficient to conclude that the benefit of a low target blood pressure differed according to the cause of kidney disease, baseline glomerular filtration rate, or degree of proteinuria.

Limitations.—The exact mechanism underlying the benefit of a low target blood pressure is unknown.

Conclusions.—Assignment to a low target blood pressure slowed the progression of nondiabetic kidney disease in patients with a moderately to severely decreased glomerular filtration rate.

► Unlike the previous Ramipril Efficacy in Nephropathy 2(REIN-2) trial, which found no benefit of lower blood pressure (BP) in nondiabetic kidney disease, and the African American Study of Kidney Disease and Hypertension (AASK), which also did demonstrate a renal benefit, this long-term follow-up of the Modification of Diet in Renal Disease (MDRD) trial demonstrates that effective control of the blood pressure (BP)(target mean arterial pressure < 92 mm Hg-130/80 mm Hg) slows the progression of renal disease and reduces mortality, even in patients with moderate and severely reduced renal function. Previous (3-year) MDRD follow-up had suggested that target BP control was most beneficial in patients with proteinuria that exceeded 1 gm/d. This longer follow-up showed that patients with a variety of kidney disorders, including non-diabetics and patients with low-grade proteinuria (under 1 gm/d), can sustain long-term benefit from 2 years of target BP control. Differences in design and length of follow-up may explain the difference between these data and those of the other studies. These long-term data certainly suggest that even patients with advanced renal disease benefit from improved BP control.

R. Garrick, MD

Independent and Additive Impact of Blood Pressure Control and Angiotensin II Receptor Blockade on Renal Outcomes in the Irbesartan Diabetic Nephropathy Trial: Clinical Implications and Limitations

Pohl MA, for the Collaborative Study Group (Cleveland Clinic Found, Ohio; et al)

J Am Soc Nephrol 16:3027-3037, 2005 30–3

Introduction.—Elevated arterial pressure is a major risk factor for progression to ESRD in diabetic nephropathy. However, the component of arterial pressure and level of BP control for optimal renal outcomes are disputed. Data from 1590 hypertensive patients with type 2 diabetes in the Irbesartan Diabetic Nephropathy Trial (IDNT), a randomized, double-blind, placebo-controlled trial performed in 209 clinics worldwide, were examined, and the effects of baseline and mean follow-up systolic BP (SBP) and diastolic BP and the interaction of assigned study medications (irbesartan, amlodipine, and placebo) on progressive renal failure and all-cause mortality were assessed. Other antihypertensive agents were added to achieve predetermined BP goals. Entry criteria included elevated baseline serum creatinine concentration up to 266 μmol/L (3.0 mg/dl) and urine protein excretion >900 mg/d. Baseline BP averaged 159/87 ± 20/11 mmHg. Median patient follow-up was 2.6 yr. Follow-up achieved SBP most strongly predicted renal outcomes. SBP >149 mmHg was associated with a 2.2-fold increase in the risk for doubling serum creatinine or ESRD compared with SBP <134 mmHg. Progressive lowering of SBP to 120 mmHg was associated with improved renal and patient survival, an effect independent of baseline renal function. Below this threshold, all-cause mortality increased. An additional renoprotective effect of irbesartan, independent of achieved SBP, was observed down to 120 mmHg. There was no correlation between diastolic BP and renal outcomes. We recommend a SBP target between 120 and 130 mmHg, in conjunction with blockade of the renin-angiotensin system, in patients with type 2 diabetic nephropathy.

► The optimal blood pressure (BP) level in this high-risk patient population continues to be defined. A previous meta-analysis in non-diabetics with proteinuria over 1 gm/d showed that a systolic BP between 110 and 129 mm Hg was reno-protective and that lower systolic levels might worsen the rate of progression of renal disease.[1] The current study in high-risk diabetics demonstrated an increase in all-cause mortality with systolic levels below 120 mm Hg. A systolic BP of 120 to 30 mm Hg with renin-angiotensin blockade appears a reasonable goal in diabetics with proteinuria of about 1 g/d or greater.

R. Garrick, MD

Reference

1. Jafar TH, Stark PC, Schmid CH, et al: Progression of chronic kidney disease: The role of blood pressure control, proteinuria, and angiotensin-converting enzyme inhibition: A patient-level meta-analysis. *Ann Intern Med* 139:244-252, 2003.

Apolipoprotein E and Progression of Chronic Kidney Disease

Hsu CC, Kao WHL, Coresh J, et al (Johns Hopkins Med Institutions, Baltimore, Md; Univ of Minnesota School of Public Health, Minneapolis; Univ of Texas—Houston Health Science Ctr)

JAMA 293:2892-2899, 2005 30–4

Context.—Apolipoprotein E (APOE) genetic variation has been implicated in diabetic nephropathy with the ϵ2 allele increasing and the ϵ4 allele decreasing risk. APOE allelic associations with chronic kidney disease beyond diabetic nephropathy are unknown, with no studies reported in high-risk African American populations.

Objective.—To quantify the risk of chronic kidney disease progression associated with APOE in a population-based study including white, African American, diabetic, and nondiabetic individuals.

Design, Setting, and Participants.—Prospective follow-up (through January 1, 2003) of Atherosclerosis Risk in Communities (ARIC) study participants, including 3859 African American and 10,661 white adults aged 45 to 64 years without severe renal dysfunction at baseline in 1987-1989, sampled from 4 US communities.

Main Outcome Measures.—Incident chronic kidney disease progression, defined as hospitalization or death with kidney disease or increase in serum creatinine level of 0.4 mg/dL (35 μmol/L) or more above baseline, examined by APOE genotypes and alleles.

Results.—During median follow-up of 14 years, chronic kidney disease progression developed in 1060 individuals (incidence per 1000 person-years: 5.5 overall; 8.8 in African Americans and 4.4 in whites). Adjusting for major chronic kidney disease risk factors, ϵ2 moderately increased and ϵ4 decreased risk of disease progression (likelihood ratio test, $P = .03$). Further adjustment for low- and high-density lipoprotein cholesterol and triglycerides did not attenuate relative risks (RRs) (ϵ2: 1.08 [95% CI, 093-1.25] and ϵ4: 0.85 [95% CI, 0.75-0.95] compared with ϵ3; likelihood ratio test, $P = .008$). ϵ4 decreased risk of end-stage renal disease (RR, 0.60 [95% CI, 0.43-0.84]). ϵ2 was associated with a decline in renal function (RR, 1.25 [95% CI, 1.02-1.53]), though not with events, such as hospitalizations or end-stage renal disease. Risks were similar stratified by race, sex, diabetes, and hypertension (all *P* values for interaction >.05). Excess risk of chronic kidney disease in African Americans was not explained by APOE alleles.

Conclusions.—APOE variation predicts chronic kidney disease progression, independent of diabetes, race, lipid, and nonlipid risk factors. Our study suggests that nonlipid-mediated pathways, such as cellular mechanisms of kidney remodeling, may be involved in the association of APOE alleles and progression of chronic kidney disease.

► This is perhaps the first large, community-population based longitudinal study to examine the association between APOE and chronic kidney disease (CKD) progression. Several aspects of the study are noteworthy. The results confirm that the ε2 allele of APOE predicts CKD progression, but suggest that alterations in the ε2 APOE allele are unlikely to explain the increased risk of CKD in African Americans. The consistency of this allele effect from participants with and without diabetes, and/or hypertension, is in keeping with the notion that the pathogenesis of CKD is multifactorial, but shares common pathways, across many different disease categories. And, the fact that the ε2 allele effect is of similar magnitude but opposite direction from that seen in coronary heart disease suggests that APOE variation may affect CKD progression through novel cellular pathways. The finding that APOE is expressed in the kidney and that the allele isoforms differentially affect mesangial cell proliferation is particularly intriguing.[1] Although the ε2 allele effect seen here is too small to allow it to be used as a predictor for progression for an individual patient, it may be that ultimately, as more information regarding the specificity of various genes becomes available, such screening panels will be possible.

R. Garrick, MD

Reference

1. Chen G, Paka L, Kaka Y: Protective role for kidney apolipoprotein E: Regulation of mesangial cell proliferation and matrix expansion. *J Biol Chem* 276:49142-49147, 2001.

Obesity and Prevalent and Incident CKD: The Hypertension Detection and Follow-up Program

Kramer H, Luke A, Bidani A, et al (Loyola Med Ctr, Maywood, IL; Florida State Univ, Tallahassee)

Am J Kidney Dis 46:587-594, 2005 30–5

Background.—Obesity is associated with increased single-nephron glomerular filtration rate, which may increase the risk for chronic kidney disease (CKD), especially when combined with hypertension. However, epidemiological data supporting an association between overweight and obesity and risk for CKD currently are limited.

Methods.—We used data from the Hypertension Detection and Follow-Up Program (HDFP) to test the hypothesis that overweight and obesity are associated with incident CKD in 5,897 hypertensive adults. Serum and spot urine samples were collected at baseline and year 5. CKD is defined as the presence of 1^+ or greater proteinuria on routine urinalysis and/or an estimated glomerular filtration rate less than 60 mL/min/1.73 m^2 (<1.0 mL/s).

Results.—In HDFP participants without CKD at baseline, the incidence of CKD at year 5 was 28% in the ideal-body-mass-index group, 31% in the overweight group, and 34% in the obese group. After adjustment for all covariates, including diabetes mellitus, mean baseline diastolic blood pressure, and slope of diastolic blood pressure, both baseline overweight (odds ratio [OR], 1.21; 95% confidence interval [CI], 1.05 to 1.41) and obesity (OR, 1.40; 95% CI, 1.20 to 1.63) were associated with increased odds of incident CKD at year 5. Similar results were noted after exclusion of participants with baseline diabetes mellitus, with both overweight (OR, 1.22; 95% CI, 1.05 to 1.43) and obesity (OR, 1.38; 95% CI, 1.17 to 1.63) remaining significantly associated with incident CKD.

Conclusion.—These results suggest that obese adults with hypertension have an increased risk for CKD.

► Several factors associated with obesity, including an increase in single-nephron glomerular filtration rate (GFR) with associated glomerular hyperfiltration and secondary glomerulosclerosis, and obesity and hypertension-induced overactivity of the sympathetic nervous and renin-angiotensin systems, I suggest that obesity per se might be a risk factor for CKD. Using the HDFP database, the present study tries to better define the associated risk between obesity and CKD. When other covariates were controlled, the incidence of CKD (defined as a GFR <60 and +1 proteinuria at year 5) was increased from 28% in the ideal body mass index (BMI) group to 34% in the obese BMI group. This study is among the first to try to quantify this risk. Given the impending obesity epidemic, it seems likely that this risk will contribute to the growing incidence of CKD unless we are able to make significant lifestyle changes. Furthermore, obesity counseling should include information regarding the risk of developing CKD.

M. Brogan, MD

Relationship of Office, Home, and Ambulatory Blood Pressure to Blood Glucose and Lipid Variables in the PAMELA Population

Mancia G, Facchetti R, Bombelli M, et al (Università Milano-Bicocca, Milan, Italy; Istituto Auxologico Italiano, Milan, Italy; Ospedale Maggiore, Milan, Italy)

Hypertension 45:1072-1077, 2005 30–6

Introduction.—Alterations in blood glucose and cholesterol are more frequently detectable in hypertensive than in normotensive conditions. However, no information exists as to whether this phenomenon involves only office or also home and 24-hour ambulatory blood pressure (ie, when values are representative of daily life). In 2045 subjects enrolled in the Pressioni Arteriose Monitorate E Loro Associazioni (PAMELA) study, we measured home, 24-hour, and office blood pressure. Measurements also included fasting blood glucose and serum total and HDL cholesterol values. Prevalence of diabetes (≥126 mg/dL or use of antidiabetic drugs), impaired fasting blood glucose (≥110 to <126 mg/dL), and hypercholesterolemia (serum total cholesterol ≥240 mg/dL or 200 mg/dL) increased progressively from "optimal" to "normal," "high-normal," and "elevated" office systolic or diastolic blood pressure. Fasting blood glucose and total serum cholesterol also increased progressively from the first to the fourth group, with HDL cholesterol values showing a concomitant progressive decrease. This was also the case for quartiles of office, home, and 24-hour blood pressure. In the whole population, there was a positive correlation between serum cholesterol or blood glucose and all blood pressure values (*P* always <0.0001), with a much smaller and less consistent relationship with heart rate. In a multivariate analysis that included gender, body mass index, age, and antihypertensive treatment, all blood pressure values remained highly significantly related to values of either metabolic variables. Thus, in the PAMELA population, glucose and lipid values are independently related to blood pressure. This is also the case when daily life blood pressure values are considered.

► These findings offer a very interesting insight into the metabolic syndrome. This large Milan population–based study showed that home blood pressure (BP) measurements and ambulatory (real life values) do track with office BP determinations, and that BP elevation is separately related to changes in the lipids and glucose. The implication of causality between BP elevations and resultant changes in lipids and glucose is certainly intriguing. If substantiated, it would provide further evidence of the value and need of BP control.

R. Garrick, MD

Essential Hypertension, Progressive Renal Disease, and Uric Acid: A Pathogenetic Link?

Johnson RJ, Segal MS, Srinivas T, et al (Univ of Florida, Gainesville; Instituto Nacional de Cardiología "Ignacio Chávez," Mexico City; Hosp Universitario and Instituto de Investigaciones Biomédicas, Maracaibo, Venezuela; et al)

J Am Soc Nephrol 16:1909-1919, 2005 30–7

Introduction.—Hypertension and hypertension-associated ESRD are epidemic in society. The mechanisms responsible for renal progression in mild to moderate hypertension and those groups most at risk need to be identified. Historic, epidemiologic, clinical, and experimental studies on the pathogenesis of hypertension and hypertension-associated renal disease are reviewed and an overview/hypothesis for the mechanisms involved in renal progression is presented. There is increasing evidence that hypertension may exist in one of two forms/stages. The first stage, most commonly observed in early or borderline hypertension, is characterized by salt-resistance, normal or only slightly decreased GFR, relatively normal or mild renal arteriolosclerosis, and normal renal autoregulation. This group is at minimal risk for renal progression. The second stage, characterized by salt-sensitivity, renal arteriolar disease, and blunted renal autoregulation, defines a group at highest risk for the development of microalbuminuria, albuminuria, and progressive renal disease. This second stage is more likely to be observed in blacks, in subjects with gout or hyperuricemia, with low level lead intoxication, or with severe obesity/metabolic syndrome. The two major mechanistic pathways for causing impaired autoregulation at mild to moderate elevations in BP appear to be hyperuricemia and/or low nephron number. Understanding the pathogenetic pathways mediating renal progression in hypertensive subjects should help identify those subjects at highest risk and may provide insights into new therapeutic maneuvers to slow or prevent progression.

► The authors review the pathology and pathophysiology of the spectrum of hypertension and renal disease. The stages of hypertension, the role of interstitial renal inflammation, and the possible clinical significance of uric acid levels are reviewed. These uric acid data are of particular interest, as the prevalence of diuretic-induced hyperuricemia will likely increase as the use of these drugs in hypertension, cardiovascular disease, and renal disease continues to increase.

R. Garrick, MD

Cystatin C Concentration as a Risk Factor for Heart Failure in Older Adults

Sarnak MJ, for the Cardiovascular Health Study (Tufts-New England Med Ctr, Boston; et al)

Ann Intern Med 142:497-505, 2005 30–8

Background.—Previous studies that evaluated the association of kidney function with incident heart failure may be limited by the insensitivity of serum creatinine concentration for detecting abnormal kidney function.

Objective.—To compare serum concentrations of cystatin C (a novel marker of kidney function) and creatinine as predictors of incident heart failure.

Design.—Observational study based on measurement of serum cystatin C from frozen sera obtained at the 1992-1993 visit of the Cardiovascular Health Study. Follow-up occurred every 6 months.

Setting.—Adults 65 years of age or older from 4 communities in the United States.

Participants.—4384 persons without previous heart failure who had measurements of serum cystatin C and serum creatinine.

Measurements.—Incident heart failure.

Results.—The mean (±SD) serum concentrations of cystatin C and creatinine were 82 ± 25 nmol/L (1.10 ± 0.33 mg/L) and 89 ± 34 μmol/L (1.01 ± 0.39 mg/dL), respectively. During a median follow-up of 8.3 years (maximum, 9.1 years), 763 (17%) participants developed heart failure. After adjustment for demographic factors, traditional and novel cardiovascular risk factors, cardiovascular disease status, and medication use, sequential quintiles of cystatin C concentration were associated with a stepwise increased risk for heart failure in Cox proportional hazards models (hazard ratios, 1.0 [reference], 1.30 [95% CI, 0.96 to 1.75], 1.44 [CI, 1.07 to 1.94], 1.58 [CI, 1.18 to 2.12], and 2.16 [CI, 1.61 to 2.91]). In contrast, quintiles of serum creatinine concentration were not associated with risk for heart failure in adjusted analysis (hazard ratios, 1.0 [reference], 0.77 [CI, 0.59 to 101], 0.85 [CI, 0.64 to 1.13], 0.97 [CI, 0.72 to 1.29], and 1.14 [CI, 0.87 to 1.49]).

Limitations.—The mechanism by which cystatin C concentration predicts risk for heart failure remains unclear.

Conclusions.—The cystatin C concentration is an independent risk factor for heart failure in older adults and appears to provide a better measure of risk assessment than the serum creatinine concentration. *For a full list of participating Cardiovascular Health Study investigators and institutions, see http://www.chs-nhlbi.org.

▶ Cohort studies, including subpopulation studies from the Antihypertensive and Lipid-Lowering Treatment to Prevent Heart Attack Trial (ALLHAT) and Valsartan in Acute Myocardial Infarction Trial (VALIANT) have demonstrated that even mild to moderate chronic kidney disease (CKD) (glomerular filtration rate [GRF] 30-59 mL/min)[1-3] increases the risk for adverse cardiovascular events and mortality. For early intervention to occur, markers of renal function need to be sensitive, easy to use and understand, and widely available. Serum creatinine is altered by factors such as age, race, and muscle mass, and alone is an insensitive marker of renal function. Derivative equations such as Cockcroft-Gault[4] and the Modification of Diet in Renal Disease equation (MDRD) are more sensitive, but both are based on creatinine, and both have limitations. Cystatin C data need to be confirmed against a gold standard measurement for GRF. If confirmed, cystatin-C may prove to be a better measurement of renal function than those currently in use. But no matter what technique is used, education regarding early detection of renal disease and appropriate intervention remains paramount.

R. Garrick, MD

References

1. Go AS, Chertow GM, Fan D, et al: Chronic kidney disease and the risks of death, cardiovascular events, and hospitalization. *N Engl J Med* 351:1296-1305, 2004.
2. Rahman M, Pressel S, Davis BR, et al: Renal outcomes in high-risk hypertensive patients treated with an angiotensin-converting enzyme inhibitor or a calcium channel blocker vs a diuretic: A report from the Antihypertensive and Lipid-Lowering Treatment to Prevent Heart Attack Trial (ALLHAT). *Arch Intern Med* 165:936-946, 2005.
3. Anavekar NS, McMurray JJ, Velazquez EJ, et al: Relation between renal dysfunction and cardiovascular outcomes after myocardial infarction. *N Engl J Med* 351:1285-1295, 2004.
4. Cockcroft DW, Gault MH: Prediction of creatinine clearance from serum creatinine. *Nephron* 16:31-41, 1976.

B-Type Natriuretic Peptide (BNP) and Amino-Terminal proBNP in Patients With CKD: Relationship to Renal Function and Left Ventricular Hypertrophy

Vickery S, Price CP, John RI, et al (East Kent Hospitals Natl Health Service Trust, Canterbury, England; Bayer HealthCare, Newbury, England)

Am J Kidney Dis 46:610-620, 2005 30–9

Background.—Most patients with chronic kidney disease (CKD) develop cardiovascular complications. Natriuretic peptides are novel markers that can be used to identify and monitor heart failure, but the effect of renal disease on these markers is not fully understood. The aim of the present study is to explore the relationship among circulating B-type natriuretic peptide (BNP) and N-terminal proBNP (NT-proBNP) concentrations and clinical variables in a cohort of patients with CKD.

Methods.—Plasma BNP and NT-proBNP concentrations and left ventricular (LV) mass index were measured in 213 predialysis patients with CKD.

Results.—Plasma BNP and NT-proBNP concentrations increased with declining estimated glomerular filtration rate (GFR; $P < 0.0001$). Estimated GFR had an independent effect on plasma BNP ($P = 0.0028$) and, to a greater extent, plasma NT-proBNP ($P < 0.0001$) concentrations: mean BNP concentration increased by 20.6% per 10-mL/min/1.73 m^2 (017-mL/s) reduction in estimated GFR compared with 37.7% for NT-proBNP. NT-proBNP/BNP ratio increased with CKD stage ($P < 0.0001$). Median plasma BNP and NT-proBNP concentrations were greater in patients with LV hypertrophy ($P < 0.0001$), and LV mass index had an independent effect on both BNP ($P = 0.0223$) and NT-proBNP ($P < 0.0017$).

Conclusion.—Estimated GFR and LV mass index have independent effects on both plasma BNP and NT-proBNP concentrations in patients with CKD. NT-proBNP appears to be affected more by declining kidney function, in keeping with the hypothesis that its clearance is predominantly renal. Our data have significant implications for application of these peptides as cardiac biomarkers in patients with CKD.

► It is often difficult to elucidate the relative contribution of LV hypertrophy (LVH), fluid overload, and LV dysfunction to high levels of BNP in predialysis and dialysis patients. This study showed that mild elevations in levels of BNP can occur solely due to LVH and varying degrees of reduction in GFR. Unlike similar studies done in the past, LV ejection fraction was documented in nearly half of the studied patients, excluding the possibility of undiagnosed heart failure. It also supports prior studies showing that endogenous renal clearance of these peptides is limited, and that very high levels of BNP are unlikely to be primarily due to reduced GFR.

F. Tedla, MD

31 Lipid Therapy in Chronic Kidney Disease and Transplantation

---

Long-term Cardiac Outcomes in Renal Transplant Recipients Receiving Fluvastatin: The ALERT Extension Study

Holdaas H, for the Assessment of LEscol in Renal Transplantation (ALERT) Study Investigators (Rikshospitalet, Oslo, Norway; et al)

Am J Transplant 5:2929-2936, 2005 31–1

Introduction.—Renal transplant recipients (RTR) have an increased risk of premature cardiovascular disease. The ALERT study is the first trial to evaluate the effect of statin therapy on cardiac outcomes following renal transplantation. Patients initially randomized to fluvastatin or placebo in the 5-6 year ALERT study were offered open-label fluvastatin XL 80 mg/day in a 2-year extension to the original study. The primary endpoint was time to first major adverse cardiac event (MACE). Of 1787 patients who completed ALERT, 1652 (92%) were followed in the extension. Mean total follow-up was 6.7 years. Mean LDL-cholesterol was 98 mg/dL (2.5 mmol/L) at last follow-up compared to a pre-study level of 159 mg/dL (4.1 mmol/L). Patients randomized to fluvastatin had a reduced risk of MACE (hazards ratio [HR] 0.79, 95% CI 0.63-0.99, $p = 0.036$), and a 29% reduction in cardiac death or definite non-fatal MI (HR 0.71, 95% CI 0.55-0.93, $p = 0.014$). Total mortality and graft loss did not differ significantly between groups. Fluvastatin produces a safe and effective reduction in LDL-cholesterol associated with reduced risk of MACE in RTR. The lipid-lowering and cardiovascular benefits of fluvastatin are comparable to those of statins in other patient groups, and support use of fluvastatin in RTR.

► An extension of a negative controlled clinical trial, this is the first study to demonstrate that statin therapy reduces the risk of major adverse cardiac events in renal transplant recipients. This study illustrates other facets of clinical studies in addition to its primary finding. First, it questions the applicability of established therapy to a unique subset of patients. The authors emphasize that the known risk of drug interactions in renal transplant recipients could have unfavorably tipped the risk-benefit scale. Second, it underlines the importance of adequate duration of follow-up, since the advantage of treatment did not become apparent until well after the initial 5 years. Third, it raises the ethical dilemma of withholding therapy that has been proven to be effective under different circumstances.

F. Tedla, MD

Atorvastatin in Patients With Type 2 Diabetes Mellitus Undergoing Hemodialysis

Wanner C, for the German Diabetes and Dialysis Study Investigators (Univ of Würzburg, Germany; et al)

N Engl J Med 353:238-248, 2005 31–2

Background.—Statins reduce the incidence of cardiovascular events in persons with type 2 diabetes mellitus. However, the benefit of statins in such patients receiving hemodialysis, who are at high risk for cardiovascular disease and death, has not been examined.

Methods.—We conducted a multicenter, randomized, double-blind, prospective study of 1255 subjects with type 2 diabetes mellitus receiving maintenance hemodialysis who were randomly assigned to receive 20 mg of atorvastatin per day or matching placebo. The primary end point was a composite of death from cardiac causes, nonfatal myocardial infarction, and stroke. Secondary end points included death from all causes and all cardiac and cerebrovascular events combined.

Results.—After four weeks of treatment, the median level of low-density lipoprotein cholesterol was reduced by 42 percent among patients receiving atorvastatin, and among those receiving placebo it was reduced by 1.3 percent. During a median follow-up period of four years, 469 patients (37 percent) reached the primary end point, of whom 226 were assigned to atorvastatin and 243 to placebo (relative risk, 0.92; 95 percent confidence interval, 0.77 to 1.10; P=0.37). Atorvastatin had no significant effect on the individual components of the primary end point, except that the relative risk of fatal stroke among those receiving the drug was 2.03 (95 percent confidence interval, 1.05 to 3.93; P=0.04). Atorvastatin reduced the rate of all cardiac events combined (relative risk, 0.82; 95 percent confidence interval, 0.68 to 0.99; P=0.03, nominally significant) but not all cerebrovascular events combined (relative risk, 1.12; 95 percent confidence interval, 0.81 to 1.55; P=0.49) or total mortality (relative risk, 0.93; 95 percent confidence interval, 0.79 to 1.08; P=0.33).

Conclusions.—Atorvastatin had no statistically significant effect on the composite primary end point of cardiovascular death, nonfatal myocardial infarction, and stroke in patients with diabetes receiving hemodialysis.

► Statin therapy for hyperlipidemic diabetics is so widely accepted that it is likely many physicians would question doing a placebo-controlled trial, as was done here, in a group of patients with type 2 diabetes who received dialysis with low-density lipoprotein levels up to 190 mg/dL. However, in this especially high-risk group that was studied for a median of 4 years, no benefit of statin treatment was found on the primary end point of death from cardiac causes, nonfatal myocardial infarction, and stroke. Indeed, there was an increase in the risk of fatal stroke, although the total mortality rate was unchanged. For these patients, it may be too late to receive the benefits of statin therapy, pointing up the importance of early diagnosis and treatment, and perhaps even more importantly, not generalizing from studies in very different populations.

S. Adler, MD

Effect of Pravastatin on Loss of Renal Function in People with Moderate Chronic Renal Insufficiency and Cardiovascular Disease

Tonelli M, for the Cholesterol and Recurrent Events (CARE) Trial Investigators (Univ of Alberta, Edmonton, Canada; et al)

J Am Soc Nephrol 14:1605-1613, 2003 31–3

Introduction.—Limited data suggest that HMG-CoA reductase inhibitors (statins) may slow loss of renal function in individuals with chronic renal insufficiency. This study was conducted to determine whether pravastatin reduced rates of loss of renal function in people with moderate chronic renal insufficiency. This was a post hoc subgroup analysis of a randomized double-blind placebo controlled trial. Data were analyzed from the CARE study (a randomized trial of pravastatin *versus* placebo in 4159 participants with previous myocardial infarction and total plasma cholesterol < 240 mg/dl). Participants with estimated GFR (MDRD-GFR) < 60 ml/min per 1.73 m^2 body surface area at baseline were considered to have moderate chronic renal insufficiency. Multivariate regression was used to calculate rates of decline in MDRD-GFR for individuals receiving pravastatin and placebo, controlling for prospectively determined covariates that might influence rates of renal function loss. Change in renal function could be calculated in 3384 individuals, of whom 690 (20.4%) had MDRD-GFR < 60 ml/min per 1.73 m^2 and were eligible for inclusion. Among all individuals with MDRD-GFR < 60 ml/min per 1.73 m^2, the MDRD-GFR decline in the pravastatin group was not significantly different from that in the placebo group (0.1 ml/min per 1.73 m^2/yr slower; 95% CI, −0.2 to 0.4; $P = 0.49$). However, there was a significant stepwise inverse relation between MDRD-GFR before treatment and slowing of renal function loss with pravastatin use, with more benefit in those with lower MDRD-GFR at baseline ($P = 0.04$). Rate of change in MDRD-GFR in the pravastatin group was 0.6 ml/min per 1.73 m^2/yr slower than placebo (95% CI, −0.1 to 1.2; $P = 0.07$) in those with MDRD-GFR < 50 ml/min, and 2.5 ml/min per 1.73 m^2/yr slower (95% CI, 1.4 to 3.6 slower; $P = 0.0001$) in those with MDRD-GFR < 40 ml/min per 1.73 $m^2$2/yr. Pravastatin also reduced rates of renal loss to a greater extent in participants with than without proteinuria at baseline ($P = 0.006$). It is concluded that pravastatin may slow renal function loss in individuals with moderate to severe kidney disease, especially those with proteinuria. These findings require confirmation by a large randomized trial conducted specifically in people with chronic renal insufficiency.

▶ Although statin treatment was disappointing in diabetic patients already on dialysis, this study examined its benefits in patients with stage 2 and 3 chronic kidney disease (CKD)(glomerular filtration rate [GFR] 30-89 mL/min). These patients already have severely increased cardiovascular risk compared with diabetic patients with normal renal function. The good news is that in this population, compared with those already on dialysis, a statin reduced the time to myocardial infarction, coronary death, or coronary revascularization. Whether this intervention will work in those with more severe CKD who are not yet on dialysis still needs to be studied, but diabetics who do not yet have severe CKD should definitely be treated.

S. Adler, MD

32 Glomerular Diseases and Renal Injury

Introduction

The renal glomerulus has both parietal and visceral epithelial cells. The parietal cells line the inner surface of Bowman's capsule. The visceral glomerular epithelial cells or podocytes form a critical component of the glomerular filtration membrane. Podocytes are intimately associated with the basal lamina of the glomerular capillary. Interdigitating foot processes of the podocyte come together to form a filtration slit. This slit is then covered by a split diaphragm, which is composed of a number of surface proteins. This filtration barrier prevents the entry of large macromolecules such as proteins and permits smaller molecules such as water, urea, and electrolytes to enter the urinary space to form an ultrafiltrate, which is modified by the tubules and excreted as the final urine. Damage to the podocyte, or the slit membrane, or diaphragm can lead to proteinuria and the nephrotic syndrome.

Renee Garrick, MD

Permanent Genetic Tagging of Podocytes: Fate of Injured Podocytes in a Mouse Model of Glomerular Sclerosis

Asano T, Niimura F, Pastan I, et al (Tokai Univ School of Medicine, Isehara, Kanagawa, Japan; Vanderbilt Univ Med Ctr, Nashville, Tenn; Tokyo Med and Dental Univ, Bunkyo, Tokyo, Japan; et al)

J Am Soc Nephrol 16:2257-2262, 2005 32–1

Introduction.—Injured podocytes lose differentiation markers. Therefore, the true identity of severely injured podocytes remains unverified. A transgenic mouse model equipped with a podocyte-selective injury induction system was established. After induction of podocyte injury, mice rapidly developed glomerulosclerosis, with downregulation of podocyte marker proteins. Proliferating epithelial cells accumulated within Bowman's space, as seen in collapsing glomerulosclerosis. In this study, the fate of injured podocytes was pursued. Utilizing Cre-loxP recombination, the podocyte lineage was genetically labeled with lacZ in an irreversible manner. After podocyte injury, the number of lacZ-labeled cells, which were often negative for synaptopodin, progressively declined, correlating with glomerular damage. Parietal epithelial cells, but not lacZ-labeled podocytes, avidly proliferated. The cells proliferating within Bowman's capsule and, occasionally, on the outer surface of the glomerular basement membrane were lacZ-negative. Thus, when podocytes are severely injured, proliferating parietal epithelial cells migrate onto the visceral site, thereby mimicking proliferating podocytes.

▶ These investigators studied a transgenic mouse model of selective podocyte injury, which is followed by secondary proteinuria and eventual glomerulosclerosis, to specifically study the effects of podocyte injury. In the current studies, they developed a permanent podocyte genetic tagging system that allowed them to definitively track the fate of the injured podocytes and the origin of the cells that proliferate post-injury. Using this model, they have clearly demonstrated that severely injured epithelial podocytes do not proliferate. Rather, proliferating parietal epithelial cells migrate onto the visceral site and continue to proliferate in that location. In this model, the visceral podocytes are not transformed to other cell types, and do not proliferate after injury.

R. Garrick, MD

Hepatocyte Growth Factor and Its Receptor Met Are Induced in Cresentic Glomerulonephritis

Rampino T, Gregorini M, Camussi G, et al (IRCCS Policlinico San Matteo and Univ, Pavia, Italy; Univ of Torino, Turin, Italy; Univ of Insubria, Varese, Italy)

Nephrol Dial Transplant 20:1066-1074, 2005 32–2

Background.—In experimental extracapillary glomerulonephritis (EG) podocytes migrate, proliferate and change phenotype, and play a pivotal role in crescent formation. Hepatocyte Growth Factor (HGF) is an injury-induced effector of tissue repair that causes cell migration, growth and transdifferentiation via its receptor Met.

Methods.—In 11 patients with EG we measured serum levels of HGF and investigated whether serum induces the release of HGF by Peripheral Blood Mononuclear Cells (PBMC). In renal biopsies we studied the expression of Met. In cultured podocytes we studied Met expression, migration, growth and morphological changes induced by recombinant (r) HGF.

Results.—In patients with EG average serum levels of HGF (0.73 ng/ml) were higher than in normal volunteers (N, 0.10 ng/ml, $p<0.01$) and in patients with non-crescentic glomerular disease (GD, 0.18 ng/ml, $p<0.01$). Serum of EG induced a significant HGF release by PBMC (mean 0.58 ng/ml) in comparison with serum of N and GD (0.07 and 0.06 ng/ml, respectively, both $p<0.001$). Met was strongly expressed in crescents. Cultured podocytes expressed Met, and rHGF induced in podocytes a time- and dose-dependent migration, growth and epithelial to mesenchymal transdifferentiation.

Conclusions.—These results suggest that HGF/Met system participates in the process of crescent formation by inducing podocyte migration, growth and mesenchymal transformation.

► Rampino and colleagues studied cultured podocytes (from a human podocytes line) exposed to HGF, an injury-induced factor that causes cell migration, growth, and transdifferentiation via its Met receptor. They demonstrated that HGF and its Met receptor are increased in patients with crescentic EG, and that after exposure to HGF, cultured podocytes expressed the Met receptor and underwent migration, growth, and epithelia-mesenchymal transformation.

The Asano model[1] is a noninflammatory model of podocytes injury and demonstrated proliferating parietal cells mimicked proliferating podocytes. The EC crescentic model of Rampino and the anti-GBM model of Moeller et al[2], which also suggested that some of the crescentic cells originated from visceral podocytes, are inflammatory models. Thus, the model of injury or the injury process itself may influence the podocyte response.

R. Garrick, MD

Reference

1. Asano T, Niimura F, Pastan I, et al: Permanent genetic tagging of podocytes: Fate of injured podocytes in a mouse model of glomerular sclerosis. *J Am Soc Nephrol* 16:2257-2262, 2005.
2. Moeller MJ, Soofi A, Hartmann I, et al: Podocytes populate cellular crescents in a murine model of inflammatory glomerulonephritis. *J Am Soc Nephrol* 15:61-67, 2004.

Insulin-like Growth Factors Inhibit Podocyte Apoptosis Through the P13 Kinase Pathway

Bridgewater DJ, Ho J, Sauro V, et al (Univ of Western Ontario, London, Canada; Univ of British Columbia, Vancouver, Canada)
Kidney Int 67:1308-1314, 2005 32–3

Background.—Abnormal podocyte development and progressive podocyte injury have been implicated in a number of human kidney diseases. Factors necessary for regulating development and maintenance of this cell type are only beginning to emerge.

Methods.—To study the role of the insulin-like growth factor (IGF) system in regulating podocyte survival, we induced human fetal podocytes to undergo apoptosis. We demonstrated a significant increase in apoptosis when these cells were incubated in the presence of etoposide, as measured by DNA fragmentation and nuclear membrane condensation and blebbing.

Results.—Podocyte apoptosis was reduced to control levels when the cells were coincubated in the presence of IGF-1. We showed that the protective effect of IGFs in this cell type was mediated through the activation of the phosphatidylinositol 3'-kinase (PI3K) pathway. IGF-1 stimulation resulted in the formation of the insulin receptor substrate (IRS)-1-p85 complex, an increase in PI3 kinase activity, and activation of protein kinase B (AKT/PKB) and the bcl-2 family member bad. Incubation of the podocytes with inhibitors of the PI3 kinase pathway resulted in a loss of this IGF-1 protective effect.

Conclusion.—These data demonstrate an important role for the IGF system in fetal podocyte survival in vitro, and suggest potential mediators to slow or alleviate the loss or damage of the podocyte in progressive renal disease.

► Bridgewater and colleagues demonstrated that they can inhibit podocyte apoptosis via the IGF through the PI3K pathway. Given the pivotal role of the podocytes in glomerular injury and sclerosis, the ability to potentially chemically alter podocyte apoptosis could lead to interventions that might slow the progression of renal injury.

R. Garrick, MD

A Mutation in the TRPC6 Cation Channel Causes Familial Focal Segmental Glomerulosclerosis

Winn MP, Conlin PJ, Lynn KL, et al (Duke Univ, Durham, NC; Beaumont Hosp, Dublin; Christchurch Hosp, New Zealand)

Science 308:1801-1804, 2005 32–4

Background.—Focal and segmental glomerulosclerosis (FSGS) is a major cause of end-stage renal disease, and up to 20% of dialysis patients have been diagnosed with this disease. There has been an annual increase in the prevalence of FSGS, with a particularly high incidence in the black population. FSGS typically manifests with proteinuria, renal insufficiency, hypertension, and eventual kidney failure. The etiology of FSGS is unknown, and no consistently effective treatments have been identified. However, the analysis of disease-causing mutations in hereditary FSGS and congenital nephrotic syndromes has provided new insights into the pathogenesis of nephrotic syndrome. Previous studies have identified at least 3 genes causing familial FSGS and hereditary nephrotic syndromes and have underscored the substantial genetic heterogeneity in FSGS. The present study was conducted in a large family with hereditary FSGS.

Overview.—It was determined that a missense mutation in the transient receptor potential cation channel 6 (*TRPC6*) gene on chromosome 11q was present in this family. It was speculated that the exaggerated calcium signaling prompted by the TRPC6 mutation disrupts glomerular cell function or causes apoptosis. It was also speculated that the mutant protein may amplify injurious signals triggered by ligands such as angiotensin II, which promote kidney injury and proteinuria. In contrast to persons with Finnish nephropathy and steroid-resistant nephrotic syndrome, who typically develop proteinuria in utero or at birth, renal disease does not manifest clinically until the third decade in persons with the TRPC6 mutation. This difference in onset may be reflective of the difference between these recessive disorders and the autosomal-dominant inheritance in the family described in this report.

Conclusions.—*TRPC6* was identified as a disease gene causing hereditary FSGS. It is suggested from these results that *TRPC6* may be useful as a therapeutic target for the treatment of chronic kidney disease.

► Distinct from the podocyte protein mutations that have been previously described in hereditary FSGS, this study has identified a novel ion channel mutation in a large family kindred with hereditary FSGS. The findings suggest that this channel mutation causes an alteration in calcium signaling with secondary disruption of glomerular function and cellular apoptosis. The possibility that the mutant protein may amplify angiotensin II with secondary cell injury suggests that, like other ion-channel disorders, some cases of familial FSGS may be amenable to pharmacologic therapies.

M. Brogan, MD

Restoration of Tubular Epithelial Cells During Repair of the Postischemic Kidney Occurs Independently of Bone Marrow–derived Stem Cells

Duffield JS, Park KM, Hsiao L-L, et al (Harvard Med School, Boston; Kyungpook Natl Univ, Daegu, Republic of Korea; Harvard Med School, Charlestown, Mass; et al)

J Clin Invest 115:1743-1755, 2005 32–5

Introduction.—Ischemia causes kidney tubular cell damage and abnormal renal function. The kidney is capable of morphological restoration of tubules and recovery of function. Recently, it has been suggested that cells repopulating the ischemically injured tubule derive from bone marrow stem cells. We studied kidney repair in chimeric mice expressing GFP or bacterial β-gal or harboring the male Y chromosome exclusively in bone marrow-derived cells. In GFP chimeras, some interstitial cells but not tubular cells expressed GFP after ischemic injury. More than 99% of those GFP interstitial cells were leukocytes. In female mice with male bone marrow, occasional tubular cells (0.06%) appeared to be positive for the Y chromosome, but deconvolution microscopy revealed these to be artifactual. In β-gal chimeras, some tubular cells also appeared to express β-gal as assessed by X-gal staining, but following suppression of endogenous (mammalian) β-gal, no tubular cells could be found that stained with X-gal after ischemic injury.

Whereas there was an absence of bone marrow-derived tubular cells, many tubular cells expressed proliferating cell nuclear antigen, which is reflective of a high proliferative rate of endogenous surviving tubular cells. Upon i.v. injection of bone marrow mesenchymal stromal cells, postischemic functional renal impairment was reduced, but there was no evidence of differentiation of these cells into tubular cells of the kidney. Thus, our data indicate that bone marrow-derived cells do not make a significant contribution to the restoration of epithelial integrity after an ischemic insult. It is likely that intrinsic tubular cell proliferation accounts for functionally significant replenishment of the tubular epithelium after ischemia.

► This article and a similar one from Lin et al[1] address the question of the source of cells that lead to kidney repair after ischemic injury. Somewhat surprisingly, there is virtually no or only about 10%, depending on the study, contribution of bone marrow–derived cells to the intensely proliferating cells that repopulate the injured tubules. These observations should serve as a caution to attempts to use stem cell therapies to treat acute renal injury.

S. Adler, MD

Reference

1. Lin F, Moran A, Igarashi P: Intrarenal cells, not bone marrow-derived cells, are the major source for regeneration in postischemic kidney. *J Clin Invest* 115:1756-1764, 2005.

Characterization of the T-cell Epitope That Causes Anti-GBM Glomerulonephritis

Robertson J, Wu J, Arends J, et al (Univ of Texas Health Science Ctr at Houston; Eastern Virginia Med School, Norfolk; La Jolla Inst for Allergy and Immunology, San Diego, Calif)
Kidney Int 68:1061-1070, 2005 32–6

Background.—We have demonstrated that a single T-cell epitope pCol (28-40) (SQTTANPSCPEGT) alone, which is derived from NC1 domain of α3 chain of type IV collagen (Col4α3 NC1), can induce severe glomerulonephritis in Wistar Kyoto rats. This study further characterized this T-cell epitope.

Methods.—A series of synthetic peptides derived from pCol (28-40) were tested in vivo and in vitro for their T-cell epitope activity and nephritogenicity. Major histocompatability complex (MHC) class II molecules in Wistar Kyoto rats were cloned, and MHC restriction of pCol(28-40) was determined.

Results.—The T-cell epitope pCol(28-40) was restricted by rat MHC class II RT.1B*l*. Ten amino acid residues (29 to 38) were mapped to be the minimum core of the T-cell epitope, which was capable of inducing the T-cell response and severe glomerulonephritis. Only three residues were identified as absolutely critical for the T-cell epitope: position 31 (T) was an anchor residue to the class II molecule, and positions 33 (N) and 34 (P) contributed to the specificity of the T-cell epitope. Thus, only substitution at those positions completely abrogated nephritogenicity of the T-cell epitope. Interestingly, pCol (28-40) also bound to human MHC class II human MHC class II molecule HLA-DRB*1501, which has been linked to human anti-glomerular basement membrane (GBM) disease, suggesting that human homologue of pCol(28-40) could be a potential human T-cell epitope.

Conclusion.—Our study demonstrated that only few residues in the nephritogenic T-cell epitope pCol(28-40) were critical. Our finding also revealed that pCol(28-40) is a potential nephritogenic T-cell epitope in Goodpasture's syndrome.

▶ This study has added much information to the complex interaction between immunity and pathology typified by anti-GBM glomerulonephritis (GN). Though it has been well known that anti-GBM GN is caused by auto-antibodies to collagen IV alpha chain NC domain (Col4α3NC), there has been suspicion that T-cell–mediated immunity may be involved as well.

Using a rat model, Robertson et al have clearly demonstrated that many of the clinical and pathological findings of Goodpasture's syndrome can be explained by antigen-specific T-cell infiltration of the glomerulus, and secondarily, via B-cell epitope spreading, by induction of autoantibodies to diverse GBM antigens. The relevant epitope is extremely small in size—only 10 amino acids long with only 3 critical residues—which may be the reason for possible molecular mimicry between the nephritogenic epitope and microbial peptides.

This study adds much new information to our understanding of this syndrome, which may help direct therapies to modification or blockade of the specific epitopes involved. In addition, it also suggests explanations for the role of microbial infection in the pathogenesis of this and other types of GN. Future immunosuppressive and/or antimicrobial therapy may ultimately be more specifically tailored based on the kind of findings described here.

M. Klein, MD

Caspase Inhibition Reduces Tubular Apoptosis and Proliferation and Slows Disease Progression in Polycystic Kidney Disease

Tao Y, Kim J, Faubel S, et al (Univ of Colorado Health Sciences Ctr, Denver; Idun Pharmaceuticals, Inc, San Diego, Calif)

Proc Natl Acad Sci U S A 102:6954-6959, 2005 32–7

Introduction.—We have previously demonstrated an increase in proapoptotic caspase-3 in the kidney of Han:SPRD rats with polycystic kidney disease (PKD). The aim of the present study was to determine the effect of caspase inhibition on tubular cell apoptosis and proliferation, cyst formation, and renal failure in the Han:SPRD rat model of PKD. Heterozygous (Cy/+) and littermate control (+/+) male rats were weaned at 3 weeks of age and then treated with the caspase inhibitor IDN-8050 (10 mg/kg per day) by means of an Alzet (Palo Alto, CA) minipump or vehicle [polyethylene glycol (PEG 300)] for 5 weeks. The two-kidney/total body weight ratio more than doubled in Cy/+ rats compared with +/+ rats. IDN-8050 significantly reduced the kidney enlargement by 44% and the cyst volume density by 29% in Cy/+ rats Cy/+ rats with PKD have kidney failure as indicated by a significant increase in blood urea nitrogen. IDN-8050 significantly reduced the increase in blood urea nitrogen in the Cy/+ rats. The number of proliferating cell nuclear antigen-positive tubular cells and apoptotic tubular cells in noncystic and cystic tubules was significantly reduced in IDN-8050-treated Cy/+ rats compared with vehicle-treated Cy/+ rats. On immunoblot, the active form of caspase-3 (20 kDa) was significantly decreased in IDN-8050-treated Cy/+ rats compared with vehicle-treated Cy/+ rats. In summary, in a rat model of PKD, caspase inhibition with IDN-8050 (*i*) decreases apoptosis and proliferation in cystic and noncystic tubules; (*ii*) inhibits renal enlargement and cystogenesis, and (*iii*) attenuates the loss of kidney function.

► The apparent benefit of caspase inhibition in the Han:SPRD rat is an exciting development in the possible management of autosomal dominant polycystic kidney disease (ADPKD), which remains largely untreatable in humans. Although the mechanism of disease in the rat is caused by different defects than the human disease, the similarities in hypertension, progression, and anemia make it a reasonable model for this condition.

In this study, caspase inhibition decreased cell proliferation and apoptosis and was associated with significant decreases in kidney size and renal cyst volume. This raises hopes that there may soon be therapies available for ADPKD which directly influence the underlying pathology rather than merely attacking the collateral effects and associated conditions of this devastating disease.

M. Klein, MD

Rapamycin Ameliorates Proteinuria-associated Tubulointerstitial Inflammation and Fibrosis in Experimental Membranous Nephropathy

Bonegio RGB, Fuhro R, Wang Z, et al (Boston Univ)

J Am Soc Nephrol 16:2063-2072, 2005 32–8

Introduction.—Proteinuria is a risk factor for progression of chronic renal failure. A model of proteinuria-associated tubulointerstitial injury was developed and was used to examine the therapeutic effect of rapamycin. Two studies were performed. In study A, proteinuric rats were given sheep anti-Fx1A to induce experimental membranous nephropathy; control rats received normal sheep serum. Four weeks later, groups were subdivided and underwent laparotomy alone (two kidneys), nephrectomy alone (one kidney), or nephrectomy with polectomy (0.6 kidney). Renal function and morphology were evaluated 4 wk later. Whereas control rats never developed proteinuria, anti-Fx1A induced severe proteinuria. Proteinuria was unaffected by renal mass reduction. Proteinuric rats developed tubulointerstitial disease that was most severe in rats with 0.6 kidneys. Renal function (GFR) was reduced by loss of renal mass and was reduced further in proteinuric rats with 0.6 kidneys. In study B, the effect of rapamycin on the expression of candidate proinflammatory and profibrotic genes and the progression of proteinuria-associated renal disease were examined. All rats received an injection of anti-Fx1A and were nephrectomized and then divided into groups to receive rapamycin or vehicle. Gene expression, renal morphology, and GFR were evaluated after 4, 8, and 12 wk. Rapamycin reduced expression of the proinflammatory and profibrotic genes (monocyte chemotactic protein-1, vascular endothelial growth factor, PDGF, TGF-β_1, and type 1 collagen). Tubulointerstitial inflammation and progression of interstitial fibrosis that were present in vehicle-treated rats were ameliorated by rapamycin. Rapamycin also completely inhibited compensatory renal hypertrophy. In summary, rapamycin ameliorates the tubulointerstitial disease associated with chronic proteinuria and loss of renal mass.

▶ It has been hypothesized that the progression of renal failure in membranous glomerulonephritis (MGN) is primarily due to the severity of proteinuria and its resultant effects on the renal tubules.

This study demonstrates, in a rat model of experimental MGN, that rapamycin in low doses can substantially reduce the degree of protein excretion; it can also reduce the resulting interstitial inflammation and fibrosis while preventing glomerular hypertrophy. This effect seems to be more than would be expected by simple reduction of proteinuria alone.

If this effect can be demonstrated in humans, this would be a major breakthrough in the management of idiopathic MGN, which is currently inadequately managed with alkylating agents, steroids, and angiotensin-converting enzyme inhibition.

M. Klein, MD

Consequences and Management of Hyperphosphatemia in Patients With Renal Insufficiency

Friedman EA (Downstate Med Ctr, Brooklyn, NY)

Kidney Int 67:S1-S7, 2005 32–9

Background.—It has been estimated that chronic kidney disease that induces a progressive decrease in renal function occurs in about 20 million persons in the United States. Chronic renal failure is a result of reduced synthesis of vitamin D by the kidneys and increased retention of phosphorus. Secondary hyperparathyroidism is a sequela of disturbances in calcium and phosphorus metabolism in patients with chronic kidney disease. This report focused on the consequences of secondary hyperparathyroidism in patients with chronic kidney disease and discussed the difficulties in treating altered mineral metabolism.

Overview.—The altered calcium and phosphorus metabolism associated with secondary hypermetabolism results in bone demineralization, which in turn results in fractures of the joint. In addition, patients with chronic kidney disease suffer limited mobility due to subcutaneous deposits of calcium pyrophosphate, which cause arthropathy, crippling joint pain, and swelling accompanied by osteoclast-induced erosion of bone. Vascular calcification, which is a marker of atherosclerosis and arterial stiffness, is commonly seen in dialysis patients and is a risk factor for mortality. It has been proposed that accelerated calcification of the coronary artery is based on the observation that patients with end-stage renal disease (ESRD) with more coronary calcification had reduced skeletal mass due to calcium mobilization from the bone. Electron beam tomography studies have suggested that cardiovascular calcification in dialysis patients is a result of lower vertebral bone mass rather than altered calcium and phosphate metabolism. Strategies designed to limit or prevent bone and joint destruction in chronic kidney disease and ESRD have focused on limiting dietary phosphorus, intra-gut binding of ingested phosphorus, enhancing calcium absorption, and limiting parathyroid hormone secretion.

Conclusions.—Controlling serum phosphorus levels in dialysis patients is important because hyperphosphatemia and the elevated calcium and phosphorus that results are correlated with cardiovascular mortality and bone disease. Both sevelamer and calcium-containing phosphate binders (calcium acetate and calcium carbonate) are acceptable first-line therapeutic agents in the treatment of patients with ESRD with hyperphosphatemia. Calcium acetate has superior efficacy in controlling serum phosphorus and a positive cost-benefit profile and is the treatment of choice for the initial treatment of patients with ESRD. Sevelamer hydrochloride is the preferred treatment for patients who develop persistent hypercalcemia during treatment with calcium-based binders; however, this treatment may result in acid loading in ESRD patients.

► Cardiovascular morbidity and mortality is increased in patients with mild to moderate renal disease. Whether renal disease is causally linked to the enhanced cardiac disease is uncertain. At present, best practices should address issues that affect the renal disease and the cardiac disease both independently and simultaneously. Hyperphosphatemia (PO4 > 5.4 mg/dL) is linked to a number of adverse events including soft tissue and vascular calcification and increased mortality. A number of new therapeutic strategies, including dietary adjustments, are available to achieve the appropriate targets for serum calcium, phosphate, parathyroid hormone, and bone parameters. These targets are important goals in both predialysis- and dialysis-dependent patients.

M. Brogan, MD

33 Selected Issues in Acute Renal Failure

Incidence and Etiology of Acute Renal Failure Among Ambulatory HIV-infected Patients

Franceschini N, Napravnik S, Eron JJ Jr, et al (Univ of North Carolina, Chapel Hill; Duke Univ, Durham, NC)

Kidney Int 67:1526-1531, 2005 33–1

Background.—Acute renal failure (ARF) is a cause of renal dysfunction in human immunodeficiency virus (HIV)-infected patients. Its incidence and causes have not been studied since the introduction of highly active antiretroviral therapy (HAART) in HIV ambulatory patients.

Methods.—This is a prospective cohort study of 754 HIV patients, 18 years or older, seen at a university-based infectious disease clinic between 2000 and 2002. ARF was identified using proportional increases in serum creatinine from baseline and by chart review. Clinical conditions were assessed at the time of the ARF event. ARF incidence rates (IR) were calculated by dividing the number of events by person time at risk. To compare patients with and without ARF, *t* test or chi-square test were used.

Results.—Patient's mean age was 40 years; 68% were male and 61% were black. One hundred-eleven ARF events occurred in 71 subjects (IR 5.9 per 100 person-years; 95% CI 4.9, 7.1). ARF was more common in men, in those with CD4 cell count <200 cells/mm^3, and HIV RNA levels >10,000 copies/mL. These patients more often had acquired immunodeficiency syndrome (AIDS), hepatitis C infection (HCV), and have received HAART. ARF was mainly community-acquired, due to prerenal causes or acute tubular necrosis, and associated with opportunistic infections and drugs. Liver disease was a cause of ARF in HCV-infected patients.

Conclusion.—ARF is common in ambulatory HIV patients. Immunosuppression, infection, and HCV are important conditions associated with ARF in the post-HAART era (Table 1).

► Since the introduction of HAART therapy, the incidence and etiologies of acute renal injury in HIV have not been well studied. This prospective cohort study demonstrates that ARF is most common in men, in those with high viral loads, in patients on HAART, and in patients with hepatitis C and concomitant

TABLE 1.—Demographic and Clinical Characteristics of Ambulatory Human Immunodeficiency Virus (HIV)-Infected Patients With and Without Acute Renal Failure (ARF), 2000-2002, North Carolina

	All Patients (*N* = 754)	ARF (*N* = 71)	Without ARF (*N* = 683)	*P* Value[a]
Male *number* (%)	510 (68)	57 (80)	453 (66)	0.02
Age *years*				
17–39	376 (50)	31 (44)	345 (51)	
40–59	356 (47)	38 (54)	318 (47)	0.75
60–71	22 (3)	2 (3)	20 (3)	
Race *number* (%)				
White	255 (34)	23 (32)	232 (34)	
Black	461 (61)	44 (62)	417 (61)	1.00
Other	38 (5)	4 (6)	34 (5)	
Hypertension *number* (%)	126 (17)	9 (13)	117 (17)	0.41
Diabetes mellitus *number* (%)	47 (6)	5 (7)	42 (6)	0.79
Hepatitis B *number* (%)	46 (6)	6 (8)	40 (6)	0.44
Hepatitis C *number* (%)	160 (21)	26 (37)	134 (21)	0.004
AIDS-defining illness *number* (%)	77 (10)	23 (32)	54 (8)	<0.0001
HAART ever *number* (%)	540 (68)	62 (87)	452 (66)	<0.0001
Serum creatinine *number* (%)				
<1.2	710 (95)	69 (97)	641 (85)	
≥1.2	40 (5)	2 (3)	38 (6)	0.83
CD4 cell count (cells/mm^3) *number* (%)				
<200	214 (29)	39 (57)	175 (27)	<0.0001
≥200	515 (71)	30 (43)	485 (73)	
HIV RNA (copies/mL) *number* (%)				
<10,000	433 (62)	24 (36)	409 (64)	<0.0001
10,000–30,000	64 (9)	9 (14)	55 (9)	
>30,000	204 (29)	33 (50)	171 (27)	

Abbreviations: AIDS, Acquired immunodeficiency syndrome; *HAART,* highly active antiretroviral therapy.
[a] *t* test or Pearson's chi-square test, comparing ARF with non-ARF.
(Courtesy of Franceschini N, Napravnik S, Eron JJ Jr, et al: Incidence and etiology of acute renal failure among ambulatory HIV-infected patients. *Kidney Int* 67:1526-1531, 2005. Reprinted by permission of Blackwell Publishing.)

liver disease. The etiology of ARF among ambulatory HIV infected patients is often related to their comorbid conditions such as hepatitis C and drug-related nephrotoxicity. Opportunistic infections and advanced HIV (AIDS) continue to be contributory causes of ARF. It is important to be cognizant of these comorbidities and their significance when assessing ARF in this population.

M. Brogan, MD

Acute Phosphate Nephropathy Following Oral Sodium Phosphate Bowel Purgative: An Underrecognized Cause of Chronic Renal Failure

Markowitz GS, Stokes MB, Radhakrishnan J, et al (Columbia College of Physicians & Surgeons, New York)
J Am Soc Nephrol 16:3389-3396, 2005 33–2

Introduction.—The findings of diffuse tubular injury with abundant tubular calcium phosphate deposits on renal biopsy are referred to as nephrocalcinosis, a condition typically associated with hypercalcemia. During the period from 2000 to 2004, 31 cases of nephrocalcinosis were identified among the 7349 native renal biopsies processed at Columbia University. Among the 31 patients, 21 presented with acute renal failure (ARF), were normocalcemic, and had a history of recent colonoscopy preceded by bowel cleansing with oral sodium phosphate solution (OSPS) or Visicol. Because the precipitant was OSPS rather than hypercalcemia, these cases are best termed *acute phosphate nephropathy*. The cohort of 21 patients with APhN was predominantly female (81.0%) and white (81.0%), with a mean age of 64.0 yr. Sixteen of the 21 patients had a history of hypertension, 14 (87.5%) of whom were receiving an angiotensin-converting enzyme inhibitor or angiotensin receptor blocker. The mean baseline serum creatinine was 1.0 mg/dl, available within 4 mo of colonoscopy in 19 (90.5%) patients. Patients presented with ARF and a mean creatinine of 3.9 mg/dl at a median of 1 mo after colonoscopy. In a few patients, ARF was discovered within 3 d of colonoscopy, at which time hyperphosphatemia was documented. Patients had minimal proteinuria, normocalcemia, and bland urinary sediment. At follow-up (mean 16.7 mo), four patients had gone on to require permanent hemodialysis. The remaining 17 patients all have developed chronic renal insufficiency (mean serum creatinine, 2.4 mg/dl). Acute phosphate nephropathy is an underrecognized cause of acute and chronic renal failure. Potential etiologic factors include inadequate hydration (while receiving OSPS), increased patient age, a history of hypertension, and concurrent use of an angiotensin-converting enzyme inhibitor or angiotensin receptor blocker.

▶ This important study demonstrates the potential renal risks of using OSPS for bowel preparations for gastrointestinal studies. Of note is that these solutions can cause renal injury in patients with normal renal function.

R. Garrick, MD

Meta-analysis: Low-Dose Dopamine Increases Urine Output but Does Not Prevent Renal Dysfunction or Death

Friedrich JO, Adhikari N, Herridge MS, et al (St Michael's Hosp, Toronto; Sunnybrook and Women's College, Toronto; Toronto Gen Hosp; et al)
Ann Intern Med 142:510-524, 2005 33–3

Background.—Surveys have documented the continued popularity of low-dose dopamine to influence renal dysfunction even though few data support it and editorials and reviews have discouraged its use.

Purpose.—To evaluate the effects of low-dose dopamine (≤5 μg/kg of body weight per minute) compared with placebo or no therapy in patients with or at risk for acute renal failure.

Data Sources.—MEDLINE (1966-January 2005), EMBASE (1980-week 5, 2005), CANCERLIT (1975-2002), CINAHL (1982-January 2005), and CENTRAL (The Cochrane Library, fourth quarter, 2004); bibliographies of retrieved publications; and additional information from 50 trials.

Study Selection.—Two reviewers independently selected parallel-group randomized and quasi-randomized controlled trials of low-dose dopamine versus control.

Data Extraction.—Study methods, clinical and renal physiologic outcomes, and adverse events (arrhythmias and myocardial, limb, and cutaneous ischemia) were extracted.

Data Synthesis.—61 trials that randomly assigned 3359 patients were identified. Meta-analyses using random-effects models showed no effect of low-dose dopamine on mortality (relative risk, 0.96 [95% CI, 0.78 to 1.19]), need for renal replacement therapy (relative risk, 0.93 [CI, 0.76 to 1.15]), or adverse events (relative risk, 1.13 [CI, 0.90 to 1.41]). Low-dose dopamine increased urine output by 24% (CI, 14% to 35%) on day 1. Improvements in serum creatinine level (4% relative decrease [CI, 1% to 7%]) and measured creatinine clearance (6% relative increase [CI, 1% to 11%]) on day 1 were clinically insignificant. There were no significant changes on days 2 and 3 of therapy.

Limitations.—Statistically significant between-study heterogeneity in physiologic but not clinical outcomes was unexplained by prespecified hypotheses.

Conclusion.—Low-dose dopamine offers transient improvements in renal physiology, but no good evidence shows that it offers important clinical benefits to patients with or at risk for acute renal failure.

► This meta-analysis of 61 controlled trials of almost 3400 patients is an excellent, systematic review. It indicates that so called "renal" low-dose dopamine does not have any meaningful effect on renal outcomes, the need for dialysis intervention, or mortality. The studies encompassed a wide range of medical and surgical settings, including cardiac surgery, contrast-induced nephropathy, and nephrotoxin-induced renal failure. The changes in urine output, serum creatinine, and creatinine clearances are transient, lasting about 24 hours. Adverse effects included a trend toward increased tachyarrhythmias. In sum, there is little to recommend this therapy.

R. Garrick, MD

34 Selected Issues in Chronic Renal Failure and Transplantation

---

General Medical Care Among Patients With Chronic Kidney Disease: Opportunities for Improving Outcomes

Kausz AT, Guo H, Pereira BJG, et al (Tufts-New England Med Ctr, Boston; Univ of Minnesota, Minneapolis)

J Am Soc Nephrol 16:3092-3101, 2005 34–1

Introduction.—Suboptimal health care during advancing chronic kidney disease (CKD) may result in greater morbidity and cost once dialysis is started and may preclude future transplantation. Medicare data were examined for the prevalence of selected general health, diabetes, and CKD interventions in a national cohort of patients in the 2 yr before dialysis initiation and compared with a contemporaneous non-CKD cohort. A total of 24,778 individuals who were aged ≥67 yr composed the CKD cohort, and 1,046,136 individuals who were aged ≥67 yr did not have CKD. Among patients with diabetes and CKD, fewer than two thirds had claims for eye examinations, 75% for HbA_{1C} testing, and 68% for lipid testing, with similar proportions in the non-CKD cohort. Among those without diabetes, 47 and 54% of the CKD and non-CKD cohorts, respectively, had claims for lipid testing. Fewer than 50 and 15% had claims for influenza and pneumococcal vaccination, respectively, with slightly lower proportions among patients with CKD. Claims for cancer tests were found for 14 to 41% and 29 to 52% of individuals with and without CKD, respectively, depending on the type of cancer. A greater proportion of patients with diabetes tended to have claims for tests in both cohorts. In the CKD cohort, claims for anemia testing and parathyroid hormone levels were available in fewer than 50 and 15%, respectively, and claims for permanent vascular access were found for only 30% of hemodialysis patients. This study provides further evidence that patients with CKD may not be receiving general health and CKD care according to current recommendations.

► For intervention to most effectively slow the progression of CKD and associated cardiovascular disease, it must begin during the early stages of renal injury. Practitioners need to be familiar with the stages of renal disease, the monitoring required, and the timing of appropriate interventions and referrals. Education, early detection, and early intervention are critical if we hope to reduce the incidence and enormous clinical-socioeconomic effects of CKD.

R. Garrick, MD

Prevalence of Family History of Kidney Disease and Perception of Risk for Kidney Disease: A Population-based Study

Jurkovitz C, Hylton TN, McClellan WM (Emory Univ, Atlanta, Ga)

Am J Kidney Dis 46:11-17, 2005 34–2

Background.—A family history of kidney disease is associated with an increased risk for end-stage renal disease (ESRD). However, it is unclear whether blacks are more likely to have a family history of ESRD than other groups independently of kidney disease risk factors. Moreover, their risk perception for kidney disease is unknown.

Methods.—The association of race with family history of ESRD and perception of risk for kidney disease was examined in a representative random sample of 402 Georgia residents who completed a telephone interview. Logistic regression analysis was used to derive adjusted odds ratios and 95% confidence intervals for the association between race and family history of ESRD, controlling for age, sex, education level, being a Georgia native, diabetes, hypertension, and personal history of kidney disease. A multinomial logit model was used to derive adjusted estimates for the association between race and perception of risk for kidney disease.

Results.—Mean age was 43.2 years, 41.0% of respondents were men, 20.1% were black, 6.6% had diabetes, 21.4% had hypertension, 1.6% had a personal history of kidney disease, and 3.7% reported a family member with ESRD. Although blacks were more likely to report a family history of ESRD (odds ratio, 6.43; 95% confidence interval, 2.02 to 20.43), their perception of risk was not greater.

Conclusion.—Although blacks are approximately 6 times as likely to report a family history of ESRD independently of a personal history of kidney disease, diabetes, or hypertension, they do not perceive themselves as more vulnerable for kidney disease.

► A family history of ESRD is a major risk factor for the occurrence of dialysis dependent renal disease in other family members. This telephone survey demonstrates that despite an awareness of the family history, black patients in the southeastern United States are unaware of their own personal risk of renal disease. Despite patient selection bias, this article emphasizes the need for educating both physicians and families regarding significance of a family history of kidney disease. The 2000 US Renal Data System estimated that the lifetime risk for developing ESRD for 20-year-old white men and women and black men and women are 2.5%, 1.8%, 7.3%, and 7.8%, respectively. Given the growing incidence and prevalence of kidney disease, best practices would include education of patients and family members regarding the risk of renal disease and the need to control the associated comorbid conditions of hypertension, diabetes, and cardiovascular disease.

M. Brogan, MD

Comparing the Risk for Death With Peritoneal Dialysis and Hemodialysis in a National Cohort of Patients With Chronic Kidney Disease

Jaar BG, Coresh J, Plantinga LC, et al (Johns Hopkins Univ, Baltimore, Md; Independent Dialysis Foundation, Baltimore, Md; Tufts-New England Med Ctr, Boston; et al)

Ann Intern Med 143:174-183, 2005 34–3

Background.—The influence of type of dialysis on survival of patients with end-stage renal disease (ESRD) is controversial.

Objective.—To compare risk for death among patients with ESRD who receive peritoneal dialysis or hemodialysis.

Design.—Prospective cohort study.

Setting.—81 dialysis clinics in 19 U.S. states.

Patients.—1041 patients starting dialysis (274 patients receiving peritoneal dialysis and 767 patients receiving hemodialysis) at baseline.

Measurements.—Patients were followed for up to 7 years and censored at transplantation or loss to follow-up. Cox proportional hazards regression stratified by clinic was used to compare the risk for death with peritoneal dialysis versus hemodialysis.

Results.—Twenty-five percent of patients undergoing peritoneal dialysis and 5% of hemodialysis patients switched type of dialysis. After adjustment, the risk for death did not differ between patients undergoing peritoneal dialysis and those undergoing hemodialysis during the first year (relative hazard, 1.39 [95% CI, 0.64 to 3.06]), but the risk became significantly higher among those undergoing peritoneal dialysis in the second year (relative hazard, 2.34 [CI, 1.19 to 4.59]). After stratification, the survival rate was no different for patients who had the highest propensity of being initially treated with peritoneal dialysis. Results were consistent with adjustment based on a propensity score model and in sensitivity analyses that used as-treated models and models in which switches in type of dialysis were treated as treatment failures. Results were similar but stronger in analyses that were restricted to patients who were treated only in clinics offering both types of dialysis.

Limitations.—Patients were not randomly assigned to their initial type of dialysis. Also, more patients undergoing peritoneal dialysis than hemodialysis switched type of dialysis over time, and the reason for switching was often a consequence of the technique.

Conclusions.—The risk for death in patients with ESRD undergoing dialysis depends on dialysis type. Further studies are needed to evaluate a possible survival benefit of a timely change from peritoneal dialysis to hemodialysis.

► The Choices for Healthy Outcomes in Caring for ESRD (CHOICE) study concluded that the risk of death in patients with ESRD depends on the dialysis type, and suggested that after the first year of treatment, hemodialysis (HD) confers a survival advantage over peritoneal dialysis (PD). These results are somewhat different from prior studies, which suggested that year-one PD survival rates are often superior to HD survival rates, and that over time the survival rates of PD decline and HD improve, nearing each other between 2 to 3 years.[1-6] Some limitations of the study are that it was not randomly controlled, as patients were allowed to choose their initial type of dialysis and were allowed to move from one dialysis modality to another over the course of the study. The primary analysis was as an "intention-to-treat model," wherein the outcome is ascribed to the initial dialysis modality. Prior studies have indicated that the survival rates of PD and HD are different over time, and this together with relatively small number of patients on PD (274), suggests that to avoid selection bias, it would be best if patients were tracked from the initial day of their first dialysis. In CHOICE, the time range from the start of dialysis to recruitment was 7 weeks to more than 4 months. In addition, data are not available regarding dialysis adequacy or the transport characteristics of the peritoneal membrane, both of which can affect patient outcome. Finally, a large number of the patients came from one particular dialysis provider (DCI, Inc), and therefore a "center effect" may be present.

Overall, while not giving us a definite answer regarding the best therapy, the study does alert us to critically monitor our patients over time, to be proactive regarding adjustments in the treatment modality, and to anticipate future studies regarding the effect of time on a treatment modality and survival.

R. Garrick, MD

References

1. Fenton SS, Schaubel DE, Desmeules M, et al: Hemodialysis versus peritoneal dialysis: A comparison of adjusted mortality rates. *Am J Kidney Dis* 30:334-342, 1997.
2. Bargman JM, Thorpe KE, Churchill DN: Relative contribution of residual renal function and peritoneal clearance to adequacy of dialysis: A reanalysis of the CANUSA study. *J Am Soc Nephrol* 12:2158-2162, 2001.
3. Foley RN, Parfrey PS, Harnett JD, et al: Mode of dialysis therapy and mortality in end-stage renal disease. *J Am Soc Nephrol* 9:267-276, 1998.
4. Collins AJ, Hao W, Xia H, et al: Mortality risks of peritoneal dialysis and hemodialysis. *Am J Kidney Dis* 34:1065-1074, 1999.
5. Xue JL, Everson SE, Constantini EG, et al: Peritoneal and hemodialysis: II. Mortality risk associated with initial patient characteristics. *Kidney Int* 61:741-746, 2002.
6. Tanna MM, Vonesh EF, Korbet SM: Patient survival among incident peritoneal dialysis and hemodialysis patients in an urban setting. *Am J Kidney Dis* 36:1175-1182, 2000.

Kidney Paired Donation and Optimizing the Use of Live Donor Organs

Segev DL, Gentry SE, Warren DS, et al (Johns Hopkins Univ School of Medicine, Baltimore, Md; Massachusetts Inst of Technology, Cambridge)

JAMA 293:1883-1890, 2005 34–4

Context.—Blood type and crossmatch incompatibility will exclude at least one third of patients in need from receiving a live donor kidney transplant. Kidney paired donation (KPD) offers incompatible donor/recipient pairs the opportunity to match for compatible transplants. Despite its increasing popularity, very few transplants have resulted from KPD.

Objective.—To determine the potential impact of improved matching schemes on the number and quality of transplants achievable with KPD.

Design, Setting, and Population.—We developed a model that simulates pools of incompatible donor/recipient pairs. We designed a mathematically verifiable optimized matching algorithm and compared it with the scheme currently used in some centers and regions. Simulated patients from the general community with characteristics drawn from distributions describing end-stage renal disease patients eligible for renal transplantation and their willing and eligible live donors.

Main Outcome Measures.—Number of kidneys matched, HLA mismatch of matched kidneys, and number of grafts surviving 5 years after transplantation.

Results.—A national optimized matching algorithm would result in more transplants (47.7% vs 42.0%, P<.001), better HLA concordance (3.0 vs 4.5 mismatched antigens; P<.001), more grafts surviving at 5 years (34.9% vs 28.7%; P<.001), and a reduction in the number of pairs required to travel (2.9% vs 18.4%; P<.001) when compared with an extension of the currently used first-accept scheme to a national level. Furthermore, highly sensitized patients would benefit 6-fold from a national optimized scheme (2.3% vs 14.1% successfully matched; P<.001). Even if only 7% of patients awaiting kidney transplantation participated in an optimized national KPD program, the health care system could save as much as $750 million.

Conclusions.—The combination of a national KPD program and a mathematically optimized matching algorithm yields more matches with lower HLA disparity. Optimized matching affords patients the flexibility of customizing their matching priorities and the security of knowing that the greatest number of high-quality matches will be found and distributed equitably.

▶ This article addresses an underutilized way of increasing the availability of live-donor kidneys. While the practical application of the tested algorithm awaits further discussion in the transplant community, the study brings to the attention of the nontransplant physician the option of paired kidney donation that is practiced in selected centers across the nation. This information may be useful in counseling patients with end-stage renal disease and their families.

F. Tedla, MD

Costimulation Blockade With Belatacept in Renal Transplantation

Vincent F, for the Belatacept Study Group (Univ of California, San Francisco; et al)

N Engl J Med 353:770-781, 2005 34–5

Background.—Renal transplantation is the standard of care for patients with end-stage renal disease. Although maintenance immunosuppression with calcineurin inhibitors yields excellent one-year survival, it is associated over the long term with high rates of death and graft loss, owing in part to the adverse renal, cardiovascular, and metabolic effects of these agents. The use of potentially less toxic agents, such as belatacept, a selective blocker of T-cell activation, may improve outcomes.

Methods.—We randomly assigned renal-transplant recipients to receive an intensive or a less-intensive regimen of belatacept or cyclosporine. All patients received induction therapy with basiliximab, mycophenolate mofetil, and corticosteroids. The primary objective was to demonstrate the noninferiority of belatacept over cyclosporine in the incidence of acute rejection at six months (with an upper bound of the 95 percent confidence interval around the treatment difference of less than 20 percent).

Results.—At six months, the incidence of acute rejection was similar among the groups: 7 percent for intensive belatacept, 6 percent for less-intensive belatacept, and 8 percent for cyclosporine. At 12 months, the glomerular filtration rate was significantly higher with both intensive and less-intensive belatacept than it was with cyclosporine (66.3, 62.1, and 53.5 ml per minute per 1.73 m^2, respectively), and chronic allograft nephropathy was less common with both regimens of belatacept than with cyclosporine (29 percent, 20 percent, and 44 percent, respectively). Lipid levels and blood-pressure values were similar or slightly lower in the belatacept groups, despite the greater use of lipid-lowering and antihypertensive medications in the cyclosporine group.

Conclusions.—Belatacept, an investigational selective costimulation blocker, did not appear to be inferior to cyclosporine as a means of preventing acute rejection after renal transplantation. Belatacept may preserve the glomerular filtration rate and reduce the rate of chronic allograft nephropathy.

▶ This agent represents a novel new immunosuppressive agent with a unique mechanism of action. It offers a new strategy in the clinical arena of immunosuppressant.

F. Tedla, MD

PART FIVE

PULMONARY DISEASE

BARBARA A. PHILLIPS, MD, MSPH

Introduction

To capture the diversity and significance of the new knowledge contained in this section, I have "headlined" some of the issues that may be of particular interest to internists. This year's pulmonary literature continues to demonstrate the importance of smoking cessation and gives us insight into how to go about it. The controversial topic of spiral CT scanning for lung cancer detection continues to receive attention in our literature (and in the lay press). The importance and long-lasting benefits of influenza and pneumococcal vaccination are becoming increasingly apparent. Gastric-acid suppressing drugs increase the risk of community-acquired pneumonia (CAP). New information about outpatient treatment and single lactam antibiotic treatment of mild CAP is also contained in this volume, as is information about the risks and outcomes of pneumonia in older people. Both the diagnosis and the treatment of thromboembolic disease continue to evolve, and a variety of disciplines (obstetrics and gynecology, emergency medicine, surgery, and cardiology) are contributing to our understanding of how to manage clots better. Sleep-disordered breathing is increasingly managed by internists. New data indicate that the in-laboratory continuous positive airway pressure titration may be unnecessary. A high percentage of commercial drivers appear to be at risk for sleep apnea, but there are some surprising risk factors for crashes in this group. Women with sleep apnea "look different" from men, and being Asian is probably an independent risk factor for sleep apnea. The surgeons have come up with yet another approach to sleep apnea that doesn't work. Reports about the sickest asthmatics give some insight into who is most at risk for repeated emergency department visits or death. More evidence accumulates that obesity increases the risk of asthma, and that gastroesophageal reflux and asthma are intertwined. Over-the-counter analgesics may increase the risk of lung disease. Finally, we still use ICUs mostly for the dying. There have been major advances in the fields of pulmonary, critical care and sleep medicine. I hope you find this section useful.

Barbara A. Phillips, MD, MSPH

35 Pulmonary

Effectiveness of Implementing the Agency for Healthcare Research and Quality Smoking Cessation Clinical Practice Guideline: A Randomized, Controlled Trial

Katz DA, for the AHRQ Smoking Cessation Guideline Study Group (Univ of Iowa, Iowa City; et al)

J Natl Cancer Inst 96:594-603, 2004 35–1

Background.—The Agency for Healthcare Research and Quality (AHRQ) Smoking Cessation Clinical Practice Guideline recommends that all clinicians strongly advise their patients who use tobacco to quit.

Methods.—We conducted a randomized, controlled trial of the effectiveness of Guideline implementation at eight community-based primary care clinics in southern Wisconsin (four test sites, four control sites) among 2163 consecutively enrolled adult patients who smoked at least one cigarette per day and presented for nonemergency care during the baseline period (June 16, 1999, to June 20, 2000) or the intervention period (from June 21, 2000, to May 3, 2001). After collecting baseline data, staff at test sites implemented the intervention over a 2-month period. The intervention included a tutorial for intake clinicians, group and individual performance feedback for intake clinicians, use of a modified vital signs stamp, an offer of free nicotine replacement therapy, and proactive telephone counseling. Staff at control sites received only general information about the AHRQ Guideline. Self-reported abstinence from smoking was determined by telephone interviews at 2- and 6-month follow-up assessments. Hierarchical logistic regression models were used to estimate the odds ratios (ORs) for treatment assignment after adjustment for patient characteristics. All statistical tests were two-sided.

Results.—There were no statistically significant differences in smoking cessation rates between participants at test and control sites during the baseline period. Among participants treated during the intervention period, those at test sites were more likely than those at control sites to report being abstinent at the 2-month (16.4% versus 5.8%; adjusted OR = 3.3, 95% confidence interval [CI] = 1.9 to 5.6; $P<.001$) and 6-month (15.4% versus 9.8%; adjusted OR = 1.7, 95% CI = 1.2 to 2.6; $P = .009$) follow-up assessments and to report continuous abstinence, that is, abstinence at both 2 and

6 months (10.9% versus 3.8%; adjusted OR = 3.4, 95% CI = 1.8 to 6.3; $P<.001$).

Conclusion.—Implementation of a guideline-based smoking cessation intervention by intake clinicians in primary care is associated with higher abstinence among smokers.

Results of a Randomized Controlled Trial of Intervention to Implement Smoking Guidelines in Veterans Affairs Medical Centers: Increased Use of Medications Without Cessation Benefit

Joseph AM, for the GIFT Research Group (VA Med Ctr, Minneapolis; et al)

Med Care 42:1100-1110, 2004 35–2

Background.—The AHRQ Clinical Practice Guideline for Treating Tobacco Use and Dependence recommends screening and treatment of all tobacco users. Effective methods to implement recommendations are needed because simple guideline dissemination does not necessarily result in changes in practice.

Objectives.—The Guideline Implementation for Tobacco (GIFT) study tested an organizational intervention to improve Guideline implementation.

Research Design.—GIFT randomized 20 Veterans Affairs medical centers to intervention or control conditions. We trained prime movers at each site to improve identification of smoking status, promote primary care interventions and increase availability of smoking cessation medications. Sites and patients were evaluated before and after intervention.

Subjects.—GIFT included 20 Veterans Affairs medical centers and 5678 subjects.

Measures.—Data regarding smoking status, delivery of treatment, medication use, and smoking cessation were collected from participant surveys, medical record review, survey of site leaders, and Pharmacy Benefits Management.

Results.—The intervention did not increase participant report of being asked about smoking status or receipt of counseling. It did increase the rate of identification of smoking status in the medical record ($P = 0.0001$) but did not increase the rate of counseling to stop smoking. Site level data showed no increase in the number of patients receiving smoking cessation medications or dollars spent on medications. Individual smoker data showed a significant increase in the use of medications for smoking cessation in intervention sites (odds ratio = 6.89, $P < 0.0001$); however, only a small minority of smokers received medication even after the intervention. There was no difference in smoking cessation rates between participants at the intervention and treatment sites.

Conclusions.—We conclude that improvements in smoking cessation rates are likely to require more intensive intervention in this population.

► Smoking cessation remains a critical public health goal in this country, as approximately 1 of every 4 American adults continues to smoke. Because an estimated 70% of smokers see a physician each year, the potential impact of physician-based interventions targeted to smoking cessation could be enormous. However, these opportunities are underused. In 2001, the National Committee for Quality Assurance reported that 66% of smokers enrolled in managed care received advice from their doctors to quit.[1] The Agency for Healthcare Research and Quality (AHRQ) published guidelines for treating tobacco use and dependence in 2000.[2] A number of studies have been published evaluating implementation of these guidelines, with variable results. These 2 studies (Abstracts 35–1 and 35–2) point out that the interventions used to promote guideline implementation will affect the success rates of smoking cessation efforts. In the study by Katz and colleagues (Abstract 35–1), guidelines were implemented in community-based primary-care clinics with a physician-focused process including the following procedures: (1) clinicians were tutored on assessment of smoking status and how to provide a brief smoking cessation message at each visit; (2) a visual chart prompt reminded physicians at each patient encounter; (3) patients were provided pharmacologic smoking cessation aids and telephone counseling; and (4) feedback that was based on patient exit interviews was given to physicians as to whether they had provided adequate counseling. At 6 months, there was a statistically significant increase in smoking abstinence (10.9% vs 3.8% in clinics where these interventions were not instituted). In contrast, the Veterans Affairs Medical Centers intervention described in the article by Joseph and colleagues (Abstract 35–2) focused on "academic detailing" of persons perceived to be "prime movers," such as directors of primary care services, smoking cessation coordinators, and primary care nurses. In this study, there was no increase in the rate of smoking cessation counseling by physicians, in the rates of provision of behavioral or pharmacologic interventions for smoking cessation, or in smoking cessation rates. These studies point out that simply having a guideline available is inadequate. Implementation of guideline recommendations may be difficult, particularly, in a primary-care setting where physician resources and time are limited, where training of physicians in smoking cessation principles may be inconsistent, and when reimbursement for preventive interventions is poor. Nonetheless, the benefit that could be realized by more successful physician-based smoking-cessation interventions justifies the effort. Further investigation is warranted on how to best make this a consistent part of patient care.

L. T. Tanoue, MD

References

1. *The State of Managed Care Quality, 2001.* National Committee for Quality Assurance, 2001, [online], http://www.ncqa.org/somc2001/advise_sm/somc_2001_advise_sm.html, accessed June 17, 2005.
2. Fiore M, Bailey W, Cohen S, et al: *Treating Tobacco Use and Dependence Clinical Practice Guideline.* Rockville, MD, US Department of Health and Human Services, Public Health Service, 2000.

Effects of Restaurant and Bar Smoking Regulations on Exposure to Environmental Tobacco Smoke Among Massachusetts Adults

Albers AB, Siegel M, Cheng DM, et al (Boston Univ)
Am J Public Health 94:1959-1964, 2004 35–3

Objectives.—We examined the association of local restaurant and bar regulations with self-reported exposure to environmental tobacco smoke among adults.

Methods.—Data were derived from a telephone survey involving a random sample of Massachusetts households.

Results.—Compared with adults from towns with no restaurant smoking restrictions, those from towns with strong regulations had more than twice the odds of reporting nonexposure to environmental tobacco smoke (odds ratio [OR]=2.74; 95% confidence interval [CI]=1.97, 3.80), and those from towns with some restrictions had 1.62 times the odds of reporting nonexposure (OR=1.62; 95% CI=1.29, 2.02). Bar smoking bans had even greater effects on exposure.

Conclusions.—Strong local clean indoor air regulations were associated with lower levels of reported exposure to environmental tobacco smoke in restaurants and bars (Table 2).

► Control of exposure to environmental tobacco smoke (ETS) is a relatively new aspect of tobacco regulation. Major government efforts to educate the public and affect national policy relating to cigarettes include such landmark events as the 1964 Surgeon General's report on the health consequences of smoking, the institution of larger federal cigarette taxes, the ban on various forms of tobacco advertising, and the Synar amendment limiting the sale of

TABLE 2.—Exposure to Environmental Tobacco Smoke in Restaurants and Bars, by Strength of Local Ordinance

Strength of Ordinance[a]	Nonexposure, % (95% CI)	Exposure, % (95% CI)	Unadjusted OR[b] (95% CI)
Restaurants[c]			
Weak	55.8 (53.3, 58.4)	44.2 (41.6, 46.7)	1.00
Medium	70.2 (66.1, 74.0)	29.8 (26.0, 33.9)	1.87* (1.50, 2.31)
Strong	81.2 (76.2, 85.4)	18.8 (14.6, 23.8)	3.42* (2.49, 4.69)
Bars[d]			
Weak	10.4 (8.4, 12.7)	89.6 (87.3, 91.6)	1.00
Strong	51.8 (41.9, 61.5)	48.2 (38.5, 58.1)	9.27* (5.85, 14.68)

[a]$P < .01$ for overall X^2 test.

[b]Reflects the likelihood of not being exposed to environmental tobacco smoke in restaurants or bars.

[c]We categorized restrictions as "weak" (no enclosed, separately ventilated areas), "medium" (smoking allowed in enclosed, separately ventilated areas only), or "strong" (smoking prohibited, including in bar areas with no variances).

[d]We categorized restrictions prohibiting smoking with no variances as "strong" and all other restriction categories as "weak."

*$P < .01$, from logistic regression analysis.

Abbreviations: OR, Odds ratio; *CI*, confidence interval.

cigarettes to minors. Advocacy against smoking should also be aimed at a local level in cities and communities. This is an interesting article in that it examines the effects of local restaurant and bar smoking regulations on exposure to ETS. It demonstrates that indoor air regulations in individual towns can have an important impact on ETS exposure. Towns were stratified by strength of local restaurant and bar ordinances pertaining to ETS. "Strong" restrictions were defined as prohibition of smoking from all areas; "medium" restrictions mandated smoking only in enclosed, separately ventilated areas; "weak" restrictions did not mandate enclosed or separately ventilated smoking areas. Table 2 shows that a graded association existed between the strength of local ordinances and ETS exposure. This supports the argument that strong local clean indoor-air regulations can have a significant positive impact on limiting ETS exposure.

L. T. Tanoue, MD

Lung Cancer Screening With Sputum Cytologic Examination, Chest Radiography, and Computed Tomography: An Update for the US Preventive Services Task Force

Humphrey LL, Teutsch S, Johnson M (Oregon Health & Science Univ, Portland; Merck & Co, West Point, Pa; Univ of Medicine and Dentistry, Newark, NJ)

Ann Intern Med 140:740-753, 2004 35–4

Background.—Lung cancer is the leading cause of cancer-related death in the United States and worldwide. No major professional organizations, including the U.S. Preventive Services Task Force (USPSTF), currently recommend screening for lung cancer.

Purpose.—To examine the evidence evaluating screening for lung cancer with chest radiography, sputum cytologic examination, and low-dose computed tomography (CT) to aid the USPSTF in updating its recommendation on lung cancer screening.

Data Sources.—MEDLINE, the Cochrane Library, reviews, editorials, and experts.

Study Selection.—Studies that evaluated mass screening programs for lung cancer involving the tests of interest were selected. All studies were reviewed, but only studies with control groups were rated in quality since these would most directly influence the USPSTF screening recommendation.

Data Extraction.—Data were abstracted to data collection forms. Studies were graded according to criteria developed by the USPSTF.

Data Synthesis.—None of the 6 randomized trials of screening for lung cancer with chest radiography alone or in combination with sputum cytologic examination showed benefit among those screened (Table 4). All studies were limited because some level of screening occurred in the control population. Five case-control studies from Japan suggested benefit to both high- and low-risk men and women. All studies were limited by potential healthy screenee bias. Six cohort studies showed that when CT was used to screen for lung cancer, lung cancer was diagnosed at an earlier stage than in

TABLE 4.—Outcomes of Lung Cancer Screening With Low-dose Computed Tomography

Study, Year (Reference)	Screening Interval	Screening Type	Screening Tests Performed	Positive Test Results	Recommendation for Follow-up Based on LDCT			Surgery for Diagnosis (Benign Nodules)	Lung Cancer†	Stage 1 Disease
					HRCT	Referral	Biopsy			
	mo		*n*	*n* (%)	←	*n*	→	*n* (*n*)	*n* (%)	%
Diederich et al., 2002 (53)		Baseline	817	350 (43)	269	29	13	1 (1)	11 (1.3) (1 interval)	58
Henschke et al., 1999, 2001 (54, 55)	6-18	Baseline								
		LDCT	1000	237 (24)	233	104	27	0	31 (3.1)	85
		Incidence								
		LDCT	1184	40	40	NR	9	NR	9 (0.9)	67
		Baseline								
		CXR	1000	68 (6.8)	33	NR	NR	0	7 (0.7)	
		CXR after LDCT		33 (3.3)						
Nawa et al., 2002 (56)	12	Baseline		2099 (26.4)						
		LDCT	7956		541	64	NR	NR	36 (0.5)	86
		Incidence							4 (0.1)	
		LDCT	5568	NR	148	7	NR	NR		100
Sone et al., 2001 (58)	12	Baseline								
		LDCT	5483	279 (5.1)	266	NR	NR	NR (7)	22 (0.4)	100
		Incidence								
		LDCT	8303†	309	297	NR	NR	NR (9)	37 (0.6)	86
Sobue et al., 2002 (59)	6	Baseline		186 (11.5)						
		LDCT	1611		186	25	21	0	13 (0.8)	77
		Incidence								
		LDCT	7891	721	721	57	35	1 (0)	19 (0.2)	79
		Baseline								
		CXR	1611	55 (3.4)	22	9	8	0	5 (0.3)	60
		Incidence								
		CXR	7891	202	89	7	4	0	3 (0.2)	0
Swensen et al., 2002, 2003 (61, 62)	12	Baseline		782 (51.4)						
		LDCT	1520		NR	NR	NR		27 (1.8)‡	
		Combined data						NR (8)		66
		Incidence							11 (0.7) (+2 interval)‡	
		LDCT	2916	336	NR	NR	NR			

*All data are presented by individual, except incidence, which refers to screening tests performed.

†Percentage of lung cancer for incidence = cases of lung cancer identified with incidence screening/cases of lung cancer in cohort minus cases of prevalence cancer.

‡One case of malignant disease diagnosed with sputum cytologic examination only.

Abbreviations: CXR, Chest radiography; *HRCT*, high-resolution computed tomography; *LDCT*, low-dose computed tomography; *NR*, not reported.

(Courtesy of Humphrey LL, Teutsch S, Johnson M: Lung cancer screening with sputum cytologic examination, chest radiography, and computed tomography: An update for the US Preventive Services Task Force. *Ann Intern Med* 140:740-753, 2004.)

usual clinical care. However, these studies did not have control groups, making mortality evaluation difficult. In addition, the studies demonstrated a high rate of false-positive findings.

Conclusions.—Current data do not support screening for lung cancer with any method. These data, however, are also insufficient to conclude that screening does not work, particularly in women. Two randomized trials of screening with chest radiography or low-dose CT are currently under way and will better inform lung cancer screening decisions.

Baseline Findings of a Randomized Feasibility Trial of Lung Cancer Screening With Spiral CT Scan vs Chest Radiograph: The Lung Screening Study of the National Cancer Institute

Gohagan J, Marcus P, Fagerstrom R, et al (Natl Cancer Inst, Bethesda, Md)

Chest 126:114-121, 2004 35–5

Background.—Low-radiation-dose spiral CT (LDCT) scanning is capable of detecting lung neoplasms in asymptomatic individuals. To determine whether such detection can reduce lung cancer mortality, a randomized controlled trial (RCT) of LDCT scanning is necessary.

Methods.—The feasibility of conducting an RCT in asymptomatic individuals who are at high risk for lung cancer was explored in the Lung Screening Study (LSS), a 12-month special project of the ongoing Prostate, Lung, Colorectal, and Ovarian (PLCO) cancer screening trial. During the fall of 2000, six PLCO screening centers recruited a total of 3,318 heavy or long-term smokers who were not participants in the PLCO trial and randomized them to receive either a screening LDCT scan (1,660 participants) or screening posteroanterior view chest radiograph (CXR) [1,658 participants].

Results.—The screens were completed on 96% of subjects in the LDCT scan arm and 93% of subjects in the CXR arm. A total of 20.5% of screened subjects in the LDCT scan arm and 9.8% of those in the CXR arm had findings that were suspicious for lung cancer. Thirty lung cancers in subjects in the LDCT arm and 7 lung cancers in patients in the CXR arm were diagnosed following a positive screening result. Additional data from the LSS indicated that, among persons who were at elevated risk for lung cancer, CT scan use was not pervasive, interest in participating in an RCT of LDCT scanning was strong, and few subjects randomized to CXR either refused their examination or sought a CT scan after their study CXR.

Interpretation.—The results of the LSS demonstrated convincingly the feasibility of an RCT of LDCT scanning in the United States.

Chest Radiography as the Comparison for Spiral CT in the National Lung Screening Trial

Church TR, for the National Lung Screening Trial Executive Committee (Univ of Minnesota, Minneapolis)

Acad Radiol 10:713-715, 2003 35–6

Background.—The prevention of lung cancer requires strategies beyond smoking prevention and cessation. No widely accepted guidelines are available regarding lung cancer screening. The National Lung Screening Trial (NLST) was designed to evaluate the effectiveness of annual screening among long-term or heavy smokers for lung cancer by using low-dose spiral CT.

Overview.—The NLST decided to use chest radiography, rather than usual care, as the most appropriate screening procedure for comparison for 3 reasons: it has not been adequately studied as a screening method for lung cancer; chest radiography and usual care are currently being compared in the Prostate, Lung, Colorectal, and Ovarian (PLCO) cancer screening trial; and a comparison of spiral CT to usual care could decrease the potential value of the NLST. A 3-arm study comparing usual care, chest radiography, and spiral CT would be the ideal approach, but the NLST is being conducted under less-than-ideal conditions, and a 3-arm study would increase the cost of the study beyond feasibility.

Conclusions.—At present, no recommendation for or against screening for lung cancer or widely accepted guidelines regarding such screening exist. Results from NLST and the Prostate, Lung, Colorectal, and Ovarian Cancer Screening Trial may provide insight into the best approach for screening lung cancer in high-risk groups and facilitate the development of guidelines for screening for lung cancer.

► Screening for lung cancer remains a controversial issue that challenges physicians on a daily basis. In stark contrast to cancers of the breast, prostate, and colon, no widely accepted guidelines regarding lung cancer screening exist. The most recent recommendation statement from the US Preventive Services Task Force concluded that "the evidence is insufficient to recommend for or against screening asymptomatic persons for lung cancer with either low-dose computerized tomography, chest x-ray, sputum cytology, or a combination of these tests."[1] This leaves the decision of whether to perform a screening evaluation of any kind for lung cancer up to physicians, with a decision made individually for each patient deemed to be at risk.

It seems intuitively obvious that diagnosing lung cancer at an earlier stage should result in improved outcomes. The controversy about screening for lung cancer exists because no studies have demonstrated satisfactorily that there is measurable benefit from screening. Three large and well-publicized randomized controlled trials in the United States in the 1970s and 1980s evaluating lung cancer screening with chest radiograph and sputum cytology (the Johns Hopkins Study, the Memorial Sloan-Kettering study, and the Mayo Lung

Project) all failed to demonstrate a reduction in deaths from lung cancer with screening.[2-4]

These studies were powered to detect large and perhaps unrealistic decreases in lung cancer mortality and were hampered by crossover contamination as well as by comparison with "usual care," which at the time of the studies typically included yearly chest radiograph.

The concept that screening should do more good than harm is a sound one. The cautions against screening with currently available techniques relate largely to the potential for harm related to false-positive findings. Compilation of the outcomes of several prominent trials of lung cancer screening with LDCT was presented in the report by Humphrey and colleagues (Abstract 35–4). Positive test results (ie, the identification of 1 or more lung nodules) were found in as few as 5.1% to as high as 51.4% of baseline screening studies, with only a small fraction of these abnormalities found to be lung cancer. False-positive results may lead to unnecessary invasive biopsy procedures, unnecessary surgeries, a staggering increase in health care costs,[5] and immeasurable emotional stress. Furthermore, repeated CT scanning may incur risks related to radiation from the screening study itself (see Abstract 35–6). Nonetheless, the fact that more than 80% of lung cancers have already spread beyond surgical resectability at the time of diagnosis makes the need to develop reliable early screening imperative.

It is clear that the question of whether lung cancer screening can improve outcomes urgently needs to be revisited. The article by Gohagan et al (Abstract 35–5) outlines the baseline findings of the Lung Screening Study (LSS) conducted by the Division of Cancer Prevention at the National Cancer Institute, which was a pilot study assessing the feasibility of performing a clinical trial of lung cancer screening. Six centers recruited 3318 heavy or long-term smokers, who were randomized to receive screening by LDCT or CXR. A total of 20.5% of subjects in the LDCT arm were found to have baseline abnormalities; cancer detection rate in this arm was 1.9%. A total of 9.8% of subjects in the CXR arm had baseline abnormalities; cancer detection rate in this group was 0.45%. Based on the findings of the LSS, the National Lung Screening Trial (NLST) is currently under way. The NLST is an enormous undertaking. It will enroll 50,000 persons deemed at risk for lung cancer based on smoking status, will monitor them for a minimum of 4.5 years, and is powered to detect a 20% reduction in lung cancer mortality rate with LDCT screening. Interim analyses should begin in 2005, with final analyses projected for 2009. This trial has no nonscreened control group. However, the efficacy of annual CXR screening versus "usual care" is being addressed separately in the ongoing Prostate, Lung, Colorectal, and Ovarian Cancer Screening Trial.[6] Hopefully the results of these trials will further our understanding of how best to screen for lung cancer in high-risk groups and provide a foundation for the development of new guidelines for lung cancer screening.

A last note: Physicians must continue to decide in conjunction with their patients whether screening examinations should be performed, understanding that false-positive tests are common and that there are currently no data demonstrating improvement in survival from screening, but hoping that there will be benefit if lung cancer can be identified at early stages.

L. T. Tanoue, MD

References

1. Lung cancer screening: Recommendation statement. *Ann Intern Med* 140:738-739, 2004.
2. Melamed MR: Lung cancer screening results in the National Cancer Institute New York study. *Cancer* 89(11 suppl):2356-2362, 2000.
3. Frost JK, Ball WC Jr, Levin ML, et al: Early lung cancer detection: Results of the initial (prevalence) radiologic and cytologic screening in the Johns Hopkins study. *Am Rev Respir Dis* 130:549-554, 1984.
4. Fontana RS: The Mayo Lung Project: A perspective. *Cancer* 89(11 suppl):2352-2355, 2000.
5. Mahadevia PJ, Fleisher LA, Frick KD, et al: Lung cancer screening with helical computed tomography in older adult smokers: A decision and cost-effectiveness analysis. *JAMA* 289:313-322, 2003.
6. Gohagan JK, Prorok PC, Hayes RB, et al: The Prostate, Lung, Colorectal and Ovarian (PLCO) Cancer Screening Trial of the National Cancer Institute: History, organization, and status. *Control Clin Trials* 21(6 suppl):251S-272S, 2003.

Cardiopulmonary Exercise Tests and Lung Cancer Surgical Outcome

Win T, Jackson A, Sharples L, et al (Addenbrooke's Hosp, Cambridge, England)
Chest 127:1159-1165, 2005 35–7

Study Objectives.—Surgical resection remains the treatment of choice for anatomically resectable non-small cell lung cancer. However, the presence of associated comorbid conditions increases the risk of death and surgical complications. Several studies have evaluated the usefulness of preoperative ex-

TABLE 4.—$\dot{V}O_2$max by Surgical Outcome

Variables	$\dot{V}O_2$max, mL/kg/min	$\dot{V}O_2$max, % Predicted	FEV_1, L
Postoperative course			
Uncomplicated	19.2 (4.5)	94.3 (32.1)	2.1 (0.6)
Complicated	17.5 (4.7)	70.7 (19.5)	2.0 (0.8)
Difference (95% CI)	1.8 (−0.3 to 3.8)	23.6 (10.0 to 37.1)	0.1 (−0.2 to 0.4)
p Value	0.10	0.001	0.58
Outcome			
Satisfactory	19.0 (4.6)	91.7 (31.5)	2.1 (0.6)
Poor	17.6 (4.5)	65.9 (16.0)	2.1(0.9)
Difference (95% CI)	1.4 (−1.3 to 4.1)	25.8 (8.1 to 43.6)	0.0 (−0.4 to 0.4)
p Value	0.29	0.005	0.98
Mortality			
Alive after operation	18.9 (4.5)	89.5 (31.1)	2.1 (0.6)
30-d mortality	16.5 (5.2)	61.3 (15.1)	1.9 (1.1)
Difference	2.4	28.2	0.2
p Value	0.43	0.2	0.8

*Data are presented as mean (SD) unless otherwise indicated.

(Courtesy of Win T, Jackson A, Sharples L, et al: Cardiopulmonary exercise tests and lung cancer surgical outcome. *Chest* 127:1159-1165, 2005.)

TABLE 5.—Positive and Negative Predictive Probabilities of Poor Outcome ($\dot{V}O_2$peak % Predicted)*

Threshold, %	Good Outcome if $\dot{V}O_2$ Is Greater Than Threshold	Poor Outcome if $\dot{V}O_2$ Is Less Than or Equal to Threshold
50	85/96 (89)	2/3 (67)
60	77/85 (91)	5/14 (36)
65	71/76 (93)	8/23 (35)
70	65/70 (93)	8/29 (28)
75	57/61 (93)	9/38 (24)

*Data are presented as No. of patients/total patients (%).

(Courtesy of Win T, Jackson A, Sharples L, et al: Cardiopulmonary exercise tests and lung cancer surgical outcome. *Chest* 127:1159-1165, 2005.)

ercise testing for predicting postoperative morbidity and mortality. The aim of this study was to establish whether exercise testing could predict poor surgical outcome in lung cancer surgery and whether the absolute value or percentage of predicted value is the better predictor of the surgical outcome.

Design.—The study was designed as a prospective study.

Patients and Setting.—One hundred thirty patients with potentially operable lung cancer at Papworth Hospital over 2 years were recruited; of these, 101 underwent curative surgery.

Interventions.—Spirometry and cardiopulmonary exercise tests were performed for every patient (n = 99), except for two patients with back problems. We also recorded the outcome of surgery, in particular, complications and mortality (Table 4).

Measurements and Results.—Mean maximum oxygen transport at peak exercise ($\dot{V}O_2$peak) was 18.3 mL/kg/min (SD, 4.7 mL/kg/min), and mean percentage of predicted $\dot{V}O_2$peak value was 84.4% (SD, 30%). Poor surgical outcome was significantly related to $\dot{V}O_2$peak percentage of predicted ($p < 0.01$) but not to the actual oxygen uptake value.

Conclusions.—The use of the percentage of predicted $\dot{V}O_2$peak value would be a better indicator of surgical outcome, since it predicts the surgical outcome better, and corrects for normal physiologic ranges (Table 5). The threshold of $\dot{V}O_2$peak for surgical intervention could be set between 50% and 60% of predicted without excess surgical mortality.

► Evaluation of operability in patients with lung cancer is a process that continues to be refined. In a population of patients whose cardiopulmonary status is often abnormal, what is the threshold level at which surgical risk is unacceptable? Deciding which patients can tolerate surgery has focused in the past on measurements of pulmonary physiology and more recently on evaluation of functional capacity as determined by cardiopulmonary exercise testing. In this report, exercise capacity measured as percent predicted $\dot{V}O_2$peak was a better predictor of surgical outcome than absolute $\dot{V}O_2$peak. This correction takes into consideration factors that are increasingly important in the demographics of lung cancer, specifically gender and age. Table 4 outlines surgical outcomes stratified by absolute and predicted $\dot{V}O_2$peak. It is somewhat sobering to note that mean absolute $\dot{V}O_2$peak in patients with complicated postoperative course or poor outcome was higher than the typically quoted "safe" threshold of 15 mL/kg per minute.[1,2] While a threshold level of "safe" percent predicted $\dot{V}O_2$peak cannot be determined on the basis of this study alone, Table 5 demonstrates a substantial increase in poor outcomes (myocardial infarction, respiratory failure, or postoperative death) in patients with percent predicted $\dot{V}O_2$peak below 50% to 60%. This parallels findings in other studies evaluating percent predicted $\dot{V}O_2$peak as a predictor of surgical outcomes for lung cancer.[3-5] It is important to note that these studies have been performed in centers with large experience in cardiopulmonary exercise testing as well as high surgical volume for lung cancer. Referral to such centers should be considered for patients deemed at high surgical risk but for whom surgery is the best therapeutic choice.

L. T. Tanoue, MD

References

1. BTS: Guidelines on the selection of patients with lung cancer for surgery. *Thorax* 56:89-108, 2001.
2. Beckles MA, Spiro SG, Colice GL, et al: The physiologic evaluation of patients with lung cancer being considered for resectional surgery. *Chest* 123(1 suppl):105S-114S, 2003.
3. Bolliger CT, Jordan P, Soler M, et al: Exercise capacity as a predictor of postoperative complications in lung resection candidates. *Am J Respir Crit Care Med* 151:1472-1480, 1995.
4. Morice RC, Peters EJ, Ryan MB, et al. Exercise testing in the evaluation of patients at high risk for complications from lung resection. *Chest* 101:356-361, 1992.
5. Richter Larsen K, Svendsen UG, Milman N, et al: Exercise testing in the preoperative evaluation of patients with bronchogenic carcinoma. *Eur Respir J* 10:1559-1565, 1997.

Annual Revaccination Against Influenza and Mortality Risk in Community-Dwelling Elderly Persons

Voordouw ACG, Sturkenboom MCJM, Dieleman JP, et al (Erasmus Univ, Rotterdam, The Netherlands; Inspectorate for Health Care, The Hague, The Netherlands; Univ of Cambridge, England)

JAMA 292:2089-2095, 2004 35–8

Context.—Although large-scale observational studies have demonstrated the effectiveness of influenza vaccination, no large studies have systematically addressed the clinical benefit of annual revaccinations.

Objective.—To investigate the effect of annual influenza revaccination on mortality in community-dwelling elderly persons.

Design, Setting, and Participants.—A population-based cohort study using the computerized Integrated Primary Care Information (IPCI) database in the Netherlands including community-dwelling individuals aged 65 years or older from 1996 through 2002. For each year, we computed the individual cumulative exposure to influenza vaccination since study start.

Main Outcome Measure.—Association between the number of consecutive influenza vaccinations and all-cause mortality vs no vaccination after adjusting for age, sex, chronic respiratory and cardiovascular disease, hypertension, diabetes mellitus, renal failure, and cancer.

Results.—The study population included 26071 individuals, of whom 3485 died during follow-up. Overall, a first vaccination was associated with a nonsignificant annual reduction of mortality risk of 10% (hazard ratio [HR], 0.90; 95% confidence interval [CI], 0.78-1.03) while revaccination was associated with a reduced mortality risk of 24% (HR, 0.76; 95% CI, 0.70-0.83). Compared with a first vaccination, revaccination was associated with a reduced annual mortality risk of 15% (HR, 0.85; 95% CI, 0.75-0.96). During the epidemic periods this reduction was 28% (HR, 0.72; 95% CI, 0.53-0.96). Similar estimates were obtained for persons with and without chronic comorbidity and those aged 70 years or older at baseline. Overall, influenza vaccination is estimated to prevent 1 death for every 302 vaccinees at a vaccination coverage that varied between 64% and 74%.

Conclusion.—Annual influenza vaccination is associated with a reduction in all-cause mortality risk in a population of community-dwelling elderly persons, particularly in older individuals.

Inpatient Computer-Based Standing Orders vs Physician Reminders to Increase Influenza and Pneumococcal Vaccination Rates: A Randomized Trial

Dexter PR, Perkins SM, Maharry KS, et al (Indiana Univ, Indianapolis; Regenstrief Inst for Health Care, Indianapolis, Ind; Richard L Roudebush VA Med Ctr, Indianapolis, Ind)

JAMA 292:2366-2371, 2004 35–9

Context.—Computerized reminder systems increase influenza and pneumococcal vaccination rates, but computerized standing order systems have not been previously described or evaluated.

Objective.—To determine the effects of computerized physician standing orders compared with physician reminders on inpatient vaccination rates.

Design, Setting, and Patients.—Randomized trial of 3777 general medicine patients discharged from 1 of 6 study wards during a 14-month period (November 1, 1998, through December 31, 1999) composed of 2 overlapping influenza seasons at an urban public teaching hospital.

Interventions.—The hospital's computerized physician order entry system identified inpatients eligible for influenza and pneumococcal vaccination. For patients with standing orders, the system automatically produced vaccine orders directed to nurses at the time of patient discharge. For patients with reminders, the computer system provided reminders to physicians that included vaccine orders during routine order entry sessions.

Main Outcome Measure.—Vaccine administration.

Results.—During the approximately 6 months of the influenza season, 50% of all hospitalized patients were identified as eligible for influenza vaccination. Twenty-two percent of patients hospitalized during the entire 14 months of the study were found eligible for pneumococcal vaccination. Patients with standing orders received an influenza vaccine significantly more often (42%) than those patients with reminders (30%) ($P<.001$). Patients with standing orders received a pneumococcal vaccine significantly more often (51%) than those with reminders (31%) ($P<.001$).

Conclusions.—Computerized standing orders were more effective than computerized reminders for increasing both influenza and pneumococcal vaccine administration. Our findings suggest that computerized standing orders should be used more widely for this purpose.

► Influenza kills. Especially the elderly. The Voordouw et al article (Abstract 35–8) reinforces information that has been published in other articles: not only does influenza vaccine reduce influenza deaths, it reduces overall mortality rates. Yet we physicians are incredibly lax in making sure our at-risk patients get the vaccine. Dexter et al, in a prospective randomized trial (Abstract 35–9), found that even with reminders or standing orders, only about half of patients received vaccine. It is true that many patients refused the vaccine; however, one cannot help but believe that a few minutes of education to dispel myths and provide documented positive data, as shown here, would change many minds and save many lives and much suffering. We need to embrace this responsibility, as the authors note, to come close to the Healthy People 2010 goal of 90% vaccination rates for patients older than 65 years in inner-city populations.

J. R. Maurer, MD

Effectiveness of β Lactam Antibiotics Compared With Antibiotics Active Against Atypical Pathogens in Non-severe Community Acquired Pneumonia: Meta-analysis

Mills GD, Oehley MR, Arrol B (Waikato Hosp, Hamilton, New Zealand; Univ of Auckland, New Zealand)

BMJ 330:456-460, 2005 35–10

Objective.—To systematically compare β lactam antibiotics with antibiotics active against atypical pathogens in the management of community acquired pneumonia.

Data Sources.—Medline, Embase, Cochrane register of controlled trials, international conference proceedings, drug registration authorities, and pharmaceutical companies.

Review Methods.—Double blind randomised controlled monotherapy trials comparing β lactam antibiotics with antibiotics active against atypical pathogens in adults with community acquired pneumonia. Primary outcome was failure to achieve clinical cure or improvement.

Results.—18 trials totalling 6749 participants were identified, with most patients having mild to moderate community acquired pneumonia. The summary relative risk for treatment failure in all cause community acquired pneumonia showed no advantage of antibiotics active against atypical pathogens over β lactam antibiotics (0.97, 95% confidence interval 0.87 to 1.07). Subgroup analysis was undertaken in those with a specific diagnosis involving atypical pathogens. We found a significantly lower failure rate in patients with *Legionella* species who were treated with antibiotics active against atypical pathogens (0.40, 0.19 to 0.85). Equivalence was seen for *Mycoplasma pneumoniae* (0.60, 0.31 to 1.17) and *Chlamydia pneumoniae* (2.32, 0.67 to 8.03).

Conclusions.—Evidence is lacking that clinical outcomes are improved by using antibiotics active against atypical pathogens in all cause non-severe community acquired pneumonia. Although such antibiotics were superior in the management of patients later shown to have legionella related pneumonia, this pathogen was rarely responsible for pneumonia within the included trials. β lactam agents should remain the antibiotics of initial choice in adults with non-severe community acquired pneumonia.

▶ Several guidelines for the treatment of community-acquired pneumonia exist, and most of them include the use of an antibiotic active against atypical organisms as first-line therapy. This meta-analysis challenges that dictum. The authors contend that little high-level evidence shows the superiority or even need for antibiotics directed against atypical organisms in oral regimens, with the exception of cases of *Legionella,* which are uncommon. This is an interesting meta-analysis, and the evidence-based findings should be taken into account in the creation of guidelines for low- and moderate-risk patients who can be treated as outpatients.

J. R. Maurer, MD

Risk of Community-Acquired Pneumonia and Use of Gastric Acid–Suppressive Drugs

Laheij RJF, Sturkenboom MCJM, Hassing R-J, et al (Univ Med Ctr St Radboud, Nijmegen, The Netherlands; Erasmus MC Univ, Rotterdam, The Netherlands)

JAMA 292:1955-1960, 2004 35–11

Context.—Reduction of gastric acid secretion by acid-suppressive therapy allows pathogen colonization from the upper gastrointestinal tract. The bacteria and viruses in the contaminated stomach have been identified as species from the oral cavity.

Objective.—To examine the association between the use of acid-suppressive drugs and occurrence of community-acquired pneumonia.

Design, Setting, and Participants.—Incident acid-suppressive drug users with at least 1 year of valid database history were identified from the Integrated Primary Care Information database between January 1, 1995, and December 31, 2002. Incidence rates for pneumonia were calculated for unexposed and exposed individuals. To reduce confounding by indication, a case-control analysis was conducted nested in a cohort of incident users of acid-suppressive drugs. Cases were all individuals with incident pneumonia during or after stopping use of acid-suppressive drugs. Up to 10 controls were matched to each case for practice, year of birth, sex, and index date. Conditional logistic regression was used to compare the risk of community-acquired pneumonia between use of proton pump inhibitors (PPIs) and H_2-receptor antagonists.

Main Outcome Measure.—Community-acquired pneumonia defined as certain (proven by radiography or sputum culture) or probable (clinical symptoms consistent with pneumonia).

Results.—The study population comprised 364,683 individuals who developed 5551 first occurrences of pneumonia during follow-up. The incidence rates of pneumonia in non–acid-suppressive drug users and acid-suppressive drug users were 0.6 and 2.45 per 100 person-years, respectively. The adjusted relative risk for pneumonia among persons currently using PPIs compared with those who stopped using PPIs was 1.89 (95% confidence interval, 1.36-2.62). Current users of H_2-receptor antagonists had a 1.63-fold increased risk of pneumonia (95% confidence interval, 1.07-2.48) compared with those who stopped use. For current PPI users, a significant positive dose-response relationship was observed. For H_2-receptor antagonist users, the variation in dose was restricted.

Conclusion.—Current use of gastric acid-suppressive therapy was associated with an increased risk of community-acquired pneumonia.

► Using a 500,000-patient, detailed electronic database in The Netherlands, the authors were able to associate development of community-acquired pneumonia with the use of gastric acid–suppressing drugs. The association between increased pH and increased colonization of the upper gastrointestinal tract has been known for many years in critically ill patients in whom acid-suppressing drugs are often used. Presumably this can facilitate airway colonization and subsequent pneumonia. While the risk is not excessive, it is another risk to note in ambulatory patients on these drugs.

J. R. Maurer, MD

Indicators of Recurrent Hospitalization for Pneumonia in the Elderly

El Solh AA, Brewer T, Okada M, et al (Univ of Buffalo, New York)

J Am Geriatr Soc 52:2010-2015, 2004 35–12

Objectives.—To identify modifiable risk factors of late unplanned readmissions for elderly with community-acquired pneumonia.

Design.—A case-control study.

Setting.—Three university-affiliated tertiary-care hospitals.

Participants.—Two hundred four case-control pairs. Case patients referred to all patients readmitted with pneumonia 30 days to 1 year after discharge. Control subjects were matched for age, admission date, and residence before admission.

Measurements.—Baseline sociodemographic information, clinical data, activity of daily living (ADLs) information, and Charlson Comorbidity Index score were obtained. The Pneumonia Severity Index was calculated with swallowing dysfunction and pattern and extent of radiographic abnormalities, antimicrobial coverage, and total duration recorded.

Results.—Median time to readmission was 123 days (interquartile range = 65-238 days). Readmission was not associated with increased severity or length of hospital stay. In a Cox proportional hazards regression model, swallowing dysfunction (hazard ratio (HR) = 2.15, 95% confidence interval (CI) = 1.46-2.97), current smoking (HR = 2.04, 95% CI = 1.48-2.82), use of tranquilizers (HR = 1.5, 95% CI = 1.02-2.22), and lower ADL scores (HR = 1.06, 95% CI = 1.02-1.10) were independently associated with readmission for pneumonia. The receipt of angiotensin-converting enzyme inhibitors (HR = 0.46, 95% CI = 0.27-0.78) and prior pneumococcal vaccination (HR = 0.59, 95% CI = 0.42-0.82) had a protective effect.

Conclusion.—Although there are limited effective measures to improve functional status, preventive strategies that include smoking cessation and pneumococcal vaccination should be actively pursued. Routine evaluation of swallowing dysfunction and use of pharmacological agents to improve the cough reflex deserve further evaluation in multicenter controlled trials.

Outcome Predictors of Pneumonia in Elderly Patients: Importance of Functional Assessment

Torres OH, Muñoz J, Ruiz D, et al (Autonomous Univ of Barcelona)
J Am Geriatr Soc 52:1603-1609, 2004 35–13

Objectives.—To evaluate the outcome of elderly patients with community-acquired pneumonia (CAP) seen at an acute-care hospital, analyzing the importance of CAP severity, functional status, comorbidity, and frailty.

Design.—Prospective observational study.

Setting.—Emergency department and geriatric medical day hospital of a university teaching hospital.

Participants.—Ninety-nine patients aged 65 and older seen for CAP over a 6-month recruitment period.

Measurements.—Clinical data were used to calculate Pneumonia Severity Index (PSI), Barthel Index (BI), Charlson Comorbidity Index, and Hospital Admission Risk Profile (HARP). Patients were then assessed 15 days later to determine functional decline and 30 days and 18 months later for mortality and readmission. Multiple logistic regression was used to analyze outcomes.

Results.—Functional decline was observed in 23% of the 93 survivors. Within the 30-day period, case-fatality rate was 6% and readmission rate 11%; 18-month rates were 24% and 59%, respectively. Higher BI was a protective factor for 30-day and 18-month mortality (odds ratio (OR) = 0.96, 95% confidence interval (CI) = 0.94-0.98 and OR = 0.97, 95% CI = 0.95-0.99, respectively; $P < .01$), and PSI was the only predictor for functional decline (OR = 1.03, 95% CI = 1.01-1.05; $P = .01$). Indices did not predict readmission. Analyses were repeated for the 74 inpatients and indicated similar results except for 18-month mortality, which HARP predicted (OR = 1.73; 95% CI = 1.16-2.57; $P < .01$).

Conclusion.—Functional status was an independent predictor for short- and long-term mortality in hospitalized patients whereas CAP severity predicted functional decline. Severity indices for CAP should possibly thus be adjusted in the elderly population, taking functional status assessment into account.

► These 2 articles (Abstracts 35–12 and 35–13) are included because they highlight the importance of functional status on outcomes in elderly patients with pneumonia. Functional status has been previously identified as a significant predictor for mortality in nursing home patients who develop pneumonia, but Torres et al (Abstract 35–13) found that it is also a powerful predictor in patients from the noninstitutionalized elderly. In addition, they found that functional status declines, at least short-term, in more than 20% of patients. El Solh and colleagues (Abstract 35–12), who studied a mixed population of noninstitutionalized and institutionalized patients, were able to associate functional status (as well as several other factors) with readmissions for pneumonia. The groups argue that pneumonia severity indices should be adjusted to better reflect functional status and that attempts should be made to improve functional status. These are good suggestions. Awareness by treating physicians of the importance of independence should help them better manage functionally impaired patients.

J. R. Maurer, MD

Outpatient Care Compared With Hospitalization for Community-Acquired Pneumonia: A Randomized Trial in Low-Risk Patients

Carratalà J, Fernández-Sabé N, Ortega L, et al (Univ of Barcelona; SCIAS-Hosp de Barcelona)

Ann Intern Med 142:165-172, 2005 35–14

Background.—The Pneumonia Severity Index (PSI) has been advocated as an objective measure of risk stratification to help determine the initial site of treatment for patients with community-acquired pneumonia.

Objective.—To determine whether outpatient care of PSI-defined low-risk patients with community-acquired pneumonia is as safe and effective as hospitalization.

Design.—Unblinded, randomized, controlled trial.

Setting.—2 tertiary care hospitals.

Patients.—224 immunocompetent adults in risk class II or III (PSI scores ≤90 points) who received a diagnosis of community-acquired pneumonia in the emergency department and had no extenuating circumstances.

Intervention.—Outpatient care with oral levofloxacin therapy or hospitalization with sequential intravenous and oral levofloxacin therapy.

Measurements.—The primary end point was the percentage of patients with an overall successful outcome at the end of treatment, according to 7 predefined criteria. Secondary end points included patients' quality of life and satisfaction.

Results.—Overall successful outcome was achieved in 83.6% of outpatients and 80.7% of hospitalized patients (absolute difference, 2.9 percentage points [95% CI, −7.1 to 12.9 percentage points]). More outpatients were satisfied with their overall care (91.2% vs. 79.1%; absolute difference, 12.1 percentage points [CI, 1.8 to 22.5 percentage points]). Quality of life and the percentages of patients with adverse drug reactions (9.1% vs. 9.6%), medical complications (0.9% vs. 2.6%), subsequent hospital admissions (6.3% vs. 7.0%), and overall mortality (0.9% vs. 0%) were similar in the outpatient and hospitalization groups.

Limitations.—The power to detect a serious complication, such as death, was limited given the relatively small sample size.

Conclusions.—In selected patients who had community-acquired pneumonia, PSI risk class II and III, and were treated with levofloxacin, outpatient care in the absence of respiratory failure, unstable comorbid conditions, complicated pleural effusions, and social problems was as safe and effective as hospitalization and provided greater patient satisfaction.

► Only about 15% of patients who develop community-acquired pneumonia each year are hospitalized. The criteria for admission focus on severity of pulmonary findings, comorbidities, and age, but they vary considerably by physician and locale. In this study, the authors looked at lower-risk disease without comorbidities and randomized patients to inpatient or outpatient management. Outcomes were similar in the groups, with outpatients expressing greater satisfaction with care. Unfortunately, the authors did not include a cost comparison of the 2 treatment groups. This could have been done very accurately, since it was a prospective trial, and would have added an important dimension to the study.

J. R. Maurer, MD

Measurements of Health-Related Quality of Life in the National Emphysema Treatment Trial

Kaplan RM, for the National Emphysema Treatment Trial Research Group (Univ of California, San Diego; et al)

Chest 126:781-789, 2004 35–15

Purposes.—To evaluate two generic and two disease-specific measures of health-related quality of life (QOL) using prerandomization data from the National Emphysema Treatment Trial (NETT).

Method.—The analyses used data collected from the 1,218 subjects who were randomized in the NETT. Patients completed evaluations before and after completion of the prerandomization phase of the NETT pulmonary rehabilitation program. Using data obtained prior to participation in the rehabilitation program, QOL measures were evaluated against physiologic and functional criteria using correlational analysis. The physiologic criteria included estimates of emphysema severity based on FEV_1 and measures of PaO_2 obtained with the subject at rest and breathing room air. Functional measures included the 6-min walk distance (6MWD), maximum work, and hospitalizations in the prior 3 months.

Results.—Correlation coefficients between QOL measures ranged from −0.31 to 0.70. In comparison to normative samples, scores on general QOL measures were low, suggesting that the NETT participants were quite ill. All QOL measures were modestly but significantly correlated with FEV_1, maximum work, and 6MWD. Patients who had stayed overnight in a hospital in the prior 3 months reported lower QOL on average than those who had not been hospitalized. There were significant improvements for all QOL measures following the rehabilitation program, and improvements in QOL were correlated with improvements in 6MWD.

► One of the secondary outcome measures in the NETT, which compared the outcomes of patients undergoing pulmonary rehabilitation followed by lung volume reduction surgery with the outcomes of those undergoing pulmonary rehabilitation only, was to evaluate QOL in the groups. However, the utility of different types of QOL instruments in chronic obstructive pulmonary disease was not well-defined when this study began, so the investigators used 4 different instruments, 2 that evaluate general well-being and 2 that are designed to be specifically used for respiratory disease. In this report, patients were studied only after undergoing rehabilitation and before half went on to lung volume reduction surgery. Thus, the data reflect changes in QOL afforded by pulmonary rehabilitation alone. Not surprisingly, all the instruments showed that the patients had a relatively low QOL and showed modest improvement after rehabilitation. The unexpected finding was that the more general instruments were nearly as sensitive as the disease-specific instruments in picking up these improvements. There may be some advantages, as the authors note, to using more general instruments, since scores can be compared with those found in other disease states to determine relative impacts. Also, general instruments that are utility based—the Quality of Well-Being Scale in this case—can be used to calculate the cost-effectiveness of interventions. This information was helpful in assisting Medicare to decide whether to cover lung volume reduction surgery. As we all know, based on the NETT study and in part on the QOL data, coverage was approved for a selected group of patients.

J. R. Maurer, MD

Thromboprophylaxis Does Not Protect Severely Injured Patients Against Pulmonary Embolism

Velmahos GC, Toutouzas KG, Brown C, et al (Univ of Southern California, Los Angeles)
Am Surg 70:893-896, 2004 35–16

Introduction.—The existing evidence on the effectiveness of thromboprophylaxis after trauma is conflicting. Although prophylaxis with heparin and/

or sequential compression devices is practiced widely, many studies failed to document a clear benefit. A recent meta-analysis suggests that prophylaxis does not reduce posttraumatic deep venous thrombosis rates compared to no prophylaxis. The objective of this prospective study is to examine if the use of thromboprophylaxis prevents posttraumatic pulmonary embolism (PE). Sixty-four critically injured patients with clinical evidence of PE were studied by computed tomographic pulmonary angiography and/or conventional pulmonary angiography. PE was diagnosed in 24 (37.5%) patients. Patients with PE were similar to patients without PE with regard to demographics, injury type and severity, operations, and mortality. Thromboprophylaxis was used with equal frequency between PE and no-PE patients (71% *vs* 80%, $P = 0.4$). The type of prophylaxis used was similar between patients with PE (17% heparin, 71% sequential compression devices, 17% combination) and patients without PE (32%, 57%, and 10%, respectively; $P = 0.16, 0.28, 0.69$, respectively). Current methods of posttraumatic thromboprophylaxis may be inadequate. Practices from nontrauma populations have been erroneously extrapolated to the unique trauma population. To reduce the rate of PE after trauma, new methods of thromboprophylaxis should be considered.

Deep Venous Thrombosis and Pulmonary Embolism in Trauma Patients: An Overstatement of the Problem?

Stawicki SP, Grossman MD, Cipolla J, et al (St Luke's Hosp, Bethlehem, Pa; Univ of Pennsylvania, Philadelphia)

Am Surg 71:387-391, 2005 35–17

Introduction.—Deep venous thrombosis (DVT) and pulmonary embolism (PE) affect high-risk trauma patients (HRTP). Accurate incidence and clinical importance of DVT and PE in HRTP may be overstated. We performed a ten-year retrospective analysis of HRTP of the Pennsylvania Trauma Outcome Study. High-risk factors (HRF) included pelvic fracture (PFx), lower extremity fracture (LEFx), severe head injury (CHI) (AIS—head ≥3), and spinal cord injury. HRF alone or in combination, age, Injury Severity Score (ISS), and Glasgow Coma Score (GCS) were examined for association with DVT/PE. A total of 73,419 HRTP were included: 1377 (1.9%) had DVT, 365 (05%) had PE. The incidence of DVT in level I trauma centers was 2.2 per cent and was 1.5 per cent in level II centers. The lowest incidence of DVT was 1.3 per cent for isolated LEFx; highest was 5.4% for combined PFx, LEFx, and CHI. Variables associated with DVT included age, ISS, and GCS (all $P < 0.001$). In logistic regression analysis, only ISS was consistently predictive for DVT and PE. Though increased during the past decade, the overall incidence of DVT in HRTP remains below 3 per cent. Only the combination of multiple injuries or an ISS >30 result in DVT incidence of ≥5 per cent. We believe that current guidelines for screening for DVT may need to be reevaluated.

► Trauma patients are a high-risk group for venous thromboembolic disorders, but no clear-cut method of thromboprophylaxis in such patients is superior. Despite the limitations of nonrandomization and low power, Velmahos et al (Abstract 35–16) did not find significant differences in the rates of several types of thromboprophylaxis between patients who developed pulmonary embolism and those who did not. These authors discussed the limitations of currently accepted methods of prophylaxis in this patient population. Pneumatic compression is difficult to apply in multitrauma patients, and it is very rarely performed effectively even when ordered. Also, trauma patients will often have reduced antithrombin III activity, leading to reduced activity of heparin-based therapy. Finally, the risk of bleeding must be considered. Recent interest and early experience with removable vena cava filters is promising.[1,2] That does not mean that widespread use of vena cava filters is being endorsed here. In fact, the study by Stawicki et al (Abstract 35–17) suggests that the reported incidence of DVT and PE in trauma patients has been overstated, and a more careful selection of who needs prophylaxis is required. This study reported an amount of venous thromboembolic disease approximately 10 times lower than previous reports. Their results cannot be ignored since over 70,000 patients were included from the Pennsylvania Trauma Registry.

K. L. Lewis, MD

References

1. Allen TL, Carter, JL, Morris BJ, et al: Retrievable vena cava filters in trauma patients for high risk prophylaxis and prevention of pulmonary embolism. *Am J Surg* 189:656-661, 2005.
2. Hoff WS, Hoey BA, Wainwright GA, et al: Early experience with retrievable inferior vena cava filters in high-risk trauma patients. *J Am Coll Surg* 199:869-874, 2004.

Thrombolysis Compared With Heparin for the Initial Treatment of Pulmonary Embolism: A Meta-Analysis of the Randomized Controlled Trials

Wan S, Quinlan DJ, Agnelli G, et al (Univ of Western Australia, Perth; King's College, London; Univ of Perugia, Italy)

Circulation 110:744-749, 2004 35–18

Background.—Randomized trials and meta-analyses have reached conflicting conclusions about the role of thrombolytic therapy for the treatment of acute pulmonary embolism.

Method and Results.—We performed a meta-analysis of all randomized trials comparing thrombolytic therapy with heparin in patients with acute pulmonary embolism. Eleven trials, involving 748 patients, were included. Compared with heparin, thrombolytic therapy was associated with a nonsignificant reduction in recurrent pulmonary embolism or death (6.7% versus 9.6%; OR 0.67, 95% CI 0.40 to 1.12, *P* for heterogeneity=0.48), a nonsignificant increase in major bleeding (9.1% versus 6.1%; OR 1.42, 95% CI 0.81 to 2.46), and a significant increase in nonmajor bleeding (22.7% versus 10.0%; OR 2.63, 95% CI 1.53 to 4.54; number needed to harm=8). Thrombolytic therapy compared with heparin was associated with a significant reduction in recurrent pulmonary embolism or death in trials that also enrolled patients with major (hemodynamically unstable) pulmonary embolism (9.4% versus 19.0%; OR 0.45, 95% CI 0.22 to 0.92; number needed to treat=10) but not in trials that excluded these patients (5.3% versus 4.8%; OR 1.07, 95% CI 0.50 to 2.30), with significant heterogeneity between these 2 groups of trials (*P*=0.10).

Conclusions.—Currently available data provide no evidence for a benefit of thrombolytic therapy compared with heparin for the initial treatment of unselected patients with acute pulmonary embolism. A benefit is suggested in those at highest risk of recurrence or death. The number of patients enrolled in randomized trials to date is modest, and further evaluation of the efficacy and safety of thrombolytic therapy for the treatment of high-risk patients with acute pulmonary embolism appears warranted.

► This study supports the current recommendations for thrombolytic therapy in acute pulmonary embolism. Thrombolytics should only be considered in the setting of massive pulmonary embolism where hemodynamic instability exists.[1] In normotensive patients, right heart strain patterns on ECG and echocardiography, elevated natriuretic peptide levels, and elevated troponin levels can predict a worse prognosis. However, evidence does not exist to support the use of any of these discriminators as a reason to start thrombolytics in the absence of hypotension.

K. L. Lewis, MD

Reference

1. Buller HR, Agnelli G, Hull RD, et al: Antithrombotic therapy for venous thromboembolic disease: The Seventh ACCP Conference on Antithrombotic and Thrombolytic Therapy. *Chest* 126(3 suppl):401S-428S, 2004.

Asthma Exacerbations in North American Adults: Who Are the "Frequent Fliers" in the Emergency Department?

Griswold SK, Nordstrom CR, Clark S, et al (Thomas Jefferson Univ, Philadelphia; Mercy Hosp of Philadelphia; Massachusetts Gen Hosp, Boston; et al)
Chest 127:1579-1586, 2005 35–19

Objective.—To characterize adult asthma patients according to frequency of emergency department (ED) visits in the past year.

Design.—Adults presenting with acute asthma to 83 US EDs underwent structured interviews in the ED and by telephone 2 weeks later.

Results.—The 3,151 enrolled patients were classified into four groups: those reporting no ED visits in the past year (27%), one to two visits (27%),

TABLE 3.—Multivariate Model of Factors Associated With Six or More ED Visits for Asthma During the Past Year

	OR	CI	*P* Value
Age (per ↑ 10 yr)	1.07	0.97-1.19	0.19
Female gender	0.81	0.65-1.01	0.06
White race	0.60	0.46-0.78	< 0.001
High school graduate	0.94	0.76-1.17	0.58
Insurance status			
Private	1.0	Reference	
Medicaid	2.79	2.08-3.73	< 0.001
Other public	1.57	1.08-2.27	0.02
None	1.56	1.14-2.12	0.005
Has primary care provider	0.82	0.65-1.04	0.10
History of hospitalization for asthma	2.56	1.97-3.33	< 0.001
History of intubation for asthma	1.53	1.19-1.96	0.001
Receiving inhaled corticosteroids during past 4 wk	2.20	1.77-2.74	< 0.001

(Courtesy of Griswold SK, Nordstrom CR, Clark S, et al: Asthma exacerbations in North American adults: Who are the "frequent fliers" in the emergency department? *Chest* 127:1579-1586, 2005.)

three to five visits (25%), and six or more visits (21%). The number of ED visits (NEDV) was associated with older age, nonwhite race, lower socioeconomic status, and several markers of chronic asthma severity (all $p < 0.001$). NEDV was strongly associated with Medicaid insurance (17% among those with no visits, 22% with one to two visits, 30% with three to five visits, 39% with six or more visits; $p < 0.001$). NEDV was unrelated to gender or having a primary care provider (PCP). In a multivariate model, independent predictors of high ED use (six or more visits a year) were nonwhite race, Medicaid, other public, and no insurance, and markers of chronic asthma severity. Patients with six or more ED visits accounted for 67% of all prior ED visits in the past year.

Conclusions.—High NEDV is associated with characteristics that may help with identification of "frequent fliers" in the ED. A better understanding of these characteristics may advance ongoing efforts to decrease asthma health-care disparities, including differential access to primary asthma care. National guidelines recommend specific ED treatments then referral to a PCP. Although longitudinal care is surely important, attempts to reduce frequent ED asthma visits may be better directed toward more specific preventive and educational needs (Table 3).

► Report of combined data from prospective cohort studies including 83 US EDs demonstrating that the NEDV (high was defined as more than 6/year) was associated with several risk factors. Contrary to previous reports, lack of a PCP was not a statistically significant predictor of a high NEDV. Statistically significant characteristics predicting a high NEDV included coverage by Medicaid ($P < .001$), history of hospitalization for asthma ($P < .001$), history of intubation for asthma ($P = .001$), and receipt of inhaled corticosteroids during the 4 weeks preceding the ED visit ($P < .001$). Being nonwhite, of lower socioeconomic status, having Medicaid insurance, and a higher chronic asthma severity also predicted a high NEDV. The message from this study is that the commonly held belief (that if "frequent flier" asthmatics could be referred to a PCP, their NEDV might be reduced) lacks support.

S. K. Willsie, DO

Risk Factors for Near-Fatal Asthma

Gelb AF, Schein A, Nussbaum E, et al (Lakewood Regional Med Ctr, Calif; Univ of Toronto; Kaiser Permanente Hosp, Harbor City, Calif; et al)

Chest 126:1138-1146, 2004 35–20

Background.—There is a paucity of lung function data in patients, both before and after episodes of near-fatal asthma (NFA), requiring transient endotracheal intubation and mechanical ventilation.

Methods.—Lung function was initially measured in 43 asthmatic patients (age range, 16 to 49 years), who were observed and treated in a tertiary referral asthma clinic and were clinically stable at the time of study. Subsequently, clinical and physiologic follow-up studies were obtained over > 5 years. The primary outcomes were to determine (1) the integrity of lung elastic recoil and (2) the severity of expiratory airflow limitation, and (3) to correlate these outcomes with adverse clinical complications.

Results.—Fourteen of 26 asthmatic patients (54%) [age range, 30 to 49 years] had significantly reduced lung elastic recoil pressures at all lung volumes compared to 3 of 17 asthmatic patients (18%); $p = 0.02$ [χ^2 test and Fisher exact test] [age range, 16 to 26 years]. In asthmatic patients between the ages of 30 and 49 years, significant loss of lung elastic recoil was noted in 4 of 10 patients with mild reduction in FEV_1 (FEV_1, > 79% predicted), 6 of 12 patients with moderate reduction in FEV_1 (FEV_1, 61 to 79% predicted), and all 4 patients with severe reduction in FEV_1 (FEV_1, < 61% predicted). In asthmatic patients between the ages of 16 and 26 years, significant loss of lung elastic recoil was noted in 0 of 11 patients with mild reduction in FEV_1, 2 of 5 patients with moderate reduction in FEV_1, and 1 of 1 patient with severe reduction in FEV_1. A subgroup of 10 asthmatic patients (7 men) [mean (± SD) age, 37 ± 11 years] were studied when clinically stable, both before and after an episode of NFA in 8 cases and only after an episode of NFA in 2 additional cases. In 1 of 10 cases, the FEV_1 was mildly reduced, in 4 cases it was moderately reduced, and in 5 cases it was severely reduced, both before and after an episode of NFA. The sensitivity was 90%, the specificity was 61%, the positive predictive value was 41%, and the negative predictive value was 95% for NFA with an $FEV_1 \leq 79\%$ predicted or FEV_1/FVC ratio of < 75%. Prior to an episode of NFA, all 8 asthmatic patients had significant loss of lung elastic recoil pressure, and afterward all 10 had significant loss of lung elastic recoil pressure (ie, less than the predicted normal mean minus 1.64 SD at a total lung capacity [TLC] of 100 to 70% predicted). The sensitivity was 100%, the specificity was 79%, the positive predictive value was 59%, and the negative predictive value was 100% for NFA with the loss of lung elastic recoil. The mean TLC measured with a plethysmograph in 10 patients with NFA was 7.2 ± 1.41 (124 ± 16% predicted). The sensitivity for TLC of > 115% predicted was 70%, the specificity was 70%, the positive predictive value was 88%, and the negative predictive value was 41% for NFA.

Conclusion.—A persistent reduction in FEV_1 of ≤ 79% predicted or an FEV_1/FVC ratio of < 75%, and, especially, the loss of lung elastic recoil and hyperinflation at TLC are risk factors for NFA. The loss of lung elastic recoil in asthmatic patients was associated with increased age, duration of disease, and progressive expiratory airflow limitation.

► This is a prospective study of lung function and CT findings in stable asthmatics who were monitored for more than 5 years. Asthmatics subsequently experiencing episode(s) of NFA were more likely to have a persistent reduction in FEV_1 of 79% or less or FEV_1/FVC ratio of less than 75%, loss of elastic recoil, and hyperinflation at total lung capacity. Aggressive monitoring during "stable" periods, with targeted interventions imposed when the FEV_1 is persistently 79% or less, the FEV_1/FVC ratio is less than 75%, or there is loss of elastic recoil and hyperinflation at total lung capacity may help to reduce morbidity/mortality in asthmatics at risk for NFA.

S. K. Willsie, DO

Obesity Increases the Risk of Incident Asthma Among Adults

Rönmark E, Andersson C, Nyström L, et al (Sunderby Central Hosp of Norrbotten, Luleå, Sweden; Karolinska Institutet, Stockholm; Univ of Umeå, Sweden)

Eur Respir J 25:282-288, 2005 35–21

Introduction.—The annual incidence of asthma in adults in northern Sweden has been estimated at 2.3 per thousand population. Risk factors for incident asthma among adults were studied in a case-referent study based on incident cases of asthma during 1995-1999. The healthcare providers reported suspected cases of incident asthma. After clinical examination, 309 (65% female) of 473 reported subjects were included. Inclusion criteria were a history of incident asthma (onset <12 months) and verified bronchial variability. Referents were randomly selected and stratified by age, sex and area of residence. The significant risk factors were hay fever, a family history of asthma, ex-smoking status and elevated body mass index (25.0-29.9 and ≥30). The risk factor pattern was similar for females and males, and increased body mass index was a significant risk factor for both males and females, as well as for allergic and nonallergic subjects. In conclusion, in addition to hay fever, a family history of asthma, allergic sensitisation and ex-smoking status, increased body mass index was a significant risk factor for incident asthma independent of sex and allergic status.

► This Swedish study investigated adult cases of reported incident asthma and their relationship to overweight and obesity. Compared with nonasthmatic referents (controls), the odds ratio for development of asthma in this study was 2.0 (95% confidence interval [CI]: 1.3-3.1) when the body mass index (BMI) ranged from 25 to 29.9 and 2.7 (95% CI: 1.5-4.7) when the BMI was more than 30. The effect of an elevated BMI on the development of asthma was judged independent of gender and allergic status.

S. K. Willsie, DO

The Association of Acetaminophen, Aspirin, and Ibuprofen With Respiratory Disease and Lung Function

McKeever TM, Lewis SA, Smit HA, et al (Univ of Nottingham, England; King's College, London; Natl Inst of Public Health, Bilthoven, The Netherlands; et al)

Am J Respir Crit Care Med 171:966-971, 2005 35–22

Rationale.—Oxidative stress may increase the risk of asthma, contribute to asthma progression, and decrease lung function. Previous research suggests that use of acetaminophen, which is hypothesized to reduce antioxidant capacity in the lung, is associated with an increased risk of asthma. We hypothesized that acetaminophen use may also be associated with chronic obstructive pulmonary disease (COPD) and decreased lung function.

Objectives.—To investigate the associations between use of pain medication, particularly acetaminophen, and asthma, COPD, and FEV_1 in adults.

Methods.—A cross-sectional analysis using the Third National Health and Nutrition Examination Survey.

Measurement and Main Results.—Increased use of acetaminophen had a positive, dose-dependent association with COPD (adjusted odds ratio for increasing category of intake, 1.16; 95% confidence interval [CI], 1.09-1.24; p value for trend < 0.001) and an inverse association with lung function (daily user compared with never users, −54.0 ml; 95% CI, −90.3 to −17.7, adjusted). Neither of these associations was explained by overlap between COPD and asthma occurrence. We confirmed a dose-response association of acetaminophen use and asthma (adjusted odds ratio, 1.20; 95% CI, 1.12-1.28; p value for trend < 0.001).

Conclusions.—This study provides further evidence that use of acetaminophen is associated with an increased risk of asthma and COPD, and with decreased lung function.

► This very interesting study using data from the Third National Health and Nutrition Examination Survey demonstrated that regular use of acetaminophen is associated with a dose-response–related increase in the incidence of COPD when compared to controls (adjusted OR for daily use 1.94 [95% CI: 1.53-2.47], with a *P* value < .001 for the OR trend). In addition, a dose-response association exists between acetaminophen and asthma adjusted OR 1.20 (95% CI: 1.12-1.28, *P* value for trend < .001). Interesting hypotheses exist regarding why acetaminophen use might be a risk factor for respiratory disease, including that in animal models, lung glutathione is reduced in the setting of high-acetaminophen doses,[1,2] and reduced levels of lung glutathione are associated with oxidant damage in the lungs.[3,4] A common suggestion to patients with chronic pain that they use regular dosing of acetaminophen as their analgesic of choice (as opposed to a nonsteroidal anti-inflammatory agent) should perhaps be rethought.

S. K. Willsie, DO

References

1. Chen TS, Richie JP, Lang CA: Life span profiles of glutathione and acetaminophen detoxification. *Drug Metab Dispos* 18:882-887, 1990.
2. Micheli L, Cerretani D, Fiaschi AI, et al: Effect of acetaminophen on glutathione levels in rat testis and lung. *Environ Health Perspect* 102(Suppl 9):63-64, 1994.
3. Jenkinson SG, Black RD, Lawrence RA: Glutathione concentrations in rat lung bronchoalveolar lavage fluid: Effects of hyperoxia. *J Lab Clin Med* 112:345-351, 1998.
4. Smith LJ, Anderson J, Shamsuddin M, et al: Effect of fasting on hyperoxic lung injury in mice: The role of glutathione. *Am Rev Respir Crit Care Med* 141:141-149, 1990.

Smoking and Asthma in Adults

Piipari R, Jaakkola JJK, Jaakkola N, et al (Univ of Helsinki; Univ of Birmingham, England)

Eur Respir J 24:734-739, 2004 35–23

Introduction.—Studies on the effect of smoking on adulthood asthma have provided contradictory results. The current authors conducted a population-based incident case-control study to assess the effects of current and past smoking on the development of asthma in adults. During a 2.5 yr study period, all new asthma cases clinically diagnosed (n=521) and randomly selected controls (n=932) from a geographically defined district in southern Finland were recruited. The risk of developing asthma was significantly higher among current smokers with an adjusted odds ratio (OR) of 1.33 (95% confidence interval 1.00-1.77) and among ex-smokers with an adjusted OR 1.49 (1.12-1.97) compared with never-smokers. Among current smokers, the risk increased up to 14 cigarettes $\cdot$ day^{-1}, and a similar trend was observed in relation to cumulative smoking. In conclusion, the current results support the hypothesis that smoking causes asthma in adulthood.

► This population-based study showed that the OR for developing asthma was elevated particularly in women smokers: OR of 2.43 for women/current smokers (143% increased risk) and 2.38 for women/ex-smokers (138% increase). This lends credence to the importance of smoking cessation/smoking prevention efforts in women.

S. K. Willsie, DO

The Prevalence of Gastroesophageal Reflux Disease in Adult Asthmatics
Kiljander TO, Laitinen JO (Tampere Univ, Finland)
Chest 126:1490-1494, 2004 35–24

Background.—Asthma and gastroesophageal reflux disease (GERD) often coexist. However, the results of the studies investigating the prevalence of GERD among patients with asthma vary greatly.

Study Objective.—To investigate the prevalence of GERD in adult patients with asthma.

Subjects and Methods.—The basic study population consisted of 2,225 asthmatic patients who were treated in six specialist-headed hospitals during 1 year. From the common computer-based discharge register, every 14th patient was randomly selected for the study. Ninety of the 149 contacted patients (60%) agreed to participate in the study. Twenty-four-hour esophageal pH monitoring was performed on all patients.

Results.—GERD was found in 32 of the patients (36%). Eight of these patients (25%) were free from classical reflux symptoms. Forty-seven of the 90 patients (52%) presented with typical reflux symptoms. Twenty-four of these patients (51%) were found to have abnormal acidic reflux.

Conclusions.—According to the current study, one third of adult patients with asthma have GERD. These patients often do not have typical reflux symptoms. However, the presence of typical reflux symptoms in an asthmatic patient does not seem to guarantee the presence of abnormal acidic reflux.

Prevalence of Gastroesophageal Reflux in Difficult Asthma: Relationship to Asthma Outcome
Leggett JJ, Johnston BT, Mills M, et al (Belfast City Hosp, England; Royal Group Hosps, Belfast, England)
Chest 127:1227-1231, 2005 35–25

Study Objectives.—To determine the prevalence of gastroesophageal reflux disease (GERD)—both symptoms and objective evidence—using 24-h dual-probe pH monitoring in difficult asthma, and the relationship between the presence and treatment of GERD to clinical outcome.

Design and Setting.—As part of a systematic evaluation protocol, 68 subjects with difficult-to-control asthma attending a difficult asthma clinic were referred for dual-probe ambulatory pH esophageal monitoring.

Results.—Esophageal probe data were available in 52 patients (76%) with difficult asthma. The prevalence of GERD/GERD-associated asthma symptoms was 75% (39 of 52 patients; 95% confidence interval [CI], 63 to 84.7%). The prevalence of GERD as evidenced by an abnormal pH profile at the distal esophageal probe was 55% (29 of 52 patients; 95% CI, 40 to 69%). The prevalence of GERD at the proximal probe was 34.6% (18 of 52 patients; 95% CI, 23.6 to 51%). The prevalence of GERD was similar in asthmatic subjects who responded to intervention and those who remained difficult to control (therapy resistant). Asymptomatic GERD was present in 9.6% (5 of 52 patients); 16% of cough episodes correlated with acid reflux.

Conclusions.—In difficult-to-control asthma, GERD is common, but identification and treatment of GERD do not appear to relate to improvement in asthma control in this population.

► GERD was documented by 24-hour esophageal-probe pH monitoring in 75% of patients with difficult-to-control asthma (Abstract 35–25). Kiljander and Laitinen (Abstract 35–24) showed that of those with GERD, 25% had no classic symptoms and 52% had typical symptoms. Identification and treatment of GERD does not appear to relate to improvement of asthma control in this population.

S. K. Willsie, DO

Internet-based Monitoring of Asthma: A Long-term, Randomized Clinical Study of 300 Asthmatic Subjects

Rasmussen LM, Phanareth K, Nolte H, et al (Univ Hosp of Copenhagen; H:S Bispebjerg Hosp, Copenhagen; H:S Frederiksberg Hosp, Copenhagen)

J Allergy Clin Immunol 115:1137-1142, 2005 35–26

Background.—Experience from other fields of internal medicine shows that Internet-based technology can be used to monitor various diseases. The new technology handles complex calculation programs easily, and it is a unique way of communicating. These advantages might be used in optimizing the treatment for asthmatic subjects because undertreatment is a common problem found in European asthmatic subjects.

Objective.—We sought to investigate the outcome of monitoring and treatment using a physician-managed online interactive asthma monitoring tool and to assess whether the outcome differs from that of monitoring and treatment in an outpatient respiratory clinic or in primary care.

Methods.—Three hundred asthmatic subjects were randomized to 3 parallel groups in a 6-month prospective study: (1) Internet-based monitoring (n = 100); (2) specialist monitoring (n = 100); and (3) general practitioner (GP) monitoring (n = 100). All the patients were examined on entry into the study and after 6 months of treatment.

Results.—The treatment and monitoring with the Internet-based management tool lead to significantly better improvement in the Internet group than in the other 2 groups regarding asthma symptoms (Internet vs specialist: odds ratio of 2.64, $P = .002$; Internet vs GP: odds ratio of 3.26; $P < .001$), quality of life (Internet vs specialist: odds ratio of 2.21, $P = .03$; Internet vs GP: odds ratio of 2.10, $P = .04$), lung function (Internet vs specialist: odds ratio of 3.26, $P = .002$; Internet vs GP: odds ratio of 4.86, $P < .001$), and airway responsiveness (Internet vs GP: odds ratio of 3.06, $P = .02$).

Conclusion.—When physicians and patients used an interactive Internet-based asthma monitoring tool, better asthma control was achieved (Tables 2 and 3).

TABLE 2.—Treatment Effect at Follow-up

Variables	Internet vs Specialist Odds Ratio (95% CI)	Internet vs Specialist *P* Value	Internet vs GP Odds Ratio (95% CI)	Internet vs GP *P* Value	Specialist vs GP Odds Ratio (95% CI)	Specialist vs GP *P* Value
Improved symptoms	2.64*(1.43-4.88)	.002	3.26*(1.71-6.19)	<.001	1.23*(0.66-2.30)	NS
Improved AQLQ	2.21†(1.09-4.47)	.03	2.10†(1.02-4.31)	.04	0.95†(0.43-2.07)	NS
Improved FEV1 ≥300 mL	3.26‡(1.50-7.11)	.002	4.86‡(1.97-11.94)	<.001	1.49‡(0.55-4.05)	NS
Improved AHR	1.26§(0.57-2.79)	NS	3.06§(1.13-8.31)	.02	2.44§(0.89-6.72)	NS

*Odds for improvement in asthma symptoms at follow-up: the improvement in symptoms was defined as improvement of one or more severity steps: 64% (Internet group), 40% (specialist group), and 35% (GP group) of the patients improved.

†Odds for improvement in AQLQ score at follow-up; improvement in AQLQ score was defined as improvement of 0.5 (minimal important change) or more in the overall score: 33% (Internet group), 18% (specialist group), and 19% (GP group) of the patients improved.

‡Odds for improvement in FEV_1 of 300 mL or more at follow-up: 32% (Internet group), 13% (specialist group), and 9% (GP group) of the patients improved.

§Odds for improvement in airway responsiveness by one or more dosage step at follow-up: 21% (Internet group), 17% (specialist group), and 8% (GP group) of the patients improved.

Abbreviations: NS, No significant difference between groups; *AHR*, airway hyperresponsiveness.

(Reprinted by permission of the publisher from Rasmussen LM, Phanareth K, Nolte H, et al: Internet-based monitoring of asthma: A long-term, randomized clinical study of 300 asthmatic subjects. *J Allergy Clin Immunol* 115:1137-1142, 2005. Copyright 2005 by Elsevier.)

TABLE 3.—Medication, Compliance, and Use of Action Plan at Baseline and at Follow-up*

Variables	Internet Group (n = 85)			Specialist Group (n = 88)			GP Group (n = 80)		
	Baseline	Follow-up	McNemar	Baseline	Follow-up	McNemar	Baseline	Follow-up	McNemar
No asthma medication	44%	0%	<.001	57%	1%	<.001	53%	26%	<.001
Take ICS	21%	91%	<.001	20%	83%	<.001	17%	29%	.04
Daily dose of ICS,† μg		866 (0-1600)			400 (0-1600)			0 (0-1200)	
Good Compliance‡	32%	87%	<.001	25%	79%	<.001	36%	54%	<.001
Use of action plan§	2%	88%	<.001	3%	66%	<.001	0%	6%	NS

*No significant difference was seen among the 3 groups at baseline.
†The daily dose of inhaled corticosteroids actually taken by the patients during the study (median [range]).
‡Good compliance is defined as use of medication always or almost always.
§The patients were asked whether they used their action plan (yes/no).
Abbreviations: NS, No significant difference between groups; *ICS*, inhaled corticosteroids.
(Reprinted by permission of the publisher from Rasmussen LM, Phanareth K, Nolte H, et al: Internet-based monitoring of asthma: A long-term, randomized clinical study of 300 asthmatic subjects. *J Allergy Clin Immunol* 115:1137-1142, 2005. Copyright 2005 by Elsevier.)

► The wave of the future? This study shows in a prospective fashion that an Internet-based monitoring program for asthma resulted in improvement (symptoms, quality of life, lung function and airway responsiveness) when compared to monitoring by a specialist or GP. Action-plan availability at baseline ranged from zero to 3%; following intervention, action-plan availability rose to 88% for Internet-based, 66% for specialist, and 6% for GP monitoring. Number of patients needed to treat to improve outcomes in 1 patient equals 6 Internet monitored versus traditional management. Patients and insurance companies will be demanding this type of care availability in the future, and rightfully so.

S. K. Willsie, DO

36 Sleep

Sleepiness, Sleep-Disordered Breathing, and Accident Risk Factors in Commercial Vehicle Drivers

Howard HE, Desai AV, Grunstein RR, et al (Univ of Melbourne, Australia; Monash Med Centre, Victoria, Australia; Royal Prince Alfred Hosp and Royal North Shore Hosps, New South Wales; et al)

Am J Respir Crit Care Med 170:1014-1021, 2004 36–1

Introduction.—Sleep-disordered breathing and excessive sleepiness may be more common in commercial vehicle drivers than in the general population. The relative importance of factors causing excessive sleepiness and accidents in this population remains unclear. We measured the prevalence of excessive sleepiness and sleep-disordered breathing and assessed accident risk factors in 2,342 respondents to a questionnaire distributed to a random sample of 3,268 Australian commercial vehicle drivers and another 161 drivers among 244 invited to undergo polysomnography. More than half (59.6%) of drivers had sleep-disordered breathing and 15.8% had obstructive sleep apnea syndrome. Twenty-four percent of drivers had excessive sleepiness. Increasing sleepiness was related to an increased accident risk. The sleepiest 5% of drivers on the Epworth Sleepiness Scale and Functional Outcomes of Sleep Questionnaire had an increased risk of an accident (odds ratio [OR] 1.91, $p = 0.02$ and OR 2.23, $p < 0.01$, respectively) and multiple accidents (OR 2.67, $p < 0.01$ and OR 2.39, $p = 0.01$), adjusted for established risk factors. There was an increased accident risk with narcotic analgesic use (OR 2.40, $p < 0.01$) and antihistamine use (OR 3.44, $p = 0.04$). Chronic excessive sleepiness and sleep-disordered breathing are common in Australian commercial vehicle drivers. Accident risk was related to increasing chronic sleepiness and antihistamine and narcotic analgesic use.

► This article is important because it gives us some easy-to-use tools to help identify which of our patients with sleep apnea might be at greatest risk for accidents. The Epworth Sleepiness Scale[1] and the Functional Outcomes of Sleep Questionnaire[2] have been around for awhile and are easy to use. In this large sample of Australian commercial drivers, these instruments were predictive of crashes.

Almost half of the drivers in this study had some degree of sleep-disordered breathing, and almost 16% had frank sleep apnea. But we know that not all patients with sleep apnea are at increased risk for accidents. This article reminds us that it is sleepiness, not sleep apnea, that puts our patients at risk, and that there are many other causes of sleepiness besides sleep apnea. In this study, use of narcotics and antihistamines also increased the risk of crashes, as did longer durations of driving, and driving on either the interstate or in the country.

We know that continuous positive airway pressure (CPAP) quickly reverses psychomotor deficits in patients with sleep apnea,[3] and that CPAP treatment reduces automobile accident risk in sleep apneics who use it.[4] But for many patients, CPAP alone may not be enough. This article warns us that patients who are sleepy (Epworth Sleepiness Score of 18 or higher for any reason) from any cause are at markedly increased risk or crashes.

B. A. Phillips, MD, MSPH

References

1. Johns MW: A new method for measuring daytime sleepiness: The Epworth sleepiness scale. *Sleep* 14:540-545, 1991.
2. Weaver TE, Laizner AM, Evans LK, et al: An instrument to measure functional status outcomes for disorders of excessive sleepiness. *Sleep* 20:835-843, 1997.
3. Turkington PM, Sircar M, Saralaya D, et al: Time course of changes in driving simulator performance with and without treatment in patients with sleep apnoea hypopnoea syndrome. *Thorax* 59:56-59, 2004.
4. George CF: Reduction in motor vehicle collisions following treatment of sleep apnoea with nasal CPAP. *Thorax* 56:508-512, 2001.

Sleep Quality and Blood Pressure Dipping in Normal Adults

Loredo JS, Nelesen R, Ancoli-Israel S, et al (Univ of California, San Diego; Veterans Affairs San Diego Healthcare System)
Sleep 27:1097-1103, 2004 36–2

Objectives.—To investigate the relationship between sleep quality and nocturnal blood pressure dipping in normal subjects. We hypothesized that sleep quality correlates with dipping.

Design.—Cross-sectional study.

Setting.—Unattended polysomnography in the home followed by a 24-hour ambulatory blood pressure measurement.

Patients.—Eighty-eight self-described normal subjects were evaluated; 26 were excluded due to an apnea-hypopnea index ≥ 10. None were taking antihypertensive medications.

Interventions: N/A.

Measurements and Results.—Subjects were divided into dippers and nondippers based on ≥ 10% drop in nocturnal mean arterial pressure (MAP). Sleep-quality variables included total sleep time; sleep latency; percentage of stages 1, 2, 3, 4, and rapid-eye-movement sleep; percentage of wake time after sleep onset (WASO); total arousal index; and sleep efficiency. Of the remaining 62 subjects, 17.7% were nondippers, and 7 were hypertensive. There was no difference in age, body mass index, apnea-hypopnea index, blood pressure, or sleep quality between groups. Stage 4 sleep correlated significantly with dipping of diastolic blood pressure and MAP ($r = 0.410$ and 0.378, respectively, $P \leq .002$), and percentage of WASO was negatively correlated with dipping of diastolic blood pressure ($r = -0.360$, $P = .004$), suggesting that greater dipping was associated with better sleep quality. On multivariate analyses, Stage 4 sleep was independently associated with dipping of diastolic blood pressure ($P = .034$) after adjusting for screening MAP, percentage of WASO, total arousal index, and Stage 1 sleep. The same link was found between Stage 4 sleep and dipping of MAP ($P = .05$) after adjusting for screening MAP, age, sex, and body mass index. Repeat analyses excluding hypertensives yielded similar findings.

Conclusion.—Our data suggest that deeper and less-fragmented sleep is associated with more blood pressure dipping in normal subjects.

► Now, *this* is interesting! We have known for awhile that sleep apnea is causally associated with hypertension,[1,2] and that continuous positive airway pressure (CPAP) can lower blood pressure in hypertensive sleep apneics.[3] This is believed to be mediated by hypoxemia and/or increased sympathetic tone. The harbinger of development of hypertension in patients with sleep apnea is loss of the normal early morning dip in blood pressure.[4] The current paper by Loredo and colleagues suggests that poor sleep quality, in and of itself, may contribute to loss of early morning dipping. Specifically, the amount of Stage 4 sleep correlated significantly with the systolic blood pressure and mean arterial pressure, and the amount of wakefulness correlated negatively with diastolic pressure.

Stage 4 is the deepest stage of non–rapid-eye-movement (NREM) sleep. Stages 3 and 4 together are sometimes called *slow-wave sleep* or *delta sleep*, and are believed to be physically restorative. The implications of this are many. For example, exercise is known both to increase stage 4 sleep and to lower blood pressure. Aging is associated both with reduced stage 4 sleep and increased blood pressure. Is slow-wave sleep the key to the fountain of youth?

B. A. Phillips, MD, MSPH

References

1. Chobanian AV, Bakris GL, Black HR, et al: The seventh report of the Joint National Committee on Prevention, Detection, Evaluation, and Treatment of High Blood Pressure: The JNC 7 report. *JAMA* 289:2560-2572, 2003.
2. Peppard PE, Young T, Palta M, et al: Prospective study of the association between sleep-disordered breathing and hypertension. *N Engl J Med* 342:1378-1384, 2000.
3. Becker HF, Jerrentrup A, Ploch T, et al: Effect of nasal continuous positive airway pressure treatment on blood pressure in patients with obstructive sleep apnea. *Circulation* 107:68-73, 2003.
4. Suzuki M, Guilleminault C, Otsuka K, et al: Blood pressure "dipping" and "non-dipping" in obstructive sleep apnea syndrome patients. *Sleep* 19:382-387, 1996.

Comparative Study of Autotitrating and Fixed-Pressure CPAP in the Home: A Randomized, Single-blind Crossover Trial

Hukins C (Princess Alexandra Hosp, Woolloongabba, QLD, Australia)

Sleep 27:1512-1517, 2004 36–3

Study Objectives.—To compare compliance and treatment response between continuous positive airway pressure (CPAP) and auto-titrating positive airway pressure (APAP) and to develop selection criteria for the use of APAP.

Design.—Randomized, single-blinded, parallel crossover study.

Setting.—Tertiary referral sleep disorders center.

Patients.—Consecutive patients with obstructive sleep apnea syndrome requiring treatment with CPAP.

Interventions.—2-month treatment each of conventional CPAP and APAP in random order comparing objective compliance, Epworth Sleepiness Score, SF-36 Health Survey, visual-analog measures of ease of and attitude to treatment, side effects, and treatment pressures or system leaks obtained from the Autoset T device.

Measurements and Results.—There were no differences between treatment modes in overall compliance (CPAP 4.86 ± 2.65, APAP 5.05 ± 2.38 hours per night, $P = .14$), Epworth Sleepiness Scale scores (baseline 12.4 ± 5.1, CPAP 8.4 ± 5.2, APAP 7.9 ± 4.8, $P < .001$ relative to baseline, NS between modes), SF-36 scores (significant improvements in Role Physical and Vitality domains relative to baseline, $P < .001$ but NS between modes). There were fewer reported side effects in APAP mode (CPAP 28, APAP 15 reports, $P = .02$) and compliance was greater with APAP in those reporting any side effect (95% confidence interval CPAP 0-6.8, APAP 2.9-7.8 hours per night, $P < .001$). APAP delivered significantly lower median and 95th centile airway pressures and fewer system leaks.

Conclusions.—Compliance, subjective sleepiness, and quality of life are similar between patients who used CPAP and APAP. APAP delivers lower pressures and results in lower-pressure leaks and fewer reported side effects. Compliance is higher with APAP in subjects reporting any side effect. APAP may be indicated in patients reporting side effects with conventional CPAP.

► This article shows that not only does autotitrating continuous positive airway pressure (CPAP) work as well as in-laboratory titrated CPAP, it also appears to result in better compliance. Organized sleep medicine opposes routine use of autotitrating CPAP,[1] despite excellent evidence that it works just as well as in-lab titrated CPAP.[2-4] The current article suggests it may even work better, since compliance is a huge clinical issue with CPAP use. Further, in the past 3 weeks, I have seen 4 patients who had sleep studies "elsewhere," and were scheduled to go back for in-lab CPAP titrations. They and/or their referring doctors appropriately questioned the cost, hassle, and delay in that approach, and these patients wound up in my office for more expedient treatment.

B. A. Phillips, MD, MSPH

References

1. Littner M, Hirskowitz M, Davila DG, et al: Practice parameters for the use of auto-titrating continuous positive airway pressure devices for titrating pressures and treating adult patients with obstructive sleep apnea syndrome. An American Academy of Sleep Medicine report. *Sleep* 25:143-147, 2002.
2. Randerath W, Schraeder O, Galetke W, et al: Autoadjusting CPAP therapy based on impedance efficacy, compliance and acceptance. *Am J Crit Care Med* 163:652-657, 2001.
3. Massie CA, McArdle N, Hart RW, et al: Comparison between automatic and fixed positive airway pressure in the home. *Am J Respir Crit Care Med* 167:20-23, 2003.
4. Ayas NT, Patel SR, Malhotra A, et al: Auto-titrating versus standard continuous positive airway pressure for the treatment of obstructive sleep apnea: Results of a meta-analysis. *Sleep* 27:249-253, 2004.

Palatal Implants for Primary Snoring: Short-term Results of a New Minimally Invasive Surgical Technique

Maurer JT, Verse T, Stuck BA, et al (Univ Hosp Mannheim, Germany)
Otolaryngol Head Neck Surg 132:125-131, 2005 36–4

Objective.—To determine the safety and efficacy of a new soft palate implant procedure for the reduction of snoring.

Study Design and Setting.—Fifteen healthy patients with primary snoring due to palatal flutter were enrolled into this prospective study after clinical and endoscopic examination and polysomnography. The average age of the patients was 41.2 ± 8.6 years with a body mass index of 26.2 ± 2.5 kg/m^2. The Anti-Snoring Device consists of a delivery tool with a cylindrical implant of braided polyester filaments. Under local anesthesia, three implants intended for permanent implantation were placed into the soft palate. Snoring-related symptoms were assessed by visual analogue scales (VAS), polysomnography, and the SNAP system at baseline and 90 days postoperatively.

Results.—All implants were placed without complications. Only minor discomfort was reported in four cases within the first three days postprocedure. At the 90-day follow-up snoring was reduced from 7.3 ± 1.6 to 2.5 ± 2.1 (VAS, $P < 0.01$) and from 347 ± 239 to 264 ± 168 snoring sounds/hour (SNAP, $P > 0.05$). Polysomnography did not show any deterioration of sleep or breathing. Speech, swallowing, and taste were unchanged.

Conclusion.—The Anti-Snoring Device is a new surgical tool offering a simple and minimally invasive procedure. Our data demonstrate that the treatment is safe and effective with good patient acceptance. Further patient follow-ups are needed to evaluate the long-term results (Figs 1 and 5).

► Stiffening the "floppy" palate is the latest surgical approach to the treatment of snoring. There are a couple of different approaches to stiffening the palate. Cautery-assisted palatal stiffening operations (CAPSO) use a "cut and coagulate" electrocautery setting to remove a segment of the midline soft palate mucosa above the uvula. The midline nasal surface of the uvula mucosa is

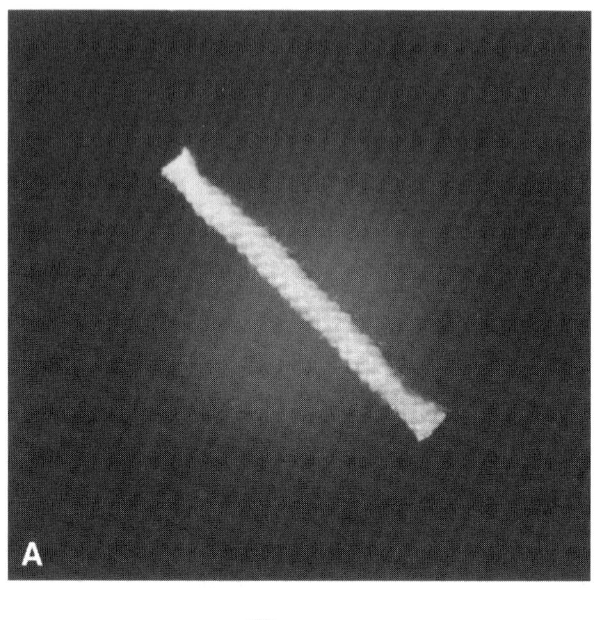

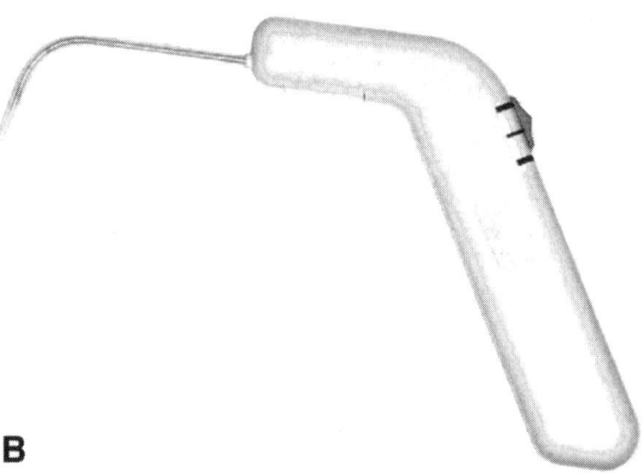

FIGURE 1.—Anti-Snoring Device Implant (A) and delivery tool (B). (Courtesy of Maurer JT, Verse T, Stuck BA, et al: Palatal implants for primary snoring: Short-term results of a new minimally invasive surgical technique. *Otolaryngol Head Neck Surg* 132:125-131, 2005. Copyright American Academy of Otolaryngology-Head and Neck Surgery Foundation, Inc.)

also cauterized. The wound is allowed to heal by secondary intention, and the resultant scarring causes stiffening of the palate after about 3 weeks.[1,2] In typical ENT fashion, studies of this technique have included small numbers of patients who had subjective improvement in snoring, insignificant falls in the apnea/hypopnea index, no improvement in nocturnal oxygen desaturation, and limited follow-up. The procedure is only supposed to be applied to snorers but is obviously being applied to those with sleep apnea as well.

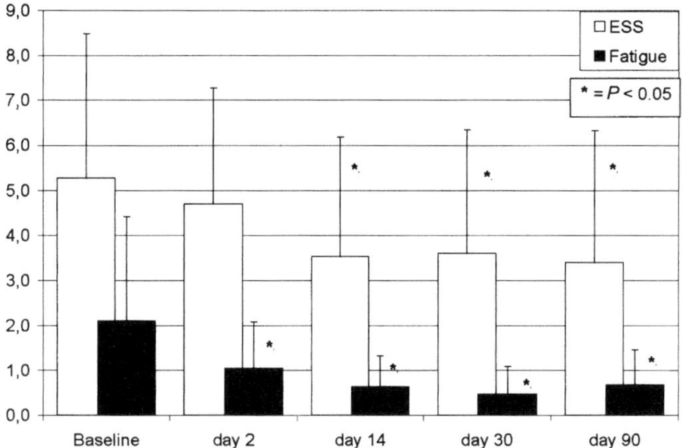

FIGURE 5.—Daytime sleepiness (*ESS*) and fatigue (*VAS*) during the study. Statistical significance is calculated compared to baseline. (Courtesy of Maurer JT, Verse T, Stuck BA, et al: Palatal implants for primary snoring: Short-term results of a new minimally invasive surgical technique. *Otolaryngol Head Neck Surg* 132:125-131, 2005. Copyright American Academy of Otolaryngology-Head and Neck Surgery Foundation, Inc.)

The technique being evaluated in this article by Maurer et al is the use of palatal implants, sometimes referred to as "palatal restoration." This technique is being aggressively marketed as the Pillar Palatal Implant System (Restore Medical, Inc, St Paul, Minn).[3] The implants consist of 3 narrow threads of braided polyester, which are inserted under the mucosa of the soft palate using a delivery tool. One is placed in the midline and one each in right and left lateral locations. The procedure can be done as an outpatient under local anesthesia. Over time, scar tissue grows around the implants, further stiffening the palate. The implants are designed to be permanent structures but can be removed if they become infected. Incredibly, on the basis of a very limited study of a very few patients, the Pillar system received market clearance from the US Food and Drug Administration in 2003.

I selected this article to review because this technique is being heavily marketed in lay publications and on the Internet, and our patients are asking about it. It is important to note that palatal implants have not been studied and are not intended for use in patients with obstructive sleep apnea. The current study is typical of the surgical literature about treatment of sleep-disordered breathing: few (15) patients were studied, no objective data were measured, and results were overstated. For example, the Epworth Sleepiness Score fell "significantly," from a normal level of 5.3 to a normal level of 3.4. This approach may be helpful for some snorers, but it is important for them to hear from you that this has *not* been tested and is *not* recommended for people with sleep apnea, and that this procedure is considered investigational by third-party payors.[4] And it should be.

B. A. Phillips, MD, MSPH

References

1. Mair EA, Day RH: Cautery-assisted palatal stiffening operation. *Otolaryngol Head Neck Surg* 122:547-556, 2000.
2. Wassmuth Z: Cautery-assisted palatal stiffening operation for the treatment of obstructive sleep apnea syndrome. *Otolaryngol Head Neck Surg* 123:55-60, 2000.
3. *The Pillar System: A new treatment for snoring—Long-term clinical results.* St Paul, Minn, Restore Medical, Inc, 2003. Available at: http://www.restoremedical.com/docs/LT_Clinical_White_Paper.pdf.
4. *Blue Cross of California Medical Policy MED.00054: Treatment for obstructive sleep apnea.* Available at: http://medpolicy.bluecrossca.com/policies/med/osa.html.

Alternative Methods of Titrating Continuous Positive Airway Pressure: A Large Multicenter Study

Masa JF, Jiménez A, Durán J, et al (San Pedro de Alcántara Hosp, Cáceres, Spain; Hosp de Valdecilla, Santander, Spain; Txagorritxu Hosp, Vitoria, Spain; et al)

Am J Respir Crit Care Med 170:1218-1224, 2004 36–5

Introduction.—Standard practice for continuous positive airway pressure (CPAP) treatment in sleep apnea and hypopnea syndrome (SAHS) requires pressure titration during attended laboratory polysomnography. However, polysomnographic titration is expensive and time-consuming. The aim of this study was to ascertain, in a large sample of CPAP-naive patients, whether CPAP titration performed by an unattended domiciliary autoadjusted CPAP device or with a predicted formula was as effective as CPAP titration performed by full polysomnography. The main outcomes were the apnea-hypopnea index and the subjective daytime sleepiness. We included 360 patients with SAHS requiring CPAP treatment. Patients were randomly allocated into three groups: standard, autoadjusted, and predicted formula titration with domiciliary adjustment. The follow-up period was 12 weeks. With CPAP treatment, the improvement in subjective sleepiness and apnea-hypopnea index was very similar in the three groups. There were no differences in the objective compliance of CPAP treatment and in the dropout rate of the three groups at the end of the follow-up. Autoadjusted titration at home and predicted formula titration with domiciliary adjustment can replace standard titration. These procedures could lead to considerable savings in cost and to significant reductions in the waiting list.

► Now, *this* article is important. Although the authors conservatively recommend an in-lab diagnostic study and a daytime continuous positive airway pressure (CPAP) trial for suspected sleep apneics, it doesn't take a great leap of imagination to understand that using a prediction formula or an autotitrating machine is an expedient, cost-effective approach to treating the obese, middle-aged man who is falling asleep and snorting himself awake in your waiting room. I am not sure how far away we are from treating patients empirically with autotitrating machines or empiric pressures, but I suspect that many well-connected or savvy consumers (including several physician colleagues of mine) are addressing their sleep apnea in just that way. This study is particularly important because of the large (n = 360) number of patients studied and their careful attention to compliance rates between the 3 groups. Please note that the vast majority of patients wound up on 8 or 9 cm H_2O CPAP. These findings are very similar to those of Stradling et al,[1] who also compared autotitrating CPAP, in-lab titrated CPAP, and algorithm-determined CPAP, and concluded, "Considerable night-to-night variation means that a one-night titration is not very precise and is subject to random variation. A one-night titration has a similar inaccuracy to that resulting from using an algorithm, based on OSA severity and neck circumference. Setting all patients with OSA at 10 cm H_2O is little worse." To drive this point home, Hukins[2] demonstrated that patients assigned to "arbitrary" CPAP pressure (ranging from 8 to 12 cm H_2O, based entirely on body mass index) did about as well as those assigned to be treated with in-lab titrated CPAP. If you are as old as I am (which means you are reading this with reading glasses), you remember when we treated acutely ill asthmatic patients with IV aminophylline, totaled up the 24-hour dose, and multiplied it times 0.85 to figure the proper dose of oral theophylline. Strangely, it nearly always worked out to 300 mg of Theo-Dur twice daily.

It is likely that most folks with sleep apnea will do extremely well on 8 to 10 cm H_2O CPAP. The ones who don't can come to the lab for a formal titration.

B. A. Phillips, MD, MSPH

References

1. Stradling JR, Hardinge M, Paxton J, et al: Relative accuracy of algorithm-based prescription of nasal CPAP in OSA. *Respir Med* 98:152-154, 2004.
2. Hukins CA: Arbitrary-pressure continuous positive airway pressure for obstructive sleep apnea syndrome. *Am J Respir Crit Care Med* 171:500-505, 2005. Epub 2004 Nov 24.

All-Cause Mortality in Males With Sleep Apnoea Syndrome: Declining Mortality Rates With Age

Lavie P, Lavie L, Herer P (Technion-Israel Inst of Technology, Haifa)
Eur Respir J 25:514-520, 2005 36–6

Introduction.—The objective of this study was to assess whether an increasing severity of sleep apnoea is associated with increased all-cause mortality hazards and to assess whether the syndrome is associated with excess mortality, in comparison with the general population. Participants included 14,589 adult males, aged 20-93 yrs, referred to the sleep clinics with suspected sleep apnoea or diagnosed with sleep apnoea. Altogether, 372 deaths were recorded after a median follow-up of 4.6 yrs. The crude all-cause mortality rate was 5.55/1,000 patient yrs, increasing with apnoea severity. Cox proportional analysis revealed that both respiratory disturbance index (RDI) and body mass index significantly influenced all-cause mortality hazard but there was no interaction between them. Males with respiratory disturbance index >30 had a significantly higher mortality hazard rate than the reference group of males with RDI ≤10. Comparing mortality rates of males with moderate/severe sleep apnoea to the general population revealed that only males aged <50 yrs showed an excess mortality rate. The hazard of mortality in sleep apnoea increases with apnoea severity as indexed by respiratory disturbance index. Moderate and severe levels of sleep apnoea are moderately associated with an increased risk of all-cause mortality, in comparison with the general population, particularly in males aged <50 yrs. The lack of information about possible confounders and treatment effects should be taken into consideration in the interpretation of these results.

► This article changes my thinking quite a bit. It is by far the largest, longest follow-up of a cohort of men who are characterized with regard to sleep-disordered breathing. The main finding is that most of the excess mortality associated with sleep apnea is in men under the age of 50. This was suggested a long time ago by the work of He et al,[1] but the study by Lavie et al includes a much larger cohort. The authors speculate on why this may be true. They consider a variety of possibilities, including referral bias in favor of older patients, more severe sleep apnea in younger patients, development of adaptive mechanisms in older patients, and treatment differences between younger and older patients. Frankly, I strongly believe the mortality differences result from treatment differences. In my experience, young men are the most resistant to medical evaluation, treatment, or lifestyle change. This article suggests that we need to work even harder with this group, because sleep-disordered breathing is particularly deadly for them, keeping them from reaching their most productive years.

B. A. Phillips, MD, MSPH

Reference

1. He J, Kryger MH, Zorick FJ, et al: Mortality and apnea index in obstructive sleep apnea. Experience in 385 patients. *Chest* 94:9-14, 1988.

Effect of Nasal Continuous Positive Airway Pressure in Uncontrolled Nocturnal Asthmatic Patients With Obstructive Sleep Apnea Syndrome

Ciftci TU, Ciftci B, Guven SF, et al (Gazi Univ, Ankara, Turkey; Ataturk Chest Disease and Chest Surgery Hosp, Ankara, Turkey)

Respir Med 99:529-534, 2005 36–7

Introduction.—The mechanisms of nocturnal asthma are intimately related to circadian rhythms, which influence inflammatory cells and mediators, hormone levels and cholinergic tone. Nocturnal airway narrowing in asthma is sometimes associated with sleep disorders, such as obstructive sleep apnea syndrome (OSAS). The aims of this study were to evaluate the association of nocturnal asthma and OSAS, and investigate the influence of continuous positive airway pressure (CPAP) therapy to improve nighttime symptoms in asthmatic patients with OSAS. Forty-three asthmatic patients who had nocturnal symptoms in spite of the optimal medical treatment according to the Global Initiative for Asthma guidelines and associated with snoring were studied. Pulmonary function tests (PFTs), asthma nighttime symptom scores, and polysomnography were performed on all patients. We treated the patients with an apnea-hypopnea index (AHI) ≥15 (moderate-severe OSAS) (n = 16) with CPAP during 2 months. After 2 months, PFT, asthma nighttime symptom scores were reperformed. There was no significant difference in PFT values before and after CPAP treatment in OSAS patients. Asthma nighttime symptom scores were improved significantly (P<0.05) after CPAP treatment. In conclusion, in some patients with nocturnal asthma, OSAS may be responsible disease for nocturnal symptoms. In this condition, CPAP improves nocturnal symptoms without amelioration in PFT abnormalities.

► A growing body of literature supports a relationship between asthma and sleep apnea.[1,2] There are many potential explanations for this, many including obesity as a common risk factor. Whatever the mechanism, this study demonstrates improvement in nighttime symptom scores (without change in body weight or pulmonary function).

B. A. Phillips, MD, MSPH

References

1. Fitzpatrick MF, Jokic R: Nocturnal asthma, in McNicholas WT (ed): *Respiratory Disorders During Sleep, Eur Respir Monograph* 3:285-302, 1998.
2. Lin CC, Lin CY: Obstructive sleep apnea syndrome and bronchial hyperreactivity. *Lung* 173:117-126, 1995.

37 Critical Care

Use of Intensive Care at the End of Life in the United States: An Epidemiologic Study

Angus DC, for the Robert Wood Johnson Foundation ICU End-of-Life Peer Group (Univ of Pittsburgh, Pa; et al)

Crit Care Med 32:638-643, 2004 37–1

Objective.—Despite concern over the appropriateness and quality of care provided in an intensive care unit (ICU) at the end of life, the number of Americans who receive ICU care at the end of life is unknown. We sought to describe the use of ICU care at the end of life in the United States using hospital discharge data from 1999 for six states and the National Death Index.

Design.—Retrospective analysis of administrative data to calculate age-specific rates of hospitalization with and without ICU use at the end of life, to generate national estimates of end-of-life hospital and ICU use, and to characterize age-specific case mix of ICU decedents.

Setting.—All nonfederal hospitals in the states of Florida, Massachusetts, New Jersey, New York, Virginia, and Washington.

Patients.—All inpatients in nonfederal hospitals in the six states in 1999.

Intervention.—None.

Measurements and Main Results.—We found that there were 552,157 deaths in the six states in 1999, of which 38.3% occurred in hospital and 22.4% occurred after ICU admission. Using these data to project nationwide estimates, 540,000 people die after ICU admission each year. The age-specific rate of ICU use at the end of life was highest for infants (43%), ranged from 18% to 26% among older children and adults, and fell to 14% for those >85 yrs. Average length of stay and costs were 12.9 days and $24,541 for terminal ICU hospitalizations and 8.9 days and $8,548 for non-ICU terminal hospitalizations.

Conclusions.—One in five Americans die using ICU services. The doubling of persons over the age of 65 yrs by 2030 will require a system-wide expansion in ICU care for dying patients unless the healthcare system pursues rationing, more effective advanced care planning, and augmented capacity to care for dying patients in other settings.

► This study underscores how important a number of issues are for society in general and for critical care manpower. Because a high percentage of patients (20%) enter the ICU in their final stages of life currently, and because the baby boomers are now beginning to age, we have some tough times ahead: "Can we as a society afford critical care for everyone or does rationing become reality? Will hospitals become a combination of ICU, rehabilitation unit, and outpatient services? Where will all the critical care practioners come from, or will care be via regional systems or telemedicine systems with the doers being nurse practitioners or physician assistants in allegiance with hospitalists?"

I for one plan to get my advanced directive written. Perhaps that is the real answer: mandated advanced directives as part of enrollment for health insurance or admission to a hospital? It would relieve a lot of surrogate decision-making family members and may also decompress our ICUs.

J. A. Barker, MD

Achieving House Staff Competence in Emergency Airway Management: Results of a Teaching Program Using a Computerized Patient Simulator

Mayo PH, Hackney JE, Mueck JT, et al (Albert Einstein College of Medicine, New York)

Crit Care Med 32:2422-2427, 2004 37–2

Objectives.—Patient simulation is emerging as a training technique in the field of medicine. It has particular application in training responses to high-risk, low-frequency clinical events, of which a typical example is in-hospital cardiac arrest. A critical element of response by the cardiac arrest team is initial airway management. In teaching hospitals, medical interns are first responders to in-hospital cardiac arrests. Our objective was to design and test a program using a computer-controlled patient simulator to train medical interns and demonstrate their competence in initial airway management.

Design.—Prospective, randomized, controlled, unblinded trial.

Setting.—Internal medicine residency training program in an urban teaching hospital.

Participants.—All 50 starting internal medicine interns in July 2002, all Advanced Cardiac Life Support certified in June 2002.

Interventions.—All interns were tested in initial airway management skills and then were randomly assigned to receive either immediate or delayed individualized training using a computer-controlled patient simulator. The computer-simulated training process consisted of a scenario of respiratory arrest. The interns were challenged with the scenario twice following testing. The interns were debriefed extensively and given hands-on training by the attending using the simulator until they achieved perfect performance.

Measurements and Main Results.—Initial airway management was divided into specific scorable steps. Individual step scores and total scores were recorded for each intern on initial and repeat testing. For 10 months following simulator training, intern airway management skills were scored in actual patient airway events. Despite recent Advanced Cardiac Life Support training and certification, all starting medical interns demonstrated poor airway management skills. The immediate training group showed significant improvement in initial airway management when tested before and 4 wks after training. In contrast, the delayed training group showed no significant improvement. Direct observation of interns in actual initial airway events revealed excellent clinical performance.

Conclusions.—Individualized training of medical interns using a computer-controlled patient simulator is an effective means of achieving and measuring competence in initial airway management skills. The improvement appears to be transferable to the bedside of real patients.

► There is tremendous interest in the movement of simulator-based education from other fields (such as the airline industry) to medicine. Despite the common requirements of basic life support and advanced cardiac life support training, residents in internal medicine are often not proficient in endotracheal intubation. Yet, these are the physicians who respond to emergencies and codes within teaching hospitals. The authors have contributed nicely to the burgeoning field of simulator use in medical education. No one wants a physician untrained in low incidence/high risk situations. Medical simulation is a very safe way to improve our skills.

J. A. Barker, MD

Ultrasonographic Evaluation of Liver/Spleen Movements and Extubation Outcome

Jiang J-R, Tsai T-H, Jerng J-S, et al (Natl Taiwan Univ Hosp, Taipei)
Chest 126:179-185, 2004 37–3

Introduction.—The diaphragm plays a pivotal role in weaning and successful extubation. We hypothesized that ultrasonographic evaluation of the movements of the diaphragm by measuring liver/spleen displacement during spontaneous breathing trials is a good predictor for extubation outcome.

Patients and Methods.—The studied subjects were intubated patients receiving mechanical ventilation who were scheduled to be extubated. The displacement of liver/spleen was measured by ultrasonography before extubation. The patients were classified into a success group (SG) or failure group according to the extubation outcome. The baseline data and organ displacements in these two groups were analyzed. The sensitivity and specificity for the mean organ displacements and weaning parameters to predict successful extubation were calculated.

Results.—We included 55 patients, 32 of whom (58%) were in the SG. The baseline data are similar for these two groups, but the mean values of liver and spleen displacements were higher in the SG. Using a cutoff value of 1.1 cm, the sensitivity and specificity to predict successful extubation were 84.4% and 82.6%, respectively, better than traditional weaning parameters in this study.

Conclusion.—The displacement of the liver/spleen, measured by ultrasonography, is a good predictor for extubation outcome.

► These authors describe a technique I have used for many years: using bedside US to assess diaphragm functionality. It is well accepted that patients with 1 or both diaphragms paralyzed will have poor outcomes with extubation and may need additional support with noninvasive ventilation. Likewise, significant literature has been published concerning diaphragm fatigue in progression to respiratory failure. Most of these studies have used techniques unavailable to practicing physicians, such as research electromyograms. In the same manner, radiologists traditionally recommend fluoroscopy of the diaphragms (sniff test), which is impractical in ICU patients.

Now we have an identified technique that should be readily available to all intensivists. I predict we will use US in the ICU for many applications in the years ahead.[1]

J. A. Barker, MD

Reference

1. Legome E, Pancu D: Future applications for emergency ultrasound. *Emerg Med Clin North Am* 22:817-827, 2004.

Steroid-Induced Myopathy in Patients Intubated Due to Exacerbation of Chronic Obstructive Pulmonary Disease

Amaya-Villar R, Garnacho-Montero J, García-García-Garmendía JL, et al (Univ Hosp Virgen del Rocío, Sevilla, Spain)
Intensive Care Med 31:157-161, 2005 37–4

Objective.—To determine incidence, risk factors and impact on various outcome parameters of the development of acute quadriplegic myopathy in a selected population of critically ill patients.

Setting.—A prospective cohort study carried out in the intensive care unit of a tertiary-level university hospital.

Patients.—All patients admitted due to acute exacerbation of chronic obstructive pulmonary disease who required intubation and mechanical ventilation, and received high doses of intravenous corticosteroids.

Interventions.—A neurophysiological study was performed in all cases at the onset of weaning. Muscular biopsy was taken when the neurophysiological study revealed a myopathic pattern.

Measurements and Results.—Twenty-six patients were enrolled in the study. Nine patients (34.6%) developed myopathy. Only seven patients were treated with muscle relaxants. Histology confirmed the diagnosis in the three patients who underwent muscle biopsy. APACHE II score at admission, the rate of sepsis and the total doses of corticosteroids were significantly higher in patients with myopathy compared with those patients that did not develop it. Myopathy is associated with an increase in the duration of mechanical ventilation [15.4 (9.2) versus 5.7 (3.9) days; $p<0.006$], the length of ICU stay [23.6 (10.7) versus 11.4 (7.05) days; $p<0.003$] and hospital stay [33.3 (19.2) versus 21.2 (16.1) days; $p<0.034$)]. Myopathy was not associated with increased mortality.

Conclusions.—In the population under study, severity of illness at admission, the development of sepsis and the total dose of corticosteroids are factors associated with the occurrence of myopathy after the administration of corticosteroids. Myopathy was associated with prolonged mechanical ventilation and in-hospital stay.

► Despite a paucity of good evidence for doses (and even usage!) of corticosteroids for patients in respiratory failure from chronic obstructive pulmonary disease (COPD), we all use them. Some physicians use them in industrial strength. These researchers from Spain have shown that up to a third of these patients may develop myopathy. Since the total dose of steroids, coupled with disease severity and use of neuromuscular blocking agents, is controllable, we physicians can make a difference in reducing this complication. I suggest low to moderate initial steroid dosing followed by rapid deescalation (as with antibiotics) be considered in every patient. Counterbalancing auto-positive end-expiratory pressure, bronchodilator therapy, attention to nutrition support, tight control of blood glucoses, and the use of noninvasive ventilation probably are much more effective for these patients' survival than is IV, high-dose solumedrol.

J. A. Barker, MD

Acinetobacter baumannii Ventilator-Associated Pneumonia: Epidemiological and Clinical Findings

Intensive Care Med 31:649-655, 2005 37–5

Objective.—To investigate prognostic factors and predictors of *Acinetobacter baumannii* isolation in ventilator-associated pneumonia (VAP). We specifically analyzed these issues for imipenem-resistant episodes.

Design and Setting.—All episodes of VAP are prospectively included in a database. Information about risk factors was retrieved retrospectively.

Patients.—Eighty-one patients exhibiting microbiologically documented VAP: 41 by *A. baumannii* (26 by imipenem-resistant) and 40 by other pathogens.

Measurements and Results.—The following variables were noted: underlying diseases, severity of illness, duration of mechanical ventilation and of hospitalization before VAP, prior episode of sepsis, previous antibiotic, corticosteroid use, type of nutrition, renal replacement therapy, reintubation, transportation out of the ICU, micro-organisms involved in VAP, concomitant bacteremia, clinical presentation, Sequential Organ Failure Assessment (SOFA) scale on the day of diagnosis, and adequacy of empirical antibiotic therapy. Prior antibiotic use was found to be associated with development of VAP by *A. baumannii* (OR 14). Prior imipenem exposure was associated with the isolation of imipenem-resistant strains (OR 4). SOFA score on the day of diagnosis was the only predictor of in-hospital mortality (OR 1.22); adequacy of empirical antibiotic therapy was a protective factor (OR 0.067).

Conclusions.—Our results confirm that prior exposure to antimicrobials is an independent predictor for the development of *A. baumannii* VAP, the prognosis of which is similar to that of infections caused by other pathogens. This study highlights the importance of initial antibiotic choice in VAP or whatever cause.

► This is another important article in the ever-expanding literature of VAP and progressive antibiotic resistance patterns. The importance of rapid de-escalation of antibiotic therapy coupled with very short (6-8 days) antibiotic courses seems the wisest way to prevent the emergence of yet another severely resistant organism, imipenim-resistant *A baumannii*.[1].

J. A. Barker, MD

Reference

1. Micek ST, Ward S, Fraser VJ, et al: A randomized controlled trial of an antibiotic discontinuation policy for clinically suspected ventilator-associated pneumonia. *Chest* 125:1791-1799, 2004.

PART SIX

HEART AND CARDIOVASCULAR DISEASE

WILLIAM H. FRISHMAN, MD

Introduction

The findings from many outstanding cardiovascular basic science and clinical research studies from the past year are reported on in this section. The articles selected for abstracting were chosen from among 5000 reviewed that related to the pathophysiology, prevention, diagnosis, and treatment of cardiovascular disease. Each selected abstract is followed by my editorial comments, and where appropriate, additional references are added.

The first chapter includes 7 selections related to cardiovascular risk factors and markers. In women, a history of hysterectomy with and without oopherectomy does not predict an increased risk of cardiovascular disease. Increased levels of oxidized phospholipids and lipoprotein a are associated with an increased risk of coronary disease. The selective cyclooxygenase-2 (COX-2) inhibitors have received a lot of attention because of reports suggesting an increased cardiovascular disease risk associated with their use. Left ventricular hypertrophy is a well-known marker of increased morbidity and mortality. A reduction in left ventricular mass with various antihypertensive treatments can improve clinical outcomes. Another marker of increased cardiovascular risk is the presence of microalbuminuria. Treatment with angiotensin-converting enzyme (ACE) inhibitors can reduce the amount of microalbuminuria, with a trend in reducing subsequent cardiovascular events. The growing epidemic of obesity is associated with various metabolic disorders and an increased cardiovascular disease risk. Elevations in glucose, insulin levels, and pro-insulin levels are independent predictors of risk. Eating disorders, with marked loss of weight, are other predictors of risk.

Acute coronary syndromes are discussed in the next chapter. Antiplatelet therapy has become a mainstay of treatment of acute coronary syndromes. The addition of clopidogrel to aspirin appears to be more efficacious than aspirin alone in reducing morbidity and mortality in patients with myocardial infarctions manifested by both ST-segment depression and elevation. On the other hand, the infusion of glucose, insulin, and potassium had no effect on the clinical course of myocardial infarction. An invasive strategy with angiography and/or stenting has been proposed as the treatment of choice for patients with myocardial infarction. However, with ST-segment depression infarcts an invasive strategy does not always provide benefit versus intensive medical therapy, except in select cases. Heart failure with left ventricular dysfunction after an acute myocardial infarction seems to predict worse sudden death mortality, especially within the first 30 days of the ischemic event. More intensive treatments may be required to reduce this risk, including the potential use of bone marrow and cardiac stem cells to stimulate myocardial regeneration and healing processes. Multiple clinical trials are now in progress regarding these types of interventions.

The next chapter discusses 4 articles related to chronic coronary artery disease (CAD). More intensive lipid lowering with statin drugs appears to be associated with fewer adverse cardiac outcomes. At this time, it is not known how low plasma lipid levels should be reduced with drug therapy and the safety of maximal lipid lowering. Similar to plasma lipid elevations, increased levels of N-terminal-pro-B-natriuretic peptides is also associated with an increased mortality risk in patients with stable CAD. Among various racial and socioeconomic groups, there are disparities in the risk of CAD, which must be taken into consideration when managing patients. Increased coronary calcification scores determined by electron beam tomography are associated with an increased risk of CAD; however, there remain questions whether this technique would be useful in screening asymptomatic individuals.

Highlighted in the next chapter are some of the major advances in the interventional management of CAD. Drug-eluting stents have been shown to be effective in reducing the rate of post-angioplasty restenosis compared with bare metal stents, with and without brachytherapy. The paclitaxel-eluting stents and sirolimus-eluting stents are both available for use in clinical practice. Angioplasty and stenting are the procedures of choice for managing patients with acute myocardial infarction, and the maximal benefit is seen if the intervention takes place within 1-2 hours of the onset of symptoms. Strategies need to be developed for rapid transfer of patients from their homes to the catheterization lab if this approach is to benefit the largest number of myocardial infarction patients. Patients with kidney disease, especially those who are dialysis dependent, appear to be at an increased risk of premature CAD. When indicated, these patients appear to benefit from both coronary artery bypass surgery and percutaneous coronary intervention. Patients who are undergoing elective vascular surgery do not appear to benefit from prophylactic coronary revascularization procedures performed to reduce operative risk. However, the use of β-blockers seems to reduce this risk and at the same time the need for an extensive preoperative CAD assessment before elective, noncoronary vascular surgery.

Patients undergoing percutaneous coronary intervention require aggressive anticoagulation. Fondaparinux, a factor Xa inhibitor, appears to provide similar efficacy and safety compared with heparin and may provide an alternative treatment in patients who are heparin intolerant.

There have been many advances in the treatment of acute and chronic heart failure. With these advances there is evidence that a specialized multidisciplinary clinical approach may reduce morbidity and mortality in the higher-risk patients with heart failure. In patients with severe left ventricular failure, left ventricular assist devices (LVAD) are being used more frequently. Transthoracic echocardiography has been shown to identify the causes of mechanical dysfunction in patients on chronic LVAD support. Women with hypertrophic cardiomyopathy appear to do worse than men. They have a higher rate of clinical heart failure and outflow obstruction. Regarding risk factors for congestive heart failure, insulin resistance appears to be associated with an increased prevalence of clinical disease, independent of diabetes. This association between obesity and heart failure may be mediated by insulin resistance. In patients with heart failure and cardiac dyssynchrony, cardiac resynchrony with biventricular pacing will improve clinical outcomes. Digoxin also appears to be of benefit in heart failure patients if the drug serum level is 0.5 to 0.9 ng/mL. Levels greater than1.2 ng/mL appear to be harmful. Left ventricular diastolic dysfunction is a common cause of clinical heart failure, and does not seem to be related to ventricular systolic dysfunction.

Valvular heart disease and its clinical complications remain major problems in cardiovascular medicine. Endocarditis is still a major cause of valvular dysfunction. In 5% of endocarditis patients, blood cultures are negative. Causes of culture-negative endocarditis include slow-growing bacteria, fungi, and right-sided endocarditis. Advances in microbiological technique may help to identify those cases due to slow-growing bacteria. Staphylococcus is now the No. 1 cause of culture-positive endocarditis. Worldwide there appears to be regional differences in the prevalence of staphylococcus endocarditis and the clinical course. There are medical and surgical approaches to the management of valvular heart disease. In patients with aortic regurgitation, β blockers have been shown to be of benefit, in addition to vasodilators. For mitral insufficiency, operative valve repair has been shown to be effective in many situations, avoiding the need for valve replacement. Recently, a percutaneous coronary sinus-based mitral annuloplasty approach has been used for mitral valve repair, avoiding the need for surgery in some patients.

The next chapter presents 3 articles that describe advances in noninvasive cardiac diagnostic testing. Three-dimensional echocardiography appears to give a more accurate determination of ventricular volumes and ejection fraction than a 2-dimensional approach. In making the diagnosis of cardiac amyloidosis, magnetic resonance imaging can be helpful. The technique can also be of benefit in following the course of the disease. Multislice computed tomography provides an excellent noninvasive method for the detection of obstructive CAD. Scanners able to acquire up to 64 slices are now available. We currently use this modality in our private practice.

There have been many advances in the diagnosis and treatment of cardiac arrhythmias. In individuals with high degree atrioventricular block, there is no difference in clinical outcomes whether s simpler single chamber or a more complicated double chamber technique is used. Atrial fibrillation remains a common problem in medical practice. The dreaded complication of systemic embolization can be prevented by anticoagulation. However, in patients who cannot tolerate anticoagulation, a percutaneous left atrial appendage transcatheter occlusion can be performed. Regarding pharmacologic conversion of atrial fibrillation, both amiodarone and sotalol appear to be effective. However, amiodarone appears to be more effective in maintaining normal sinus rhythm after medical cardioversion. Lone atrial fibrillation (no structural abnormality associated with the arrhythmia) may not have the benign course that was initially thought to occur. These patients are still at risk for thromboembolism and anticoagulation should be used. Implantable defibrillators (ICDs) are now recommended for patients who are postinfarction with diminished left ventricular dysfunction. Compared with medical therapy alone, ICDs provide a greater survival advantage despite the increased cost.

In the last chapter, articles are presented on various topics not included in the previous chapters. Perioperative β-adrenergic blockade appears to reduce mortality in high-risk patients undergoing major noncardiac surgery. In older individuals, there is a definite decline in aerobic capacity with age. Exercise appears to decelerate the rate of decline, but does not prevent it.

More and more patients are surviving to adulthood with a history of corrected congenital heart defects. With some defects, normal exercise capacity is achieved after surgery; with other defects, exercise capacity remains depressed. With the new cardiac resuscitation guidelines, induced hypothermia appears to facilitate the response to defibrillation. The use of mild-moderate hypothermia by using intravenous saline or an ice bath will improve resuscitation outcomes.

William H. Frishman, MD

38 Risk Factors

Risk of Cardiovascular Disease by Hysterectomy Status, With and Without Oophorectomy: The Women's Health Initiative Observational Study

Howard BV, Kuller L, Langer R, et al (MedStar Research Inst, Washington, DC; Univ of Pittsburgh, Pa; Univ of California San Diego, La Jolla; et al)

Circulation 111:1462-1470, 2005 38–1

Background.—Cardiovascular disease (CVD) is a leading cause of morbidity and mortality in women and may vary by hysterectomy (or oophorectomy) status. This study compared CVD risk factors and rates between postmenopausal women who had and had not undergone hysterectomy, with or without oophorectomy.

Method and Results.—This analysis was conducted on 89 914 women in the Women's Health Initiative (WHI) Observational Study. Participants reported demographic characteristics, medical history, dietary habits, physical activity, medications, and previous hysterectomy (with or without oophorectomy). Baseline weight, height, waist circumference, and blood pressure were measured. CVD events were ascertained during 5.1 years of mean follow-up and adjudicated with standard criteria. Black, Hispanic, and American Indian women had higher rates of hysterectomy than white women (52.9%, 44.6%, and 49.2% versus 40.0%, respectively), and Asian/Pacific Islander women had lower rates (33.8%). Women with a hysterectomy (regardless of oophorectomy status) had an adverse risk profile at baseline compared with women with no hysterectomy, including a higher proportion of hypertension, diabetes, high cholesterol, obesity, and lower education, income, and physical activity (all $P<0.01$). Total mortality and fatal and nonfatal CVD were higher among women with a hysterectomy. Hysterectomy (regardless of oophorectomy status) was a significant predictor of CVD (HR: 1.26, $P<0.001$). After adjustment for demographic variables and CVD risk factors, the effect was reduced and nonsignificant.

Conclusions.—Women with a hysterectomy had a worse risk profile and higher prevalence and incidence of CVD in this cohort. Multivariate models suggest that hysterectomy is not the major determinant of this outcome; rather, CVD risk may be due to the more adverse initial risk profile of women who had undergone hysterectomy.

► CVD is the leading cause of death among women in the United States. The risk factors for coronary artery disease (CAD) in women are similar to those found in men.[1] Markers of inflammation, such as C-reactive protein, also indicate an increased risk of CAD in both men and women.[1-3] The presence of systemic lupus erythematosus appears to provide a particular risk in women.[4] Older women appear to benefit from exercise training with improvement in quality of life.[5] A nomogram has been established for predicting exercise capacity on the basis of age.[6] In contrast to the findings in men, exercise testing as a diagnostic modality in women with suspected CAD is of less value.[7] However, several resting 12-lead ECG parameters, such as QRS angle and the QRS and QTrr duration may be predictive of future cardiovascular outcomes in women with suspected myocardial ischemia.[8]

W. H. Frishman, MD

References

1. Ridker PM, Rifai N, Cook NR, et al: Non-HDL cholesterol, apolipoproteins A-1 and B100, standard lipid measures, lipid ratios and CRP as risk factors for cardiovascular disease in women. *JAMA* 294:326-333, 2005.
2. Cushman M, Arnold AM, Psaty BM, et al: C-reactive protein and the 10-year incidence of coronary heart disease in older men and women. The Cardiovascular Health Study. *Circulation* 112:25-31, 2005.
3. Pai JK, Pischon T, Ma J, et al: Inflammatory markers and the risk of coronary heart disease in men and women. *N Engl J Med* 351:2599-2610, 2004.
4. El-Magadmi M, Bodill H, Ahmad Y, et al: Systemic lupus erythematosus. An independent risk factor for endothelial dysfunction in women. *Circulation* 110:399-404, 2004.
5. Hung C, Daub B, Black B, et al: Exercise training improves overall physical fitness and quality of life in older women with coronary artery disease. *Chest* 126:1026-1031, 2004.
6. Gulati M, Black HR, Shaw LJ, et al: The prognostic value of a nomogram for exercise capacity in women. *N Engl J Med* 353:468-475, 2005.
7. Lewis JF, McGorray S, Lin L, et al: Exercise treadmill testing using a modified exercise protocol in women with suspected myocardial ischemia: Findings from the National Heart, Lung and Blood Institute-sponsored Women's Ischemia Syndrome Evaluation (WISE). *Am Heart J* 149:527-533, 2005.
8. Triola B, Olson MB, Reis SE, et al: Electrocardiographic predictors of cardiovascular outcome in women. *J Am Coll Cardiol* 46:51-56, 2005.

Oxidized Phospholipids, Lp(a) Lipoprotein, and Coronary Artery Disease

Tsimikas S, Brilakis ES, Miller ER, et al (Univ of California, San Diego; Mayo Clinic, Rochester, Minn; Interleukin Genetics, Waltham, Mass; et al)

N Engl J Med 353:46-57, 2005 38–2

Background.—Lp(a) lipoprotein binds proinflammatory oxidized phospholipids. We investigated whether levels of oxidized low-density lipoprotein (LDL) measured with use of monoclonal antibody E06 reflect the presence and extent of obstructive coronary artery disease, defined as a stenosis of more than 50 percent of the luminal diameter.

Methods.—Levels of oxidized LDL and Lp(a) lipoprotein were measured in a total of 504 patients immediately before coronary angiography. Levels of oxidized LDL are reported as the oxidized phospholipid content per particle of apolipoprotein B-100 (oxidized phospholipid:apo B-100 ratio).

Results.—Measurements of the oxidized phospholipid:apo B-100 ratio and Lp(a) lipoprotein levels were skewed toward lower values, and the values for the oxidized phospholipid:apo B-100 ratio correlated strongly with those for Lp(a) lipoprotein ($r=0.83$, $P<0.001$). In the entire cohort, the oxidized phospholipid:apo B-100 ratio and Lp(a) lipoprotein levels showed a strong and graded association with the presence and extent of coronary artery disease (i.e., the number of vessels with a stenosis of more than 50 percent of the luminal diameter) ($P<0.001$). Among patients 60 years of age or younger, those in the highest quartiles for the oxidized phospholipid:apo B-100 ratio and Lp(a) lipoprotein levels had odds ratios for coronary artery disease of 3.12 ($P<0.001$) and 3.64 ($P<0.001$), respectively, as compared with patients in the lowest quartile. The combined effect of hypercholesterolemia and being in the highest quartiles of the oxidized phospholipid:apo B-100 ratio (odds ratio, 16.8; $P<0.001$) and Lp(a) lipoprotein levels (odds ratio, 14.2; $P<0.001$) significantly increased the probability of coronary artery disease among patients 60 years of age or younger. In the entire study group, the association of the oxidized phospholipid:apo B-100 ratio with obstructive coronary artery disease was independent of all clinical and lipid measures except one, Lp(a) lipoprotein. However, among patients 60 years of age or younger, the oxidized phospholipid:apo B-100 ratio remained an independent predictor of coronary artery disease.

Conclusions.—Circulating levels of oxidized LDL are strongly associated with angiographically documented coronary artery disease, particularly in patients 60 years of age or younger. These data suggest that the atherogenicity of Lp(a) lipoprotein may be mediated in part by associated proinflammatory oxidized phospholipids.

▶ Abnormalities in plasma lipids remain a major risk factor for the development of coronary artery disease. Therapy with cholesterol-lowering drugs, especially with statins, appears to reverse this risk[1] and has been shown to reduce the progression of atherosclerosis, but not coronary calcium scores.[2] More aggressive reduction of LDL-cholesterol to levels less than 70 mg/dL with statins appears to provide maximal protection as well as pharmacologic strategies to raise high-density lipoprotein (HDL)-cholesterol.[3,4] The protective effects of statins appear to go beyond that which one would expect of lipid-lowering alone,[5] and the long-term safety record of statins has been favorable.[6,7] The risk of rhabdomyolysis with statins appears to be increased in older diabetic patients on combined statin-fibrate therapy.[8]

W. H. Frishman, MD

References

1. Nissen SE, for the Reversal of Atherosclerosis with Aggressive Lipid Lowering (REVERSAL) Investigators: Statin therapy, LDL cholesterol, C-reactive protein, and coronary artery disease. *N Engl J Med* 352:29-38, 2005.

2. Arad Y, Spadaro LA, Roth M, et al: Treatment of asymptomatic adults with elevated coronary calcium scores with atorvastatin, vitamin C, and vitamin E. *J Am Coll Cardiol* 46:166-172, 2005.
3. Ridker PM, Morrow DA, Rose LM, et al: Relative efficacy of atorvastatin 80 mg and pravastatin 40 mg in achieving the dual goals of low-density lipoprotein cholesterol <70 mg/dl and C-reactive protein <2 mg/l. An analysis of the PROVE-IT TIMI-22 Trial. *J Am Coll Cardiol* 45: 1644-1648, 2005.
4. Whitney EJ, Krasuski RA, Personius BE, et al: A randomized trial of a strategy for increasing high-density lipoprotein cholesterol levels: Effects on progression of coronary heart disease and clinical events. *Ann Intern Med* 142:95-104, 2005.
5. Landmesser U, Bahlmann F, Mueller M, et al: Simvastatin versus ezetimibe. Pleiotropic and lipid-lowering effects on endothelial function in humans. *Circulation* 111:2356-2363, 2005.
6. Alsheikh-Ali AA, Ambrose MS, Kuvin JT, et al: The safety of rosuvastatin as used in common clinical practice. A postmarketing analysis. *Circulation* 111:3051-3057, 2005.
7. Pedersen TR, for the Incremental Decrease in End Points Through Aggressive Lipid Lowering (IDEAL) Study Group: High-dose atorvastatin vs usual-dose simvastatin for secondary prevention after myocardial infarction. The IDEAL Study: a randomized controlled trial. *JAMA* 294:2437-2445, 2005.
8. Graham DJ, Staffa JA, Shatin D, et al: Incidence of hospitalized rhabdomyolysis in patients treated with lipid-lowering drugs. *JAMA* 292:2585-2590, 2004.

Cardiovascular Risk Associated With Celecoxib in a Clinical Trial for Colorectal Adenoma Prevention

Solomon SD, for the Adenoma Prevention with Celecoxib (APC) Study Investigators (Brigham and Women's Hosp, Boston; et al)
N Engl J Med 352:1071-1080, 2005 38–3

Background.—Selective cyclooxygenase-2 (COX-2) inhibitors have come under scrutiny because of reports suggesting an increased cardiovascular risk associated with their use. Experimental research suggesting that these drugs may contribute to a prothrombotic state provides support for this concern.

Methods.—We reviewed all potentially serious cardiovascular events among 2035 patients with a history of colorectal neoplasia who were enrolled in a trial comparing two doses of celecoxib (200 mg or 400 mg twice daily) with placebo for the prevention of colorectal adenomas. All deaths were categorized as cardiovascular or noncardiovascular, and nonfatal cardiovascular events were categorized in a blinded fashion according to a prespecified scheme.

Results.—For all patients except those who died, 2.8 to 3.1 years of follow-up data were available. A composite cardiovascular end point of death from cardiovascular causes, myocardial infarction, stroke, or heart failure was reached in 7 of 679 patients in the placebo group (1.0 percent), as compared with 16 of 685 patients receiving 200 mg of celecoxib twice daily (2.3 percent; hazard ratio, 2.3; 95 percent confidence interval, 0.9 to 5.5) and with 23 of 671 patients receiving 400 mg of celecoxib twice daily (3.4 percent; hazard ratio, 3.4; 95 percent confidence interval, 1.4 to 7.8). Similar trends were observed for other composite end points. On the basis of these observations, the data and safety monitoring board recommended early discontinuation of the study drug.

Conclusions.—Celecoxib use was associated with a dose-related increase in the composite end point of death from cardiovascular causes, myocardial infarction, stroke, or heart failure. In light of recent reports of cardiovascular harm associated with treatment with other agents in this class, these data provide further evidence that the use of COX-2 inhibitors may increase the risk of serious cardiovascular events.

► There is growing evidence that the long-term use of COX-2 inhibitors can increase the risk of myocardial infarction, stroke and heart failure, while also increasing the risk of cardiovascular events after cardiac surgery.[1] The cause for this increased risk with COX-2 inhibitors is not known, and various mechanisms have been proposed that include a potentiation of thromboxane's effect over that of prostacyclin and increases in systemic blood pressure.[2] Aspirin may mitigate some of this risk when it is used with lower doses of COX-2 inhibitors.[3] This increased risk with COX-2 inhibitors may also be seen with all NSAIDS, so these drugs need to be used with caution in individuals at risk for cardiovascular disease and should probably not be given long term. Whether it is safe to use aspirin along with all NSAIDS has not been established.

W. H. Frishman, MD

References

1. Nussmeier NA, Whelton AA, Brown MT, et al: Complications of the COX-2 inhibitors parecoxib and valdecoxib after cardiac surgery. *N Engl J Med* 352:1081-1091, 2005.
2. Frishman WH: Effects of non-steroidal anti-inflammatory drug therapy on blood pressure and peripheral edema. *Am J Cardiol* 89:18D-25D, 2002.
3. Lévesque LE, Brophy JM, Zhang B: The risk for myocardial infarction with cyclo-oxygenase-2 inhibitors: A population study of elderly adults. *Ann Intern Med* 142:481-489, 2005.

Prognostic Significance of Left Ventricular Mass Change During Treatment of Hypertension

Devereux RB, Wachtell K, Gerdts E, et al (Cornell Med Ctr, New York; Glostrup Univ, Denmark; Haukeland Univ, Bergen, Norway; et al)
JAMA 292:2350-2356, 2004 38–4

Context.—Increased baseline left ventricular (LV) mass predicts cardiovascular (CV) complications of hypertension, but the relation between lower LV mass and outcome during treatment for hypertension is uncertain.

Objective.—To determine whether reduction of LV mass during antihypertensive treatment modifies risk of major CV events independent of blood pressure change.

Design, Setting, and Participants.—Prospective cohort substudy of the Losartan Intervention For Endpoint Reduction in Hypertension (LIFE) randomized clinical trial, conducted from 1995 to 2001. A total of 941 prospectively identified patients aged 55 to 80 years with essential hypertension and electrocardiographic LV hypertrophy had LV mass measured by echocardiography at enrollment in the LIFE trial and thereafter were followed up annually for a mean (SD) of 4.8 (1.0) years for CV events.

Main Outcome Measures.—Composite end point of CV death, fatal or nonfatal myocardial infarction, and fatal or nonfatal stroke.

Results.—The composite end point occurred in 104 patients (11%). The multivariable Cox regression model showed a strong association between lower in-treatment LV mass index and reduced rate of the composite CV end point (hazard ratio [HR], 0.78 per 1-SD (25.3) decrease in LV mass index; 95% confidence interval [CI], 0.65-0.94; $P = .009$) over and above that predicted by reduction in blood pressure. There were parallel associations between lower in-treatment LV mass index and lower CV mortality (HR, 0.62; 95% CI, 0.47-0.82; $P = .001$), stroke (HR, 0.76; 95% CI, 0.60-0.96; $P = .02$), myocardial infarction (HR, 0.85; 95% CI, 0.62-1.17, $P = .33$), and all-cause mortality (HR, 0.72; 95% CI, 0.59-0.88, $P = .002$), independent of systolic blood pressure and assigned treatment. Results were confirmed in analyses adjusting for additional CV risk factors, electrocardiographic changes, or when only considering events after the first year of study treatment.

Conclusion.—In patients with essential hypertension and baseline electrocardiographic LV hypertrophy, lower LV mass during antihypertensive treatment is associated with lower rates of clinical end points, additional to effects of blood pressure lowering and treatment modality.

▶ The presence of LV hypertrophy by ECG criteria or by its development increases the risk of clinical morbidity and mortality in hypertensive patients.[1] Regression of hypertrophy appears to reduce this risk.[2-5]

Various blood pressure-lowering drugs can improve clinical outcomes even in normotensive patients.[6] Diuretics appear to provide equal or superior effects on morbidity and mortality rates in hypertensive patients when used as monotherapy. Certain combination antihypertensive regimens also seem to provide better clinical outcomes.[7]

W. H. Frishman, MD

References

1. Frishman WH: Diagnosis and treatment of systolic heart failure in the elderly. *Am J Geriatr Cardiol* 7:10-16, 1998.
2. Okin PM, for the LIFE Study Investigators: Regression of electrocardiographic left ventricular hypertrophy during antihypertensive treatment and the prediction of major cardiovascular events. *JAMA* 292:2343-2349, 2004.
3. Devereux RB, Agabiti-Rosei E, Dahlöf B, et al: Regression of left ventricular hypertrophy as a surrogate end point for morbid events in hypertension treatment trials. *J Hypertens* 14:95S-102S, 1996.
4. Muiesan ML, Salvetti M, Rizzoni D, et al: Association of change in left ventricular mass with prognosis during long-term antihypertensive treatment. *J Hypertens* 13:1091-1095, 1995.

5. Mathew J, Sleight P, Lonn E, et al: Reduction of cardiovascular risk by regression of electrocardiographic markers of left ventricular hypertrophy by the angiotensin-converting enzyme inhibitor ramipril. *Circulation* 104:1615-1621, 2001.
6. Nissen SE, for the CAMELOT Investigators: Effect of antihypertensive agents on cardiovascular events in patients with coronary disease and normal blood pressure. The CAMELOT Study: a randomized controlled trial. *JAMA* 292:2217-2226, 2004.
7. Wassertheil-Smoller S, Psaty B, Greenland P, et al: Association between cardiovascular outcomes and antihypertensive drug treatment in older women. *JAMA* 292:2849-2859, 2004.

Urine Albumin Excretion and Subclinical Cardiovascular Disease: The Multi-Ethnic Study of Atherosclerosis

Kramer H, Jacobs DR Jr, Bild D, et al (Loyola Univ, Maywood, Ill; Univ of Minnesota, Minneapolis; Univ of Oslo, Norway; et al)

Hypertension 46:38-43, 2005 38–5

Introduction.—We examined the association between urine albumin excretion (UAE) and common and internal carotid artery intima-media thickness (IMT), end-diastolic left ventricular (LV) mass, and coronary artery calcification (CAC) scores using data from the Multi-Ethnic Study of Atherosclerosis (MESA), a population-based study of 6814 adults aged 45 to 85 years without clinical cardiovascular disease (CVD). The mean age of the MESA participants was 62.7 years, 47% were male, and 15% had diabetes mellitus (DM). Sex-specific spot urine albumin/creatinine ratios were used to define 4 UAE categories: normal, high normal, microalbuminuria, and macroalbuminuria. CAC scores were log-transformed after adding 1 to all scores. Mean values of subclinical CVD measures were computed by level of UAE after adjustment for blood pressure, DM, and other covariates. After adjustment for all covariates, geometric mean CAC scores were higher among participants with high normal UAE (8.8; $P=0.07$), microalbuminuria (9.9; $P=0.002$), and macroalbuminuria (13.1; $P=0.02$) compared with normal UAE (7.4), but only microalbuminuria reached statistical significance. Mean LV mass (g/$m^{2.7}$) was significantly higher in participants with high normal UAE (37.0; $P=0.001$), microalbuminuria (38.3; $P\leq0.0001$), and macroalbuminuria (42.3; $P\leq0.0001$) compared with normal UAE (36.0) after adjustment for all covariates. No significant difference in mean carotid IMT was found after adjustment for all covariates. Similar results were noted in MESA participants with and without DM. In conclusion, higher UAE, including levels below microalbuminuria, may reflect the presence of subclinical CVD among adults without established CVD.

► Patients with chronic kidney disease have an increased risk of CV morbidity and mortality that goes well and beyond what one might expect from traditional risk factors for CAD.[1,2] Subclinical renal disease manifested by microalbuminuria and/or a decreased glomerular filtration rate[3-6] is also associated with an increased risk of symptomatic CAD.[3,4] The use of angiotensin converting enzyme inhibitor drugs appears to reduce the risk of CV events in patients with renal disease.[5] The exact mechanism for the advanced vasculopathy of renal disease in both patients on and off dialysis has not been determined.[1]

W. H. Frishman, MD

References

1. Shlipak MG, Fried LF, Cushman M, et al: Cardiovascular mortality risk in chronic kidney disease. *JAMA* 293:1727-1745, 2005.
2. Varma R, Garrick R, McClung J, et al: Chronic renal dysfunction as an independent risk factor for the development of cardiovascular disease. *Cardiol Rev* 13:98-107, 2005.
3. Koulouris S, Lekatsas I, Karabinos I, et al: Microalbuminuria: A strong predictor of 3-year adverse prognosis in nondiabetic patients with acute myocardial infarction. *Am Heart J* 149: 840-845, 2005.
4. Arnlöv J, Evans JC, Meigs JB, et al: Low-grade albuminuria and incidence of cardiovascular disease events in nonhypertensive and nondiabetic individuals. The Framingham Heart Study. *Circulation* 112:969-975, 2005.
5. Tokmakova MP, Skali H, Kenchaiah S, et al: Chronic kidney disease, cardiovascular risk, and response to angiotensin-converting enzyme inhibition after myocardial infarction. The Survival and Ventricular Enlargement (SAVE) Study. *Circulation* 110:3667-3673, 2004.
6. Asselbergs FW, Diercks GF, Hillege HL, et al: Effects of fosinopril and pravastatin on cardiovascular events in subjects with microalbuminuria. *Circulation* 110:2809-2816, 2004.

Proinsulin Concentration Is an Independent Predictor of All-Cause and Cardiovascular Mortality: An 11-Year Follow-up of the Hoorn Study

Alssema M, Stehouwer CDA, Dekker JM, et al (VU Univ, Amsterdam; Academic Hosp Maastricht, the Netherlands)

Diabetes Care 28:860-865, 2005 38–6

Objective.—High proinsulin concentration may be a better predictor for cardiovascular disease (CVD) mortality than insulin concentration. Previous observations may have been confounded by glucose tolerance status or lack of precision because of high intraindividual variability. We investigated the longitudinal relation of means of duplicate measurements of insulin and proinsulin with all-cause and CVD mortality in a population-based cohort taking glucose tolerance status into account.

Research Design and Methods.—Fasting and post-75-g glucose-load (2-h) glucose, insulin, and proinsulin values were determined in duplicate on separate days in 277 participants with normal glucose metabolism, 208 participants with impaired glucose metabolism, and 119 newly detected patients with type 2 diabetes of the Hoorn Study. Insulin resistance and β-cell function were estimated by homeostasis model assessment (HOMA-IR and HOMA-B, respectively), and the fasting proinsulin-to-insulin ratio was calculated. Subjects were followed with respect to mortality until January 2003.

Results.—Fasting proinsulin levels were significantly associated with all-cause and CVD mortality. The hazard ratios (HRs) per increase in interquartile range adjusted for age and sex were 1.21 (95% CI 1.04-1.42) for all-cause mortality and 1.33 (1.06-1.66) for CVD mortality. Adjustment for glucose tolerance status and HOMA-IR did not substantially change the associations.

Conclusions.—Fasting proinsulin was associated with all-cause and CVD mortality, independent of glucose tolerance status and insulin resistance and largely independent of other CVD risk factors. Proinsulin might play a role in the relationship between insulin resistance and CVD.

► Insulin resistance, hyperinsulinemia and hyperglycemia are associated with an increased risk of CVD.[1-4] Even in the normal range, higher levels of blood glucose are predictive of increased CV risk compared to lower levels.[5] Agents that can cause hyperglycemia, such as glucocorticoids, especially in high amounts, can also increase the risk of CVD.[6,7] In diabetic patients, low levels of lower toenail chromium are seen more frequently in patients with CVD.[8] Whether chromium supplementation in diabetic patients will improve outcomes is not known. Hypoglycemic agents seem to favorably affect the levels of CV risk factors independent of glucose control.[9] The risk factors for CVD, along with hyperglycemia, appear to be associated with an increased risk of peripheral neuropathy in diabetic patients.[10] Whether risk factor treatment interventions beyond that of glycemic control will modify the course of peripheral neuropathy has yet to be determined.

W. H. Frishman, MD

References

1. Ragucci E, Zonszein J, Frishman WH: Pharmacotherapy of diabetes mellitus: Implications for the prevention and treatment of cardiovascular disease. *Heart Dis* 5:18-33, 2003.
2. Pyorala M, Miettinen H, Laakso M, et al: Plasma insulin and all-cause, cardiovascular, and noncardiovascular mortality: The 22-year follow-up results of the Helsinki Policemen Study. *Diabetes Care* 23:1097-1102, 2000.
3. Hu G, Qiao Q, Tuomilehto J, et al: Plasma insulin and cardiovascular mortality in non-diabetic European men and women: A meta-analysis of data from eleven prospective studies. *Diabetologia* 47:1245-1256, 2004.
4. Lakka HM, Lakka TA, Tuomilehto J, et al: Hyperinsulinemia and the risk of cardiovascular death and acute coronary and cerebrovascular events in men: The Kuopio Ischaemic Heart Disease Risk Factor Study. *Arch Intern Med* 160:1160-1168, 2000.
5. Port SC, Goodarzi MO, Boyle NG, et al: Blood glucose: A strong risk factor for mortality in nondiabetic patients with cardiovascular disease. *Am Heart J* 150:209-214, 2005.
6. Wei L, MacDonald TM, Walker BR: Taking glucocorticoids by prescription is associated with subsequent cardiovascular disease. *Ann Intern Med* 141:764-770, 2004.
7. Smith GD, Ben-Shlomo Y, Beswick A, et al: Cortisol, testosterone, and coronary heart disease. Prospective evidence from the Caerphilly Study. *Circulation* 112:332-340, 2005.
8. Rajpathak S, Rimm EB, Li T, et al: Lower toenail chromium in men with diabetes and cardiovascular disease compared with healthy men. *Diabetes Care* 27:2211-2216, 2004.

9. Pfutzner A, Marx N, Lubben G, et al: Improvement of cardiovascular risk markers by pioglitazone is independent from glycemic control. *J Am Coll Cardiol* 45:1925-1931, 2005.
10. Tesfaye S, for the EURODIAB Prospective Complications Study Group: Vascular risk factors and diabetic neuropathy. *N Engl J Med* 352: 341-350, 2005.

Excess Deaths Associated With Underweight, Overweight, and Obesity

Flegal KM, Graubard BI, Williamson DF, et al (Ctrs for Disease Control and Prevention; Hyattsville, Md; Univ of California at Berkeley; Natl Cancer Inst, Bethesda, Md; et al)
JAMA 293:1861-1867, 2005 38–7

Context.—As the prevalence of obesity increases in the United States, concern over the association of body weight with excess mortality has also increased.

Objective.—To estimate deaths associated with underweight (body mass index [BMI] <18.5), overweight (BMI 25 to <30), and obesity (BMI ≥30) in the United States in 2000.

Design, Setting, and Participants.—We estimated relative risks of mortality associated with different levels of BMI (calculated as weight in kilograms divided by the square of height in meters) from the nationally representative National Health and Nutrition Examination Survey (NHANES) I (1971-1975) and NHANES II (1976-1980), with follow-up through 1992, and from NHANES III (1988-1994), with follow-up through 2000. These relative risks were applied to the distribution of BMI and other covariates from NHANES 1999-2002 to estimate attributable fractions and number of excess deaths, adjusted for confounding factors and for effect modification by age.

Main Outcome Measures.—Number of excess deaths in 2000 associated with given BMI levels.

Results.—Relative to the normal weight category (BMI 18.5 to <25), obesity (BMI ≥30) was associated with 111 909 excess deaths (95% confidence interval [CI], 53 754-170 064) and underweight with 33,746 excess deaths (95% CI, 15 726-51 766). Overweight was not associated with excess mortality (−86 094 deaths; 95% CI, −161 223 to −10 966). The relative risks of mortality associated with obesity were lower in NHANES II and NHANES III than in NHANES I.

Conclusions.—Underweight and obesity, particularly higher levels of obesity, were associated with increased mortality relative to the normal weight category. The impact of obesity on mortality may have decreased over time, perhaps because of improvements in public health and medical care. These findings are consistent with the increases in life expectancy in the United States and the declining mortality rates from ischemic heart disease.

► The prevalence of obesity is increasing in the United States and with it are higher rates of diabetes mellitus, hypertension, and hyperlipidemia, factors associated with an increased cardiovascular disease risk.[1,2] Epidemiologic data suggest that weight extremes at either end, and a BMI less than 18.5 and more than 35 are associated with an increased mortality rate. It appears that both extreme overeating and undereating may be harmful.

Childhood obesity is associated with an increased risk of left ventricular hypertrophy in adults.[3] In adult women, elevated triglycerides and an enlarged waist size predict an increased risk of atherogenesis and cardiovascular mortality.[4] Recently, a syndrome has been described in women who have both truncal obesity and insulin resistance and other metabolic abnormalities.[5]

Regarding various long-term dietary approaches (Atkins, Ornish, Weight Watchers, Zone Diets) to weight loss, poor adherence results in only modest weight loss and cardiac risk factor reduction.[6] Cardiac risk factor reductions are similar with either dietary approach. The results of the Women's Health Initiative dietary study, where a low-fat diet is compared to a regular diet in tens of thousands of subjects, should shed more light on the cardiovascular and noncardiovascular effects of diet.

W. H. Frishman, MD

References

1. Klein S, Burke LE, Bray GA, et al: Clinical implications of obesity with specific focus on cardiovascular disease. A statement for professionals from the American Heart Association Council on Nutrition, Physical Activity, and Metabolism. *Circulation* 110:2952-2967, 2004.
2. Gregg EW, Cheng YJ, Cadwell BL, et al: Secular trends in cardiovascular disease risk factors according to body mass index in US adults. *JAMA* 293:1868-1874, 2005.
3. Li X, Li S, Ulusoy E, et al: Childhood adiposity as a predictor of cardiac mass in adult-hood. The Bogalusa Heart Study. *Circulation* 110:3488-3492, 2004.
4. Tankó LB, Bagger YZ, Qin G, et al: Enlarged waist combined with elevated triglycerides is a strong predictor of accelerated atherogenesis and related cardiovascular mortality in postmenopausal women. *Circulation* 111:1883-1890, 2005.
5. Mogul HR: *Syndrome W. A Woman's Guide to Reversing Midlife Weight Gain.* New York, M. Evans & Co. Inc., 2005.
6. Dansinger ML, Gleason JA, Griffith JL, et al: Comparison of the Atkins, Ornish, Weight Watchers, and Zone Diets for weight loss and heart disease risk reduction. A randomized trial. *JAMA* 293:43-53, 2005.

39 Acute Coronary Syndromes

Addition of Clopidogrel to Aspirin and Fibrinolytic Therapy for Myocardial Infarction With ST-Segment Elevation

Sabatine MS, for the CLARITY–TIMI 28 Investigators (Harvard Med School, Boston; et al)

N Engl J Med 352:1179-1189, 2005 39–1

Background.—A substantial proportion of patients receiving fibrinolytic therapy for myocardial infarction with ST-segment elevation have inadequate reperfusion or reocclusion of the infarct-related artery, leading to an increased risk of complications and death.

Methods.—We enrolled 3491 patients, 18 to 75 years of age, who presented within 12 hours after the onset of an ST-elevation myocardial infarction and randomly assigned them to receive clopidogrel (300-mg loading dose, followed by 75 mg once daily) or placebo. Patients received a fibrinolytic agent, aspirin, and when appropriate, heparin (dispensed according to body weight) and were scheduled to undergo angiography 48 to 192 hours after the start of study medication. The primary efficacy end point was a composite of an occluded infarct-related artery (defined by a Thrombolysis in Myocardial Infarction flow grade of 0 or 1) on angiography or death or recurrent myocardial infarction before angiography.

Results.—The rates of the primary efficacy end point were 21.7 percent in the placebo group and 15.0 percent in the clopidogrel group, representing an absolute reduction of 6.7 percentage points in the rate and a 36 percent reduction in the odds of the end point with clopidogrel therapy (95 percent confidence interval, 24 to 47 percent; P<0.001). By 30 days, clopidogrel therapy reduced the odds of the composite end point of death from cardiovascular causes, recurrent myocardial infarction, or recurrent ischemia leading to the need for urgent revascularization by 20 percent (from 14.1 to 11.6 percent, P=0.03) (Fig 2). The rates of major bleeding and intracranial hemorrhage were similar in the two groups.

Conclusions.—In patients 75 years of age or younger who have myocardial infarction with ST-segment elevation and who receive aspirin and a standard fibrinolytic regimen, the addition of clopidogrel improves the patency rate of the infarct-related artery and reduces ischemic complications.

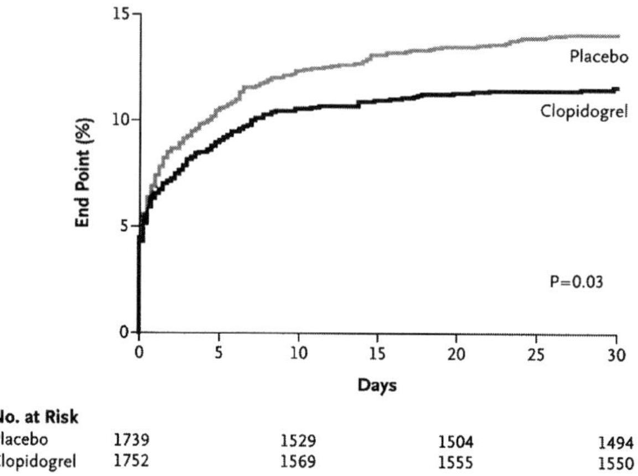

FIGURE 2.—Cumulative incidence of the end point of death from cardiovascular causes, recurrent myocardial infarction, or recurrent ischemia leading to the need for urgent revascularization. The odds ratio for this end point was significantly lower in the clopidogrel group than in the placebo group at 30 days (11.6 percent vs. 14.1 percent, odds ratio, 0.80 [95 percent confidence interval, 0.65 to 0.97]; P=0.03). (Reprinted by permission of *The New England Journal of Medicine* from Sabatine MS, for the CLARITY–TIMI 28 Investigators: Addition of clopidogrel to aspirin and fibrinolytic therapy for myocardial infarction with ST-segment elevation. *N Engl J Med* 352:1179-1189, 2005. Copyright 2005, Massachusetts Medical Society. All rights reserved.)

▶ The combination of early and sustained dual oral antiplatelet therapy with aspirin and clopidogrel has also been shown to be beneficial in patients with acute coronary syndromes without ECG ST-segment elevation and in patients who have undergone a percutaneous coronary intervention.[1,2]

Controversy still exists regarding the loading dose of clopidogrel and whether concurrent triple-antiplatelet therapy with aspirin, clopidogrel, and a glycoprotein IIb/IIIa inhibitor would provide greater clinical benefit in acute coronary syndromes.[3] There is also a question whether recent withdrawal of oral antiplatelet agents can precipitate unstable coronary syndromes.[4]

W. H. Frishman, MD

References

1. The Clopidogrel in Unstable Angina to Prevent Recurrent Ischemic Events Trial Investigators: Effects of clopidogrel in addition to aspirin patients with acute coronary syndromes without ST-segment elevation. *N Engl J Med* 345:494-502, 2001 (Erratum 345:1506, 1716, 2001).
2. Beinart SC, Kolm P, Veledar E, et al: Long-term cost effectiveness of early and sustained dual oral antiplatelet therapy with clopidogrel given for up to one year after percutaneous coronary intervention. *J Am Coll Cardiol* 46:761-769, 2005.
3. Gurbel PA, Bliden KP, Zaman KA, et al: Clopidogrel loading with eptifibatide to arrest the reactivity of platelets. Results of the Clopidogrel Loading with Eptifibatide to Arrest the Reactivity of Platelets (CLEAR PLATELETS) Study. *Circulation* 111:1153-1159, 2005.
4. Collet JP, Montalescot G, Blanchet B, et al: Impact of prior use or recent withdrawal of oral antiplatelet agents on acute coronary syndromes. *Circulation* 110:2361-2367, 2004.

Effect of Glucose-Insulin-Potassium Infusion on Mortality in Patients With Acute ST-Segment Elevation Myocardial Infarction: The CREATE-ECLA Randomized Controlled Trial

Mehta SR, for the CREATE-ECLA Trial Group Investigators (McMaster Univ, Hamilton, Ont, Canada; et al)

JAMA 293:437-446, 2005 39–2

Context.—Glucose-insulin-potassium (GIK) infusion is a widely applicable, low-cost therapy that has been postulated to improve mortality in patients with acute ST-segment elevation myocardial infarction (STEMI). Given the potential global importance of GIK infusion, a large, adequately powered randomized trial is required to determine the effect of GIK on mortality in patients with STEMI.

Objective.—To determine the effect of high-dose GIK infusion on mortality in patients with STEMI.

Design, Setting, and Participants.—Randomized controlled trial conducted in 470 centers worldwide among 20,201 patients with STEMI who presented within 12 hours of symptom onset. The mean age of patients was 58.6 years, and evidence-based therapies were commonly used.

Intervention.—Patients were randomly assigned to receive GIK intravenous infusion for 24 hours plus usual care (n = 10,091) or to receive usual care alone (controls; n = 10,110).

Main Outcome Measures.—Mortality, cardiac arrest, cardiogenic shock, and reinfarction at 30 days after randomization.

Results.—At 30 days, 976 control patients (9.7%) and 1004 GIK infusion patients (10.0%) died (hazard ratio [HR], 1.03; 95% confidence interval [CI], 0.95-1.13; P = .45). There were no significant differences in the rates of cardiac arrest (1.5% [151/10 107] in control and 1.4% [139/10,088] in GIK infusion; HR, 0.93; 95% CI, 0.74-1.17; *P* = .51), cardiogenic shock (6.3% [640/10 107] vs 6.6% [667/10 088]; HR, 1.05; 95% CI, 0.94-1.17; *P* = .38), or reinfarction (2.4% [246/10,107] vs 2.3% [236/10,088]; HR, 0.98; 95% CI, 0.82-1.17; *P* = .81). The rates of heart failure at 7 days after randomization were also similar between the groups (16.9% [1711/10,107] vs 17.1% [1721/10,088]; HR, 1.01; 95% CI, 0.95-1.08; *P* = .72). The lack of benefit of GIK infusion on mortality was consistent in prespecified subgroups, including in those with and without diabetes, in those presenting with and without heart failure, in those presenting early and later after symptom onset, and in those receiving and not receiving reperfusion therapy (thrombolysis or primary percutaneous coronary intervention).

Conclusion.—In this large, international randomized trial, high-dose GIK infusion had a neutral effect on mortality, cardiac arrest, and cardiogenic shock in patients with acute STEMI.

► The concept of a metabolic manipulation with a GIK infusion to modify the course of acute myocardial infarction dates back to 1962.[1] Although experimental evidence would suggest a benefit with this treatment,[2] clinical studies done to date do not show benefit.[3] Metabolic factors do play an unfavorable role in the course of myocardial infarction, especially diabetes and reactive hyperglycemia.[4] Whether specific therapy for hyperglycemia will make a difference in the clinical outcome of myocardial infarction needs to be determined.[5]

Adjunctive therapies with antiplatelet drugs, antithrombin drugs, and fibrinolytic agents have definitely improved the outcomes of myocardial infarction.[6-8]

W. H. Frishman, MD

References

1. Sodi-Pallares D, Testelli MR, Fishleder BL, et al: Effects of an intravenous infusion of potassium-glucose-insulin solution on the electrocardiographic signs of myocardial infarction: a preliminary clinical report. *Am J Cardiol* 9:166-181, 1962.
2. Apstein CS, Tacgtmeyer H: Glucose-insulin-potassium in acute myocardial infarction: the time has come for a large, prospective trial. *Circulation* 96:1074-1077, 1997.
3. van der Horst ICC, et al on behalf of the GIPS Investigators: Glucose-insulin-potassium and reperfusion in acute myocardial infarction: rationale and design of the glucose-insulin-potassium study-2 (GIPS-2). *Am Heart J* 149:585-591, 2005.
4. Kosiborod M, Rathore SS, Inzucchi SE, et al: Admission glucose and mortality in elderly patients hospitalized with acute myocardial infarction. Implications for patients with and without recognized diabetes. *Circulation* 111:3078-3086, 2005.
5. Ragucci E, Zonszein J, Frishman WH: Pharmacotherapy of diabetes mellitus: implications for the prevention and treatment of cardiovascular disease. *Heart Dis* 5:18-33, 2003.
6. De Luca G, Suryapranata H, Stone GW, et al: Abciximab as adjunctive therapy to reperfusion in acute ST-segment elevation myocardial infarction. A meta-analysis of randomized trials. *JAMA* 293:1759-1765, 2005.
7. The CREATE Trial Group Investigators: Effects of reviparin, a low-molecular-weight heparin, on mortality, reinfarction, and strokes in patients with acute myocardial infarction presenting with ST-segment elevation. *JAMA* 293:427-436, 2005.
8. Rebeiz AG, Johanson P, Green CL, et al: Comparison of ST-segment resolution with combined fibrinolytic and glycoprotein IIb/IIIa inhibitor therapy versus fibrinolytic alone (data from four clinical trials). *Am J Cardiol* 95:611-614, 2005.

Early Invasive Versus Selectively Invasive Management for Acute Coronary Syndromes

de Winter RJ, for the Invasive versus Conservative Treatment in Unstable Coronary Syndromes (ICTUS) Investigators (Academisch Medisch Centrum, Amsterdam; et al)

N Engl J Med 353:1095-1104, 2005 39–3

Background.—Current guidelines recommend an early invasive strategy for patients who have acute coronary syndromes without ST-segment elevation and with an elevated cardiac troponin T level. However, randomized trials have not shown an overall reduction in mortality, and the reduction in the rate of myocardial infarction in previous trials has varied depending on the definition of myocardial infarction.

Methods.—We randomly assigned 1200 patients with acute coronary syndrome without ST-segment elevation who had chest pain, an elevated

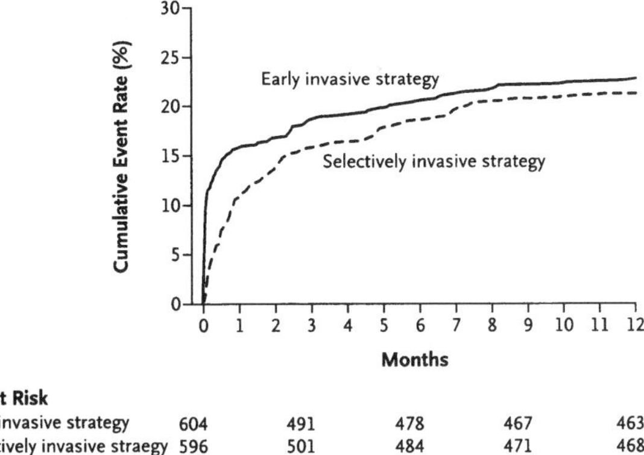

FIGURE 1.—Kaplan–Meier estimates of the cumulative rate of the composite primary end point of death, nonfatal myocardial infarction, or rehospitalization for anginal symptoms within one year. The rate of a composite primary end point within one year was 22.7 percent in the group assigned to an early invasive strategy and 21.2 percent in the group assigned to a selectively invasive strategy (relative risk, 1.07; 95 percent confidence interval, 0.87 to 1.33; P=0.33). (Reprinted by permission of *The New England Journal of Medicine* from de Winter RJ, for the Invasive versus Conservative Treatment in Unstable Coronary Syndromes (ICTUS) Investigators: Early invasive versus selectively invasive management for acute coronary syndromes. *N Engl J Med* 353:1095-1104, 2005. Copyright 2005, Massachusetts Medical Society. All rights reserved.)

cardiac troponin T level (≥0.03 μg per liter), and either electrocardiographic evidence of ischemia at admission or a documented history of coronary disease to an early invasive strategy or to a more conservative (selectively invasive) strategy. Patients received aspirin daily, enoxaparin for 48 hours, and abciximab at the time of percutaneous coronary intervention. The use of clopidogrel and intensive lipid-lowering therapy was recommended. The primary end point was a composite of death, nonfatal myocardial infarction, or rehospitalization for anginal symptoms within one year after randomization.

Results.—The estimated cumulative rate of the primary end point was 22.7 percent in the group assigned to early invasive management and 21.2 percent in the group assigned to selectively invasive management (relative risk, 1.07; 95 percent confidence interval, 0.87 to 1.33; P=0.33) (Fig 1). The mortality rate was the same in the two groups (2.5 percent). Myocardial infarction was significantly more frequent in the group assigned to early invasive management (15.0 percent vs. 10.0 percent, P=0.005), but rehospitalization was less frequent in that group (7.4 percent vs. 10.9 percent, P=0.04).

Conclusions.—We could not demonstrate that, given optimized medical therapy, an early invasive strategy was superior to a selectively invasive strategy in patients with acute coronary syndromes without ST-segment elevation and with an elevated cardiac troponin T level.

► With improvements in the medical therapy of acute coronary syndromes, an early invasive treatment approach may not be appropriate for all patients.[1] Regarding the ability to carry out invasive procedures in a timely manner, such as on nights and weekends, interventions take place much later with catheter-based treatment compared with fibrinolytic therapy.[2] There are definite situations, such as cardiogenic shock, where timely intervention is necessary, and this is why specialized myocardial infarction centers are being planned that can provide, when necessary, 7 days a week, 24 hours a day, catheter laboratory coverage.[3]

W. H. Frishman, MD

References

1. Stukel TA, Lucas FL, Wennberg DE: Long-term outcomes of regional variations in intensity of invasive vs medical management of Medicare patients with acute myocardial infarction. *JAMA* 293:1329-1337, 2005.
2. Magid DJ, Wang Y, Herrin J, et al: Relationship between time of day, day of week, timeliness of reperfusion, and in-hospital mortality for patients with acute ST-segment elevation myocardial infarction. *JAMA* 294:803-812, 2005.
3. Babaev A, et al for the NRMI Investigators: Trends in management and outcomes of patients with acute myocardial infarction complicated by cardiogenic shock. *JAMA* 294:448-454, 2005.

Sudden Death in Patients With Myocardial Infarction and Left Ventricular Dysfunction, Heart Failure, or Both

Solomon SD, for the Valsartan in Acute Myocardial Infarction Trial (VALIANT) Investigators (Brigham and Women's Hosp, Boston; et al)

N Engl J Med 352:2581-2588, 2005 39–4

Background.—The risk of sudden death from cardiac causes is increased among survivors of acute myocardial infarction with reduced left ventricular systolic function. We assessed the risk and time course of sudden death in high-risk patients after myocardial infarction.

Methods.—We studied 14,609 patients with left ventricular dysfunction, heart failure, or both after myocardial infarction to assess the incidence and timing of sudden unexpected death or cardiac arrest with resuscitation in relation to the left ventricular ejection fraction.

Results.—Of 14,609 patients, 1067 (7 percent) had an event a median of 180 days after myocardial infarction: 903 died suddenly, and 164 were resuscitated after cardiac arrest. The risk was highest in the first 30 days after myocardial infarction—1.4 percent per month (95 percent confidence interval, 1.2 to 1.6 percent)—and decreased to 0.14 percent per month (95 percent confidence interval, 0.11 to 0.18 percent) after 2 years. Patients with a left ventricular ejection fraction of 30 percent or less were at highest risk in this early period (rate, 2.3 percent per month; 95 percent confidence interval, 1.8 to 2.8 percent). Nineteen percent of all sudden deaths or episodes of cardiac arrest with resuscitation occurred within the first 30 days after myocardial infarction, and 83 percent of all patients who died suddenly did so in the first 30 days after hospital discharge. Each decrease of 5 percentage points in the left ventricular ejection fraction was associated with a 21 percent adjusted increase in the risk of sudden death or cardiac arrest with resuscitation in the first 30 days.

Conclusions.—The risk of sudden death is highest in the first 30 days after myocardial infarction among patients with left ventricular dysfunction, heart failure, or both. Thus, earlier implementation of strategies for preventing sudden death may be warranted in selected patients.

► Peri-infarction survival is influenced by multiple risk factors and disease markers. Included among factors associated with increased mortality risk from myocardial infarction are anemia,[1] azotemia,[2] β_2-adrenergic receptor genotype,[3] T-helper-1 lymphocyte activation,[4] specific CD14 C(-260)T promoter polymorphisms,[5] and an increased level of circulating endothelial cells.[6] Recently a serum marker of coronary plaque instability has been identified (soluble lectin-like oxidized low-density lipoprotein receptor-1 levels).[6]

W. H. Frishman, MD

References

1. Sabatine MS, Morrow DA, Giugliano RP, et al: Association of hemoglobin levels with clinical outcomes in acute coronary syndromes. *Circulation* 111:2042-2049, 2005.
2. Kirtane AJ, et al for the TIMI Study Group: Serum blood urea nitrogen as an independent marker of subsequent mortality among patients with acute coronary syndromes and normal to mildly reduced glomerular filtration rates. *J Am Coll Cardiol* 45:1781-1786, 2005.
3. Lanfear DE, Jones PG, Marsh S, et al: β_2-adrenergic receptor genotype and survival among patients receiving β-blocker therapy after an acute coronary syndrome. *JAMA* 294:1526-1533, 2005.
4. Methe H, Brunner S, Wiegand D, et al: Enhanced T-helper-1 lymphocyte activation patterns in acute coronary syndromes. *J Am Coll Cardiol* 45:1939-1945, 2005.
5. Arroyo-Espliguero R, El-Sharnouby K, Vasquez-Rey E, et al: CD14 C(-260)T promoter polymorphism and prevalence of acute coronary syndromes. *Int J Cardiol* 98:307-312, 2005.
6. Werner N, Kosiol S, Schiegl T, et al: Circulating endothelial progenitor cells and cardiovascular outcomes. *N Engl J Med* 353:999-1007, 2005.

Stem Cells in the Dog Heart Are Self-Renewing, Clonogenic, and Multipotent and Regenerate Infarcted Myocardium, Improving Cardiac Function

Linke A, Müller P, Nurzynska D, et al (New York Med College, Valhalla; Univ of Saarland, Homburg, Germany)

Proc Natl Acad Sci U S A 102:8966-8971, 2005 39–5

Introduction.—The purpose of this study was to determine whether the heart in large mammals contains cardiac progenitor cells that regulate organ homeostasis and regenerate dead myocardium after infarction. We report that the dog heart possesses a cardiac stem cell pool characterized by undifferentiated cells that are self-renewing, clonogenic, and multipotent. These clonogenic cells and early committed progeny possess a hepatocyte growth factor (HGF)-c-Met and an insulin-like growth factor 1 (IGF-1)-IGF-1 receptor system that can be activated to induce their migration, proliferation, and survival. Therefore, myocardial infarction was induced in chronically instrumented dogs implanted with sonomicrometric crystals in the region of the left ventricular wall supplied by the occluded left anterior descending coronary artery. After infarction, HGF and IGF-1 were injected intramyocardially to stimulate resident cardiac progenitor cells. This intervention led to the formation of myocytes and coronary vessels within the infarct. Newly generated myocytes expressed nuclear and cytoplasmic proteins specific of cardiomyocytes: MEF2C was detected in the nucleus, whereas α-sarcomeric actin, cardiac myosin heavy chain, troponin I, and α-actinin were identified in the cytoplasm. Connexin 43 and N-cadherin were also present. Myocardial reconstitution resulted in a marked recovery of contractile performance of the infarcted heart. In conclusion, the activation of resident primitive cells in the damaged dog heart can promote a significant restoration of dead tissue, which is paralleled by a progressive improvement in cardiac function. These results suggest that strategies capable of activating the growth reserve of the myocardium may be important in cardiac repair after ischemic injury.

► Investigators from our department of medicine made the original observations regarding the regenerative capacity of the heart. Recently endothelial progenitor cells, mononuclear bone marrow cells, skeletal myoblasts, and unfractionated bone marrow cells have been used both in animals and human beings to treat patients with acute myocardial infarction.[1,2] In addition, a cardiac stem cell has been identified that can be delivered by an intravascular route in infarcted dogs with evidence for myocardial regeneration and improved cardiac function.[3] Various interventions using growth factors and modified bone marrow cells may improve the regenerative capacity of the heart.[4,5] The era of stem cell therapy for the treatment of myocardial infarction, chronic congestive heart failure, and myocardial aging is here.[6] The results of ongoing controlled human trials using stem cells are being awaited with great interest.

W. H. Frishman, MD

References

1. Rosenthal N: Prometheus's vulture and the stem-cell promise. *N Engl J Med* 349:267-274, 2003.
2. Anversa P, Sussman MA, Bolli R: Molecular genetic advances in cardiovascular medicine. Focus on the myocyte. *Circulation* 109:2832-2838, 2004.
3. Dawn B, Stein AB, Urbanek K, et al: Cardiac stem cells delivered intravascularly traverse the vessel barrier, regenerate infracted myocardium, and improve cardiac function. *Proc Natl Acad Sci U S A* 102:3766-3771, 2005.
4. Kofidis T, de Bruin JL, Yamane T, et al: Stimulation of paracrine pathways with growth factors enhances embryonic stem cell engraftment and host-specific differentiation in the heart after ischemic myocardium injury. *Circulation* 111:2486-2493, 2005.
5. Li T-S, Hayashi M, Ito H, et al: Regeneration of infarcted myocardium by intramyocardial implantation of ex vivo transforming growth factor: Preprogrammed bone marrow stem cells. *Circulation* 111:2438-2445, 2005.
6. Urbanek K, Torella D, Sheikh F, et al: Myocardial regeneration by activation of multipotent cardiac stem cells in ischemic heart failure. *Proc Natl Acad Sci* 102:8692-8697, 2005.

40 Chronic Coronary Artery Disease

N-Terminal Pro–B-Type Natriuretic Peptide and Long-term Mortality in Stable Coronary Heart Disease

Kragelund C, Grønning B, Køber L, et al (Frederiksberg Hosp, Denmark; Rigshospitalet, Copenhagen; Hillerød Univ Hosp, Copenhagen)

N Engl J Med 352:666-675, 2005 40–1

Background.—The level of the inactive N-terminal fragment of pro–brain (B-type) natriuretic peptide (BNP) is a strong predictor of mortality among patients with acute coronary syndromes and may be a strong prognostic marker in patients with chronic coronary heart disease as well. We assessed the relationship between N-terminal pro-BNP (NT-pro-BNP) levels and long-term mortality from all causes in a large cohort of patients with stable coronary heart disease.

Methods.—NT-pro-BNP was measured in baseline serum samples from 1034 patients referred for angiography because of symptoms or signs of coronary heart disease. The rate of death from all causes was determined after a median follow-up of nine years.

Results.—At follow-up, 288 patients had died. The median NT-pro-BNP level was significantly lower among patients who survived than among those who died (120 pg per milliliter [interquartile range, 50 to 318] vs. 386 pg per milliliter [interquartile range, 146 to 897], $P<0.001$). Patients with NT-pro-BNP levels in the highest quartile were older, had a lower left ventricular ejection fraction (LVEF) and a lower creatinine clearance rate, and were more likely to have a history of myocardial infarction, clinically significant coronary artery disease, and diabetes than patients with NT-pro-BNP levels in the lowest quartile. In a multivariable Cox regression model, the hazard ratio for death from any cause for the patients with NT-pro-BNP levels in the fourth quartile as compared with those in the first quartile was 2.4 (95 percent confidence interval, 1.5 to 4.0; $P<0.001$); the NT-pro-BNP level added prognostic information beyond that provided by conventional risk factors, including the patient's age; sex; family history with respect to ischemic heart disease; the presence or absence of a history of myocardial infarction, angina, hypertension, diabetes, or chronic heart failure; creatinine clearance rate; body-mass index; smoking status; plasma lipid levels; LVEF; and the

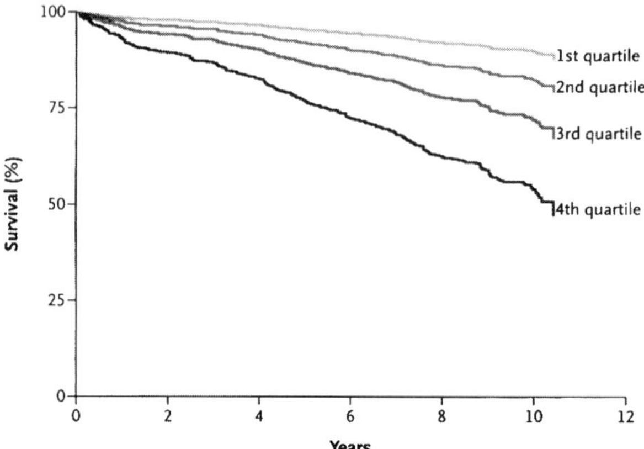

FIGURE 2.—Adjusted estimates of overall survival among patients with stable coronary disease, according to quartiles of N-terminal pro–B-type natriuretic peptide (NT-pro-BNP). The survival estimates have been adjusted for age, presence or absence of diabetes, smoking status, left ventricular ejection fraction, presence or absence of suspected heart failure, and severity of angiographic coronary disease. The NT-pro-BNP levels were as follows: first quartile, less than 64 pg per milliliter; second quartile, 64 to 169 pg per milliliter; third quartile, 170 to 455 pg per milliliter; and fourth quartile, more than 455 pg per milliliter. $P<0.001$ by the log-rank test for the overall comparison among the groups. (Reprinted by permission of *The New England Journal of Medicine* from Kragelund C, Grønning B, Køber L, et al: N-terminal pro–B-type natriuretic peptide and long-term mortality in stable coronary heart disease. *N Engl J Med* 352:666-675, 2005. Copyright 2005, Massachusetts Medical Society. All rights reserved.)

presence or absence of clinically significant coronary artery disease on angiography (Fig 2).

Conclusions.—NT-pro-BNP is a marker of long-term mortality in patients with stable coronary disease and provides prognostic information above and beyond that provided by conventional cardiovascular risk factors and the degree of left ventricular systolic dysfunction.

► Measurements of serum natriuretic peptide levels appear to be useful as a prognostic indicator in patients with stable coronary heart disease.[1,2] Elevations in natriuretic peptide can also predict the anatomic and hemodynamic severity of coronary artery disease.[3] In addition, natriuretic peptide elevations can identify high-risk patients with a history of unstable coronary artery disease.[4]

W. H. Frishman, MD

References

1. Omland T, Richard AM, Wergeland R, et al: B-type natriuretic peptide and long-term survival in patients with stable coronary artery disease. *Am J Cardiol* 95:24-28, 2005.
2. de Winter RJ, Stroobants A, Koch KT, et al: Plasma N-terminal pro-B-type natriuretic peptide for prediction of death or nonfatal myocardial infarction following percutaneous coronary intervention. *Am J Cardiol* 94:1481-1485, 2004.
3. Ndrepepa G, Braun S, Mehilli J, et al: Plasma levels of N-terminal pro-brain natriuretic peptide in patients with coronary artery disease and relation to clinical presentation, angiographic severity, and left ventricular ejection fraction. *Am J Cardiol* 95:553-557, 2005.

4. Morrow DA, for the A to Z Investigators: Prognostic value of serial B-type natriuretic peptide testing during follow-up of patients with unstable coronary artery disease. *JAMA* 294:2866-2871, 2005.

State of Disparities in Cardiovascular Health in the United States

Mensah GA, Mokdad AH, Ford ES, et al (Centers for Disease Control, Atlanta, Ga)

Circulation 111:1233-1241, 2005 40–2

Background.—Reducing health disparities remains a major public health challenge in the United States. Having timely access to current data on disparities is important for policy and program development. Accordingly, we assessed the current magnitude of disparities in cardiovascular disease (CVD) and its risk factors in the United States.

Method and Results.—Using national surveys, we determined CVD and risk factor prevalence and indexes of morbidity, mortality, and overall quality of life in adults ≥18 years of age by race/ethnicity, sex, education level, socioeconomic status, and geographic location. Disparities were common in all risk factors examined. In men, the highest prevalence of obesity (29.2%) was found in Mexican Americans who had completed a high school education. Black women with or without a high school education had a high prevalence of obesity (47.3%). Hypertension prevalence was high among blacks (39.8%) regardless of sex or educational status. Hypercholesterolemia was high among white and Mexican American men and white women in both groups of educational status. Ischemic heart disease and stroke were inversely related to education, income, and poverty status. Hospitalization was greater in men for total heart disease and acute myocardial infarction but greater in women for congestive heart failure and stroke. Among Medicare enrollees, congestive heart failure hospitalization was higher in blacks, Hispanics, and American Indians/Alaska Natives than among whites, and stroke hospitalization was highest in blacks. Hospitalizations for congestive heart failure and stroke were highest in the southeastern United States. Life expectancy remains higher in women than men and higher in whites than blacks by approximately 5 years. CVD mortality at all ages tended to be highest in blacks.

Conclusions.—Disparities in CVD and related risk factors remain pervasive. The data presented here can be invaluable for policy development and in the planning, implementation, and evaluation of interventions designed to eliminate health disparities.

► There are wide disparities in cardiovascular health and health care delivery between various ethnic groups. Many cardiovascular specialists are unaware of these disparities.[1] Black patients who often have more CVD risk factors than white patients are less likely to receive many of the evidence-based treatments.[2-4] It is an obligation of all physicians to ensure that the best possible care is provided to patients, regardless of ethnic differences and financial status.

W. H. Frishman, MD

References

1. Lurie N, Fremont A, Jain AK, et al: Racial and ethnic disparities in care. The perspectives of cardiologists. *Circulation* 111:1264-1269, 2005.
2. Kaul P, Lytle BL, Spertus JA, et al: Influence of racial disparities in procedure use on functional status outcomes among patients with coronary artery disease. *Circulation* 111:1284-1290, 2005.
3. Sonel AF, for the CRUSADE Investigators: Racial variations in treatment and outcomes of black and white patients with high-risk non–ST-elevation acute coronary syndromes. Insights from CRUSADE (Can Rapid Risk Stratification of Unstable Angina Patients Suppress Adverse Outcomes with Early Implementation of the ACC/AHA Guidelines?) *Circulation* 111:1225-1232, 2005.
4. Sabatine MS, Blake GJ, Drazner MH, et al: Influence of race on death and ischemic complications in patients with non–ST-elevation acute coronary syndromes despite modern, protocol-guided treatment. *Circulation* 111:1217-1224, 2005.

Coronary Calcification Improves Cardiovascular Risk Prediction in the Elderly

Vliegenthart R, Oudkerk M, Hofman A, et al (Erasmus Med Ctr, Rotterdam, The Netherlands; Univ Hosp Groningen, The Netherlands)
Circulation 112:572-577, 2005 40–3

Background.—Coronary calcification detected by electron beam tomography may improve cardiovascular risk prediction. The technique is particularly promising in the elderly because the predictive power of cardiovascular risk factors weakens with age. We investigated the prognostic value of coronary calcification for cardiovascular events and mortality in a general, asymptomatic population of elderly subjects.

Method and Results.—From 1997 to 2000, electron beam tomography scanning to assess coronary calcification was performed in subjects of the population-based Rotterdam Study. Risk factors were measured by standardized procedures. Coronary calcium scores were available for 1795 asymptomatic participants (mean age, 71 years; range, 62 to 85 years). During a mean follow-up of 3.3 years, 88 cardiovascular events, including 50 coronary events, occurred. The risk of coronary heart disease increased with increasing calcium score. The multivariate-adjusted relative risk of coronary events was 3.1 (95% CI, 1.2 to 7.9) for calcium scores of 101 to 400, 4.6 (95% CI, 1.8 to 11.8) for calcium scores of 401 to 1000, and 8.3 (95% CI, 3.3 to 21.1) for calcium scores >1000 compared with calcium scores of 0 to 100. The predictive value in subjects >70 years of age was similar. Risk prediction based on the cardiovascular risk factors improved when coronary calcification was added.

Conclusions.—Coronary calcification is a strong and independent predictor of coronary heart disease, also in the elderly. Coronary calcification improves prediction of coronary events based on cardiovascular risk factors.

Risk stratification by assessment of coronary calcification may have an important role in the primary prevention of coronary heart disease events in the elderly.

► Coronary calcification assessed by electron beam tomography (EBT) may be useful for identifying individuals at risk for coronary artery disease.[1] There is an ongoing debate regarding the utility of this technique as a screening test in asymptomatic individuals.[2] The use of EBT has identified a familial disposition to premature coronary artery disease related to siblings rather than parents.[3] In addition, there appears to be ethnic differences in the rate of EBT calcification of the coronary circulation that is not explained by known coronary risk factors.[4] There is a substantially lower prevalence of coronary calcification in blacks and Hispanics compared with whites.

W. H. Frishman, MD

References

1. Greenland P, LaBree L, Azen SP, et al: Coronary artery calcium score combined with Framingham score for risk prediction in asymptomatic individuals. *JAMA* 291:210-215, 2004.
2. Mozaffarian D: Electron-beam computer tomography for coronary calcium. A useful test to screen for coronary heart disease? *JAMA* 294:2897-2901, 2005.
3. Nasir K, Michos ED, Rumberger JA, et al: Coronary artery calcification and family history of premature coronary heart disease. Sibling history is more strongly associated than parental history. *Circulation* 110:2150-2156, 2004.
4. Bild DE, Detrano R, Peterson D, et al: Ethnic differences in coronary calcification. The multi-ethnic study of atherosclerosis (MESA). *Circulation* 111:1313-1320, 2005.

41 Coronary Intervention Procedures

Sirolimus-Eluting and Paclitaxel-Eluting Stents for Coronary Revascularization

Windecker S, Remondino A, Eberli FR, et al (Univ Hosp Bern, Switzerland; Univ Hosp Zurich; Univ of Bristol, England)

N Engl J Med 353:653-662, 2005 41–1

Background.—Sirolimus-eluting stents and paclitaxel-eluting stents, as compared with bare-metal stents, reduce the risk of restenosis. It is unclear whether there are differences in safety and efficacy between the two types of drug-eluting stents.

Methods.—We conducted a randomized, controlled, single-blind trial comparing sirolimus-eluting stents with paclitaxel-eluting stents in 1012 patients undergoing percutaneous coronary intervention. The primary end point was a composite of major adverse cardiac events (death from cardiac causes, myocardial infarction, and ischemia-driven revascularization of the target lesion) by nine months. Follow-up angiography was completed in 540 of 1012 patients (53.4 percent).

Results.—The two groups had similar baseline clinical and angiographic characteristics. The rate of major adverse cardiac events at nine months was 6.2 percent in the sirolimus-stent group and 10.8 percent in the paclitaxel-stent group (hazard ratio, 0.56; 95 percent confidence interval, 0.36 to 0.86; P=0.009). The difference was driven by a lower rate of target-lesion revascularization in the sirolimus-stent group than in the paclitaxel-stent group (4.8 percent vs. 8.3 percent; hazard ratio, 0.56; 95 percent confidence interval, 0.34 to 0.93; P=0.03). Rates of death from cardiac causes were 0.6 percent in the sirolimus-stent group and 1.6 percent in the paclitaxel-stent group (P=0.15); the rates of myocardial infarction were 2.8 percent and 3.5 percent, respectively (P=0.49); and the rates of angiographic restenosis were 6.6 percent and 11.7 percent, respectively (P=0.02) (Fig 1).

Conclusions.—As compared with paclitaxel-eluting stents, the use of sirolimus-eluting stents results in fewer major adverse cardiac events, primarily by decreasing the rates of clinical and angiographic restenosis.

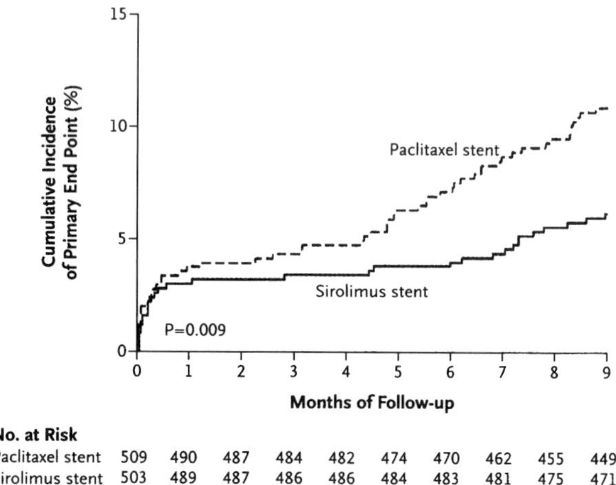

FIGURE 1.—Kaplan–Meier cumulative-event curves for the primary end point of death from cardiac causes, myocardial infarction, or ischemia-driven revascularization of the target lesion. (Reprinted by permission of *The New England Journal of Medicine* from Windecker S, Remondino A, Eberli FR, et al: Sirolimus-Eluting and Paclitaxel-Eluting Stents for Coronary Revascularization. *N Engl J Med* 353:653-662, 2005.)

► In patients with coronary artery disease, drug-eluting stents have been shown to be effective in reducing the rate of restenosis compared with bare metal stents.[1-6] Among the available drug-eluting stents, the sirolimus-eluting device appears to be more effective than the paclitaxel-eluting device in reducing restenosis.[7,8] Drug-eluting stents have been shown to be effective in treating patients with vein graft lesions,[9] diabetes,[7] and left main coronary artery disease.[10,11] Insertion of drug-eluting stents has been shown to be effective without the need for angioplasty,[12] and long-term follow up studies (3 years) have shown the benefit of the drug-eluting stent on restenosis and cardiovascular events.[13] It is still not known, even with improved microcirculatory protection,[14] if stenting of multiple vessels will be more advantageous than coronary bypass surgery.[15]

W. H. Frishman, MD

References

1. Morice M-C, Serruys PW, Sousa JE, et al: A randomized comparison of a sirolimus-eluting stent with a standard stent for coronary revascularization. *N Engl J Med* 346: 1773-1780, 2002.
2. Moses JW, Leon MB, Popma JJ, et al: Sirolimus-eluting stents versus standard stents in patients with stenosis in a native coronary artery. *N Engl J Med* 349:1315-1323, 2003.
3. Stone GW, Ellis SG, Cox DA, et al: A polymer-based, paclitaxel-eluting stent in patients with coronary artery disease. *N Engl J Med* 350:221-231, 2004.
4. Gruchalla KJA, Nawarskas JJ: The paclitaxel-eluting stent in percutaneous coronary intervention. Part I: Background and clinical comparison to bare metal stents. *Cardiol Rev.* 14:88-98, 2006.
5. Gruchalla KJA, Nawarskas JJ: The paclitaxel-eluting stent in percutaneous coronary intervention. Part II: Comparison to the sirolimus-eluting stent and considerations for use. *Cardiol Rev.* In press.

6. Cheng-Lai A, Frishman WH: Sirolimus-eluting coronary stents: Novel devices for the management of coronary artery disease. *Am J Ther* 11:218-228, 2004.
7. Dibra A, et al for the ISAR-DIABETES Study Investigators: Paclitaxel-eluting or sirolimus-eluting stents to prevent restenosis in diabetic patients. *N Engl J Med* 353:663-670, 2005.
8. Kastrati A, et al for the ISAR-DESIRE Study Investigators: Sirolimus-eluting stent or paclitaxel-eluting stent vs balloon angioplasty for prevention of recurrences in patients with coronary in-stent restenosis. A randomized controlled trial. *JAMA* 293:165-171, 2005.
9. Ge L, Iakovou I, Sangiorgi GM, et al: Treatment of saphenous vein graft lesions with drug-eluting stents. *J Am Coll Cardiol* 45:989-994, 2005.
10. Valgimigli M, van Mieghem CAG, Ong ATL, et al: Short- and long-term clinical outcome after drug-eluting stent implantation for the percutaneous treatment of left main coronary artery disease. Insights from the Rapamycin-Eluting and Taxus Stent Evaluated at Rotterdam Cardiology Hospital Registries (RESEARCH and T-SEARCH). *Circulation* 111:1383-1389, 2005.
11. Chieffo A, Stankovic G, Bonizzoni E, et al: Early and mid-term results of drug-eluting stent implantation in unprotected left main. *Circulation* 111:791-795, 2005.
12. Schlüter M, et al for the E- and C-SIRIUS Investigators: Direct stenting of native de novo coronary artery lesions with the sirolimus-eluting stent. A post hoc subanalysis of the pooled E- and C-SIRIUS Trials. *J Am Coll Cardiol* 45:10-13, 2005.
13. Fajadet J, Morice M-C, Bode C, et al: Maintenance of long-term clinical benefit with sirolimus-eluting coronary stents. Three-year results of the RAVEL trial. *Circulation* 111:1040-1044, 2005.
14. Stone GW, et al for the Enhanced Myocardial Efficacy and Recovery by Aspiration of Liberated Debris (EMERALD) Investigators: Distal microcirculatory protection during percutaneous coronary intervention in acute ST-segment elevation myocardial infarction. A randomized controlled trial. *JAMA* 293:1063-1072, 2005.
15. Mercado N, Wijns W, Serruys PW, et al: One-year outcomes of coronary artery bypass graft surgery versus percutaneous coronary intervention with multiple stenting for multi-system disease: A meta-analysis of individual patient data from randomized clinical trials. *J Thorac Cardiovasc Surg* 130:512-519, 2005.

Times to Treatment in Transfer Patients Undergoing Primary Percutaneous Coronary Intervention in the United States: National Registry of Myocardial Infarction (NRMI)-3/4 Analysis

Nallamothu BK, for the NRMI Investigators (Ann Arbor VA Med Ctr, Mich; et al)
Circulation 111:761-767, 2005 41–2

Background.—Treatment delays in patients with ST-segment–elevation myocardial infarction (STEMI) transferred for primary percutaneous coronary intervention (PCI) may decrease the advantage of this strategy over on-site fibrinolytic therapy that has been demonstrated in recent clinical trials. Accordingly, we sought to describe patterns of times to treatment in patients undergoing interhospital transfer for primary PCI in the United States.

Method and Results.—We analyzed patients with STEMI undergoing interhospital transfer for primary PCI between January 1999 and December 2002 in the National Registry of Myocardial Infarction. The primary outcome was "total" door-to-balloon time measured from time of arrival at the initial hospital to time of balloon inflation at the PCI hospital. Multivariable hierarchical models were used to assess the relationship of total door-to-balloon time with patient and hospital characteristics. Among 4278 patients transferred for primary PCI at 419 hospitals, the median total door-to-balloon time was 180 minutes, with only 4.2% of patients treated within 90 minutes, the benchmark recommended by national quality guidelines. Comorbid conditions, absence of chest pain, delayed presentation after symptom onset, less specific ECG findings, and hospital presentation during off-hours were associated with longer total door-to-balloon times. Patients at teaching hospitals in rural areas also had significantly longer times to treatment.

Conclusions.—Total door-to-balloon times for transfer patients undergoing primary PCI in the United States rarely achieve guideline-recommended benchmarks, and current decision making should take these times into account. For the full benefits of primary PCI to be realized in transfer patients, improved systems are urgently needed to minimize total door-to-balloon times.

► The successful use of a percutaneous coronary intervention to treat acute myocardial infarction is said to depend on a short time interval from the onset of symptoms to procedure. Within a window of 1 hour a coronary artery percutaneous intervention would obviate the need for fibrinolysis.[1] There are data to suggest that an invasive strategy based on coronary stenting might still be of benefit 12 to 48 hours after symptom onset.[2]

W. H. Frishman, MD

References

1. Machecourt J, Bonnefoy E, Vanzetto G, et al: Primary angioplasty is cost-minimizing compared with pre-hospital thrombolysis for patients within 60 min of a percutaneous coronary intervention center. *J Am Coll Cardiol* 45:515-524, 2005.
2. Schömig A, et al for the Beyond 12 hours Reperfusion Alternative Evaluation (BRAVE-2) Trial Investigators: Mechanism reperfusion in patients with acute myocardial infarction presenting more than 12 hours from symptom onset. A randomized controlled trial. *JAMA* 293:2865-2872, 2005.

Survival After Coronary Revascularization Among Patients With Kidney Disease

Hemmelgarn BR, for the Alberta Provincial Project for Outcomes Assessment in Coronary Heart Disease (APPROACH) Investigators (Univ of Calgary, Alta, Canada)

Circulation 110:1890-1895, 2004 41–3

Background.—The optimal approach to revascularization in patients with kidney disease has not been determined. We studied survival by treatment group (CABG, percutaneous coronary intervention [PCI], or no revascularization) for patients with 3 categories of kidney function: dialysis-dependent kidney disease, non–dialysis-dependent kidney disease, and a reference group (serum creatinine <2.3 mg/dL).

Method and Results.—Data were derived from the Alberta Provincial Project for Outcomes Assessment in Coronary Heart Disease (APPROACH), which captures information on all patients undergoing cardiac catheterization in Alberta, Canada. Characteristics and patient survival in 662 dialysis patients (1.6%) and 750 non–dialysis-dependent kidney disease patients (1.8%) were compared with the remainder of the 40,374 patients (96.6%). For the reference group, the adjusted 8-year survival rates for CABG, PCI, and no revascularization (NR) were 85.5%, 80.4%, and 72.3%, respectively ($P<0.001$ for CABG versus NR; $P<0.001$ for PCI versus NR). Adjusted survival rates were 45.9% for CABG, 32.7% for PCI, and 29.7% for NR in the nondialysis kidney disease group (P<0.001 for CABG versus NR; P=0.48 for PCI versus NR) and 44.8% for CABG, 41.2% for PCI, and 30.4% for NR in the dialysis group ($P=0.003$ for CABG versus NR; $P=0.03$ for PCI versus NR).

Conclusions.—Compared with no revascularization, CABG was associated with better survival in all categories of kidney function. PCI was also associated with a lower risk of death than no revascularization in reference patients and dialysis-dependent kidney disease patients but not in patients with non–dialysis-dependent kidney disease. The presence of kidney disease or dependence on dialysis should not be a deterrent to revascularization, particularly with CABG.

▶ There are multiple clinical factors that can adversely affect the outcome of coronary bypass surgery and percutaneous coronary interventions. These factors include diabetes mellitus,[1,2] anemia,[3] female sex,[4] and endothelin levels.[5] Troponin elevations after a percutaneous coronary intervention suggest myocardial damage that is proportional to the height of the elevation.[6]

W. H. Frishman, MD

References

1. Woods SE, Smith JM, Sohail S, et al: The influence of type 2 diabetes mellitus in patients undergoing coronary artery bypass graft surgery. An 8-year prospective cohort study. *Chest* 126:1789-1795, 2004.
2. Robertson BJ, Gascho JA, Gabbay RA, et al: Usefulness of hyperglycemia in predicting renal and myocardial injury in patients with diabetes mellitus undergoing percutaneous coronary intervention. *Am J Cardiol* 94:1027-1029, 2004.
3. Nikolsky E, Mehran R, Aymong ED, et al: Impact of anemia on outcomes of patients undergoing percutaneous coronary interventions. *Am J Cardiol* 94:1023-1027, 2004.
4. Lansky AJ, Pietras C, Costa RA, et al: Gender differences in outcomes after primary angioplasty versus primary stenting with and without abciximab for acute myocardial infarction. Results of the Controlled Abciximab and Device Investigation to Lower Late Angioplasty Complications (CADILLAC) Trial. *Circulation* 111:1611-1618, 2005.
5. Yip H-K, Wu C-J, Chang H-W, et al: Prognostic value of circulating levels of endothelin-1 in patients after acute myocardial infarction undergoing primary coronary angioplasty. *Chest* 127:1491-1497, 2005.
6. Selvanayagam JB, Porto I, Channon K, et al: Troponin elevation after percutaneous coronary intervention directly represents the extent of irreversible myocardial injury. Insights from cardiovascular magnetic resonance imaging. *Circulation* 111:1027-1032, 2005.

Coronary-Artery Revascularization Before Elective Major Vascular Surgery

McFalls EO, Ward HB, Moritz TE, et al (Univ of Minnesota, Minneapolis; VA Med Ctr, Hines, Ill; Univ of Arizona, Tucson; et al)
N Engl J Med 351:2795-2804, 2004 41–4

Background.—The benefit of coronary-artery revascularization before elective major vascular surgery is unclear.

Methods.—We randomly assigned patients at increased risk for perioperative cardiac complications and clinically significant coronary artery disease to undergo either revascularization or no revascularization before elective major vascular surgery. The primary end point was long-term mortality.

Results.—Of 5859 patients scheduled for vascular operations at 18 Veterans Affairs medical centers, 510 (9 percent) were eligible for the study and were randomly assigned to either coronary-artery revascularization before surgery or no revascularization before surgery. The indications for a vascular operation were an expanding abdominal aortic aneurysm (33 percent) or arterial occlusive disease of the legs (67 percent). Among the patients assigned to preoperative coronary-artery revascularization, percutaneous coronary intervention was performed in 59 percent, and bypass surgery was performed in 41 percent. The median time from randomization to vascular surgery was 54 days in the revascularization group and 18 days in the group not undergoing revascularization (P<0.001). At 2.7 years after randomization, mortality in the revascularization group was 22 percent and in the no-revascularization group 23 percent (relative risk, 0.98; 95 percent confidence interval, 0.70 to 1.37; P=0.92) (Fig 1). Within 30 days after the vascular operation, a postoperative myocardial infarction, defined by el-

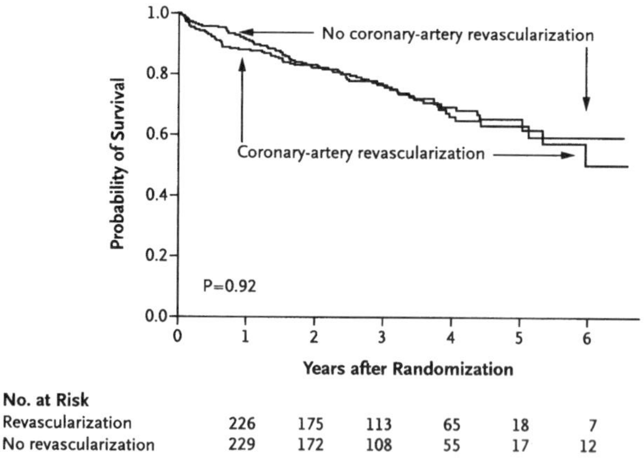

FIGURE 1.—Long-term survival among patients assigned to undergo coronary-artery revascularization or no coronary-artery revascularization before elective major vascular surgery. (Reprinted by permission of *The New England Journal of Medicine* from McFalls EO, Ward HB, Moritz TE, et al: Coronary-artery revascularization before elective major vascular surgery. *N Engl J Med* 351:2795-2804, 2004. Copyright 2004, Massachusetts Medical Society. All rights reserved.)

evated troponin levels, occurred in 12 percent of the revascularization group and 14 percent of the no-revascularization group (P=0.37).

Conclusions.—Coronary-artery revascularization before elective vascular surgery does not significantly alter the long-term outcome. On the basis of these data, a strategy of coronary-artery revascularization before elective vascular surgery among patients with stable cardiac symptoms cannot be recommended.

► Patients with suspected coronary artery disease are at an increased risk of cardiovascular morbidity and mortality when undergoing noncardiac surgery.[1] The prophylactic utilization of β-blocker therapy seems to reduce this risk and eliminates the need for an extensive preoperative coronary artery disease assessment with a subsequent coronary revascularization.[2-4]

W. H. Frishman, MD

References

1. Goldman L, Caldera DL, Nussbaum SR, et al: Multifactorial index of cardiac risk in noncardiac surgical procedures. *N Engl J Med* 297:845-850, 1977.
2. Mangano DT, Layug EL, Wallace A, et al: Effect of atenolol on mortality and cardiovascular morbidity after noncardiac surgery. *N Engl J Med* 335:1713-1720, 1996.
3. Poldermans D, Boersma E, Bax JJ, et al: The effect of bisoprolol on perioperative mortality and myocardial infarction in high-risk patients undergoing vascular surgery. *N Engl J Med* 341:1789-1794, 1993.
4. Devereaux PJ, Beattie WS, Choi PT-L, et al: How strong is the evidence for the use of perioperative β blockers in non-cardiac surgery? Systematic review and meta-analysis of randomized controlled trials. *BMJ* 331:313-316, 2005.

Randomized, Blinded Trial Comparing Fondaparinux With Unfractionated Heparin in Patients Undergoing Contemporary Percutaneous Coronary Intervention: Arixtra Study in Percutaneous Coronary Intervention: A Randomized Evaluation (ASPIRE) Pilot Trial

Mehta SR, for the ASPIRE Investigators (McMaster Univ, Hamilton, Ont, Canada; et al)

Circulation 111:1390-1397, 2005 41–5

Background.—Factor Xa plays a central role in the generation of thrombin, making it a novel target for treatment of arterial thrombosis. Fondaparinux is a synthetic factor Xa inhibitor that has been shown to be superior to standard therapies for the prevention of venous thrombosis. We performed a randomized trial to determine the safety and feasibility of fondaparinux in the percutaneous coronary intervention (PCI) setting.

Method and Results.—A total of 350 patients undergoing elective or urgent PCI were randomized in a blinded manner to receive unfractionated heparin (UFH), 2.5 mg fondaparinux IV, or 5.0 mg fondaparinux IV. Randomization was stratified for planned or no planned use of glycoprotein (GP) IIb/IIIa antagonists. The primary safety outcome was total bleeding, which was a combination of major and minor bleeding events. The incidence of total bleeding was 7.7% in the UFH group and 6.4% in the combined fondaparinux groups (hazard ratio, 0.81; 95% confidence interval, 0.35 to 1.84; P=0.61). Bleeding was less common in the 2.5-mg fondaparinux group compared with the 5-mg fondaparinux group (3.4% versus 9.6%, P=0.06). The composite efficacy outcome of all-cause mortality, myocardial infarction, urgent revascularization, or need for a bailout GPIIb/IIIa antagonist was 6.0% in the UFH group and 6.0% in the fondaparinux group, with no significant difference in efficacy among the fondaparinux doses compared with UFH. Coagulation marker analysis at 6 and 12 hours after PCI demonstrated that fondaparinux was superior to UFH in inducing a sustained reduction in markers of thrombin generation, as measured by prothrombin fragment F1.2 (P=0.02).

Conclusions.—In this pilot study of patients undergoing contemporary PCI, factor Xa inhibition with the synthetic anticoagulant fondaparinux in doses of 2.5 and 5.0 mg was comparable to UFH for clinical safety and efficacy outcomes. These data form the basis for further evaluation of fondaparinux in arterial thrombosis.

► Adjunctive antithrombotic drugs have been shown to favorably alter the clinical course of patients undergoing PCI.[1,2] These drugs include antiplatelet and antithrombin agents. Regarding antiplatelet drugs, it is still not known what the loading dose of clopidogrel should be because of interpatient variability in response.[3,4]

W. H. Frishman, MD

References

1. Gurm HS, Sarembock IJ, Kereiakes DJ, et al: Use of bivalirudin during percutaneous coronary intervention in patients with diabetes mellitus. *J Am Coll Cardiol* 45: 1932-38, 2005.
2. Frishman WH, Lerner RG, Klein MD, et al: Antiplatelet and antithrombotic drugs. In Frishman WH, Sonnenblick EH, Sica DA, editors: *Cardiovascular Pharmacotherapeutics*, ed 2, New York, 2003, McGraw Hill, pp 259-299.
3. Gurbel PA, Bliden KP, Hayes KM, et al: The relation of dosing to clopidogrel responsiveness and the incidence of high post-treatment platelet aggregation in patients undergoing coronary stenting. *J Am Coll Cardiol* 45:1392-1396, 2005.
4. Nguyen T, Frishman WH, Nawarskas J, et al: Variability of response to clopidogrel: Possible mechanisms and clinical implications. *Cardiol Rev* 14:136-142, 2006.

42 Cardiomyopathy

Impact of Care at a Multidisciplinary Congestive Heart Failure Clinic: A Randomized Trial

Ducharme A, Doyon O, White M, et al (McGill Univ, Montréal)

CMAJ 173:40-45, 2005 42–1

Background.—Although multidisciplinary congestive heart failure clinics in the United States appear to be effective in reducing the number of hospital readmissions, it is unclear whether the same benefit is seen in countries such as Canada, where access to both general and specialized medical care is free and unrestricted. We sought to determine the impact of care at a multidisciplinary specialized outpatient congestive heart failure clinic compared with standard care.

Methods.—We randomly assigned 230 eligible patients who had experienced an acute episode of congestive heart failure to standard care (n = 115) or follow-up at a multidisciplinary specialized heart failure outpatient clinic (n = 115). The intervention consisted of a structured outpatient clinic environment with complete access to cardiologists and allied health professionals. The primary outcomes were all-cause hospital admission rates and total number of days in hospital at 6 months. The secondary outcomes were total number of emergency department visits, quality of life and total mortality.

Results.—At 6 months, fewer patients in the intervention group had required readmission to hospital than patients in the control group (45 [39%] v. 66 [57%], crude hazard ratio [HR] 0.59, 95% confidence interval [CI] 0.38-0.92. Patients in the intervention group stayed in hospital for 514 days compared with 815 days required by patients in the control group (adjusted HR 0.56, 95% CI 0.35-0.89). The number of patients seen in the emergency department and the total number of emergency department visits were similar in the intervention and control groups. At 6 months, quality of life, which was self-assessed using the Minnesota Living with Heart Failure questionnaire, was unchanged in the control group but improved in the intervention group ($p < 0.001$). No difference in mortality was observed, with 19 deaths in the control group and 12 in the intervention group (HR 0.61, 95% CI 0.24-1.54).

Interpretation.—Compared with usual care, care at a multidisciplinary specialized congestive heart failure outpatient clinic reduced the number of hospital readmissions and hospital days and improved quality of life. When our results are integrated with those from other, similar trials, multidisciplinary disease management strategies for congestive heart failure are associated with clinically worthwhile improvements in survival.

► There is growing evidence that a specialized multidisciplinary approach to heart failure can reduce morbidity and mortality rates in high-risk patients, and at the same time be cost effective.[1-3] In contrast, in patients with heart failure who are at low risk, a multidisciplinary case management program provides little or no additional benefit on clinical outcomes.[4]

W. H. Frishman, MD

References

1. Tsuyuki RT for the REACT Investigators: A multicenter disease management program for hospitalized patients with heart failure. *J Card Fail* 10:473-480, 2004.
2. Gregory D, DeNofrio D, Konstam MA: The economic effect of a tertiary hospital-based heart failure program. *J Am Coll Cardiol* 46: 660-666, 2005.
3. Lee DS, Tu JV, Juurlink DN, et al: Risk-treatment mismatch in the pharmacotherapy of heart failure. *JAMA* 294:1240-1247, 2005.
4. DeBusk RF, Houston Miller N, Parker KM, et al: Care management for low-risk patients with heart failure. A randomized, controlled trial. *Ann Intern Med* 141: 606-613, 2004.

Left Ventricular Assist Device Malfunction: An Approach to Diagnosis by Echocardiography

Horton SC, Khodaverdian R, Chatelain P, et al (Univ of Utah, Salt Lake City)
J Am Coll Cardiol 45:1435-1440, 2005 42–2

Objectives.—A protocol using transthoracic echocardiography was designed to diagnose the common malfunctions of patients on chronic support with a left ventricular assist device (LVAD).

Background.—Mechanical circulatory support, primarily with a LVAD, is increasingly used for treatment of advanced heart failure as a bridge to transplant and for long-term treatment of heart failure. The LVAD dysfunction is a recognized complication. To date, no studies have defined the role of transthoracic echocardiography in evaluating long-term mechanical complications of chronic LVAD support.

Methods.—Transthoracic echocardiography was used in a protocol designed to detect the common types of mechanical malfunction. Patients were followed up with serial echocardiograms, and clinical validations were made with findings from a catheter-based protocol and inspection at the time of cardiac transplant or corrective surgery.

Results.—Thirty-two patients with 44 LVADs were followed up during a four-year period using this protocol that correctly identified 11 patients with inflow valve regurgitation, 2 with intermittent inflow conduit obstruction, 1 with severe kinking of the outflow graft, and 9 with new insufficiency of the native aortic valve.

Conclusions.—As LVAD use for end-stage heart failure becomes widespread, and durations of support are extended, dysfunction will be increasingly prevalent. Transthoracic echocardiography provides a practical method to accurately identify the causes of mechanical dysfunction with patients on chronic LVAD support.

► Circulatory support with an LVAD is being used frequently to treat advanced heart failure. Both hemodynamic and histopathology improvement is seen with these devices. With long-term use, aortic stenosis will develop on a native valve, and total occlusive thrombus on an aortic prosthetic valve.[1] An increased risk of unifocal ventricular tachycardia is seen with no adverse effect on the incidence of ventricular fibrillation.[2] A noninvasive approach to treat heart failure with enhanced external counterpulsation is now under investigation.[3]

W. H. Frishman, MD

References

1. Rose AG, Park SJ: Pathology in patients with ventricular assist devices. A study of 21 autopsies, 24 ventricular apical core biopsies, and 24 explanted hearts. *Cardiovasc Pathol* 14:19-23, 2005.
2. Ziv O, Dizon J, Thosani A, et al: Effects of left ventricular assist device therapy on ventricular arrhythmias. *J Am Coll Cardiol* 45: 1428-1434, 2005.
3. Feldman AM, Silver MA, Francis GS, et al: Treating heart failure with enhanced external counterpulsation (EECP): Design of the Prospective Evaluation of EECP in Heart Failure (PEECH) trial. *J Card Fail* 11:240-245, 2005.

Gender-related Differences in the Clinical Presentation and Outcome of Hypertrophic Cardiomyopathy

Olivotto I, Maron MS, Adabag AS, et al (Universitaria Careggi, Florence, Italy: Minneapolis Heart Inst; Tufts-New England Med Ctr, Boston)

J Am Coll Cardiol 46:480-487, 2005 42–3

Objectives.—The goal of this study was to assess gender-related differences in a multicenter population with hypertrophic cardiomyopathy (HCM).

Background.—Little is known regarding the impact of gender on the heterogeneous clinical profile and clinical course of HCM.

Methods.—We studied 969 consecutive HCM patients from Italy and the U.S. followed over 6.2 ± 6.1 years.

Results.—Male patients had a 3:2 predominance (59%), similar in Italy and the U.S. ($p = 0.24$). At initial evaluation, female patients were older and more symptomatic than male patients (47 ± 23 years vs. 38 ± 18 years; $p < 0.001$; mean New York Heart Association [NYHA] functional class 1.8 ± 0.8 vs. 1.4 ± 0.6; $p < 0.001$), and more frequently showed left ventricular outflow obstruction (37% vs. 23%; $p < 0.001$). Moreover, female patients were less often diagnosed fortuitously by routine medical examination (23% vs. 41% in male patients, $p < 0.001$). Female gender was independently associated with the risk of symptom progression to NYHA functional classes III/IV or death from heart failure or stroke compared with male gender (independent relative hazard 1.5; $p < 0.001$), particularly patients ≥50 years of age and with resting outflow obstruction ($p < 0.005$). Hypertrophic cardiomyopathy-related mortality and risk of sudden death were similar in men and women.

Conclusions.—Women with HCM were under-represented, older, and more symptomatic than men, and showed higher risk of progression to advanced heart failure or death, often associated with outflow obstruction. These gender-specific differences suggest that social, endocrine, or genetic factors may affect the diagnosis and clinical course of HCM. A heightened suspicion for HCM in women may allow for timely implementation of treatment strategies, including relief of obstruction and prevention of sudden death or stroke.

► Obstructive HCM is associated with considerable cardiac morbidity and mortality rates. Surgical myectomy performed to relieve obstruction and symptoms can provide a long-term survival rate equivalent to that of the general population.[1] Specific preoperative clinical and echocardiographic variables are associated with a worse surgical outcome, and include female sex, atrial fibrillation, and a large left atrium by echo.[2]

Myocardial disarray is a structural abnormality seen in HCM and may be associated with adrenergic stress.[3] An unusual course of HCM is glycogen storage disease, which is associated with preexcitation.[4]

W. H. Frishman, MD

References

1. Ommen SR, Maron BJ, Olivotto I, et al: Long-term effects of surgical septal myectomy on survival in patients with obstructive hypertrophic cardiomyopathy. *J Am Coll Cardiol* 46:470-476, 2005.
2. Woo A, Williams WG, Choi R, et al: Clinical and echocardiographic determinants of long-term survival after surgical myectomy in obstructive hypertrophic cardiomyopathy. *Circulation* 111:2033-2041, 2005.
3. Fineschi V, Silver MD, Karch SB, et al: Myocardial disarray: An architectural disorganization linked with adrenergic stress? *Int J Cardiol* 99:277-282, 2005.
4. Arad M, Maron BJ, Gorham JM, et al: Glycogen storage diseases presenting as hypertrophic cardiomyopathy. *N Engl J Med* 352:362-372, 2005.

Insulin Resistance and Risk of Congestive Heart Failure

Ingelsson E, Sundström J, Ärnlöv J, et al (Uppsala Univ, Sweden; Astra Zeneca R&D, Mölndal, Sweden)

JAMA 294:334-341, 2005 42–4

Context.—Diabetes and obesity are established risk factors for congestive heart failure (CHF) and are both associated with insulin resistance.

Objective.—To explore if insulin resistance may predict CHF and may provide the link between obesity and CHF.

Design, Setting, and Participants.—The Uppsala Longitudinal Study of Adult Men, a prospective, community-based, observational cohort in Uppsala, Sweden. We investigated 1187 elderly (≥70 years) men free from CHF and valvular disease at baseline between 1990 and 1995, with follow-up until the end of 2002. Variables reflecting insulin sensitivity (including euglycemic insulin clamp glucose disposal rate) and obesity were analyzed together with established risk factors (prior myocardial infarction, hypertension, diabetes, electrocardiographic left ventricular hypertrophy, smoking, and serum cholesterol level) as predictors of subsequent incidence of CHF, using Cox proportional hazards analyses.

Main Outcome Measure.—First hospitalization for heart failure.

Results.—One hundred four men developed CHF during a median follow-up of 8.9 (range, 0.01-11.4) years. In multivariable Cox proportional hazards models adjusted for established risk factors for CHF, increased risk of CHF was associated with a 1-SD increase in the 2-hour glucose value of an oral glucose tolerance test (hazard ratio [HR], 1.44; 95% confidence interval [CI], 1.08-1.93), fasting serum proinsulin level (HR, 1.29; 95% CI, 1.02-1.64), body mass index (HR, 1.35; 95% CI, 1.11-1.65), and waist circumference (HR, 1.36; 95% CI, 1.10-1.69), whereas a 1-SD increase in clamp glucose disposal rate decreased the risk (HR, 0.66; 95% CI, 0.51-0.86). When adding clamp glucose disposal rate to these models as a covariate, the obesity variables were no longer significant predictors of subsequent CHF.

Conclusions.—Insulin resistance predicted CHF incidence independently of established risk factors including diabetes in our large community-based sample of elderly men. The previously described association between obesity and subsequent CHF may be mediated largely by insulin resistance.

▶ Multiple factors and biomarkers have been identified that predict an increased risk for the development of heart failure. Lower levels of kidney function are an independent risk factor for heart failure.[1] The serum cystatin C concentration may provide a better measure of risk assessment than serum creatinine level.[2] An elevation in the erythrocyte sedimentation rate, an elevated endothelin level, a low serum sodium, and retinopathy have also been shown to be independent predictors of heart failure.[3-6] Of interest, the level of plasma natriuretic peptide, serum C-reactive protein, and the presence of mucosal congestion on gastrointestinal endoscopy are also predictive of a worse outcome.[7-9]

Regarding mortality from acute heart failure, the most predictive factors are a blood urea nitrogen level of more than 43 mg/dL, a serum creatinine more than 2.75 mmol/L, and a systolic blood pressure more than 115 mm Hg.[10] Sex is not a factor.[11]

Phonocardiographic third and fourth heart sounds are not sensitive markers of left ventricular dysfunction.[12]

W. H. Frishman, MD

References

1. Smith GL, Shlipak MG, Havranek EP, et al: Race and renal impairment in heart failure. Mortality in blacks versus whites. *Circulation* 111:1270-1277, 2005.

2. Sarnak MJ, Katz R, Stehman-Breen CO, et al: Cystatin C concentration as a risk factor for heart failure in older adults. *Ann Intern Med* 142:497-505, 2005.
3. Klein L for the OPTIME-CHF Investigators: Lower serum sodium is associated with increased short-term mortality in hospitalized patients with worsening heart failure. Results from the Outcomes of a Prospective Trial of Intravenous Milrinone for Exacerbations of Chronic Heart Failure (OPTIME-CHF) Study. *Circulation* 111:2454-2460, 2005.
4. Ingelsson E, Ärnlöv J, Sundström J, et al: Inflammation, as measured by the erythrocyte sedimentation rate, is an independent predictor for the development of heart failure. *J Am Coll Cardiol* 45:1802-1806, 2005.
5. Van Beneden R, Gurné O, Selvais PL, et al: Superiority of big endothelin-1 and endothelin-1 over natriuretic peptides in predicting survival in severe congestive heart failure: A 7-year follow-up study. *J Card Fail* 10:490-495, 2004.
6. Wong TY, Rosamond W, Chang PP, et al: Retinopathy and risk of congestive heart failure. *JAMA* 293:63-69, 2005.
7. Watanabe J, Shiba N, Shinozaki T, et al: Prognostic value of plasma brain natriuretic peptide combined with left ventricular dimensions in predicting sudden death of patients with chronic heart failure. *J Card Fail* 11:50-55, 2005.
8. Chirinos JA, Zambrano JP, Chakko S, et al: Usefulness of C-reactive protein as an independent predictor of death in patients with ischemic cardiomyopathy. *Am J Cardiol* 95:88-90, 2005.
9. Raja K, Kochhar R, Sethy PK, et al: An endoscopic study of upper-GI mucosal changes in patients with congestive heart failure. *Gastrointest Endosc* 60:887-893, 2004.
10. Fonarow GC, for the ADHERE Scientific Advisory Committee, Study Group, and Investigators: Risk stratification for in-hospital mortality in acutely decompensated heart failure. Classification and regression tree analysis. *JAMA* 293:572-580, 2005.
11. Lee WY, for the Epidemiology, Practice Outcomes, and Cost of Heart Failure (EPOCH) Study: Gender and risk of adverse outcomes in heart failure. *Am J Cardiol* 94:1147-1152, 2004.
12. Marcus GM, Gerber IL, McKeown BH, et al: Association between phonocardiographic third and fourth heart sounds and objective measures of left ventricular function. *JAMA* 293:2238-2244, 2005.

The Effect of Cardiac Resynchronization on Morbidity and Mortality in Heart Failure

Cleland JGF, for the Cardiac Resynchronization—Heart Failure (CARE-HF) Study Investigators (Castle Hill Hosp, Kingston-upon-Hull, England; et al)
N Engl J Med 352:1539-1549, 2005 42–5

Background.—Cardiac resynchronization reduces symptoms and improves left ventricular function in many patients with heart failure due to left ventricular systolic dysfunction and cardiac dyssynchrony. We evaluated its effects on morbidity and mortality.

Methods.—Patients with New York Heart Association class III or IV heart failure due to left ventricular systolic dysfunction and cardiac dyssynchrony who were receiving standard pharmacologic therapy were randomly assigned to receive medical therapy alone or with cardiac resynchronization. The primary end point was the time to death from any cause or an unplanned hospitalization for a major cardiovascular event. The principal secondary end point was death from any cause.

Results.—A total of 813 patients were enrolled and followed for a mean of 29.4 months. The primary end point was reached by 159 patients in the cardiac-resynchronization group, as compared with 224 patients in the medical-therapy group (39 percent vs. 55 percent; hazard ratio, 0.63; 95 percent confidence interval, 0.51 to 0.77; P<0.001). There were 82 deaths in the cardiac-resynchronization group, as compared with 120 in the medical-therapy group (20 percent vs. 30 percent; hazard ratio 0.64; 95 percent confidence interval, 0.48 to 0.85; P<0.002). As compared with medical therapy, cardiac resynchronization reduced the interventricular mechanical delay, the end-systolic volume index, and the area of the mitral regurgitant jet; increased the left ventricular ejection fraction; and improved symptoms and the quality of life (P<0.01 for all comparisons).

Conclusions.—In patients with heart failure and cardiac dyssynchrony, cardiac resynchronization improves symptoms and the quality of life and reduces complications and the risk of death. These benefits are in addition to those afforded by standard pharmacologic therapy. The implantation of a cardiac-resynchronization device should routinely be considered in such patients.

► Various adjunctive modalities have improved the clinical outcomes of patients with heart failure and include cardiac resynchronization therapy and the use of implantable cardioverter defibrillators.[1,2] The use of cardiac resynchronization therapy can also allow for higher β-blocker doses to be used.[3] Compared to amiodarone, the use of implantable defibrillators will reduce mortality rates in class II or III patients with heart failure.[1]

W. H. Frishman, MD

References

1. Bardy GH, for the Sudden Cardiac Death in Heart Failure Trial (SCD-HeFT) Investigators: Amiodarone or an implantable cardioverter-defibrillator for congestive heart failure. *N Engl J Med* 352:225-237, 2005.
2. De Cock CC, Van Campen LMC, Jessurun ER, et al: Long-term follow-up of patients with refractory heart failure and myocardial ischemia treated with cardiac resynchronization therapy. *Pacing Clin Electrophysiol* 28:8S-10S, 2005.
3. Aranda JM Jr, Woo GW, Conti JB, et al: Use of cardiac resynchronization therapy to optimize beta blocker therapy in patients with heart failure and prolonged QRS duration. *Am J Cardiol* 95:889-891, 2005.

Relationship of Serum Digoxin Concentration to Mortality and Morbidity in Women in the Digitalis Investigation Group Trial: A Retrospective Analysis

Adams KF Jr, Patterson JH, Gattis WA, et al (Univ of North Carolina at Chapel Hill; Duke Univ, Durham, NC; Northwestern Univ, Chicago)

J Am Coll Cardiol 46:497-504, 2005 42–6

Objectives.—The purpose of this study was to investigate the relationship of serum digoxin concentration (SDC) and outcomes in women with heart failure (HF).

Background.—Controversy continues concerning the clinical utility of digoxin in women with HF.

Methods.—Our analysis was retrospective with data from the Digitalis Investigation Group (DIG) trial. The principal study analysis reviewed 4,944 patients with HF due to systolic dysfunction who survived for at least 4 weeks (all 3,366 patients randomized to placebo and the 1,578 of 3,372 patients randomized to digoxin who had serum concentration measured 6 to 30 h [inclusive] after the last dose of study drug at 4 weeks).

Results.—Continuous multivariable analysis demonstrated a significant linear relationship between SDC and mortality in women ($p = 0.008$) and men ($p = 0.002$, $p = 0.766$ for gender interaction). Averaging hazard ratios

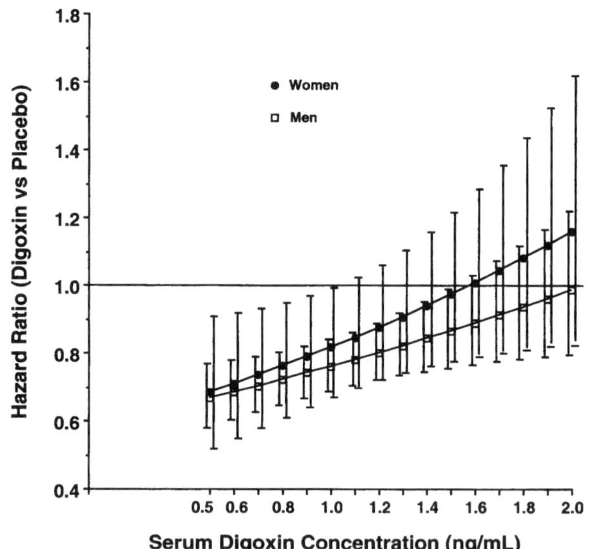

FIGURE 4.—Plot of the adjusted point estimates and 95% confidence intervals of women and men for the hazard ratio for the combined study end point (of all-cause mortality or first hospitalization due to worsening heart failure) on digoxin versus placebo at various serum digoxin concentrations (ng/ml) with concentration modeled as a continuous variable. The 95% confidence intervals for the women are offset to allow better depiction of results. (Courtesy of Adams KF Jr, Patterson JH, Gattis WA, et al: Relationship of serum digoxin concentration to mortality and morbidity in women in the digitalis investigation group trial: A retrospective analysis. *J Am Coll Cardiol* 46:497-504, 2005. Reprinted with permission from the American College of Cardiology.)

(HRs) across serum concentrations from 0.5 to 0.9 ng/ml in women produced a HR for death of 0.8 (95% confidence interval [CI] 0.62 to 1.13, p = 0.245) and for death or hospital stay for worsening HF of 0.73 (95% CI 0.58 to 0.93, p = 0.011). In contrast, SDCs from 1.2 to 2.0 ng/ml were associated with a HR for death for women of 1.33 (95% CI 1.001 to 1.76, p = 0.049).

Conclusions.—Retrospective analysis of data from the DIG trial indicates a beneficial effect of digoxin on morbidity and no excess mortality in women at serum concentrations from 0.5 to 0.9 ng/ml, whereas serum concentrations ≥1.2 ng/ml seem harmful (Fig 4).

► The current drug treatment paradigm for patients with chronic congestive HF includes diuretics, β-adrenergic blockers, digoxin, and inhibitors of the renin-angiotensin-aldosterone system. Adjunctive treatment with aspirin is also of benefit,[1] but it is not being used as much as it should, especially in older patients. Spironolactone is probably not being used to its maximal extent in elderly patients because of a concern about hyperkalemia and the need for more frequent electrolyte monitoring.[2,3]

Innovative drug treatments under investigation in HF include the use of gherlin,[4] a growth hormone-releasing peptide, use of rho-kinase inhibitors,[5] and both selective and nonselective vasopressin antagonists.[6]

Of great interest is the use of stem cells to regenerate the heart and blood vessels.[7-13] In patients with HF, various stem cell strategies have been suggested, including the use of bone marrow cells, skeletal myoblasts, cardiac stem cells, and embryonal stem cells, which can be delivered by direct intramyocardial ejection or infusion. Preliminary studies in humans suggest a clinical benefit on ventricular function, but larger blinded trials are needed. In addition to stem cell therapy, various gene therapy strategies are under investigation.[14]

W. H. Frishman, MD

References

1. Masoudi FA, Wolfe P, Havranek EP, et al: Aspirin use in older patients with heart failure and coronary artery disease. *J Am Coll Cardiol* 46:955-962, 2005.
2. Svensson M, Gustafsson F, Galatius S, et al: How prevalent is hyperkalemia and renal dysfunction during treatment with spironolactone in patients with congestive heart failure? *J Card Fail* 10:297-303, 2004.
3. Masoudi FA, Gross CP, Wang Y, et al: Adoption of spironolactone therapy for older patients with heart failure and left ventricular systolic dysfunction in the United States, 1998-2001. *Circulation* 112:39-47, 2005.
4. Nagaya N, Moriya J, Yasumura Y, et al: Effects of gherlin administration on left ventricular function, exercise capacity, and muscle wasting in patients with chronic heart failure. *Circulation* 110: 3674-3679, 2004.
5. Kishi T, Hirooka Y, Masumoto A, et al: Rho-kinase inhibitor improves increased vascular resistance and impaired vasodilation of the forearm in patients with heart failure. *Circulation* 111:2741-2747, 2005.
6. Frishman WH, Klapholz M, Acharya N, et al: Vasopression and vasopressin-receptor antagonists in the treatment of cardiovascular disease, in Frishman WH, Sonnenblick EH, Sica DA (eds): *Cardiovascular Pharmacotherapeutics*, ed 2. New York, McGraw Hill, 2003, pp 601-616.

7. Min J-Y, Chen Y, Malek S, et al: Stem cell therapy in the aging hearts of Fisher 344 rats: Synergistic effects on myogenesis and angiogenesis. *J Thorac Cardiovasc Surg* 130:547-553, 2005.
8. Fiaccavento R, Carotenuto F, Minieri M, et al: Stem cell activation sustains hereditary hypertrophy in hamster cardiomyopathy. *J Pathol* 205:397-407, 2005.
9. Strauer BE, Brehm M, Zeus T, et al: Regeneration of human infracted heart muscle by intracoronary autologus bone marrow cell transplantation in chronic coronary artery disease. *J Am Coll Cardiol* 46:1651-1658, 2005.
10. Bolli R, Jneid H, Dawn B: Bone marrow cell-mediated cardiac regeneration. A veritable revolution (editorial comment). *J Am Coll Cardiol* 46:1659-1661, 2005.
11. Kajstura J, Rota M, Whang B, et al: Bone marrow cells differentiate in cardiac cell lineages after infarction independently on cell fusion. *Circ Res* 96:127-137, 2005.
12. Anversa P, Sussman MA, Bolli R: Molecular genetic advances in cardiovascular medicine. Focus on the myocyte. *Circulation* 109: 2832-2838, 2004.
13. Beltrami AP, Torella D, Limana F, et al: Adult cardiac stem cells are multipotent and support myocardial regeneration. *Cell* 114:763-776, 2003.
14. Okada H, Takemura G, Kosai K-I, et al: Postinfarction gene therapy against transforming growth factor signal modulates infarct tissue dynamics and attenuates left ventricular remodeling and heart failure. *Circulation* 111:2430-2437, 2005.

Left Ventricular Systolic Performance, Function, and Contractility in Patients With Diastolic Heart Failure

Baicu CF, Zile MR, Aurigemma GP, et al (Med Univ of South Carolina, Charleston; Univ of Massachusetts, Worcester; Lahey Clinic, Burlington, Mass)
Circulation 111:2306-2312, 2005 42–7

Background.—Patients with diastolic heart failure (DHF) have significant abnormalities in left ventricular (LV) diastolic function, including slow and delayed relaxation and increased chamber stiffness. Whether and to what extent these abnormalities in diastolic function occur in association with abnormalities in LV systolic performance, function, and contractility has not been investigated thoroughly.

Methods and Results.—The systolic properties of the LV were examined in 75 patients with heart failure and a normal ejection fraction (ie, DHF) and 75 normal control subjects with no evidence of cardiovascular disease. LV systolic properties were assessed with echocardiographic and cardiac catheterization data. Stroke work (an index of LV systolic performance), preload recruitable stroke work and ejection fraction (indices of LV systolic function), systolic stress-shortening relationship, end-systolic pressure-volume relationship, and peak (+)dP/dt (indices of LV contractility) were examined. The systolic properties of the LV were normal in patients with DHF. Stroke work was 8.4±2.3 in DHF versus 8.8±2.5 kg·cm in controls ($P=0.26$). Preload recruitable stroke work was 99±22 in DHF versus 109±18 g/cm^2 in controls ($P=0.13$). The relationship between stroke work and end-diastolic volume was similar in DHF and controls. Peak (+) dP/dt was 1596±362 in DHF versus 1664±305 mm Hg/s in controls ($P=0.54$). The end-systolic pressure-volume relationship was increased in DHF. The systolic stress versus endocardial fractional shortening relationship was similar in DHF and controls.

Conclusions.—Patients with DHF had normal LV systolic performance, function, and contractility. The pathophysiology of DHF does not appear to be related to significant abnormalities in these systolic properties of the LV.

► LV diastolic dysfunction is a common cause of clinical heart failure and carries with it an unfavorable prognosis. Diastolic dysfunction can also contribute to left atrial remodeling and increased atrial size.[1] Unlike systolic heart failure where there is a plethora of pharmacologic agents and devices for treatment, diastolic dysfunction has limited treatment options. There is a suggestion that inhibitors of the renin-angiotensin system and calcium blockers may be of benefit in patients with diastolic dysfunction.[2]

W. H. Frishman, MD

References

1. Pritchett AM, Mahoney DW, Jacobsen SJ, et al: Diastolic dysfunction and left atrial volume. A population-based study. *J Am Coll Cardiol* 45: 87-92, 2005.
2. Yusuf S, Pfeffer MA, Swedberg K, et al: Effects of candesartan in patients with chronic heart failure and preserved left ventricular ejection fraction: the CHARM Preserved trial. *Lancet* 362:777-781, 2003.

43 Valvular Heart Disease

Blood Culture-Negative Endocarditis in a Reference Center: Etiologic Diagnosis of 348 Cases

Houpikian P, Raoult D (Université de la Méditerranée, Marseille Cedex, France)

Medicine 84:162-173, 2005 43–1

Introduction.—To identify the current etiologies of blood culture-negative infective endocarditis and to describe the epidemiologic, clinical, laboratory, and echocardiographic characteristics associated with each etiology, as well as with unexplained cases, we tested samples from 348 patients suspected of having blood culture-negative infective endocarditis in our diagnostic center, the French National Reference Center for Rickettsial Diseases, between 1983 and 2001. Serology tests for *Coxiella burnettii, Bartonella* species, *Chlamydia* species, *Legionella* species, and *Aspergillus* species; blood culture on shell vial; and, when available, analysis of valve specimens through culture, microscopic examination, and direct PCR amplification were performed. Physicians were asked to complete a questionnaire, which was computerized. Only cases of definite infective endocarditis, as defined by the modified Duke criteria, were included. A total of 348 cases were recorded—to our knowledge, the largest series reported to date. Of those, 167 cases (48%) were associated with *C. burnetii*, 99 (28%) with *Bartonella* species, and 5 (1%) with rare, fastidious bacterial agents of endocarditis (*Tropheryma whipplei, Abiotrophia elegans, Mycoplasma hominis, Legionella pneumophila*). Among 73 cases without etiology, 58 received antibiotic drugs before the blood cultures. Six cases were right-sided endocarditis and 4 occurred in patients who had a permanent pacemaker. Finally, no explanatory factor was found for 5 remaining cases (1%), despite all investigations.

Q fever endocarditis affected males in 75% of cases, between 40 and 70 years of age. Ninety-one percent of patients had a previous valvulopathy, 32% were immunocompromised, and 70% had been exposed to animals. Our study confirms the improved clinical presentation and prognosis of the disease observed during the last decades. Such an evolution could be related to earlier diagnosis due to better physician awareness and more sensitive diagnostic techniques. As for *Bartonella* species, *B. quintana* was recorded more frequently than *B. henselae* (53 vs 17 cases). For 18 patients with *Bartonella* endocarditis, the responsible species was not identified. Species determination was achieved through culture and/or PCR in 49 cases and through Western immunoblotting in 22. Comparison of *B. quintana* and *B. henselae* endocarditis revealed distinct epidemiologic patterns. The 2 cases due to *T. whipplei* reflect the emerging role of this agent as a cause of infective endocarditis. Because identification of the bacterium was possible only through analysis of excised valves by histologic examination, PCR, and culture on shell vial, the prevalence of the disease might be underestimated. Among patients who received antibiotic drugs before blood cultures, 4 cases (7%) were found to be associated with *Streptococcus* species (2 *S. bovis* and 2 *S. mutans*) through 16S rDNA gene amplification directly from the valve, which shows the usefulness of this technique in overcoming the limitations of previous antibiotic treatment. Right-sided endocarditis occurred classically in young patients (mean age, 36 yr), intravenous drug users in 50% of cases, and suffering more often from embolic complications. Finally, 5 cases without etiology or explaining factors were all immunocompetent male patients with previous aortic valvular lesions, and 3 of the 5 presented with an aortic abscess. Further investigations should be focused on this group to identify new agents of infective endocarditis.

► Blood culture-negative endocarditis makes up 5% of all endocarditis cases. Causes for culture-negative endocarditis include the presence of fastidious slow-growing bacteria (eg, *Coxiella burnetii* and *Bartonella* species), fungi, antibiotic administration before obtaining blood cultures, right-sided endocarditis, and endocarditis in a patient with a permanent pacemaker.[1-3] Culture-independent molecular methods can improve the diagnostic outcome of the microbiological examination of excised heart valves, including the detection of fastidious slow-growing organisms.[4]

W. H. Frishman, MD

References

1. Hoen B, Selton-Suty C, Lacassin F, et al: Infective endocarditis in patients with negative blood culture: Analysis of 88 cases from a one-year nationwide survey in France. *Clin Infect Dis* 21:501-506, 1995.
2. Hogevik H, Olaison L, Andersson R, et al: Epidemiologic aspects of infective endocarditis in an urban population. A 5-year prospective study. *Medicine (Baltimore)* 74:324-339, 1995.
3. Gandelman G, Frishman WH, Wiese C, et al: Intravascular device infections: Epidemiology, diagnosis, and management. *Cardiol Rev* 2006 (in press).
4. Breitkopf C, Hammel D, Scheld HH, et al: Impact of molecular approach to improve the microbiological diagnosis of infective heart valve endocarditis. *Circulation* 111:1415-1421, 2005.

Staphylococcus aureus Endocarditis: A Consequence of Medical Progress

Fowler VG Jr, for the ICE Investigators (Duke Univ, Durham, NC; et al)
JAMA 293:3012-3021, 2005 43–2

Context.—The global significance of infective endocarditis (IE) caused by *Staphylococcus aureus* is unknown.

Objectives.—To document the international emergence of health care-associated *S aureus* IE and methicillin-resistant *S aureus* (MRSA) IE and to evaluate regional variation in patients with S aureus IE.

Design, Setting, and Participants.—Prospective observational cohort study set in 39 medical centers in 16 countries. Participants were a population of 1779 patients with definite IE as defined by Duke criteria who were enrolled in the International Collaboration on Endocarditis-Prospective Cohort Study from June 2000 to December 2003.

Main Outcome Measure.—In-hospital mortality.

Results.—*S aureus* was the most common pathogen among the 1779 cases of definite IE in the International Collaboration on Endocarditis Prospective-Cohort Study (558 patients, 31.4%). Health care-associated infection was the most common form of *S aureus* IE (218 patients, 39.1%), accounting for 25.9% (Australia/New Zealand) to 54.2% (Brazil) of cases. Most patients with health care-associated *S aureus* IE (131 patients, 60.1%) acquired the infection outside of the hospital. MRSA IE was more common in the United States (37.2%) and Brazil (37.5%) than in Europe/Middle East (23.7%) and Australia/New Zealand (15.5%, $P<.001$). Persistent bacteremia was independently associated with MRSA IE (odds ratio, 6.2; 95% confidence interval, 2.9-13.2). Patients in the United States were most likely to be hemodialysis dependent, to have diabetes, to have a presumed intravascular device source, to receive vancomycin, to be infected with MRSA, and to have persistent bacteremia ($P<.001$ for all comparisons).

Conclusions.—*S aureus* is the leading cause of IE in many regions of the world. Characteristics of patients with *S aureus* IE vary significantly by region. Further studies are required to determine the causes of regional variation.

► *S aureus*, including methicillin resistant *S aureus*, is becoming an important cause of endocarditis worldwide. Surgical treatment appears to provide better clinical outcomes than medical approaches.[1] Some studies have shown that a mitral valve repair rather than a valve replacement may be a suitable surgical approach.[2]

In the United States, *S viridans* is more common than *S aureus* as a cause of endocarditis.[3] During the past 30 years, the incidence of endocarditis has not changed.[4]

W. H. Frishman, MD

References

1. Remadi JP, Najdi G, Brahim A, et al: Superiority of surgical versus medical treatment in patients with *Staphylococcus aureus* infective endocarditis. *Int J Cardiol* 99:195-199, 2005.
2. Zegdi R, Debipeche M, Latrémouille C, et al: Long-term results of mitral valve repair in active endocarditis. *Circulation* 111:2532-2536, 2005.
3. Gandelman G, Frishman WH, Wiese C, et al: Intravascular device infections: Epidemiology, diagnosis, and management. *Cardiol Rev* 2006 (in press).
4. Tleyjeh IM, Steckelberg JM, Murad HS, et al: Temporal trends in infective endocarditis. A population-based study in Olmsted County, Minnesota. *JAMA* 293:3022-3028, 2005.

Effectiveness of β-Blockade in Experimental Chronic Aortic Regurgitation

Plante E, Lachance D, Gaudreau M, et al (Université Laval, Quebec)
Circulation 110:1477-1483, 2004 43–3

Background.—Past studies have suggested that the adrenergic system becomes abnormally activated in chronic volume overload, such as in severe aortic valve regurgitation (AR). However, the effectiveness of agents directed against this adrenergic activation has never been adequately tested in chronic AR. We therefore tested the effects of metoprolol treatment on the left ventricular (LV) function and remodeling in severe chronic AR in rats.

Methods and Results.—Severe AR was created in adult male Wistar rats by retrograde puncture of the aortic leaflets under echocardiographic guidance. Two weeks later, some animals received metoprolol treatment (25 mg/kg) orally for 24 weeks, and some were left untreated. LV dimensions, ejection fraction, and filling parameters were evaluated by echocardiography. Hearts were harvested at 1, 2, 14, and 180 days for the evaluation of hypertrophy, β-adrenergic receptor status, and extracellular matrix remodeling. We found that metoprolol treatment prevented LV dilatation and preserved the ejection fraction and filling parameters compared with untreated animals. Metoprolol increased the expression of β_1-adrenoreceptor mRNA and reduced G protein receptor kinase 2 levels. Collagen I and III mRNA levels were reduced. Cardiac myocyte hypertrophy was also prevented.

Conclusions.—In our experimental model of severe AR, metoprolol treatment had a significant beneficial global effect on LV remodeling and function. These results suggest that the adrenergic system is important in the development of volume-overload cardiomyopathy in AR and that adrenergic-blocking agents may play a role in the treatment of this disease.

► Various medical therapies including vasodilators have been used to treat valvular insufficiency. In mitral regurgitation, angiotensin-converting enzyme inhibitors favorably reduce LV dimensions while preserving ventricular function.[1] Doppler imaging can help in the noninvasive assessment of ventricular function in patients on medical therapy.[2]

Regarding innovative therapies to treat valve disease, stem-cell tissue-engineered heart valves can be created from mesenchymal cells in combination with a biodegradable scaffold.[3]

W. H. Frishman, MD

References

1. Sampaio RO, Grinberg M, Leite JJ, et al: Effect of enalapril on left ventricular diameters and exercise capacity in asymptomatic or mildly symptomatic patients with regurgitation secondary to mitral valve prolapse or rheumatic heart disease. *Am J Cardiol* 96:117-121, 2005.
2. Diwan A, McCulloch M, Lawrie GM, et al: Doppler estimation of left ventricular filling pressures in patients with mitral valve disease. *Circulation* 111:3281-3289, 2005.
3. Sutherland FWH, Perry TE, Yu Y, et al: From stem cells to viable autologous semilunar heart valve. *Circulation* 111:2783-2791, 2005.

Percutaneous Mitral Valve Repair for Chronic Ischemic Mitral Regurgitation: A Real-Time Three-Dimensional Echocardiographic Study in an Ovine Model

Daimon M, Shiota T, Gillinov AM, et al (Cleveland Clinic Found, Ohio; Beth Israel Med Ctr, Boston; Massachusetts Gen Hosp, Boston; et al)

Circulation 111:2183-2189, 2005 43–4

Background.—Although surgical annuloplasty is the standard repair for ischemic mitral regurgitation (IMR), its application is limited by high morbidity and mortality. Using 2D and real-time 3D echocardiography in an ovine model of chronic IMR, we evaluated the geometric impact and short-term efficacy of a percutaneous transvenous catheter-based approach for mitral valve (MV) repair using a novel annuloplasty device placed in the coronary sinus.

Methods and Results.—Six sheep developed IMR 8 weeks after induced posterior myocardial infarction. An annuloplasty device optimized to reduce anterior-posterior (A-P) mitral annular dimension and MR was placed percutaneously in the coronary sinus. Mitral annular A-P and commissure-commissure dimensions and MV tenting area (MVTa) in 3 parallel A-P planes (medial, central, and lateral) were assessed by real-time 3D echocardiography with 3D software. The annuloplasty device reduced MR jet area from 5.4±2.6 to 1.3±0.9 cm^2 ($P<0.01$), mitral annular A-P dimension in both systole and diastole (24.3±2.5 to 19.7±2.4 mm; $P<0.03$; 31.0±3.9 to 24.7±2.1 mm; $P<0.001$), and MVTa at mid systole in all 3 planes (153±46 to 93±24 mm^2, $P<0.01$; 140±47 to 88±23 mm^2, $P<0.03$; and 103±23 to 87±26 mm^2, $P<0.03$).

Conclusions.—Percutaneous coronary sinus-based mitral annuloplasty reduces chronic IMR by reducing mitral annular A-P diameter and MVTa.

This suggests the potential clinical application of a new nonsurgical therapeutic approach in patients with IMR.

► Innovative percutaneous catheter-based techniques are being evaluated to treat valvular disease. Catheter-based commissurotomy techniques have been used to treat both mitral and aortic stenosis, with greater benefit seen with the mitral approach. Repeat balloon valvuloplasty is a potential strategy in nonsurgical patients with calcific aortic stenosis with good long-term palliation.[1]

W. H. Frishman, MD

Reference

1. Agarwal A, Kini AS, Attanti S, et al: Results of repeat balloon valvuloplasty for treatment of aortic stenosis in patients aged 59 to 104 years. *Am J Cardiol* 95:43-47, 2005.

44 Noninvasive Testing

Real-Time Three-Dimensional Echocardiography: A Novel Technique to Quantify Global Left Ventricular Mechanical Dyssynchrony

Kapetanakis S, Kearney MT, Siva A, et al (King's College, London)

Circulation 112:992-1000, 2005 44–1

Background.—Left ventricular (LV) mechanical dyssynchrony (LVMD) has emerged as a therapeutic target using cardiac resynchronization therapy (CRT) in selected patients with chronic heart failure. Current methods used to evaluate LVMD are technically difficult and do not assess LVMD of the whole LV simultaneously. We developed and validated real-time 3D echocardiography (RT3DE) as a novel method to assess global LVMD.

Method and Results.—Eighty-nine healthy volunteers and 174 unselected patients referred for routine echocardiography underwent 2D echocardiography and RT3DE. RT3DE data sets provided time-volume analysis for global and segmental LV volumes. A systolic dyssynchrony index (SDI) was derived from the dispersion of time to minimum regional volume for all 16 LV segments. Healthy subjects and patients with normal LV systolic function had highly synchronized segmental function (SDI, 3.5±1.8% and 4.5±2.4%; P=0.7). SDI increased with worsening LV systolic function regardless of QRS duration (mild, 5.4±0.83%; moderate, 10.0±2%; severe LV dysfunction, 15.6±1%; P for trend <0.001). We found that 37% of patients with moderate to severe LV systolic dysfunction had significant dyssynchrony with normal QRS durations (SDI, 14.7±1.2%). Twenty-six patients underwent CRT. At long-term follow-up, responders demonstrated reverse remodeling after CRT with a significant reduction in SDI (16.9±1.1% to 6.9±1%; P<0.0001) and end-diastolic volume (196.6±17.3 to 132.1±13.5 mL; P<0.0001) associated with an increase in LV ejection fraction (17±2.2% to 31.6±2.9%; P<0.0001).

Conclusions.—RT3DE can quantify global LVMD in patients with and without QRS prolongation. RT3DE represents a novel technique to identify chronic heart failure patients who may otherwise not be considered for CRT.

► Compared with 2-dimensional echocardiography, 3-dimensional echocardiography can give more accurate measurements of diastolic and systolic volumes and ejection fractions.[1,2] There are some technical problems with the procedure when tissue Doppler is done concomitantly. On the other hand, the procedure is quick, does not exclude certain patient subgroups, and requires no patient preparation.

Transesophageal echocardiography remains the gold standard technique for estimating the risk of embolism in patients with endocarditis,[3] atrial fibrillation,[4] and the antiphospholipid syndrome.[5] It is especially useful for assessing the left atrial appendage.[5]

W. H. Frishman, MD

References

1. Fleming SM, Cumberledge B, Kiesewetter C, et al: Usefulness of real-time three-dimensional echocardiography for reliable measurement of cardiac output in patients with ischemic or idiopathic dilated cardiomyopathy. *Am J Cardiol* 95:308-310, 2005.
2. Corsi C, Lang RM, Veronesi F, et al: Volumetric quantification of global and regional left ventricular function from real-time three-dimensional echocardiographic images. *Circulation* 112:1161-1170, 2005.
3. Thuny F, Disalvo G, Belliard O, et al: Risk of embolism and death in infective endo-carditis: Prognostic value of echocardiography. A prospective multicenter study. *Circulation* 112:69-75, 2005.
4. DiAngelantonio E, Ederhy S, Benyounes N, et al: Comparison of transesophageal echocardiographic identification of embolic risk markers in patients with lone versus non-lone atrial fibrillation. *Am J Cardiol* 95:592-596, 2005.
5. Erdogan D, Goren T, Diz-Kucukkaya R, et al: Assessment of cardiac structure and left atrial appendage functions in primary antiphospholipid syndrome. A transesophageal echocardiographic study. *Stroke* 36:592-596,

Cardiovascular Magnetic Resonance in Cardiac Amyloidosis

Maceira AM, Joshi J, Prasad SK, et al (Royal Brompton Hosp, London; Royal Free Hosp, London; Istituto di Cardiologia, Bologna, Italy; et al)

Circulation 111:186-193, 2005 44–2

Background.—Cardiac amyloidosis can be diagnostically challenging. Cardiovascular magnetic resonance (CMR) can assess abnormal myocardial interstitium.

Method and Results.—Late gadolinium enhancement CMR was performed in 30 patients with cardiac amyloidosis. In 22 of these, myocardial gadolinium kinetics with T_1 mapping was compared with that in 16 hypertensive controls. One patient had CMR and autopsy only. Subendocardial T_1 in amyloid patients was shorter than in controls (at 4 minutes: 427±73 versus 579±75 ms; $P<0.01$), was shorter than subepicardium T_1 for the first 8 minutes ($P\leq0.01$), and was correlated with markers of increased myocardial amyloid load, as follows: left ventricular (LV) mass ($r=-0.51$, $P=0.013$); wall thickness ($r=-0.54$ to -0.63, $P<0.04$); interatrial septal thickness ($r=-0.52$, $P=0.001$); and diastolic function ($r=-0.42$, $P=0.025$). Global subendocardial late gadolinium enhancement was found in 20 amyloid patients (69%); these patients had greater LV mass (126±30 versus 93±25 g/m^2; $P=0.009$) than unenhanced patients. Histological quantification showed substantial interstitial expansion with amyloid (30.5%)

but only minor fibrosis (1.3%). Amyloid was dominantly subendocardial (42%) compared with midwall (29%) and subepicardium (18%). There was 97% concordance in diagnosis of cardiac amyloid by combining the presence of late gadolinium enhancement and an optimized T_1 threshold (191 ms at 4 minutes) between myocardium and blood.

Conclusions.—In cardiac amyloidosis, CMR shows a characteristic pattern of global subendocardial late enhancement coupled with abnormal myocardial and blood-pool gadolinium kinetics. The findings agree with the transmural histological distribution of amyloid protein and the cardiac amyloid load and may prove to have value in diagnosis and treatment follow-up.

► Cardiac MRI is a noninvasive modality that helps to diagnose conditions which otherwise require an invasive approach. Molecular MRI can selectively visualize acute coronary, cardiac, and pulmonary thrombi.[1] It can be useful in the assessment of myocardial viability,[2] and for determining ventricular hemodynamics with an accuracy similar to Doppler imaging and invasive measurements.[3] It also has been used as a noninvasive method to detect patent foramen ovale and septal aneurysm.[4]

W. H. Frishman, MD

References

1. Spuentrup E, Buecker A, Katoh M, et al: Molecular magnetic resonance imaging of coronary thrombosis and pulmonary emboli with a novel fibrin-targeted contrast agent. *Circulation* 111:1377-1382, 2005.
2. Jansen MA, Van Emous JG, Nederhoff MGJ, et al: Asssessment of myocardial viability by intracellular ^{23}Na magnetic resonance imaging. *Circulation* 110:3457-3464, 2004.
3. Paelinck BP, deRoos A, Bax JJ, et al: Feasibility of tissue magnetic resonance imaging. A pilot study in comparison with tissue Doppler imaging and invasive measurement. *J Am Coll Cardiol* 45:1109-1116, 2005.
4. Mohrs OK, Petersen SE, Erkapic D, et al: Diagnosis of patent foramen ovale using contrast-enhanced dynamic MRI: A pilot study. *Am J Roentgenol* 184:232-240, 2005.

Noninvasive Coronary Angiography With Multislice Computed Tomography

Hoffmann MHK, Shi H, Schmitz BL, et al (Univ Hosp, Ulm, Germany; Heart-Center, Ulm, Germany)

JAMA 293:2471-2478, 2005 44–3

Context.—Multislice computed tomography (MSCT) has recently evolved as a modality for noninvasive coronary imaging.

Objective.—To assess the accuracy and robustness of MSCT vs the criterion standard of invasive coronary angiography for detection of obstructive coronary artery disease.

Design, Setting, and Patients.—Prospective, single-center study conducted in a referral center setting in Germany and enrolling 103 consecutive patients (mean age, 61.5 [SD, 9.7] years) from November 2003–August 2004 who were undergoing both invasive coronary angiography and MSCT using a scanner with 16 detector rows.

Main Outcome Measures.—Blinded results for both modalities compared using the patient as the primary unit of analysis, with supplementary segment- and vessel-based analyses.

Results.—One thousand three hundred eighty-four segments (≥1.5 mm diameter) were identified by invasive coronary angiography; nondiagnostic image quality of MSCT was identified for only 88 (6.4%) of these segments, mainly due to faster heart rates. Compared with invasive coronary angiography for detection of significant lesions (>50% stenosis), segment-based sensitivity, specificity, and positive and negative predictive values of MSCT were 95%, 98%, 87%, and 99%, respectively. Quantitative comparison of MSCT and invasive coronary angiography showed good correlation (r=0.87, P<.001), with MSCT systematically measuring greater-percentage stenoses (bias, +12%). In the patient-based analysis, the area under the receiver operating characteristic curve was 0.97 (95% confidence interval, 0.90-1.00), indicating high discriminative power to identify patients who might be candidates for revascularization (>50% left main artery stenosis and/or >70% stenosis in any other epicardial vessel). Threshold optimization allowed either detection of these patients with 100% sensitivity at a reasonable false-positive rate (specificity, 76.5%; MSCT stenosis, >66%) or optimization of both the sensitivity and specificity (>90%; MSCT stenosis, >76%).

Conclusions.—Multislice computed tomography provides high accuracy for noninvasive detection of suspected obstructive coronary artery disease. This promising technology has potential to complement diagnostic invasive coronary angiography in routine clinical care.

▶ MSCT is a useful and reliable contrast-based noninvasive modality for visualizing the coronary circulation. The technique has also been shown to be useful in patients with hypertension for assessing both left ventricular function and the presence of concomitant coronary artery disease.[1,2] As the technology has evolved, the images from MSCT have become more refined,[3] allowing for a qualitative assessment of coronary artery plaque burden and the ability to identify calcified, noncalcified, and mixed lesions.[4] MSCT can also allow for accurate assessment of venous and arterial conduits.[5]

Scanners able to acquire up to 64 slices (we currently have one in our outpatient cardiology practice), with a slice thickness of less than 0.5 mm, are now available. This updated MSCT version reduces the time for breath holding and reduces motion artifacts. It also reduces the amount of contrast needed for the scan. These advances will translate into clinically significant improvements in accuracy, making this modality a powerful screening tool for ruling in or ruling out coronary artery disease.[6]

W. H. Frishman, MD

References

1. Schuijf JD, Bax JJ, Jukema JW, et al: Noninvasive evaluation of the coronary arteries with multislice computed tomography in hypertensive patients. *Hypertension* 45:227-232, 2005.
2. Schuijf JD, Bax JJ, Salm LP, et al: Noninvasive coronary imaging and assessment of left ventricular function using 16-slice computed tomography. *Am J Cardiol* 95:571-574, 2005.
3. Maruyama T, Yoshizumi T, Tamura R, et al: Comparison of eight-versus 16-slice multidetector-row computed tomography for visibility and image quality of coronary segments. *Am J Cardiol* 94:1539-1543, 2004.
4. Mollet NR, Cademartiri F, Nieman K, et al: Noninvasive assessment of coronary plaque burden using multislice computed tomography. *Am J Cardiol* 95:1165-1169, 2005.
5. Martuscelli E, Romagnoli A, D'Eliseo A, et al: Evaluation of venous and arterial conduit patency by 16-slice spiral computed tomography. *Circulation* 110:3234-3238, 2004.
6. Moore RK, Sampson C, MacDonald S, et al: Coronary artery bypass graft imaging using ECG-gated multislice computed tomography: Comparison with catheter angiography. *Clin Radiol* 60:990-998, 2005.

45 Arrhythmias

Single-Chamber Versus Dual-Chamber Pacing for High-Grade Atrioventricular Block

Toff WD, for the United Kingdom Pacing and Cardiovascular Events (UKPACE) Trial Investigators (Univ of Leicester, England; et al)

N Engl J Med 353:145-155, 2005 45–1

Background.—In the treatment of atrioventricular block, dual-chamber cardiac pacing is thought to confer a clinical benefit as compared with single-chamber ventricular pacing, but the supporting evidence is mainly from retrospective studies. Uncertainty persists regarding the true benefits of dual-chamber pacing, particularly in the elderly, in whom it is used less often than in younger patients.

Methods.—In a multicenter, randomized, parallel-group trial, 2021 patients 70 years of age or older who were undergoing their first pacemaker implant for high-grade atrioventricular block were randomly assigned to receive a single-chamber ventricular pacemaker (1009 patients) or a dual-chamber pacemaker (1012 patients). In the single-chamber group, patients were randomly assigned to receive either fixed-rate pacing (504 patients) or rate-adaptive pacing (505 patients). The primary outcome was death from all causes. Secondary outcomes included atrial fibrillation, heart failure, and a composite of stroke, transient ischemic attack, or other thromboembolism.

Results.—The median follow-up period was 4.6 years for mortality and 3 years for other cardiovascular events. The mean annual mortality rate was 7.2 percent in the single-chamber group and 7.4 percent in the dual-chamber group (hazard ratio, 0.96; 95 percent confidence interval, 0.83 to 1.11). We found no significant differences between the group with single-chamber pacing and that with dual-chamber pacing in the rates of atrial fibrillation, heart failure, or a composite of stroke, transient ischemic attack, or other thromboembolism.

Conclusions.—In elderly patients with high-grade atrioventricular block, the pacing mode does not influence the rate of death from all causes during the first five years or the incidence of cardiovascular events during the first three years after implantation of a pacemaker (Fig 2).

► In elderly patients with high degree atrioventricular block, the mode of pacing has no long-term influence on mortality or morbidity. Single-chamber pac-

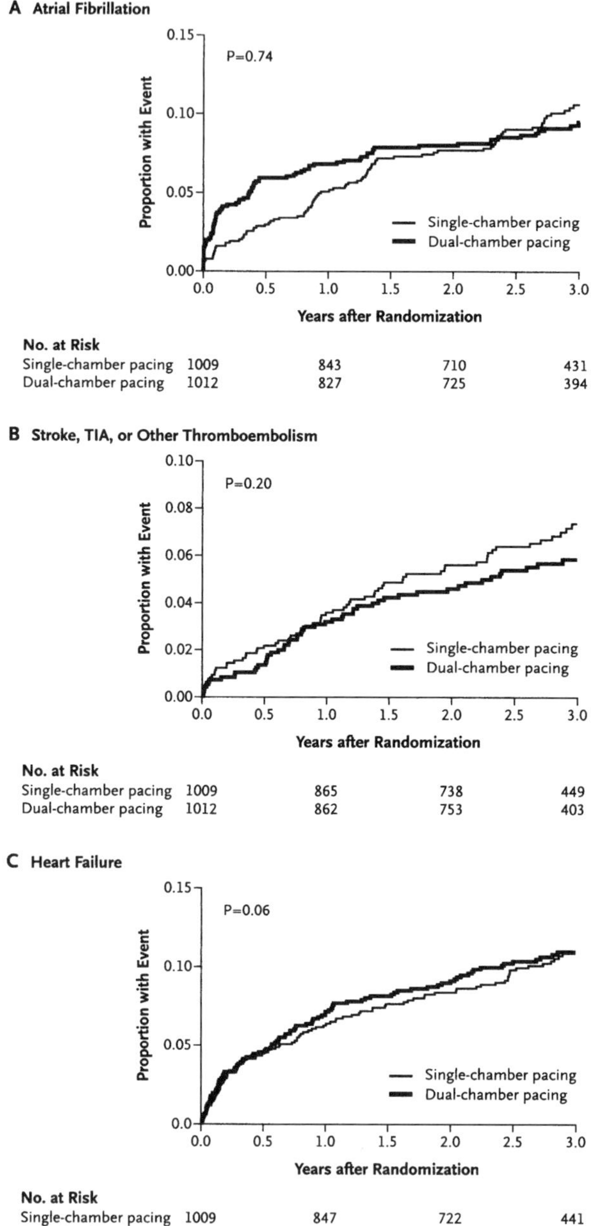

FIGURE 2.—Cumulative risk of cardiovascular events according to the mode of pacing. TIA denotes transient ischemic attack. Reprinted by permission of *The New England Journal of Medicine* from Toff WD, for the United Kingdom Pacing and Cardiovascular Events (UKPACE) Trial Investigators: Single-chamber versus dual-chamber pacing for high-grade atrioventricular block. *N Engl J Med* 353:145-155, 2005.

ing devices are less prone to complications than dual-chamber pacers, and are also less expensive.

Questions have been raised about possible adverse effects of mobile phones on pacemaker function. These phones might have adverse effects on pacemaker function, especially with older pacing devices.[1]

In patients receiving pacemakers for sinus node dysfunction, the presence of a prolonged ECG QRS duration before pacer implantation is associated with an increased risk of death. This finding suggests that patients with a prolonged QRS duration who need to be paced should have an implantable cardioverter defibrillator.[2]

W. H. Frishman, MD

References

1. Tandogan I, Temizhan A, Yetkin E, et al: The effects of mobile phones on pacemaker function. *Int J Cardiol* 103:51-58, 2005.
2. Sweeney MO, for the Mode Selection Trial (MOST) Investigators: Association of prolonged QRS duration with death in a clinical trial of pacemaker therapy for sinus node dysfunction. *Circulation* 111:2418-2423, 2005.

Percutaneous Left Atrial Appendage Transcatheter Occlusion (PLAATO System) to Prevent Stroke in High-Risk Patients With Non-rheumatic Atrial Fibrillation: Results From the International Multi-Center Feasibility Trials

Ostermayer SH, Reisman M, Kramer PH, et al (CardioVascular Ctr Frankfurt, Germany; Swedish Cardiovascular Research Inst, Seattle; Shawnee Mission Med Ctr, Kan; et al)

J Am Coll Cardiol 46:9-14, 2005 45–2

Objectives.—These studies were conducted to evaluate the feasibility of percutaneous left atrial appendage (LAA) occlusion using the PLAATO system (ev3 Inc., Plymouth, Minnesota).

Background.—Patients with atrial fibrillation (AF) have a five-fold increased risk for stroke. Other studies have shown that more than 90% of atrial thrombi in patients with non-rheumatic AF originate in the LAA. Transvenous closure of the LAA is a new approach in preventing embolism in these patients.

Methods.—Within two prospective, multi-center trials, LAA occlusion was attempted in 111 patients (age 71 ± 9 years). All patients had a contraindication for anticoagulation therapy and at least one additional risk factor for stroke. The primary end point was incidence of major adverse events (MAEs), a composite of stroke, cardiac or neurological death, myocardial infarction, and requirement for procedure-related cardiovascular surgery within the first month.

Results.—Implantation was successful in 108 of 111 patients (97.3%, 95% confidence interval [CI] 92.3% to 99.4%) who underwent 113 procedures. One patient (0.9%, 95% CI 0.02% to 4.9%) experienced two MAEs within the first 30 days: need for cardiovascular surgery and in-hospital neurological death. Three other patients underwent in-hospital pericardiocentesis due to a hemopericardium. Average follow-up was 9.8 months. Two patients experienced stroke. No migration or mobile thrombus was noted on transesophageal echocardiogram at one and six months after device implantation.

Conclusions.—Closing the LAA using the PLAATO system is feasible and can be performed at acceptable risk. It may become an alternative in patients with AF and a contraindication for lifelong anticoagulation treatment.

► AF is associated with an increased risk of stroke from cardiac emboli.[1] Echocardiography and autopsy studies have shown that thrombi form in the left atrial appendage,[2,3] suggesting that occlusion of the appendage might prevent thrombotic and embolic complications. The PLAATO system is a percutaneous transseptal device for closing off the LAA and consists of a self-expanding nitinol cage covered with expanded polytetrafluoroethylene to close off blood flow from the remaining part of the appendage. Three rows of anchors along the struts help stabilize the occluder in the appendage.

This technique could become an alternative treatment approach for patients with AF at risk for stroke who cannot tolerate long-term anticoagulation.[4]

W. H. Frishman, MD

References

1. Kimura K, for the Japan Multicenter Stroke Investigators Collaboration (J-MUSIC). *J Neurol Neurosurg Psychiatry* 76:679-683, 2005.
2. Stoddard MF, Dawkins PR, Prince CR, et al: Left atrial appendage thrombus is not uncommon in patients with acute atrial fibrillation and a recent embolic event: A transesophageal echocardiographic study. *J Am Coll Cardiol* 25:452-459, 1995.
3. Blackshear JL, Odell JA: Appendage obliteration to reduce stroke in cardiac surgical patients with atrial fibrillation. *Ann Thorac Surg* 61:755-759, 1996.
4. Hanna IR, Kolm P, Martin R, et al: Left atrial structure and function after percutaneous left atrial appendage transcatheter occlusion (PLAATO): Six-month echocardiographic follow up. *J Am Coll Cardiol* 43:1868-1872, 2004.

Amiodarone Versus Sotalol for Atrial Fibrillation

Singh BN, for the Sotalol Amiodarone Atrial Fibrillation Efficacy Trial (SAFE-T) Investigators (Veterans Affairs Med Ctr of West Los Angeles; et al)

N Engl J Med 352:1861-1872, 2005 45–3

Background.—The optimal pharmacologic means to restore and maintain sinus rhythm in patients with atrial fibrillation remains controversial.

Methods.—In this double-blind, placebo-controlled trial, we randomly assigned 665 patients who were receiving anticoagulants and had persistent atrial fibrillation to receive amiodarone (267 patients), sotalol (261 patients), or placebo (137 patients) and monitored them for 1 to 4.5 years. The primary end point was the time to recurrence of atrial fibrillation beginning on day 28, determined by means of weekly transtelephonic monitoring.

Results.—Spontaneous conversion occurred in 27.1 percent of the amiodarone group, 24.2 percent of the sotalol group, and 0.8 percent of the placebo group, and direct-current cardioversion failed in 27.7 percent, 26.5 percent, and 32.1 percent, respectively. The median times to a recurrence of atrial fibrillation were 487 days in the amiodarone group, 74 days in the sotalol group, and 6 days in the placebo group according to intention to treat and 809, 209, and 13 days, respectively, according to treatment received. Amiodarone was superior to sotalol ($P<0.001$) and to placebo ($P<0.001$), and sotalol was superior to placebo ($P<0.001$). In patients with ischemic heart disease, the median time to a recurrence of atrial fibrillation was 569 days with amiodarone therapy and 428 days with sotalol therapy ($P=0.53$). Restoration and maintenance of sinus rhythm significantly improved the quality of life and exercise capacity. There were no significant differences in major adverse events among the three groups.

Conclusions.—Amiodarone and sotalol are equally efficacious in converting atrial fibrillation to sinus rhythm. Amiodarone is superior for maintaining sinus rhythm, but both drugs have similar efficacy in patients with ischemic heart disease. Sustained sinus rhythm is associated with an improved quality of life and improved exercise performance (Fig 2).

▶ Studies have shown that therapy to convert atrial fibrillation to normal sinus rhythm provided no survival advantage over rate control with anticoagulation.[1-3] If one contemplates a medical cardioversion, the drugs amiodarone and sotalol are comparable in efficacy; however, amiodarone has an advantage over sotalol regarding long-term maintenance of sinus rhythm, especially in patients without ischemic heart disease. Amiodarone may have a greater risk of toxicity over time.

Amiodarone prophylaxis has also been shown to decrease the risk of atrial fibrillation, ventricular tachyarrhythmias, and stroke after cardiac surgery.[4] Magnesium has been shown to have similar efficacy.[5]

Postoperative atrial fibrillation appears to be associated with a decreased level of triiodothyronine.[6] Whether thyroid hormone replacement in the postoperative state might be beneficial to prevent atrial fibrillation is a question that needs to be resolved.

W. H. Frishman, MD

References

1. Wyse DG, Waldo AL, DiMarco JP, et al: A comparison of rate control and rhythm control in patients with atrial fibrillation. *N Engl J Med* 347:1825-1833, 2002.
2. Hohnloser SH, Kuck KH, Lilienthal J: Rhythm or rate control in atrial fibrillation—Pharmacological Intervention in Atrial Fibrillation (PIAF): A randomized trial. *Lancet* 356:1789-1794, 2000.
3. Van Gelder IC, Hagens VE, Bosker HA, et al: A comparison of rate control and rhythm control in patients with recurrent persistent atrial fibrillation. *N Engl J Med* 347:1834-1840, 2002.
4. Aasbo JD, Lawrence AT, Krishnan K, et al: Amiodarone prophylaxis reduces major cardiovascular morbidity and length of stay after cardiac surgery: A meta-analysis. *Ann Intern Med* 143:327-336, 2005.

FIGURE 2.

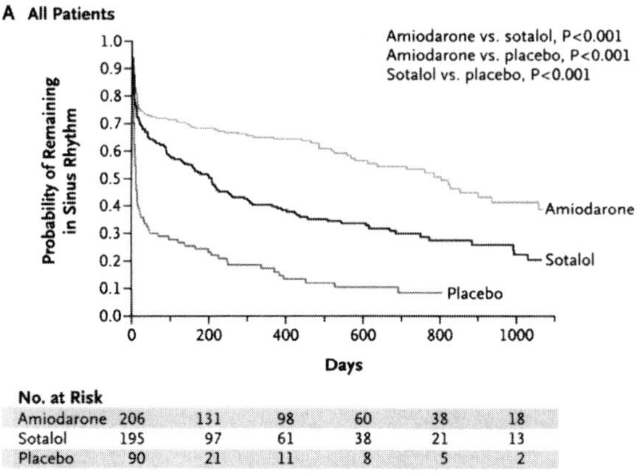

No. at Risk

Amiodarone	206	131	98	60	38	18
Sotalol	195	97	61	38	21	13
Placebo	90	21	11	8	5	2

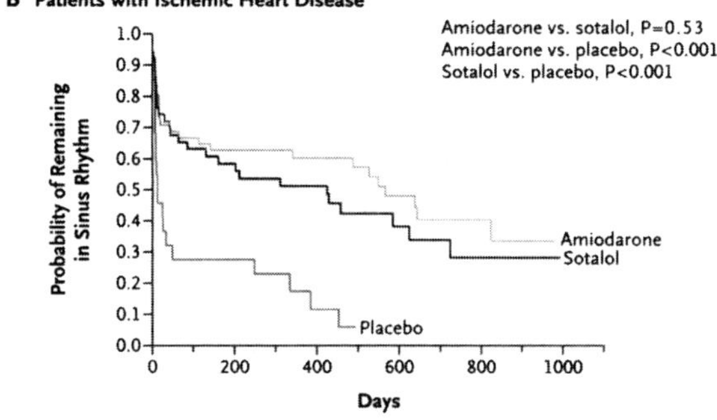

No. at Risk

Amiodarone	51	30	24	15	7	2
Sotalol	47	26	19	10	6	4
Placebo	22	7	3	0		

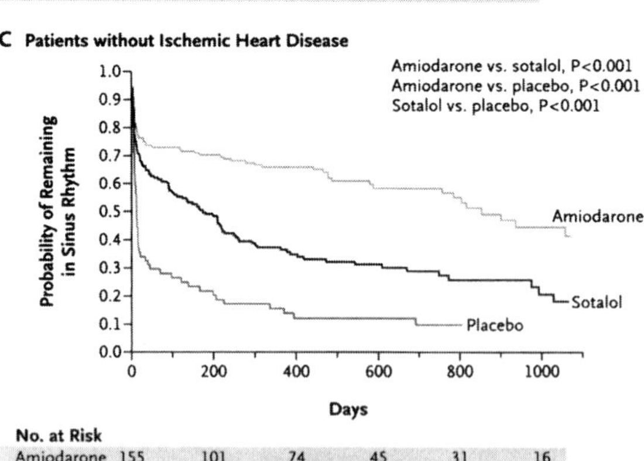

No. at Risk

Amiodarone	155	101	74	45	31	16
Sotalol	148	71	42	28	15	9
Placebo	68	14	8	5	2	

(Continued)

5. Miller S, Crystal E, Garfinkle M, et al: Effects of magnesium on atrial fibrillation after cardiac surgery: A meta-analysis. *Heart* 91: 618-623, 2005.
6. Kokkonen L, Majahalme S, Kööbi T, et al: Atrial fibrillation in elderly patients after cardiac surgery: Postoperative hemodynamics and low postoperative serum triiodothyronine. *J Cardiothorac Vasc Anesth* 19:182-187, 2005.

Clinical Characteristics of Persistent Lone Atrial Fibrillation in the RACE Study

Rienstra M, for the RAte Control versus Electrical cardioversion for persistent atrial fibrillation Study Group (Univ Hosp Groningen, The Netherlands; Rijnstate Hosp, Arnheim, The Netherlands; Academic Med Ctr, Amsterdam)
Am J Cardiol 94:1486-1490, 2004 45–4

Introduction.—In the RAte Control versus Electrical cardioversion for persistent atrial fibrillation (RACE) study, 522 patients were randomized to either rate or rhythm control therapy. Lone atrial fibrillation (AF) was present in 89 patients. Demographics, cardiovascular mortality and morbidity, and quality of life were compared between patients with lone AF and those with underlying structural heart disease. Patients with lone AF were significantly younger (65 ± 10 vs 69 ± 8 years) and had fewer complaints of fatigue ($p = 0.01$) and dyspnea ($p = 0.005$). With lone AF, quality-of-life scores were higher on almost all 8 Medical Outcomes Study Short-Form health survey questionnaire subscales, and comparable to healthy, age- and gender-matched controls. Mean follow-up was 2.3 ± 0.6 years. Cardiovascular end points occurred in 9 patients with lone AF (10%), consisting of death (all bleedings) 3%, thromboembolic complications in 3%, nonfatal bleeding in 2%, and pacemaker implantation in 2%, but no heart failure and severe adverse effects due to antiarrhythmic drugs occurred. End points occurred in 95 patients (22%) with underlying diseases. Heart failure and severe adverse effects from drugs did not occur in patients with lone AF in this study. Despite the absence of demonstrable cardiovascular and cerebrovascular disease, lone AF is associated with bleeding and thromboembolism.

► In 15% to 30% of patients with AF there is no known, apparent structural etiology for the arrhythmia,[1,2] a condition known as "lone" AF, which allegedly carries with it a benign clinical course. More recent studies suggest that older patents with lone AF might be at risk for thromboembolism because atrial remodeling may occur over time.

FIGURE 2.—Kaplan-Meier estimates of the time to recurrence of atrial fibrillation among patients in whom sinus rhythm was restored on day 28. Estimates of the time to recurrence of atrial fibrillation are shown for all patients with conversion to sinus rhythm (Panel A) and in subgroups of patients with conversion to sinus rhythm according to the presence or absence of ischemic heart disease (Panels B and C, respectively). (Reprinted with permission of *The New England Journal of Medicine* from Singh BN, for the Sotalol Amiodarone Atrial Fibrillation Efficacy Trial (SAFE-T) Investigators: Amiodarone versus sotalol for atrial fibrillation. *N Engl J Med* 352:1861-1872, 2005.

Clinical subtypes of lone AF appear to exist, including a familial type, an exercise-induced type, and a type associated with conduction disease.[3] A relationship may be present between lone AF and personality, socioeconomic factors, and life stresses.[4] Younger individuals with AF appear to have foci for the arrhythmia in the pulmonary vein and may benefit from catheter ablation.[5,6] In addition, discordant natriuretic peptide levels have been observed in patients with lone AF.[7] This biomarker is also present in individuals with normal sinus rhythm and may identify individuals who are prone to lone AF.[7]

W. H. Frishman, MD

References

1. Oral H: Mechanisms of atrial fibrillation: Lessons from studies in patients. *Prog Cardiovasc Dis* 48:29-40, 2005.
2. Kopecky SL, Gersh BJ, McGoon MD, et al: The natural history of lone atrial fibrillation. A population-based study over three decades. *N Engl J Med* 317:669-674, 1987.
3. Patton KK, Zacks ES, Chang JY, et al: Clinical subtypes of lone atrial fibrillation. *Pacing Clin Electrophysiol* 28:630-638, 2005.
4. Mattioli AV, Bonatti S, Zennaro M, et al: The relationship between personality, socioeconomic factors, acute life stress, and the development, spontaneous conversion, and recurrences of acute lone atrial fibrillation. *Europace* 7:211-220, 2005.
5. Nanthakumar K, Lau YR, Plumb VJ, et al: Electrophysiological findings in adolescents with atrial fibrillation who have structurally normal hearts. *Circulation* 110:117-123, 2004.
6. Lazar S, Dixit S, Marchlinski FE, et al: Presence of left-to-right atrial frequency gradient in paroxysmal but not persistent atrial fibrillation in humans. *Circulation* 110:3181-3186, 2004.
7. Ellinor PT, Low AF, Patton KK, et al: Discordant atrial natriuretic peptide and brain natriuretic peptide levels in lone atrial fibrillation. *J Am Coll Cardiol* 45:82-86, 2005.

Clinical and Economic Implications of the Multicenter Automatic Defibrillator Implantation Trial-II

Al-Khatib SM, Anstrom KJ, Eisenstein EL, et al (Duke Clinical Research Inst, Durham, NC)

Ann Intern Med 142:593-600, 2005 45–5

Background.—The Multicenter Automatic Defibrillator Implantation Trial (MADIT)-II demonstrated that implantable cardioverter defibrillators (ICDs) save lives when used in patients with a history of myocardial infarction (MI) and an ejection fraction of 0.3 or less.

Objective.—To investigate the cost-effectiveness of implanting ICDs in patients who met MADIT-II eligibility criteria and were enrolled in the Duke Cardiovascular Database between 1 January 1986 and 31 December 2001.

Design.—Cost-effectiveness analysis.

Data Sources.—Published literature, databases owned by Duke University Medical Center, and Medicare data.

Target Population.—Adults with a history of MI and an ejection fraction of 0.3 or less.

Time Horizon.—Lifetime.

Perspective.—Societal.

Interventions.—ICD therapy versus conventional medical therapy.

Outcomes Measures.—Cost per life-year gained and incremental cost-effectiveness.

Results.—Compared with conventional medical therapy, ICDs are projected to result in an increase of 1.80 discounted years in life expectancy and an incremental cost-effectiveness ratio of 50 500 dollars per life-year gained. Cost-effectiveness varied dramatically with changes in time horizon: The cost-effectiveness ratio increased to 67 800 dollars per life-year gained, 79 900 dollars per life-year gained, 100 000 dollars per life-year gained, 167 900 dollars per life-year gained, and 367 200 dollars per life-year gained for 15-year, 12-year, 9-year, 6-year, and 3-year time horizons, respectively. Changing the frequency of follow-up visits, complication rates, and battery replacements had less of an effect on the cost-effectiveness ratios than reducing the cost of ICD placement and leads.

Limitations.—The study was limited by the completeness of the data, referral bias, difference in medical therapy between the Duke cohort and the MADIT-II cohort, and not addressing potential upgrades to biventricular devices.

Conclusions.—The economic expense of defibrillator implantation in all patients who meet MADIT-II eligibility criteria is substantial. However, in the range of survival benefit observed in MADIT-II, ICD therapy for these patients is economically attractive by conventional standards.

▶ Treatment with implantable defibrillators should be considered in patients having heart failure and left ventricular ejection fractions less than 30% who are expected to live for longer than 1 year.[1]

Regarding concomitant antiarrhythmic therapy, β-blockers appear to have a favorable effect on survival; sotalol and amiodarone have a neutral effect. There appears to be an unfavorable effect on survival with concomitant digoxin use.[2]

In patients receiving implantable defibrillators for the secondary prevention of death from ventricular tachyarrhythmias, an 80% 1-year survival rate has been observed after a successful defibrillation with the device. These patients appear to be at an increased risk of heart failure and nonsudden cardiac death.[3]

W. H. Frishman, MD

References

1. ACC/AHA 2006 guideline update for the diagnosis and management of chronic heart failure in the adult—summary article. A report of the American College of Cardiology/American Heart Association Task Force on Practice Guidelines (Writing Committee to Update the 2001 Guidelines for the Evaluation and Management of Heart Failure). *J Am Coll Cardiol* 46:1116-1143, 2005. and *Circulation* 112:1825-1852, 2005.

2. Ho AT, Pai SM, Timothy P, et al: Effect of concomitant antiarrhythmic therapy on survival in patients with implantable cardioverter defibrillators. *Pacing Clin Electrophysiol* 28:647-653, 2005.
3. Moss AJ, for the Multicenter Automatic Defibrillator Implantation Trial-II (MADIT-II) Research Group: Long-term clinical course of patients after termination of ventricular tachyarrhythmia by an implanted defibrillator. *Circulation* 110:3760-3765, 2004.

46 Other Topics

Perioperative Beta-Blocker Therapy and Mortality After Major Noncardiac Surgery

Lindenauer PK, Pekow P, Wang K, et al (Baystate Med Ctr, Springfield, Mass; Tufts Univ, Boston; Univ of Massachusetts at Amherst; et al)

N Engl J Med 353:349-361, 2005 46–1

Background.—Despite limited evidence from randomized trials, perioperative treatment with beta-blockers is now widely advocated. We assessed the use of perioperative beta-blockers and their association with in-hospital mortality in routine clinical practice.

Methods.—We conducted a retrospective cohort study of patients 18 years of age or older who underwent major noncardiac surgery in 2000 and 2001 at 329 hospitals throughout the United States. We used propensity-score matching to adjust for differences between patients who received perioperative beta-blockers and those who did not receive such therapy and compared in-hospital mortality using multivariable logistic modeling.

Results.—Of 782,969 patients, 663,635 (85 percent) had no recorded contraindications to beta-blockers, 122,338 of whom (18 percent) received such treatment during the first two hospital days, including 14 percent of patients with a Revised Cardiac Risk Index (RCRI) score of 0 and 44 percent with a score of 4 or higher. The relationship between perioperative beta-blocker treatment and the risk of death varied directly with cardiac risk; among the 580,665 patients with an RCRI score of 0 or 1, treatment was associated with no benefit and possible harm, whereas among the patients with an RCRI score of 2, 3, or 4 or more, the adjusted odds ratios for death in the hospital were 0.88 (95 percent confidence interval, 0.80 to 0.98), 0.71 (95 percent confidence interval, 0.63 to 0.80), and 0.58 (95 percent confidence interval, 0.50 to 0.67), respectively.

Conclusions.—Perioperative beta-blocker therapy is associated with a reduced risk of in-hospital death among high-risk, but not low-risk, patients undergoing major noncardiac surgery. Patient safety may be enhanced by increasing the use of beta-blockers in high-risk patients.

► The preoperative assessment of patients regarding their risk for perioperative cardiovascular complications of surgery is an important part of medical practice. Starting or maintaining β-adrenergic blockers clearly reduces the incidence of cardiovascular mortality and morbidity in high-risk patients undergoing cardiac and noncardiac surgical procedures.[1-7] The Agency for Healthcare Research and Quality has identified the perioperative use of β-blockers among high-risk patients as an important practice for safe health care.[8]

The preoperative utilization of β-blockers has also reduced the need for expensive preoperative cardiovascular disease screening methods and the need for prophylactic coronary revascularization for patients undergoing noncardiac surgery.

W. H. Frishman, MD

References

1. Auerbach AD, Goldman L: Beta blockers and reduction of cardiac events in noncardiac surgery: Scientific review. *JAMA* 287:1435-1444, 2002.
2. Fleisher LA, Eagle KA: Lowering cardiac risk in noncardiac surgery. *N Engl J Med* 345:1677-1682, 2001.
3. Oka Y, Frishman W, Becker RM, et al: Clinical pharmacology of the new beta-adrenergic blocking drugs. Part 10: Beta-adrenoceptor blockade and coronary artery surgery. *Am Heart J* 99:255-269, 1980.
4. Selzman CH, Miller SA, Zimmerman MA, et al: The case for β-adrenergic blockade as prophylaxis against perioperative cardiovascular morbidity and mortality. *Arch Surg* 136:286-290, 2001.
5. Grayburn PA, Hillis LD: Cardiac events in patients undergoing noncardiac surgery: Shifting the paradigm from noninvasive risk stratification to therapy. *Ann Intern Med* 138:506-511, 2003.
6. Mangano DT, Layug EL, Wallace A, et al: Effect of atenolol on mortality and cardiovascular morbidity after noncardiac surgery. *N Engl J Med* 335:1713-1720, 1996 (Erratum 336:1039, 1997).
7. Poldermans D, Boersma E, Bax JJ, et al: The effect of bisoprolol on perioperative mortality and myocardial infarction in high-risk patients undergoing vascular surgery. *N Engl J Med* 341:1789-1794, 1999.
8. Shojkania KG, Duncan BW, McDonald KM, et al (eds): Making health care safer: A critical analysis of patient safety practices. Evidence report/technology assessment No 43, Rockville, Md, Agency for Healthcare Research and Quality, July 2001 (AHRQ publication #01-E058).

Accelerated Longitudinal Decline of Aerobic Capacity in Healthy Older Adults

Fleg JL, Morrell CH, Bos AG, et al (NIH, Baltimore, Md; Loyola College in Maryland, Baltimore; Uniformed Services Univ of the Health Sciences, Bethesda, Md)

Circulation 112:674-682, 2005 46–2

Background.—The ability of older persons to function independently is dependent largely on the maintenance of sufficient aerobic capacity and strength to perform daily activities. Although peak aerobic capacity is widely recognized to decline with age, its rate of decline has been estimated primarily from cross-sectional studies that may provide misleading, overly optimistic estimates of aging changes.

Method and Results.—To determine longitudinal rate of change in aerobic capacity and the influence of age, gender, and physical activity on these changes, we performed serial measurements of peak treadmill oxygen consumption (peak $\dot{V}O_2$) in 375 women and 435 men ages 21 to 87 years from the Baltimore Longitudinal Study of Aging, a community-dwelling cohort free of clinical heart disease, over a median follow-up period of 7.9 years. A linear mixed-effects regression model was used to calculate the predicted longitudinal 10-year rate of change in peak $\dot{V}O_2$, expressed in milliliters per minute, for each age decade from the 20s through the 70s after adjustment for self-reported leisure-time physical activity. A longitudinal decline in peak $\dot{V}O_2$ was observed in each of the 6 age decades in both sexes; however, the rate of decline accelerated from 3% to 6% per 10 years in the 20s and 30s to >20% per 10 years in the 70s and beyond. The rate of decline for each decade was larger in men than in women from the 40s onward. Similar longitudinal rates of decline prevailed when peak $\dot{V}O_2$ was indexed per kilogram of body weight or per kilogram of fat-free mass and in all quartiles of self-reported leisure-time physical activity. When the components of peak $\dot{V}O_2$ were examined, the rate of longitudinal decline of the oxygen pulse (ie, the O_2 utilization per heart beat) mirrored that of peak $\dot{V}O_2$, whereas the longitudinal rate of heart rate decline averaged only 4% to 6% per 10 years, and accelerated only minimally with age.

Conclusions.—The longitudinal rate of decline in peak $\dot{V}O_2$ in healthy adults is not constant across the age span in healthy persons, as assumed by cross-sectional studies, but accelerates markedly with each successive age decade, especially in men, regardless of physical activity habits. The accelerated rate of decline of peak aerobic capacity has substantial implications with regard to functional independence and quality of life, not only in healthy older persons, but particularly when disease-related deficits are superimposed.

► Graying of the hair and changes in vision are part of the normative aging process. Similarly, there are normative changes in cardiovascular function in men and women that include a decrease in chronotropic capacity and a decrease in aerobic capacity. The rate of decrease in aerobic capacity accelerates over each decade, especially over the age of 50. Aerobic exercise in the elderly can deaccelerate this process; however, it cannot prevent it. Strength training in the elderly can increase endurance and prevent falls, but will not impact on aerobic capacity.[1,2]

Orthostatic hypotension and vasovagal syncope are also common in aging populations. Physical countermaneuvers can abort or delay an impending faint, including the use of leg crossing for 2 minutes combined with muscle tensing (skeletal muscles of leg, abdomen, and buttocks) for 1 minute.[3]

W. H. Frishman, MD

References

1. Ades PA, Ballor DL, Ashikaga T, et al: Weight training improves walking endurance in healthy elderly persons. *Ann Intern Med* 124:568-572, 1996.

2. Hickson RC, Rosenkoetter MA, Brown MM: Strength training effects on aerobic power and short-term endurance. *Med Sci Sports Exerc* 12:336-339, 1980.
3. van Dijk N, de Bruin IGJM, Gisolf J, et al: Hemodynamic effects of leg crossing and skeletal muscle tensing during free standing in patients with vasovagal syncope. *J Appl Physiol* 98:584-590, 2005.

Exercise Intolerance in Adult Congenital Heart Disease: Comparative Severity, Correlates, and Prognostic Implication

Diller G-P, Dimopoulos K, Okonko D, et al (Royal Brompton Hosp, London; Imperial College, London; St Mary's Hosp, London)
Circulation 112:828-835, 2005 46–3

Background.—Although some patients with adult congenital heart disease (ACHD) report limitations in exercise capacity, we hypothesized that depressed exercise capacity may be more widespread than superficially evident during clinical consultation and could be a means of assessing risk.

Method and Results.—Cardiopulmonary exercise testing was performed in 335 consecutive ACHD patients (age, 33±13 years), 40 non–congenital heart failure patients (age, 58±15 years), and 11 young (age, 29±5 years) and 12 older (age, 59±9 years) healthy subjects. Peak oxygen consumption (peak $\dot{V}O_2$) was reduced in ACHD patients compared with healthy subjects of similar age (21.7±8.5 versus 45.1±8.6; $P<0.001$). No significant difference in peak $\dot{V}O_2$ was found between ACHD and heart failure patients of corresponding NYHA class (P=NS for each NYHA class). Within ACHD subgroups, peak $\dot{V}O_2$ gradually declined from aortic coarctation (28.7±10.4) to Eisenmenger (11.5±3.6) patients ($P<0.001$). Multivariable correlates of peak $\dot{V}O_2$ were peak heart rate ($r=0.33$), forced expiratory volume ($r=0.33$), pulmonary hypertension ($r=-0.26$), gender ($r=-0.23$), and body mass index ($r=-0.19$). After a median follow-up of 10 months, 62 patients (18.5%) were hospitalized or had died. On multivariable Cox analysis, peak $\dot{V}O_2$ predicted hospitalization or death (hazard ratio, 0.937; $P=0.01$) and was related to the frequency and duration of hospitalization ($P=0.01$ for each).

Conclusions.—Exercise capacity is depressed in ACHD patients (even in allegedly asymptomatic patients) on a par with chronic heart failure subjects. Lack of heart rate response to exercise, pulmonary arterial hypertension, and impaired pulmonary function are important correlates of exercise capacity, as is underlying cardiac anatomy. Poor exercise capacity identifies ACHD patients at risk for hospitalization or death.

► Most congenital heart lesions can be corrected in childhood with operative procedures. However, exercise capacity may often be depressed, even in asymptomatic patients. Certain corrections will have a good long-term functional result, such as correction of an aortic coarctation[1] and a transcatheter closure of an atrial septal defect.[2]

W. H. Frishman, MD

References

1. Carr JA, Amato JJ, Higgins RSD: Long-term results of surgical coarctectomy in the adolescent and young adult with 18-year follow up. *Ann Thorac Surg* 79:1950-1956, 2005.
2. Salehian O, Horlick E, Schwerzmann M, et al: Improvements in cardiac form and function after transcatheter closure of secundum atrial septal defects. *J Am Coll Cardiol* 45:499-504, 2005.

Hypothermia Improves Defibrillation Success and Resuscitation Outcomes From Ventricular Fibrillation

Boddicker KA, Zhang Y, Zimmerman MB, et al (Univ of Iowa, Iowa City)
Circulation 111:3195-3201, 2005 46–4

Background.—Induced hypothermia is recommended to improve neurological outcomes in unconscious survivors of out-of-hospital ventricular fibrillation (VF) cardiac arrest. Patients resuscitated from a VF arrest are at risk of refibrillation, but there are few data on the effects of already existing hypothermia on defibrillation and resuscitation.

Method and Results.—Thirty-two swine (mean±SE weight, 23.0±0.6 kg) were divided into 4 groups: normothermia (n=8), mild hypothermia (35°C) (n=8), moderate hypothermia (33°C) (n=8), and severe hypothermia (30°C) (n=8). Hypothermia was induced by surrounding the animal with ice, and VF was electrically induced. After 8 minutes of unsupported VF (no CPR), the swine were defibrillated (biphasic waveform) with successive shocks as needed and underwent CPR until resumption of spontaneous circulation or no response (≥10 minutes). First-shock defibrillation success was higher in the moderate hypothermia group (6 of 8 hypothermia versus 1 of 8 normothermia; *P*=0.04). The number of shocks needed for late defibrillation (≥1 minute after initial shock) was less in all 3 hypothermia groups compared with normothermia (all *P*<0.05). None of the 8 animals in the normothermia group achieved resumption of spontaneous circulation compared with 3 of 8 mild hypothermia (*P*=NS), 7 of 8 moderate hypothermia (*P*=0.001), and 5 of 8 severe hypothermia (*P*=0.03) animals. Coronary perfusion pressure during CPR was not different between the groups.

Conclusions.—When VF was induced in the setting of moderate or severe hypothermia, resuscitative measures were facilitated with significantly improved defibrillation success and resuscitation outcome. The beneficial effect of hypothermia was not due to alteration of coronary perfusion pressure, which suggests that changes in the mechanical, metabolic, or electrophysiological properties of the myocardium may be responsible.

► The most recent cardiac resuscitation guidelines from the American Heart Association summarize the major advances that have taken place in the treatment of cardiac arrest.[1] Innovative approaches, which include the use of mild-moderate hypothermia by using IV saline or an ice bath, appear to improve resuscitation outcomes.[2] Adjunctive use of isovolumic high-volume hemofiltration has also been used with hypothermia to improve the overall prognosis of cardiac resuscitation.[3]

Many survivors of resuscitation continue to exhibit both neurologic and cognitive sequelae,[4] and a coagulopathy similar to that seen with severe sepsis.[5]

During out-of-hospital resuscitation, chest compression is not performed half of the time, which seriously compromises outcome.[6] The new guidelines recommend an increased chest compression–to-breath ratio.[1]

W. H. Frishman, MD

References

1. ECC Committee, Subcommittees and Task Forces of the American Heart Association: 2005 American Heart Association Guidelines for Cardiopulmonary Resuscitation and Emergency Cardiovascular Care. *Circulation* 112(24 Suppl):IV1-IV203, 2005.
2. Kim F, Olsufka M, Carlbom D, et al: Pilot study of rapid infusion of 2L of 4°C normal saline for induction of mild hypothermia in hospitalized, comatose survivors of out-of-hospital cardiac arrest. *Circulation* 112:715-719, 2005.
3. Laurent I, Adrie C, Vinsonneau C, et al: High-volume hemofiltration after out-of-hospital cardiac arrest. A randomized study. *J Am Coll Cardiol* 46:432-437, 2005.
4. Lim C, Alexander MP, LaFleche G, et al: The neurological and cognitive sequelae of cardiac arrest. *Neurology* 63:1774-1778, 2004.
5. Adrie C, Monchi M, Laurent I, et al: Coagulopathy after successful cardiopulmonary resuscitation following cardiac arrest. *J Am Coll Cardiol* 46:21-28, 2005.
6. Wik L, Kramer-Johansen J, Myklebust H, et al: Quality of cardiopulmonary resuscitation during out-of-hospital cardiac arrest. *JAMA* 293:299-304, 2005.

PART SEVEN

THE DIGESTIVE SYSTEM

JAMIE S. BARKIN, MD

Introduction

The best practice of medicine is based on continuity in updating our knowledge base. My goal, therefore, is to focus on new and significant advances that will impact on our approach to patient care.

Eosinophilic esophagitis is increasingly recognized as causing the entire spectrum of symptoms of esophageal disease and accounts for medical refractory gastroesophageal reflux disease in some patients. Diagnosis and treatment are highlighted in the esophagus chapter.

Gastrointestinal mucosal side effects of clopidogrel (Plavix) are recurrent bleeding in patients who had ulcer bleeding; this is more so than in those who received aspirin and esomeprazole. The incidence of ulcer bleeding in patients treated with clopidogrel compared with patients receiving aspirin plus esomeprazole is discussed.

Travelers' diarrhea is becoming an increasing public health concern as more and more people are visiting exotic countries. This diarrhea may be complicated by the development of irritable bowel syndrome. Prevention and treatment approaches are highlighted.

Hopefully, my goal of providing new and beneficial information to the readers for the benefit of their patients has been met.

Jamie S. Barkin, MD

47 Esophagus

Early Heartburn Relief With Proton Pump Inhibitors: A Systematic Review and Meta-analysis of Clinical Trials

McQuaid KR, Laine L (Veterans Affairs Med Ctr, San Francisco; Univ of California San Francisco; Univ of Southern California, Los Angeles)

Clin Gastroenterol Hepatol 3:553-563, 2005 47–1

Background & Aims.—Proton pump inhibitors (PPIs) are often taken for short-term treatment of heartburn. We performed a systematic review of the efficacy of PPIs for heartburn relief within the first 1-2 days of therapy.

Methods.—Bibliographic databases were searched for clinical trials of PPIs in patients with heartburn that provided information about the proportion with heartburn relief at day 1-2. The sample size-weighted pooled proportions of patients with complete or sustained (7 consecutive days) relief were calculated. Meta-analyses of randomized comparisons of PPIs were also performed.

Results.—Eighteen trials met inclusion criteria. At day 1 of PPI therapy, complete 24-hour, daytime, nighttime, and sustained heartburn relief occurred in 0.31 (95% confidence interval [CI], 0.30-0.32), 0.49 (95% CI, 0.48-0.50), 0.55 (95% CI, 0.53-0.56), and 0.21 (95% CI, 0.20-0.22) of patients. Up to 37% of the heartburn relief achievable with 28 days of PPIs occurred on day 1. Placebo was significantly less effective than PPIs for 24-hour relief on day 1 (relative risk [RR], 0.41; 95% CI, 0.29-0.58), and single-dose PPI therapy was less effective than double-dose therapy (RR, 0.82; 95% CI, 0.74-0.92).

Conclusions.—Complete heartburn relief for the entire day occurs in approximately 30% of patients after their first PPI dose and 9% of patients after their first placebo (RR for relief on day 1 for placebo versus PPI was 0.41 [95% CI, 0.28-0.58]). Although PPIs might provide benefit from the first day of therapy, most patients will not have symptom relief with 1 or 2 days of PPI therapy.

► PPIs are the drug of choice for long-term heartburn management. In patients with occasional and/or intermittent symptoms, the use of antacids or histamine 2 receptor antagonists are utilized for acute symptom relief. McQuaid et al evaluated the benefits of PPIs for relief of heartburn in the first day or 2 of therapy. They found that acute PPI therapy yields complete heartburn relief in 31% of patients at day 1 versus 9% with placebo and 35% on day

2. While initial bioavailability varies among PPI drugs with repeated daily dosing of gastric acid inhibitor, as the authors emphasize, gastric acid inhibition increases during the first 5 days.

This review found that omeprazole was less effective than lansoprazole 30 mg and esomeprazole 40 mg for achieving sustained heartburn relief during the first day of treatment. The latter 2 drugs were equivalent after 1 day of therapy. Therefore, clinically it is reasonable to encourage patients to continue use of their usual non-PPI medications for the initial day of PPI use. My caveats with PPI use are:

1. Reinforce the need to take a PPI 15 to 30 minutes before breakfast and, if twice daily, 15 to 20 minutes before dinner.
2. All PPIs last less than 14 hours; therefore, patients with both day and night heartburn may need twice-daily dosing.
3. If symptoms of gastroesophageal reflux disease only occur nocturnally, use 1 dose of PPI before the evening meal.
4. The most common reason for failure, as with other chronically taken medication, is noncompliance.

J. S. Barkin, MD

Pill-Induced Esophageal Injury: Endoscopic Features and Clinical Outcomes

Abid S, Mumtaz K, Jafri W, et al (Aga Khan Univ , Karachi, Pakistan; Univ of Missouri, Kansas City)

Endoscopy 37:740-744, 2005 47–2

Background and Study Aims.—Pill-induced esophageal injury is a common but under-reported problem. The purpose of this study was to explore the clinical and endoscopic features, and the outcome of pill-related esophageal injury.

Patients and Methods.—Endoscopy records for the period from January 1997 to June 2003 were searched for reports of esophageal pathology. The records of patients with pill-induced esophageal injury were evaluated.

Results.—A total of 92 patients with pill-induced esophageal injury were identified (33 men, 59 women; mean age 59, range 25-87). Common symptoms were odynophagia (n = 69, 75%), chest pain (n = 55, 60%), vomiting (n = 53, 58%), dysphagia (n = 31, 33%), and hematemesis (n = 14, 15%). The endoscopic findings in the esophagus were: erythema in 76 patients (83%), erosions in 53 patients (58%), ulcers in 24 patients (26%), seven of which were "kissing" ulcers, esophageal ulcer with bleeding in 17 patients (18%), and esophageal strictures in seven patients (8%). The causative pills were nonsteroidal anti-inflammatory drugs in 38 patients (41%), tetracyclines in 20 patients (22%), potassium chloride tablets in nine patients (10%), alendronate in eight patients (9%), and other drugs in 17 patients (18%). Underlying diseases included diabetes in 60 patients (65%), ischemic heart disease in 39 patients (42%), and hypothyroidism in four patients

(4%). The mean hospital stay was 1.94 days; 14 patients (15%) required injection of epinephrine 1:10 000 to control bleeding; and two patients died.

Conclusions.—Pill-induced injury may present as erosions, kissing ulcers, and multiple small areas of ulceration with bleeding, mainly in the middle third of the esophagus. Advanced age, female gender, diabetes, and ischemic heart disease were common associations. The majority of patients made an uneventful recovery.

► In our patients with acute onset of retrosternal discomfort, odynophagia, and dysphagia, our primary diagnosis is gastroesophageal reflux disease. Our differential diagnoses must include infectious causes, ie, herpes simplex virus eosinophilic esophagitis and pill-induced esophageal injuries. There are a plethora of medications that can cause esophageal injury. These include some of the most common drugs that our patients ingest such as tetracycline, alendronate, quinidine, vitamin C, potassium chloride, ferrous sulfate, and erythromycin.

Abid et al reviewed those patients who came to endoscopy because of suspected pill-induced injury. Their history duration was less than 3 days with symptoms of heartburn, chest pain, dysphagia, and odynophagia. The population included 92 patients with probable pill-induced esophageal injury. Their symptoms included odynophagia in 72%, chest pain in 59%, vomiting in 58%, dysphagia in 33%, and hematemesis in 15%. Recall that this is the most severe group of patients as they were referred for endoscopy. Our therapeutic approach to most patients with mild to moderate symptoms is clinical recognition that pill-induced injury is the likely cause, stopping its intake, and prescribing a proton pump inhibitor and Xylocaine Viscous for symptom relief.

The most common etiologic agents in the authors' population were intake of nonsteroidal anti-inflammatory drugs, with or without aspirin, followed by the antibiotic group, commonly the tetracycline group including doxycycline and minocycline and use of ampicillin, and clarithromycin. Our role as physicians should focus on the prevention of pill-induced esophageal injury, reminding our patient to take the pill in the upright position and remain upright for 15 to 30 minutes, drinking at least 2 glasses of water with intake of a pill. In addition, we must focus on those patients who have a propensity for esophageal pill hang-up, ie, those with enlarged left ventricles and those with esophageal dysmotility—ie, scleroderma and diabetes mellitus—and remind them regarding preventing pill-induced esophageal injury.

J. S. Barkin, MD

Predictors of Heartburn During Sleep in a Large Prospective Cohort Study

Fass R, Quan SF, O'Connor GT, et al (Univ of Arizona, Tucson; Boston Univ; Johns Hopkins Univ, Baltimore, Md; et al)

Chest 127:1658-1666, 2005 47–3

Background and Aims.—Nocturnal gastroesophageal reflux, which may result in nocturnal heartburn, has been demonstrated to be associated with a more severe form of gastroesophageal reflux disease (GERD). The aim of this study was to determine the clinical predictors of heartburn during sleep in a large prospective cohort study.

Methods.—Study subjects were members of the parent cohorts from which the Sleep Heart Health Study (SHHS) recruited participants. SHHS is a multicenter, longitudinal, cohort study of the cardiovascular consequences of sleep-disordered breathing. As part of the recruitment process, parent cohort members completed a questionnaire that permitted an assessment of the relationships between heartburn during sleep, and patient demographics, sleep abnormalities, medical history, and social habits in nine community-based parent cohorts across the United States. All variables, significant at the $p < 0.05$ level, were included as independent variables in multivariate logistic regression models with heartburn during sleep status included as the dependent variable.

Results.—A total of 15,314 subjects completed the questions about heartburn during sleep, and of these, 3,806 subjects (24.9%) reported having this symptom. In four increasingly comprehensive multivariate models, increased body mass index (BMI), carbonated soft drink consumption, snoring and daytime sleepiness (Epworth sleepiness scale score), insomnia, hypertension, asthma, and usage of benzodiazepines were strong predictors of heartburn during sleep. In contrast, college education decreased the risk of reporting heartburn during sleep.

Conclusions.—Heartburn during sleep is very common in the general population. Reports of this type of symptom of GERD are strongly associated with increased BMI, carbonated soft drink consumption, snoring and daytime sleepiness, insomnia, hypertension, asthma, and usage of benzodiazepines. Overall, heartburn during sleep may be associated with sleep complaints and excessive daytime sleepiness.

► GERD occurs both at daytime and during sleep. Nocturnal reflux is more damaging to the esophagus as gravity, one of the protective factors for upright GERD, is negated during sleeping horizontally. Therefore, esophageal contact time of the erosive acid—and other, ie, bile injurious substances—with the esophageal mucosa is increased. In addition, loss of gravity may allow more proximal migration of the gastric contents into the pharynx, resulting in aspiration pneumonia, asthma, and laryngitis. Nocturnal reflux adversely affects quality of life, more so than daytime reflux.

Fass et al determined, in a prospective study, the demographic, social, and medical factors predictive of nocturnal heartburn. They found that college education was found to decrease the risk of reporting heartburn and, as the authors point out, may be a surrogate for differences in lifestyle and diet and more knowledge of the precipitating factors of GERD. The top 2 quartiles of BMI were associated with increased reports of heartburn during sleep (see Abstract 47–5 by Hampel et al). Dietary factors associated with nocturnal reflux were ingestion of carbonated soft drinks, which may be related to the acidic pH. They also found that snoring and sleepiness were associated with heartburn during sleep.

These symptoms are surrogate, as the authors point out, for the presence of obstructive sleep apnea. We should therefore counsel our patients with obstructive sleep apnea regarding the avoidance of behavior that predisposes to GERD, ie, development of obesity and alcohol intake and use of benzodiazepines, which decrease basal lower esophageal pressure and therefore increase the number of gastroesophageal events. This effect may be related to their use as a hypnotic.

It is important for us to attempt to eliminate the factors that predispose to nocturnal reflux in our patients. If successful, this will significantly improve their quality of life, which is adversely affected by sleep disturbance that occurs with nocturnal heartburn.

J. S. Barkin, MD

Association of Eosinophilic Inflammation With Esophageal Food Impaction in Adults

Desai TK, Stecevic V, Chang C-H, et al (Beaumont Hosp, Royal Oak, Mich; Massachusetts Gen Hosp, Boston; Harvard Med School, Boston)

Gastrointest Endosc 61:795-801, 2005 47–4

Introduction.—Esophageal food impaction is a common presentation of eosinophilic esophagitis. The prevalence of eosinophilic esophagitis among patients with food impaction is unknown. To address this, we evaluated clinicopathologic features of adults with food impaction.

Methods.—For a 3-year period, patients from a single, adult, community-based gastroenterology practice with esophageal food impaction were evaluated. Histories were assessed and esophageal biopsy specimens were evaluated by routine and immunohistochemical techniques.

Results.—Thirty-one patients with food impaction were evaluated. Seventeen of 31 patients had >20 eosinophils/high power field (HPF) without gender predilection. Thirteen of these 17 patients had been treated with proton pump inhibitors at the time biopsy specimens were obtained. Patients with >20 eosinophils/HPF were significantly younger (mean age 42 ± 4 years) than patients with <20 eosinophils/HPF (mean age 70 + 3 years). Superficial white exudates and eosinophilic microabscesses in the squamous epithelium were features observed only in patients with >20 eosinophils/HPF. Immunopathologic analysis demonstrated increased CD8 lymphocytes and major basic protein deposition in their squamous epithelium.

Conclusions.—More than half of patients with esophageal food impaction in a primary gastroenterology practice have >20 eosinophils/HPF. Based on clinicopathologic features, a significant number likely have eosinophilic esophagitis.

► Eosinophilic esophagitis has been increasingly recognized as causing the entire spectrum of symptoms of esophageal disease. These include symptoms of resistant gastroesophageal reflux disease (GERD) and range from esophageal-induced chest pain to odynophagia, dysphagia, and food impaction. Our goal in the latter group of patients is to eliminate the obstruction and does not routinely involve esophageal biopsy. However, food impaction occurs in >50% of patients affected with eosinophilic esophagitis.[1-3]

Our differential diagnosis of the causes of food impaction focus upon GERD and its complications including esophageal stricture and Schatzki's ring. However, we must realize that eosinophilic esophagitis must be considered in these patients and that mucosal esophageal biopsies need to be obtained in all patients with GERD-like symptoms and/or food impaction.

We as internists must insist that esophageal biopsies be obtained in all of our patients with this symptom, despite a normal-appearing esophageal mucosa, and if eosinophilia is present in the biopsy—especially >20%/pHPF—then the diagnosis is eosinophilic esophagitis. Eosinophilic esophagitis is associated with atopic allergy or peripheral eosinophilia. It can be suspected with the presence of esophageal symptoms and the associated symptoms. Its diagnosis requires histologic confirmation.

Interestingly, eosinophilic esophagitis can coexist with GERD, and patients may require therapy for GERD as well as eosinophilic esophagitis. The treatment of eosinophilic esophagitis is swallowed fluticasone. This disease is easily diagnosed and treated, but the key to diagnosis is obtaining an esophageal biopsy in all patients with esophageal symptoms.

J. S. Barkin, MD

References

1. Straumann A, Spichtin HP, Grize L, et al: Natural history of primary eosinophilic esophagitis: A follow-up of 30 adult patients for up to 11.5 years. *Gastroenterology* 125:1660-1669, 2003.
2. Potter JW, Saeian K, Staff D, et al: Eosinophilic esophagitis in adults: An emerging problem with unique esophageal features. *Gastrointest Endosc* 59:355-361, 2004.
3. Croese J, Fairley SK, Masson JW, et al: Clinical and endoscopic features of eosinophilic esophagitis in adults. *Gastrointest Endosc* 58:516-522, 2003.

Meta-analysis: Obesity and the Risk for Gastroesophageal Reflux Disease and Its Complications

Hampel H, Abraham NS, El-Serag HB (Baylor College of Medicine, Houston)

Ann Intern Med 143:199-211, 2005 47–5

Background.—The association of body mass index and gastroesophageal reflux disease (GERD), including its complications (esophagitis, Barrett esophagus, and esophageal adenocarcinoma), is unclear.

Purpose.—To conduct a systematic review and meta-analysis to estimate the magnitude and determinants of an association between obesity and GERD symptoms, erosive esophagitis, Barrett esophagus, and adenocarcinoma of the esophagus and of the gastric cardia.

Data Sources.—MEDLINE search between 1966 and October 2004 for published full studies.

Study Selection.—Studies that provided risk estimates and met criteria on defining exposure and reporting outcomes and sample size.

Data Extraction.—Two investigators independently performed standardized search and data abstraction. Unadjusted and adjusted odds ratios for individual outcomes were obtained or calculated for each study and were pooled by using a random-effects model.

Data Synthesis.—Nine studies examined the association of body mass index (BMI) with GERD symptoms. Six of these studies found statistically significant associations. Six of 7 studies found significant associations of BMI with erosive esophagitis, 6 of 7 found significant associations with esophageal adenocarcinoma, and 4 of 6 found significant associations with gastric cardia adenocarcinoma. In data from 8 studies, there was a trend toward a dose-response relationship with an increase in the pooled adjusted odds ratios for GERD symptoms of 1.43 (95% CI, 1.158 to 1.774) for BMI of 25 kg/m^2 to 30 kg/m^2 and 1.94 (CI, 1.468 to 2.566) for BMI greater than 30 kg/m^2. Similarly, the pooled adjusted odds ratios for esophageal adenocarcinoma for BMI of 25 kg/m^2 to 30 kg/m^2 and BMI greater than 30 kg/m^2 were 1.52 (CI, 1.147 to 2.009) and 2.78 (CI, 1.850 to 4.164), respectively.

Limitations.—Heterogeneity in the findings was present, although it was mostly in the magnitude of statistically significant positive associations. No studies in this review examined the association between Barrett esophagus and obesity.

Conclusion.—Obesity is associated with a statistically significant increase in the risk for GERD symptoms, erosive esophagitis, and esophageal adenocarcinoma. The risk for these disorders seems to progressively increase with increasing weight.

► Each day we are seeing more patients with complaints of heartburn, as it affects between 10% and 20% of adults in the United States. Their complications of GERD include erosive esophagitis, development of Barrett's esophagus, and esophageal adenocarcinoma. The known risk factors for GERD include smoking; dietary intake such as chocolate, mint, and large meals; and prescription medications such as theophylline and calcium channel blockers.

There may be a role in GERD of the declining prevalence of *Helicobacter pylori* infection and obesity, which has also increased in our population. The question is whether obesity is a risk factor for GERD.

Hampel et al performed a meta-analysis to summarize the association of obesity with GERD and its complications. They found that the risk for GERD symptoms and its complications of erosive esophagitis or esophageal adenocarcinoma increased with overweight or obesity, compared with normal BMI. They did not report a relationship of increased BMI with squamous cell carcinoma of the esophagus. The mechanism by which obesity causes GERD is unclear, as it does not seem to be related to extrinsic gastric compression with subsequent relaxation of the lower esophageal sphincter, nor the amount or type of dietary intake, although large meals induce more transient lower esophageal sphincter relaxation, which increases GERD. It is unclear if there is an increased prevalence of hiatal hernias in obese patients.

The authors found that overweight and obesity are risk factors for acid-related esophageal disease. Conversely, weight loss occurring after bariatric surgery for morbid obesity is associated with an improvement in GERD symptoms.[1,2] Therefore, I am not sure of why patients with GERD feel better with weight loss, whether it is their intake of smaller meals or less fatty foods or less chocolate is unclear. However, it is important for us as health care professionals to emphasize a role of weight loss in the management of GERD symptoms.

J. S. Barkin, MD

References

1. Frezza EE, Ikramuddin S, Gourash W, et al: Symptomatic improvement in gastroesophageal reflux disease (GERD) following laparoscopic Roux-en-Y gastric bypass. *Surg Endosc* 16:1027-1031, 2002.
2. Jones KB Jr: Roux-en-Y gastric bypass: An effective antireflux procedure in the less than morbidly obese. *Obese Surg* 8:35-38, 1998.

48 Stomach

A Nationwide Study of Mortality Associated With Hospital Admission Due to Severe Gastrointestinal Events and Those Associated With Nonsteroidal Antiinflammatory Drug Use

Lanas A, for the Investigators of the Asociación Española de Gastroenterología (AEG) (Hosp Clínico Zaragoza, Spain; et al)

Am J Gastroenterol 100:1685-1693, 2005 48–1

Background.—The worst outcome of gastrointestinal complications is death. Data regarding those associated with nonsteroidal antiinflammatory drug (NSAID) or aspirin use are scarce.

Aim.—To determine mortality associated with hospital admission due to major gastrointestinal (GI) events and NSAID/aspirin use.

Methods.—The study was based on actual count of deaths from two different data sets from 2001. Study 1 was carried out in 26 general hospitals serving 7,901,198 people. Study 2 used a database from 197 general hospitals, representative of the 269 hospitals in the Spanish National Health System. Information regarding gastrointestinal complications and deaths was obtained throughout the Minimum Basic Data Set (CIE-9-MC) provided by participating hospitals. Deaths attributed to NSAID/aspirin use were estimated on the basis of prospectively collected data from hospitals of study 1.

Results.—The incidence of hospital admission due to major GI events of the entire (upper and lower) gastrointestinal tract was 121.9 events/100,000 persons/year, but those related to the upper GI tract were six times more frequent. Mortality rate was 5.57% (95% CI=4.9-6.7), and 5.62% (95% CI=4.8-6.8) in study 1 and study 2, respectively. Death rate attributed to NSAID/aspirin use was between 21.0 and 24.8 cases/million people, respectively, or 15.3 deaths/100,000 NSAID/aspirin users. Up to one-third of all NSAID/aspirin deaths can be attributed to low-dose aspirin use.

Conclusion.—Mortality rates associated with either major upper or lower GI events are similar but upper GI events were more frequent. Deaths attributed to NSAID/ASA use were high but previous reports may have provided an overestimate and one-third of them can be due to low-dose aspirin use.

► GI bleeding, perforation, and obstruction are the severe complications of peptic ulcer disease (PUD). PUD and its complications are decreasing in incidence. However, the GI complications secondary to acetylsalicylic acid and NSAID intake are increasing. A United Kingdom model quantified the results of these complications and concluded that one in 1200 patients who were chronic NSAIDs users die.[1] We now realize that lower gastrointestinal events are associated with chronic NSAID intake, including an increase in risk of lower GI bleeding, perforation, obstruction, and diverticular disease.[2-4]

Lanas et al reported an observational study conducted in the Spanish National Health Service to provide an estimate of mortality of all GI events (upper and lower). They found that the proportion of deaths from either upper or lower GI complications were equal, although the actual number of deaths associated with upper GI complications were 6.2 times higher. The vast majority of persons who died as a result of GI complications were the elderly and patients with concomitant diseases.

This emphasizes the importance of prophylactic use of gastroprotection in those who are at greater risk for developing complications, including those aged 60 or greater; with concomitant disease, eg, congenital heart failure; use of anticoagulants; history of PUD, especially its complications of bleeding; and use of multiple NSAIDs. Unfortunately, we do not routinely follow these guidelines as shown. The proportion of NSAID users who should be on gastroprotective agents was only 40% in a US-VA population.

J. S. Barkin, MD

References

1. Tramer MR, Moore RA, Reynolds DJ, et al: Quantitative estimation of rare adverse events which follow a biological progression: A new model applied to chronic NSAID use. *Pain* 85:169-182, 2000.
2. Lanas A, Serrano P, Bajador E, et al: Evidence of aspirin use in both upper and lower gastrointestinal perforation. *Gastroenterology* 112:683-689, 1997.
3. Langman MJ, Morgan L, Worrall A: Use of anti-inflammatory drugs by patients admitted with small or large bowel perforations and hemorrhage. *BMJ* 290:347-349, 1985.
4. Wilcox CM, Alexander LN, Cotsonis GA, et al: Nonsteroidal anti-inflammatory drugs are associated with both upper and lower gastrointestinal bleeding. *Dig Dis Sci* 42:990-997, 1997.

Clopidogrel Versus Aspirin and Esomeprazole to Prevent Recurrent Ulcer Bleeding

Chan FKL, Ching JYL, Hung LCT, et al (Chinese Univ of Hong Kong; United Christian Hosp, Hong Kong)
N Engl J Med 352:238-244, 2005 48–2

Background.—Concurrent therapy with a proton-pump inhibitor is a standard treatment for patients receiving aspirin who are at risk for ulcer. Current U.S. guidelines also recommend clopidogrel for patients who have major gastrointestinal intolerance of aspirin. We compared clopidogrel with aspirin plus esomeprazole for the prevention of recurrent bleeding from ulcers in high-risk patients.

Methods.—We studied patients who took aspirin to prevent vascular diseases and who presented with ulcer bleeding. After the ulcers had healed, we randomly assigned patients who were negative for *Helicobacter pylori* to receive either 75 mg of clopidogrel daily plus esomeprazole placebo twice daily or 80 mg of aspirin daily plus 20 mg of esomeprazole twice daily for 12 months. The end point was recurrent ulcer bleeding.

Results.—We enrolled 320 patients (161 patients assigned to receive clopidogrel and 159 to receive aspirin plus esomeprazole). Recurrent ulcer bleeding occurred in 13 patients receiving clopidogrel and 1 receiving aspirin plus esomeprazole. The cumulative incidence of recurrent bleeding during the 12-month period was 8.6 percent (95 percent confidence interval, 4.1 to 13.1 percent) among patients who received clopidogrel and 0.7 percent (95 percent confidence interval, 0 to 2.0 percent) among those who received aspirin plus esomeprazole (difference, 7.9 percentage points; 95 percent confidence interval for the difference, 3.4 to 12.4; P=0.001).

Conclusions.—Among patients with a history of aspirin-induced ulcer bleeding whose ulcers had healed before they received the study treatment, aspirin plus esomeprazole was superior to clopidogrel in the prevention of recurrent ulcer bleeding. Our finding does not support the current recommendation that patients with major gastrointestinal intolerance of aspirin be given clopidogrel.

► Aspirin use is increasing in our graying population, both for cardiovascular prophylaxis and arthritis. Aspirin increases the risk of upper gastrointestinal bleeding, especially with increased acetylsalicylic acid dosing. Aspirin-induced bleeding can be prevented by concomitant use of proton pump inhibitors.[1-3] Clopidogrel is an alternative acute platelet function–inhibiting drug that does not induce ulcer and has been utilized to prevent ischemic events.

Chan et al reported a prospective, randomized, double-blind trial that compared 75 mg clopidogrel with 80 mg aspirin plus, twice daily, 20 mg of esomeprazole for patients whose ulcer had healed and who had previous aspirin-induced ulcer bleeding—the most important risk factor for subsequent GI bleeding. They found that the incidence of ulcer bleeding was 8.6% with clopidogrel in a 12-month period compared to only 0.7% of patients receiving aspirin plus esomeprazole. Their recurrent bleeding was a result of recurrent ulcers, with none having recurrent *Helicobacter pylori* infection.

The mechanism of bleeding from the recurrent ulcers (71.4%) in previously damaged gastric mucosa is possibly from suppressing release of platelet-derived growth factors.[4] As predicted, the cardiology guidelines that recommend clopidogrel for patients who are unable to take acetylsalicylic acid because of previous gastrointestinal intolerance need to be reviewed in view of the study's findings. Whether all patients who are at high risk for bleeding and who are on Plavix should be treated with a protein pump inhibitor remains to be determined. However, I would favor such an approach.

J. S. Barkin, MD

References

1. Lai KC, Lam SK, Chu KM, et al: Lansoprazole for the prevention of recurrences of ulcer complications from long-term low-dose aspirin use. *N Engl J Med* 346:2033-2038, 2002.
2. Garcia Rodriguez LA, Ruigomez A: Secondary prevention of upper gastrointestinal bleeding associated with maintenance acid-suppressing treatment in patients with peptic ulcer bleed. *Epidemiology* 10:228-232, 1999.
3. Chan FK, Chung SC, Suen BY, et al: Preventing recurrent upper gastrointestinal bleeding in patients with *Helicobacter pylori* infection who are taking low-dose aspirin or naproxen. *N Engl J Med* 344:967-973, 2001.
4. Ma L, Elliott SN, Cirino G, et al: Platelets modulate gastric ulcer healing: Role of endostatin and vascular endothelial growth factor release. *Proc Natl Acad Sci USA* 98:6470-6475, 2001.

49 Small Bowel

Post-Diarrhea Chronic Intestinal Symptoms and Irritable Bowel Syndrome in North American Travelers to Mexico

Okhuysen PC, Jiang ZD, Carlin L, et al (Univ of Texas, Houston; School of Public Health, Houston; St Luke's Episcopal Hosp, Houston; et al)

Am J Gastroenterol 99:1774-1778, 2004 49–1

Objectives.—Irritable bowel syndrome (IBS) has been reported to complicate bacterial diarrhea. Because of the frequency of international travel and the common occurrence of bacterial diarrhea, we studied the occurrence of chronic gastrointestinal complaints and post-diarrhea IBS in North U.S. travelers to Mexico.

Methods.—One hundred and sixty-nine healthy students were followed prospectively for 5 wk for the occurrence and etiology of diarrhea while studying for 5 wk in Mexico. Subjects recorded their symptoms during travel and completed a gastrointestinal symptom questionnaire 6 months after returning to the United States to determine the presence of IBS using the Rome II criteria.

Results.—Ninety-seven (57%) subjects returned a completed questionnaire. Sixty-one (63%) developed diarrhea while in Mexico, mostly due to enterotoxigenic and enteroaggregative *Escherichia coli.* Six months after travel the following chronic symptoms were reported: loose stools, abdominal pain, and fecal urgency in 17 (18%), 17 (18%), and 9 (9%) respectively. Of the 60 patients surveyed who had acquired diarrhea in Mexico, 7 (11%) met the criteria for IBS 6 months later of which 6 (10%) were newly diagnosed. No identified pathogen in the initial illness was associated with the development of IBS.

Conclusions.—Chronic gastrointestinal complaints including IBS are common in returning travelers having experienced diarrhea. Postinfectious complications of traveler's diarrhea require further study for etiology and strategy for prevention.

► IBS is defined by a conglomerate of symptoms, primarily abdominal pain occurring for 3 of 12 months nonconsecutively and a change in bowel habits with either constipation or diarrhea and associated visceral hypersensitivity. IBS is felt to be a motility disorder which may be complicated by small intestinal bacterial overgrowth. Its underlying pathogenesis is unclear. However, it is postulated that it is secondary to our inflammatory response from a GI infection.

The increasing amount of travel by our population to more exotic locations results in the frequent occurrence of travelers' diarrhea. Thus, postinfectious IBS is becoming a major public health concern. Okhuysen et al conducted a prospective study in North American travelers to Mexico and assessed their gastrointestinal symptoms by a questionnaire 6 months upon return to the United States. They found that travelers' diarrhea occurred in approximately two thirds, thus interfering with their travel, enjoyment, and/or itinerary. Of these, 10% reported the new onset of chronic symptoms compatible with IBS. This association has been reported previously after *Salmonella* infection and *Campylobacter jejuni* infections.

In the Okhuysen study, the authors found that patients who developed postinfectious IBS had more symptoms from their initial infectious episode than those that did not develop postinfectious IBS. The subsequent IBS may be related to persistent inflammation in the mucosa of the gastrointestinal tract and/or a resulting motility disturbance. A similar syndrome, postinfectious dyspepsia, and irritable bowel syndrome occurring 1 year after *Salmonella* gastroenteritis outbreak was reported by Mearin.[1] Thus, there is a postinfectious IBS syndrome that occurs after gastroenteritis, and we must be aware of its existence.

J. S. Barkin, MD

Reference

1. Mearin F, Perez-Oliveras M, Perello A, et al: Dyspepsia and irritable bowel syndrome after a *Salmonella* gastroenteritis outbreak: One-year follow-up cohort study. *Gastroenterology* 129:98-104, 2005.

A Randomized, Double-blind, Placebo-controlled Trial of Rifaximin to Prevent Travelers' Diarrhea

DuPont HL, Jiang Z-D, Okhuysen PC, et al (Univ of Texas-Houston; Baylor College of Medicine, Houston; St Luke's Episcopal Hosp, Houston; et al)
Ann Intern Med 142:805-812, 2005 49–2

Background.—Travelers' diarrhea causes substantial morbidity and postinfectious irritable bowel syndrome.

Objective.—To evaluate nonabsorbable rifaximin for prevention of travelers' diarrhea.

Design.—Randomized, double-blind, placebo-controlled clinical trial.

Setting.—Guadalajara, Mexico.

Participants.—U.S. students.

Intervention.—On arrival in Guadalajara, Mexico, 210 U.S. adults received rifaximin (200 mg/d, 200 mg twice daily, or 200 mg 3 times daily) or placebo for 2 weeks.

Measurements.—Participants were followed daily for 3 weeks for enteric disease and symptoms and daily for 5 weeks for drug side effects. Changes in intestinal coliform flora were studied.

Results.—Travelers' diarrhea developed in 14.74% of participants taking rifaximin and 53.70% of those taking placebo (rate ratio, 0.27 [95% CI, 0.17 to 0.43]). Rifaximin provided 72% and 77% protection against travelers' diarrhea and antibiotic-treated travelers' diarrhea, respectively ($P < 0.001$ for both), and all rifaximin doses were superior to placebo. In the groups that did not report travelers' diarrhea, rifaximin significantly reduced the occurrence of mild diarrhea ($P = 0.02$) and moderate and severe intestinal problems ($P = 0.009$ for pain or cramps; $P = 0.02$ for excessive gas). Rates of adverse events were comparable in the rifaximin and placebo groups. Minimal changes in coliform flora were found during rifaximin therapy.

Limitations.—Rifaximin safely prevented travelers' diarrhea in Mexico, where most cases are caused by diarrhea-producing *Escherichia coli*. A study is needed in Asia to determine whether rifaximin can prevent diarrhea caused by invasive bacterial pathogens.

Conclusions.—Rifaximin prevents travelers' diarrhea with minimal changes in fecal flora, and more liberal chemoprophylaxis against this disease should be considered. Future studies should evaluate whether rifaximin is effective in preventing postinfectious irritable bowel syndrome.

▶ The importance of travelers' diarrhea is related to one immediate effect on all patients. It is estimated that 40% of international travelers from industrialized countries to warm climates have diarrhea and, as we have discussed, the long-term development of irritable bowel symptoms and dyspepsia.[1] Travelers' diarrhea is becoming an increasing public health concern with increasing travelers to more exotic locations.

DuPont et al performed a randomized, double-blind, placebo-controlled study of students attending classes and eating in local homes in Guadalajara, Mexico. Rifaximin, a nonabsorbable antibiotic, was utilized as the active compound for prevention. Diarrhea during the first 2 weeks in Mexico developed in 23 of 156 (14.7%) rifaximin-treated versus 29 of 59 (53.7%) of those taking placebo. The authors emphasized that this protection rate of approximately 72% is similar to that with intake of absorbable antibiotics[2-4] and with no side effects. Obviously, this drug needs to be taken for the entire period that one is in the country and seems to prevent travelers' diarrhea caused by *Escherichia coli* and enteroaggregative *Escheichea coli*, which are the major pathogens causing travelers' diarrhea in Mexico.

Whether these results with intake of rifaximin 200 mg twice daily are generalized to travelers in other areas of the world where other pathogens are major causes of travelers' diarrhea remains to be determined. An initial approach to traveling patients must be their education on lifestyle change to avoid travelers' diarrhea.

Gorbach[5], in the accompanying editorial, points out the relationship between a number of dietary mistakes and risks of travelers' diarrhea. Whether all travelers should undergo prophylaxis is debatable, as overwhelmingly they are healthy individuals. Gorbach points out that we do not have safety data for this regime for the estimated 50 million travelers. Travelers who should undergo antibiotic prophylaxis, as pointed out by DuPont and Ericsson,[6] include business travelers and those with a history of frequent travelers' diarrhea and, possibly, those with chronic medical conditions. If prophylaxis is not utilized, we need to educate and prescribe medications to treat mild travelers' diarrhea with loperipimide or moderate disease by adding a fluoroquinolone.[5]

J. S. Barkin, MD

References

1. DuPont HL, Ericsson CD: Prevention and treatment of travelers' diarrhea. *N Engl J Med* 328:1821-1827, 1993.
2. DuPont HL, Evans DG, Rios N, et al: Prevention of travelers' diarrhea with trimethoprim-sulfamethoxazole. *Rev Infect Dis* 4:533-539, 1982.
3. Sack DA, Kaminsky DC, Sack RB, et al: Prophylactic doxycycline for travelers' diarrhea: Results of a prospective double-blind study of Peace Corps volunteers in Kenya. *N Engl J Med* 298:758-763, 1978.
4. Johnson PC, Ericsson CD, Morgan DR, et al: Lack of emergence of resistant fecal flora during successful prophylaxis of travelers' diarrhea with norfloxacin. *Antimicrob Agents Chemother* 30:671-674, 1986.
5. Gorbach SL: How to hit the runs for fifty million travelers at risk. *Ann Intern Med* 142:861-862, 2005
6. DuPont HL, Ericsson CD: Prevention and treatment of travelers' diarrhea. *N Engl J Med* 328:1821-1827, 1993.

Physician Awareness of Celiac Disease: A Need for Further Education

Zipser RD, Farid M, Baisch D, et al (Harbor-UCLA Med Ctr, Torrance, Calif; West Los Angeles VA Hosp; Celiac Disease Found, Studio City, Calif)

J Gen Intern Med 20:644-646, 2005 49–3

Background.—Celiac disease is a common disorder (up to 0.7%); however, it is uncommonly diagnosed in the United States.

Objective.—We sought to determine physician awareness of celiac disease.

Design.—Surveys completed by 2,440 (47%) of 5,191 patients in a support group were analyzed for frequency of diagnosis by physician specialties. Questionnaires were then sent to primary care physicians (PCPs) (n=132) in a southern California county to assess knowledge of celiac disease.

Results.—In patient surveys, only 11% were diagnosed by PCPs (internists and family physicians) versus 65% by gastroenterologists. Physician surveys (70% response) showed that only 35% of PCPs had ever diagnosed celiac disease. Almost all physicians (95%) knew of wheat intolerance, but few (32%) knew that onset of symptoms in adulthood is common. Physicians were well aware (90%) of diarrhea as a symptom, but fewer knew of common symptoms of irritable bowel syndrome (71%), chronic abdominal pain (67%), fatigue (54%), depression and irritability (24%) or of associations with diabetes (13%), anemia (45%) or osteoporosis (45%), or of diagnosis by endomysial antibody tests (44%).

Conclusions.—Lack of physician awareness of adult onset of symptoms, associated disorders, and use of serology testing may contribute to the underdiagnosis of celiac disease.

► Our understanding of celiac disease has recently changed from a disease that presents with diarrhea and malnutrition in childhood to one that has a wide spectrum of presentations which are seen daily by every internist. It is the most common hereditary gastrointestinal disease and occurs in 1 of 150 adults in the United States. Unfortunately, diagnosis is usually delayed for up to 10 years.[1,2]

Zipser et al presented a study on the awareness of the presentations and diagnosis of celiac disease among community physicians. The basis of their report was a nationwide celiac disease foundation database of celiac patients. They found that celiac disease is diagnosed primarily by gastroenterologists and uncommonly by PCPs. Diagnosis, when suspected, can be almost made with the use of blood tests using endomysial antibody (AEA) and tissue transglutaminase tests which have a sensitivity of 75% to 98%, a specificity of 96% to 100%, a positive predictive value of 98% to 100%, and a negative predictive value of 80% to 95%.[3,4]

The authors found that in the survey area, only one third of PCPs had ever diagnosed a patient with celiac disease, and only 44% were aware that AEA can be used for diagnosis. The authors emphasized that while the majority of patients first present with symptoms as adults, only one third of their PCPs were aware of this fact. In addition, and as we expected, while diarrhea was a common presentation, physicians were often not aware of its other presentations (Table).

TABLE.—Presentations of Celiac Disease

Diarrhea—May simulate irritable bowel syndrome
Fatigue
Depression
Iron deficiency anemia and folate deficiency anemia
Osteoporosis
Chronic abdominal pain
Muscle aches
Infertility and adverse fetal outcome
Liver disease—Elevated liver function tests secondary to autoimmune disease
Skin rash—Dermatitis herpetiformis
Undiagnosed celiac disease predisposed to malignant lymphoma, small bowel adenocarcinoma, oropharyngeal tumor

We have recognized predisposing conditions for celiac disease including diabetes mellitus, Sjögren's syndrome, and family history of celiac disease. Overall, celiac disease is underdiagnosed, according to the National Institutes of Health, and education about this disease, which emulates a wide variety of diseases, is mandatory In addition, serologic tests allow us to screen asymptomatic individuals.

Stevenson et al performed a prospective screening trial for the presence of celiac disease in osteoporotic and nonosteoporotic individuals.[5] Celiac disease in adults has low bone mineral density, which is increased by dietary therapy (gluten-free diet). This article's aim was to answer the question as to whether all adults with osteoporosis should be screened for celiac disease. The authors found a 2.9% prevalence of celiac disease in osteoporotic white women compared to 0.2% without osteoporosis.

The use of serologic tests, AEA, tissue transglutaminase and intestinal biopsy are the gold standard for diagnosing celiac disease. Immunoglobulin(Ig)-A–deficiency occurs in 1 in 500 individuals and they would have negative IgA, AEA, and tissue transglutaminase. Thus, it is important to obtain an IgA level when screening these individuals. The authors feel that all individuals with osteoporosis should undergo serologic screening for celiac disease.

J. S. Barkin, MD

References

1. Green PHR, Stavros SN, Panagi SG, et al: Characteristics of adult celiac disease in the USA: Results of a national survey. *Am J Gastroenterol* 96:126-131, 2001.
2. Zipser RD, Patel S, Yahya KZ, et al: Presentations of adult celiac disease in a nationwide patient support group. *Dig Dis Sci* 48:761-764, 2003.
3. Fasano A, Catassi C: Current approaches to diagnosis and treatment of celiac disease: An evolving spectrum: *Gastroenterology* 120:636-651, 2001.
4. Farrell RJ, Kelly CP: Current concepts: Celiac sprue. *N Engl J Med* 346:180-188, 2002.
5. Stenson WF, Newberry R, Lorenz R, et al: Increased prevalence of celiac disease and need for routine screening among patients with osteoporosis. *Arch Intern Med* 165:393-399, 2005.

Celiac Disease and Risk of Adverse Fetal Outcome: A Population-Based Cohort Study

Ludvigsson JF, Montgomery SM, Ekbom A (Örebro Univ, Sweden; Karolinska Inst, Stockholm; Örebro Univ, Linkoping, Sweden; et al)
Gastroenterology 129:454-463, 2005 49–4

Background & Aims.—Studies of maternal celiac disease (CD) and fetal outcome are inconsistent, and low statistical power is likely to have contributed to this inconsistency. We investigated the risk of adverse outcomes in women with CD diagnosed prior to pregnancy and in women who did not receive a diagnosis of CD until after the delivery.

Methods.—A national register-based cohort study restricted to women aged 15-44 years with singleton live born infants was used. We identified 2078 offspring to women who had received a diagnosis of CD (1964-2001): 1149 offspring to women diagnosed prior to birth and 929 offspring to women diagnosed after infant birth. Main outcome measures were: intrauterine growth retardation, low birth weight (<2500 g), very low birth weight (<1500 g), preterm birth (<37 gestational weeks), very preterm birth (<30 gestational weeks), and caesarean section.

Results.—Undiagnosed CD was associated with an increased risk of intrauterine growth retardation (OR = 1.62; 95% CI: 1.22-2.15), low birth weight (OR = 2.13; 95% CI: 1.66-2.75), very low birth weight (OR = 2.45; 95% CI: 1.35-4.43), preterm birth (OR = 1.71; 95% CI: 1.35-2.17), and caesarean section (OR = 1.82; 95% CI: 1.27-2.60). In contrast, a diagnosis of CD made before the birth was not associated with these adverse fetal outcomes.

Conclusions.—Undiagnosed maternal CD is a risk factor for unfavorable fetal outcomes, but the risks are reduced when CD has been diagnosed. CD diagnosed prior to pregnancy does not constitute as great a risk as undiagnosed CD.

► CD affects 1 of 100 pregnant women and maternal CD may influence fetal development. Ludvigsson et al reported the impact of CD in the mother and risk of adverse fetal outcome. They found that women with undiagnosed CD—which is likely, given our misdiagnosis (see Abstract 49–3)—were more likely to have a preterm birth, cesarean section, or an offspring with intrauterine growth retardation, low birth weight, or very low birth weight. However, in mothers previously diagnosed with CD, who had presumably been on a gluten-free diet, there was no association with adverse fetal outcomes. The authors advocate screening for CD among women of reproductive age, as 1% of young women may have CD[1-5] and treatment decreases pregnancy complications.[1-5]

J. S. Barkin, MD

References

1. Ivarsson A, Persson LA, Juto P, et al: High prevalence of undiagnosed celiac disease in adults: A Swedish population-based study. *J Intern Med* 245:63-68, 1999.
2. Bingley PJ, Williams AJ, Norcross AJ, et al: Undiagnosed celiac disease at age seven: Population-based prospective birth cohort study. *BMJ* 328:322-323, 2004.
3. Greco L, Veneziano A, Di Donato L, et al: Undiagnosed celiac disease does not appear to be associated with unfavorable outcome of pregnancy. *Gut* 53:149-151, 2004.
4. Maki M, Mustalahti K, Kokkonen J, et al: Prevalence of celiac disease among children in Finland. *N Engl J Med* 348:2517-2524, 2003.
5. Martinelli P, Troncone R, Paparo F, et al: Celiac disease and unfavorable outcome of pregnancy. *Gut* 46:332-335, 2000.

Anti-Tissue Transglutaminase Antibodies in Patients With Abnormal Liver Tests: Is It Always Coeliac Disease?

Iacono OL, Petta S, Venezia G, et al (Univ of Palermo, Italy)

Am J Gastroenterol 100:2472-2477, 2005 49–5

Background.—Coeliac disease (CD) is found in 5-10% of patients with chronically abnormal liver tests and no obvious cause of liver disease. In this population the efficacy of screening for CD by anti-tissue transglutaminase (anti-tTG) may be impaired by the high rate of positive anti-tTG found in chronic liver disease.

Aims.—To evaluate the prevalence of coeliac disease and the role of anti-tTG in patients with non-viral, non-autoimmune chronic and no obvious cause of liver damage.

Methods.—Out of 2,512 consecutive patients with abnormal liver tests, 168 (118 men, 50 women; mean age 40.7 ± 12.6 years) were defined, on the basis of clinical data and liver biopsy, as NAFLD or cryptogenic chronic hepatitis. All were tested by recombinant IgA and IgG anti-tissue transglutaminase. Patients with a positive serology underwent endoscopy with duodenal biopsies.

Results.—NAFLD was diagnosed in 121 patients, in 6 associated with cirrhosis, while 47 patients were considered as cryptogenic hepatitis in the absence of steatosis. Anti-tTG were positive in 20/168 patients (3 IgA alone; 11 IgG alone; 6 both IgA and IgG). Coeliac disease was found at endoscopy and confirmed by histopathology only in the 6 patients (3.6%) with both IgA and IgG anti-tTG positivity. Four of the patients with CD had NAFLD (3.3%), in 2 of them associated with cirrhosis; while 2 of those with cryptogenic hepatitis (4.2%) had CD.

Conclusions.—The prevalence of CD in patients with chronically abnormal liver tests of unexplained etiology is 4%, with no relation with the degree of liver steatosis. Screening should be done by testing for IgA and IgG antibodies and then evaluating by endoscopy and biopsy only patients positive for both.

► CD is the most common inherited gastrointestinal disease. Its prevalence ranges from 1 in 100 to 1 in 300.[1,2] We commonly think of CD through its primary manifestations in the gastrointestinal tract, ie, diarrhea and weight loss. However, we need to recall that it affects multiple organ systems (Table).

TABLE

Skin	• Dermatitis Herpetiformis
Neurologic	• Cerebral ataxia • Peripheral neuropathy
Hematologic	• Iron deficiency anemia
Hepatic	• Elevated LFTs • Primary biliary cirrhosis • Primary sclerosing cholangitis • Autoimmune hepatitis • Fatty liver • End-stage liver disease

There is an association between patients with CD and various forms of liver disease, and these patients may not have overt gastrointestinal symptoms. Iacono et al studied 2512 consecutive patients with abnormal liver tests to evaluate the prevalence of CD and to determine the role of anti-tTG in patients with nonviral, nonautoimmune chronic hepatitis who had no obvious cause of liver damage. They performed viral testing; an autoimmune panel including ANA, AMA, SMA, and LKM assay; metabolic evaluation of patients with a body mass index less than 30 kg/m^2, who had normal ceruloplasma, α1-antitrypsin, and transferrin saturation and who had no toxic exposure, including alcohol intake less than 20 g per day and no chronic drug use or work exposure to hepatotoxins.

They found that the most common reason for elevated liver function tests (LFTs) was nonalcoholic fatty liver disease in 121 patients, while 47 had cryptogenic hepatitis. Anti-tTG was positive in 2 of these 168 patients, but only confirmed by histopathology in 6. Thus, the authors found a 4% prevalence of CD in patients with chronically abnormal liver tests and unexplained etiology. In other studies, CD has been found in up to 9% of patients with elevated enzyme levels.[3,4]

The importance of testing for CD and then confirming it by duodenal biopsy in patients with unexplained elevation of liver test is that institution of a gluten-free diet leads to normalization of liver enzyme levels.[4] Therefore, we must screen for CD in patients with unexplained elevations of liver enzyme.

J. S. Barkin, MD

References

1. Volta U, Bellentani S, Bianchi FB, et al: High prevalence of coeliac disease in Italian general population. *Dig Dis Sci* 46:1500-1505, 2001.
2. Maki M, Mustalahti K, Kokkonen J, et al: Prevalence of coeliac disease among children in Finland. *N Engl J Med* 348:25172524, 2003.
3. Volta U, De Franceschi L, Lari F, et al: Coeliac disease hidden by cryptogenic hypertransaminasemia. *Lancet* 352:26-29, 1998
4. Bardella MT, Vecchi M, Conte D, et al: Chronic unexplained hypertransaminasemia may be caused by occult celiac disease. *Hepatology* 29:654-657, 1999.

50 Colon

Validation of a Clinical Prediction Rule for Severe Acute Lower Intestinal Bleeding

Strate LL, Saltzman JR, Ookubo R, et al (Brigham and Women's Hosp, Boston; Faulkner Hosp, Boston; Dana Farber Cancer Inst, Boston; et al)

Am J Gastroenterol 100:1821-1827, 2005 50–1

Objectives.—Acute lower intestinal bleeding is a heterogeneous disorder and identification of high-risk patients is challenging. We previously retrospectively identified predictors of severity in patients with acute lower intestinal bleeding. The aim of this study was to prospectively validate a clinical prediction rule for severe acute lower intestinal bleeding.

Methods.—This was a prospective, observational cohort study of consecutive patients admitted to an academic, tertiary care or a community-based teaching hospital for management of acute lower intestinal bleeding. Data were collected on seven previously identified predictors of severe bleeding: heart rate ≥ 100/min, systolic blood pressure ≤ 115 mmHg, syncope, nontender abdominal exam, rectal bleeding in the first 4 h of evaluation, aspirin use, and >2 comorbid conditions. Severe bleeding was defined as transfusion of ≥2 units of red blood cells, and/or a decrease in hematocrit of ≥20% in the first 24 h, and/or recurrent rectal bleeding after 24 h of stability (accompanied by a further decrease in hematocrit of ≥20%, and/or additional blood transfusions, and/or readmission for acute lower intestinal bleeding within 1 wk of discharge). Patients were stratified into 3 risk groups according to the previously developed prediction rule: low (no risk factors), moderate (1-3 risk factors), and high (>3 risk factors).

Results.—A total of 275 patients with acute lower intestinal bleeding were identified. The risk of severe bleeding in each risk category was similar in the validation and derivation cohorts (p values >0.05): low risk 6% versus 9%, moderate risk 43% versus 43%, and high risk 79% versus 84%. The area under the receiver operating characteristic curve was 0.754 for the validation cohort and 0.761 for the derivation cohort. The magnitude of the risk score was significantly correlated with major clinical outcomes including surgery, death, blood transfusions, and length of stay.

Conclusion.—We have developed and prospectively validated a clinical prediction rule for acute severe lower intestinal bleeding. This prediction rule could improve the triage of patients to appropriate levels of care and interventions, and guide a more standardized approach to acute lower intestinal bleeding.

► Acute lower intestinal bleeding is a common problem and may result from hemorrhoidal bleeding, with minor bleeding to life-threatening bleeding from diverticula or tumors. Strate et al, in a prospective observational cohort study, determined a clinical prediction role for patients with severe acute lower intestinal bleeding. They could stratify patients into 3 risk categories, depending on the presence of 3 of 7 risk factors (Table). Three of these 7 factors affect hemodynamic instability (hypotension, tachycardia, and syncope), and 1 reflects ongoing bleeding (bleeding within 4 hours of admission), and acetylsalicylic acid and nonsteroidal anti-inflammatory use are associated with diverticular hemorrhage.[1]

TABLE

Heart Rate	≥100/min
Systolic Blood Pressure	≤ 155 mm Hg
	Nontender abdominal examination
	Rectal bleeding during the first 4 hours of evaluation
Syncope	Acetylsalicylic acid use

A nontender abdominal examination reflects absence of transmural colitis. Patients with 3 or more factors had an 80% risk of severe bleeding; those with 1 to 3 had a 45% risk; and those with no risk factors had less than 10%. In patients with upper gastrointestinal bleeding, similar guidelines facilitate selection of high-risk patients for emergent intervention. In the high-risk patients, urgent colonoscopy with rapid preparation via a nasogastric tube or angiogram should be considered.

Urgent colonoscopy performed within 12 hours of admission and utilizing rapid purge has the ability to detect lesions, eg, bleeding diverticula that are not detected on routine colonoscopy. Endoscopic treatment of these bleeding lesions may result in decreased surgical and bleeding rates.[2-6] Thus, use of this simple scoring system will direct appropriate patient care.

J. S. Barkin, MD

References

1. Laine L, Connors LG, Reicin A, et al: Serious lower gastrointestinal clinical events with nonselective NSAID or coxib use. *Gastroenterology* 124:288-292, 2004.
2. Jensen DM, Machicado GA, Jutabha R, et al: Urgent colonoscopy for the diagnosis and treatment of severe diverticular hemorrhage. *N Engl J Med* 342:78-82, 2000.
3. Jensen DM, Machicado GA: Colonoscopy for diagnosis and treatment of severe lower gastrointestinal bleeding: Routine outcomes and cost analysis. *Gastrointest Endosc Clin North Am* 7:477-498, 1997.
4. Richter JM, Christensen MR, Kaplan LM, et al: Effectiveness of current technology in the diagnosis and management of lower gastrointestinal hemorrhage. *Gastrointest Endosc* 41:93-98, 1995.
5. Strate LL, Syngal S: Timing of colonoscopy: Impact on length of hospital stay in patients with acute lower intestinal bleeding. *Am J Gastroenterol* 98:317-322, 2003.
6. Jensen DM, Machicado GA: Diagnosis and treatment of severe hematochezia: The role of urgent colonoscopy after purge. *Gastroenterology* 95:1569-1574, 1988.

Increased Risk of Rectal Cancer After Prostate Radiation: A Population-Based Study

Baxter NN, Tepper JE, Durham SB, et al (Univ of Minnesota, Minneapolis; Univ of North Carolina, Chapel Hill)
Gastroenterology 128:819-824, 2005 50–2

Background & Aims.—Radiation therapy for prostate cancer has been associated with an increased rate of pelvic malignancies, particularly bladder cancer. The association between radiation therapy and colorectal cancer has not been established.

Methods.—We conducted a retrospective cohort study using Surveillance, Epidemiology, and End Results (SEER) registry data from 1973 through 1994. We focused on men with prostate cancer, but with no previous history of colorectal cancer, treated with either surgery or radiation who survived at least 5 years. We evaluated the effect of radiation on development of cancer for 3 sites: definitely irradiated sites (rectum), potentially irradiated sites (rectosigmoid, sigmoid, and cecum), and nonirradiated sites (the rest of the colon). Using a proportional hazards model, we evaluated the effect of radiation on development of colorectal cancer over time.

Results.—A total of 30,552 men received radiation, and 55,263 underwent surgery only. Colorectal cancers developed in 1437 patients: 267 in irradiated sites, 686 in potentially irradiated sites, and 484 in nonirradiated sites. Radiation was independently associated with development of cancer over time in irradiated sites but not in the remainder of the colon. The adjusted hazards ratio for development of rectal cancer was 1.7 for the radiation group, compared with the surgery-only group (95% CI: 1.4-2.2).

Conclusions.—We noted a significant increase in development of rectal cancer after radiation for prostate cancer. Radiation had no effect on development of cancer in the remainder of the colon, indicating that the effect is specific to directly irradiated tissue.

► Radiation-induced secondary malignancies include leukemias and thyroid and lung carcinoma.[1,2] Baxter et al have shown that prostate radiation is associated with an increased risk of rectal cancer. The magnitude of this problem is significant in that approximately one quarter of a million men will be diagnosed with nonmetastatic prostate carcinoma. Their therapy will include external beam radiation therapy or surgery. These patients have an 80% 10-year survival and thus will be alive within the period of development of solid organ neoplasms from radiation, which is 5 to 15 years.[3-7]

Prostate irradiation encompasses the urinary bladder, pelvis, and rectum. An increase in bladder carcinoma and sarcoma have previously been reported after prostate radiation.[8-10] Baxter's study is important because of its large population and 9-year follow-up period, thus including those at a risk for development of colorectal cancer and excluding those whose cancers develop within 5 years.

The risk for development of cancer was increased and, as Baxter relates, was similar to having a first-degree relative with colorectal cancer. This translates into an adjusted hazard ratio for rectal cancer of 1.7 in men surviving more than 5 years after radiation treatment of prostate cancer, compared with men with prostate cancer treated with surgery. This increased incidence was only evident in the colon within the irradiated site.

The limitation of this report is that it is a retrospective study and, as Grady points out, does not take into account the types and methods of radiation delivery, dosage, or fields of radiation.[11] Newer radiation techniques that limit extraneous radiation may change the risk of secondary malignancies.

How does this new information affect our approach to cancer screening in this group of patients? I agree that they should undergo colonoscopy beginning 5 years after completing their radiation and colonoscopy every 5 years thereafter. These high-risk patients should also be considered for colorectal chemoprevention with calcium and possibly acetylsalicylic acid/nonsteroidal anti-inflammatory drug intake.

J. S. Barkin, MD

References

1. Boice JD Jr, Day NE, Andersen A, et al: Second cancers following radiation treatment for cervical cancer: An international collaboration among cancer registries. *J Natl Cancer Inst* 74:955-975, 1985.
2. Neugut AI, Ahsan H, Robinson E, et al: Bladder carcinoma and other second malignancies after radiotherapy for prostate carcinoma. *Cancer* 79:1600-1604, 1997.
3. Brenner H: Long-term survival rates of cancer patients achieved by the end of the 20th century: A period analysis. *Lancet* 360:1131-1135. 2002.
4. Thompson DE, Mabuchi K, Ron E, et al: Cancer incidence in atomic bomb survivors. Part II: Solid tumors, 1958-1987. *Radiat Res* 137:S17-S67, 1994.
5. Jao SW, Beart RW Jr, Reiman HM, et al: Colon and anorectal cancer after pelvic irradiation. *Dis Colon Rectum* 30:953-958, 1987.
6. Boice JD Jr, Lubin JH: Occupational and environmental radiation and cancer. *Cancer Causes Control* 8:309-322, 1997.
7. Boice JD Jr: Cancer following irradiation in childhood and adolescence. *Med Pediatr Oncol* 1:29S-34S, 1996.
8. Brenner DJ, Curtis RE, Hall EJ, et al: Second malignancies in prostate carcinoma patients after radiotherapy compared with surgery. *Cancer* 88:398-408, 2000.
9. Neugut AI, Ahsan H, Robinson E, et al: Bladder carcinoma and other second malignancies after radiotherapy for prostate carcinoma. *Cancer* 79:1600-1604, 1997.
10. Pickles T, Phillips N: The risk of second malignancy in men with prostate cancer treated with or without radiation in British Columbia, 1984-2000. *Radiother Oncol* 65:145-151, 2002.
11. Grady WM, Russell K: Ionizing radiation and rectal cancer: Victims of our own success. *Gastroenterology* 128:1114-1129, 2005.

Meta-analysis: Computed Tomographic Colonoscopy

Mulhall BP, Veerappan GR, Jackson JL (Walter Reed Army Med Ctr, Washington, DC; Uniformed Services Univ, Washington, DC)

Ann Intern Med 142:635-650, 2005 50–3

Background.—Computed tomographic (CT) colonography, also called virtual colonoscopy, is an evolving technology under evaluation as a new method of screening for colorectal cancer. However, its performance as a test has varied widely across studies, and the reasons for these discrepancies are poorly defined.

Purpose.—To systematically review the test performance of CT colonography compared to colonoscopy or surgery and to assess variables that may affect test performance.

Data Sources.—The PubMed, MEDLINE, and EMBASE databases and the Cochrane Controlled Trials Register were searched for English-language articles published between January 1975 and February 2005.

Study Selection.—Prospective studies of adults undergoing CT colonography after full bowel preparation, with colonoscopy or surgery as the gold standard, were selected. Studies had to have used state-of-the-art technology, including at least a single-detector CT scanner with supine and prone positioning, insufflation of the colon with air or carbon dioxide, collimation smaller than 5 mm, and both 2-dimensional and 3-dimensional views during scan interpretation. The evaluators of the colonogram had to be unaware of the findings from use of the gold standard test.

Data Abstraction.—Data on sensitivity and specificity overall and for detection of polyps less than 6 mm, 6 to 9 mm, and greater than 9 mm in size were abstracted. Sensitivities and specificities weighted by sample size were calculated, and heterogeneity was explored by using stratified analyses and meta-regression.

Data Synthesis.—33 studies provided data on 6393 patients. The sensitivity of CT colonography was heterogeneous but improved as polyp size increased (48% [95% CI, 25% to 70%] for detection of polyps <6 mm, 70% [CI, 55% to 84%] for polyps 6 to 9 mm, and 85% [CI, 79% to 91%] for polyps >9 mm). Characteristics of the CT colonography scanner, including width of collimation, type of detector, and mode of imaging, explained some of this heterogeneity. In contrast, specificity was homogenous (92% [CI, 89% to 96%] for detection of polyps <6 mm, 93% [CI, 91% to 95%] for polyps 6 to 9 mm, and 97% [CI, 96% to 97%] for polyps >9 mm).

Limitations.—The studies differed widely, and the extractable variables explained only a small amount of the heterogeneity. In addition, only a few studies examined the newest CT colonography technology.

Conclusions.—Computed tomographic colonography is highly specific, but the range of reported sensitivities is wide. Patient or scanner characteristics do not fully account for this variability, but collimation, type of scanner, and mode of imaging explain some of the discrepancy. This heterogeneity raises concerns about consistency of performance and about technical variability. These issues must be resolved before CT colonography can be advocated for generalized screening for colorectal cancer.

▶ Colorectal cancer results in 60,000 deaths yearly. Unfortunately, colorectal cancer screening is only performed in approximately 40% of eligible patients 50 years or greater. Colorectal carcinoma screening allows early detection, which translates into diagnosis at early stages and 5-year survival rates exceeding 90%.[1,2]

The most recent radiologic modality that may have a role for colorectal carcinoma screening is CT colonoscopy, also known as virtual colonoscopy. The most recent technical advancement is multi-detector CT with single-breath hold and 3-dimensional reconstruction. CT colonoscopy requires full bowel cleansing and infiltration of air into the colon with creation of pneumocolon.[3]

Mulhall et al presented a review of the test performance of CT colonography computed with colonoscopy or surgery. They found that while CT colonography is highly specific for polyps 9 mm or larger, its sensitivities vary widely. Overall, therefore, it is a poor screening test. The technical factors that may explain this wide sensitivity range include scanners using different collimation widths overall. Recall that thinner is better and multiple detectors are more sensitive than single detectors and mode of imagery.

Other sources of false-negative studies, as the authors indicated, may include poor bowel distention, poor preparation, and perceptive or reading errors. Nine millimeter polyps can be consistently detected using CT colonography, which incorporates multi-detector scanners, low collimation, and an optional mode of imaging. Unfortunately, if these are not encompassed, high sensitivity cannot be assessed. I would agree with the authors that virtual colonoscopy presently cannot be recommended for general use. However, it may have a role for patients who refuse colonoscopy.

J. S. Barkin, MD

References

1. Roncucci L, Fante R, Losi L, et al: Survival for colon and rectal cancer in a population-based cancer registry. *Eur J Cancer* 32A:295-302, 1996.
2. Ponz de Leon M, Benatti P, Di Gregorio C, et al: Staging and survival of colorectal cancer: Are we making progress? The 14-year experience of a specialized cancer registry. *Dig Liver Dis* 32:312-317, 2000.
3. Johnson CD, Dachman AH: CT colonography: The next colon screening examination? *Radiology* 216:331-341, 2000.

Colonoscopic Screening of Average-Risk Women for Colorectal Neoplasia

Schoenfeld P, for the CONCeRN Study Investigators (niv of Michigan, Ann Arbor; et al)

N Engl J Med 352:2061-2068, 2005 50–4

Background.—Veterans Affairs (VA) Cooperative Study 380 showed that some advanced colorectal neoplasias (i.e., adenomas at least 1 cm in diameter, villous adenomas, adenomas with high-grade dysplasia, or cancer) in men would be missed with the use of flexible sigmoidoscopy but detected by colonoscopy. In a tandem study, we examined the yield of screening colonoscopy in women.

Methods.—To determine the prevalence and location of advanced neoplasia, we offered colonoscopy to consecutive asymptomatic women referred for colon-cancer screening. The diagnostic yield of flexible sigmoidoscopy was calculated by estimating the proportion of patients with advanced neoplasia whose lesions would have been identified if they had undergone flexible sigmoidoscopy alone. Lesions were considered detectable by flexible sigmoidoscopy if they were in the distal colon or if they were in the proximal colon in patients who had concurrent small adenomas in the distal colon, a finding that would have led to colonoscopy. The results were compared with the results from VA Cooperative Study 380 for age-matched men and women with negative fecal occult-blood tests and no family history of colon cancer.

Results.—Colonoscopy was complete in 1463 women, 230 of whom (15.7 percent) had a family history of colon cancer. Colonoscopy revealed advanced neoplasia in 72 women (4.9 percent). If flexible sigmoidoscopy alone had been performed, advanced neoplasia would have been detected in 1.7 percent of these women (25 of 1463) and missed in 3.2 percent (47 of 1463). Only 35.2 percent of women with advanced neoplasia would have had their lesions identified if they had undergone flexible sigmoidoscopy alone, as compared with 66.3 percent of matched men from VA Cooperative Study 380 ($P<0.001$).

Conclusions.—Colonoscopy may be the preferred method of screening for colorectal cancer in women.

► Colorectal cancer is a major health concern as it is the second most common cause of cancer deaths. Colorectal carcinoma is preventable if colon polyps are removed and can be found at an early curable stage if patients more than 50 years of age are screened. Unfortunately, only 40% of patients are being effectively screened.

Various screening methods for asymptomatic individuals are available, including Hemoccult stool testing, radiologic contrast studies, sigmoidoscopy, colonoscopy, and CT colonography. These modalities will be influenced by the distribution of the adenomas and carcinomas that are, in turn, influenced by gender.

Schoenfeld et al's study objective was to assess the predictive value of finding distal colon neoplasia with respect to advanced colonic neoplasia in the proximal colon of women. The objective was also to compare prevalence of advanced colonic neoplasia in age-matched low-risk men and women, thus determining if sigmoidoscopy is a "reasonable" alternative to colonoscopy in a symptomatic woman. The authors found that almost twice as many cases of advanced colorectal neoplasia (adenomas with advanced lesions 1 cm or greater, villous adenomas, adenomas with high-grade dysplasia or colon cancer) were detected in men as derived from the VA Cooperative Study.

The diagnostic yield of flexible sigmoidoscopy for advanced neoplasia is much lower among women than men, (35% vs 66%; $P < .001$). Therefore, there is a right-sided colon shift for advanced neoplasia in women as compared with men. Thus, sigmoidoscopy is not an acceptable screening modality in women aged 50 to 59 as it will miss two thirds of advanced lesions. Colonoscopy, therefore, is the preferred method for colorectal cancer screening.

J. S. Barkin, MD

Fecal DNA Versus Fecal Occult Blood for Colorectal-Cancer Screening in an Average-Risk Population

Imperiale TF, for the Colorectal Cancer Study Group (Indiana Univ, Indianapolis; et al)

N Engl J Med 351:2704-2714, 2004 50–5

Background.—Although fecal occult-blood testing is the only available noninvasive screening method that reduces the risk of death from colorectal cancer, it has limited sensitivity. We compared an approach that identifies abnormal DNA in stool samples with the Hemoccult II fecal occult-blood test in average-risk, asymptomatic persons 50 years of age or older.

Methods.—Eligible subjects submitted one stool specimen for DNA analysis, underwent standard Hemoccult II testing, and then underwent colonoscopy. Of 5486 subjects enrolled, 4404 completed all aspects of the study. A subgroup of 2507 subjects was analyzed, including all those with a diagnosis of invasive adenocarcinoma or advanced adenoma plus randomly chosen subjects with no polyps or minor polyps. The fecal DNA panel consisted of 21 mutations.

Results.—The fecal DNA panel detected 16 of 31 invasive cancers, whereas Hemoccult II identified 4 of 31 (51.6 percent vs. 12.9 percent, P=0.003). The DNA panel detected 29 of 71 invasive cancers plus adenomas with high-grade dysplasia, whereas Hemoccult II identified 10 of 71 (40.8 percent vs. 14.1 percent, P<0.001). Among 418 subjects with advanced neoplasia (defined as a tubular adenoma at least 1 cm in diameter, a polyp with a villous histologic appearance, a polyp with high-grade dysplasia, or cancer), the DNA panel was positive in 76 (18.2 percent), whereas Hemoccult II was positive in 45 (10.8 percent). Specificity in subjects with negative findings on colonoscopy was 94.4 percent for the fecal DNA panel and 95.2 percent for Hemoccult II.

Conclusions.—Although the majority of neoplastic lesions identified by colonoscopy were not detected by either noninvasive test, the multitarget analysis of fecal DNA detected a greater proportion of important colorectal neoplasia than did Hemoccult II without compromising specificity.

► One of the latest noninvasive screening methods for detecting colorectal cancer is fecal DNA which, in theory, detects tumor-specific products. This could be utilized to screen patients who are unwilling to undergo more sensitive but more invasive tests.

Colorectal cancers arise from chromosomal instability in 85% and in loss of genes involved in DNA-mismatch repair manifested by microsatellite instability in 15%. Imperiale et al performed a head-to-head comparison of a fecal-based multi-targeted DNA panel with Hemoccult II in patients 50 years or older with average risk for colorectal cancer, for detection of colorectal cancer alone or plus adenomas with high-grade dysplasia.

The authors reported that the sensitivity of the fecal DNA panel was 4 times that of Hemoccult II for invasive cancer and more than twice as sensitive for adenomas containing high-grade dysplasia. They found that the fecal DNA panel detected 18.2% versus 10.8% with Hemoccult II of advanced neoplasia.

The low sensitivity of both these noninvasive tests are unacceptable to me for use as a 1-time test for cancer. The take-home message is that screening for colorectal cancer is mostly determined by our efforts to inform our patients of its importance, and the use of colonoscopy or possibly CT colonography are the best modalities.

J. S. Barkin, MD

Long-term Use of Aspirin and Nonsteroidal Anti-inflammatory Drugs and Risk of Colorectal Cancer

Chan AT, Giovannucci EL, Meyerhardt JA, et al (Harvard Med School, Boston; Dana-Farber/Harvard Cancer Ctr, Boston; Harvard School of Public Health, Boston)

JAMA 294:914-923, 2005 50–6

Context.—Randomized trials of short-term aspirin use for prevention of recurrent colorectal adenoma have provided compelling evidence of a causal relationship between aspirin and colorectal neoplasia. However, data on long-term risk of colorectal cancer according to dose, timing, or duration of therapy with aspirin and other nonsteroidal anti-inflammatory drugs (NSAIDs) remain limited.

Objective.—To examine the influence of aspirin and NSAIDs in prevention of colorectal cancer.

Design, Setting, and Participants.—Prospective cohort study of 82 911 women enrolled in the Nurses' Health Study providing data on medication use biennially since 1980 and followed up through June 1, 2000.

Main Outcome Measure.—Incident colorectal cancer.

Results.—Over a 20-year period, we documented 962 cases of colorectal cancer. Among women who regularly used aspirin (≥standard [325-mg] tablets per week), the multivariate relative risk (RR) for colorectal cancer was 0.77 (95% confidence interval [CI], 0.67-0.88) compared with nonregular users. However, significant risk reduction was not observed until more than 10 years of use ($P \leq .001$ for trend). The benefit appeared related to dose: compared with women who reported no use, the multivariate RRs for cancer were 1.10 (95% CI, 0.92-1.31) for women who used 0.5 to 1.5 standard aspirin tablets per week, 0.89 (95% CI, 0.73-1.10) for 2 to 5 aspirin per week, 0.78 (95% CI, 0.62-0.97) for 6 to 14 aspirin per week, and 0.68 (95% CI, 0.49-0.95) for more than 14 aspirin per week ($P < .001$ for trend). Notably, women who used more than 14 aspirin per week for longer than 10 years in the past had a multivariate RR for cancer of 0.47 (95% CI, 0.31-0.71). A similar dose-response relationship was found for nonaspirin NSAIDs ($P = .007$ for trend). The incidence of reported major gastrointestinal bleeding events per 1000 person-years also appeared to be dose-related: 0.77 among women who denied any aspirin use; 1.07 for 0.5 to 1.5 standard aspirin tablets per week; 1.07 for 2 to 5 aspirin per week; 1.40 for 6 to 14 aspirin per week; and 1.57 for more than 14 aspirin per week.

Conclusions.—Regular, long-term aspirin use reduces risk of colorectal cancer. Nonaspirin NSAIDs appear to have a similar effect. However, a significant benefit of aspirin is not apparent until more than a decade of use, with maximal risk reduction at doses greater than 14 tablets per week. These results suggest that optimal chemoprevention for colorectal cancer requires long-term use of aspirin doses substantially higher than those recommended for prevention of cardiovascular disease, but the dose-related risk of gastrointestinal bleeding must also be considered.

► One of the goals of medicine today is prevention rather than treatment of patients with advanced diseases. This is especially relevant for prevention of colorectal carcinoma, which claims 60,000 lives annually. We have accepted that colorectal carcinomas mostly arise from colonic adenoma, and regular use of aspirin reduces the risk of recurrent adenoma in patients with a history of colorectal cancer or adenoma.[1-3] Thus, aspirin intake should decrease the risk of colorectal cancer; however, this is undocumented. Chan et al prospectively examined the influence of aspirin and NSAID use on the risk of sporadic colorectal cancer in a large cohort of women enrolled in the Nurses' Health Study. The study population encompassed 20 years of follow-up with 962 documented cases of colorectal carcinoma. This study found that long-term regular aspirin use (≥2 standard tablets per week) was associated with a significant reduction of colorectal carcinoma in the average-risk population. Interestingly, the most reduction occurred with intake of more than 14 standard tablets weekly and not until use was sustained for more than 10 years. Similar results were found with intake of NSAIDs in a dose-dependent manner. Chan et al demonstrated in this cohort study that the strongest reduction in risk of sporadic adenoma was also with more than 14 aspirin tablets weekly.[14] The dose of aspirin for prevention is important, as this and previous studies have shown no effect of aspirin with 100 mg 4 times daily. They had only a limited number of rectal cancers, and they did not observe any risk reduction. The authors observed an increased incidence of reported major gastrointestinal bleeding with increased aspirin dose.[5-8] This group that received a high dose of aspirin should be evaluated for concomitant risk factors for gastrointestinal bleeding and use of proton pump inhibitors for preventing bleeding.

J. S. Barkin, MD

References

1. Baron JA, Cole BF, Sandler RS, et al: A randomized trial of aspirin to prevent colorectal adenomas. *N Engl J Med* 348:891-899, 2003.
2. Sandler RS, Halabi S, Baron JA, et al: A randomized trial of aspirin to prevent colorectal adenomas in patients with previous colorectal cancer. *N Engl J Med* 348:883-890, 2003.
3. Benamouzig R, Deyra J, Martin A, et al: Daily soluble aspirin and prevention of colorectal adenoma recurrence: One-year results of the APACC trial. *Gastroenterology* 125:328-336, 2003.

4. Chan AT, Giovannucci EL, Schernhammer ES, et al: A prospective study of aspirin use and the risk of colorectal adenoma. *Ann Intern Med* 140:157-166, 2004.
5. Dutch TIA Trial Study Group: A comparison of two doses of aspirin (30 mg versus 283 mg daily) in patients after a transient ischemic attack or minor ischemic stroke. *N Engl J Med* 325:1261-1266, 1991.
6. Farrell B, Godwin J, Richards S, et al: The United Kingdom transient ischemic attack (UK-TIA) aspirin trial: Final results. *J Neurol Neurosurg Psychiatry* 54:1044-1054, 1991.
7. Roderick PJ, Wilkes HC, Meade TW: The gastrointestinal toxicity of aspirin: An overview of randomized control trials. *Br J Clin Pharmacol* 35:219-226, 1993.
8. Weil J, Colin-Jones D, Langman M, et al: Prophylactic aspirin and risk of peptic ulcer bleeding. *BMJ* 310:827-830, 1995.

Body Size and Composition and Colon Cancer Risk in Men

MacInnis RG, English DR, Hopper JL, et al (Cancer Council Victoria, Melbourne, Australia; Univ of Melbourne, Victoria, Australia; Monash Univ, Melbourne, Victoria, Australia)

Cancer Epidemiol Biomarkers Prev 13:553-559, 2004 50–7

Background.—Several studies of male colon cancer have found positive associations with body size and composition. It is uncertain whether this relationship is due to non-adipose mass, adipose mass, distribution of adipose mass such as central adiposity, or all three.

Methods.—In a prospective cohort study of men aged 27–75 at recruitment in 1990–1994, body measurements were taken by interviewers. Fat mass and fat-free mass (FFM) were estimated from bioelectrical impedance analysis. Waist circumference and waist-to-hips ratio (WHR) estimated central adiposity. Incident colon cancers were ascertained via the population cancer registry. Altogether, 16,556 men contributed 145,433 person-years and 153 colon cancers.

Results.—Rate ratios (RRs) comparing men in the fourth quartile with those in the first quartile were as follows: FFM 2.3 [95% confidence interval (CI) 1.4–3.7]; height 1.9 (95% CI 1.1–3.1); waist circumference 2.1 (95% CI 1.3–3.5); WHR 2.1 (95% CI 1.3–3.4); fat mass 1.8 (95% CI 1.1–3.0); and body mass index 1.7 (95% CI 1.1–2.8). When continuous measures of FFM and WHR were modeled together, the RR for FFM per 10 kg was 1.37 (95% CI 1.04–1.80) and the RR for WHR per 0.1 unit was 1.65 (95% CI 1.28–2.13). After adjustment for FFM and WHR, the RRs for fat mass and body mass index were no longer statistically significant.

Conclusion.—Male colon cancer appears to be related to body size and composition by two different pathways, via central adiposity and via non-adipose mass.

Type 2 Diabetes Mellitus and the Risk of Colorectal Cancer

Yang Y-X, Hennessy S, Lewis JD (Univ of Pennsylvania School of Medicine, Philadelphia)

Clin Gastroenterol Hepatol 3:587-594, 2005 50–8

Background & Aims.—Type 2 diabetes mellitus might increase the risk of colorectal cancer on the basis of chronic hyperinsulinemia and hyperglycemia. However, epidemiologic evidence for this association is inconclusive. We conducted a population-based study to clarify this association.

Methods.—We conducted a case-control study in the United Kingdom General Practice Research Database. Cases included all patients with incident colorectal cancer diagnoses (n = 10,447). Up to 10 control subjects were selected for each case, matching on year of birth, enrollment date, and duration of database follow-up. The exposure of interest was type 2 diabetes mellitus. Odds ratios (ORs) were calculated by using conditional logistic regression.

Results.—A prior diagnosis of type 2 diabetes mellitus was associated with a modestly increased risk of colorectal cancer (OR, 1.42; 95% confidence interval [CI], 1.25–1.62). The association between type 2 diabetes mellitus and colorectal cancer was observed in both men (OR, 1.36; 95% CI, 1.16–1.61) and women (OR, 1.38; 95% CI, 1.14–1.67). The risk increase was observed in both colon (OR, 1.45; 95% CI, 1.25–1.70) and rectal (OR, 1.34; 95% CI, 1.08–1.68) cancers.

Conclusions.—Type 2 diabetes mellitus is associated with an increased risk of colorectal cancer. The risk increase is present in both sexes, as well as in both colonic and rectal cancers.

► Increased body mass index (BMI) is positively associated with colon cancer. BMI measures weight independent of height but does not distinguish between adipose and nonadipose body mass.[1] This relationship, therefore, could be due to any one or combination of adipose/nonadipose body mass or distribution of adipose mass, that is, central obesity. MacInnis et al (Abstract 50–8) prospectively assessed the relationship between estimates of body size and the composition and risk of colon cancer. They found an approximate 2-fold greater risk of male colon cancer with increase for height, weight, waist circumference, and waist-to-height rate as well as for FFM. Modeling confirmed FFM nonadipose mass WHR (central obesity). The previous association of colorectal cancer with BMI was not present once the data were adjusted for WHR. They found that the risk was most pronounced in men with a waist circumference that equaled or exceeded their hip circumference, thus emphasizing the importance of central obesity. Increased plasma insulin level results especially from central obesity.[2] Physical activity should be stressed in men to avoid or reduce central adiposity and increase in insulin sensitivity.[2] If the effects of central obesity are mediated by hyperinsulinemia, then the presence of type 2 diabetes mellitus, which is characterized by chronic hyperinsulinemia and hyperglycemia, could increase the risk of colorectal cancer.

Yang et al (Abstract 50–9) clarified whether prior diagnosis of type 2 diabetes mellitus is associated with higher incidents of colorectal cancer. They reported that type 2 diabetes mellitus in both sexes is associated with a modestly increased risk for subsequent development of colorectal cancer. This substantiated the finding of the Nurses' Health Study, which reported a 43% increase in women with type 2 diabetes mellitus for colon, not rectal, cancer.[3] There is a report of a strong correlation between glycosylated hemoglobin levels and increased colorectal cancer risk.[4] The positive association between type 2 diabetes mellitus and colorectal cancer was strongest for those within the initial 8 years after diagnosis of type 2 diabetes mellitus. Subsequently over time, in those 2 populations the risk of colorectal cancer became comparable. Thus, we must now add central obesity and type 2 diabetes mellitus to those populations with an increased risk of colorectal cancer, which includes those (1) with a positive family history of colorectal cancer; (2) with a genetic syndrome such as familial adenomatous polyposis, Gardner's syndrome, or Peutz-Jeghers syndrome; (3) with a personal history of colorectal cancer or colonic polyps; and (4) who are black. As the American College of Gastroenterology has shown, African Americans have the highest incidence of colorectal cancer of any racial or ethnic group and, when compared with whites, have a younger mean age at diagnosis.[5]

J. S. Barkin, MD

References

1. Roubenoff R: Applications of bioelectrical impedance analysis for body composition to epidemiologic studies. *Am J Clin Nutr* D64:459S-462S, 1996.
2. Vainio H, Bianchini F, editors: *IARC Handbooks of cancer prevention, volume 6: Weight control and physical activity,* Lyon, France, 2002, IARC Press.
3. Hu FB, Mason JE, Liu S, et al: Prospective study of adult-onset diabetes mellitus (type II) and risk of colorectal cancer in women. *J Natl Cancer Inst* 91:542-547, 1999.
4. Khaw KT, Wareham N, Bingham S, et al: Preliminary communication; glycated hemoglobin, diabetes, and incident of colorectal cancer in men and women: a prospective analysis from the European Prospective Investigation into Cancer, Norfolk Study. *Cancer Epidemiol Biomarkers Prev* 13:915-919, 2004.
5. Agrawal S, Bhupinderjit A, Bhutani MS, et al: Colorectal cancer in African-Americans. *Am J Gastroenterol* 100:515-523, 2005.

Magnesium Intake in Relation to Risk of Colorectal Cancer in Women

Larsson SC, Bergkvist L, Wolk A (Karolinska Institutet, Stockholm; Central Hosp, Västerås, Sweden)

JAMA 293:86-89, 2005 50–9

Context.—Animal studies have suggested that dietary magnesium may play a role in the prevention of colorectal cancer, but data in humans are lacking.

Objective.—To evaluate the hypothesis that a high magnesium intake reduces the risk of colorectal cancer in women.

Design, Setting, and Participants.—The Swedish Mammography Cohort, a population-based prospective cohort of 61,433 women aged 40 to 75 years without previous diagnosis of cancer at baseline from 1987 to 1990.

Main Outcome Measure.—Incident invasive colorectal cancer.

Results.—During a mean of 14.8 years (911 042 person-years) of follow-up, 805 incident colorectal cancer cases were diagnosed. After adjustment for potential confounders, we observed an inverse association of magnesium intake with the risk of colorectal cancer (*P* for trend = .006). Compared with women in the lowest quintile of magnesium intake, the multivariate rate ratio (RR) was 0.59 (95% confidence interval [CI], 0.40-0.87) for those in the highest quintile. The inverse association was observed for both colon (RR, 0.66; 95% CI, 0.41-1.07) and rectal cancer (RR, 0.45; 95% CI, 0.22-0.89).

Conclusion.—This population-based prospective study suggests that a high magnesium intake may reduce the occurrence of colorectal cancer in women.

► If divalent calcium intake decreases the risk of colorectal cancer (CRC), could magnesium intake have similar effects? Larsson et al conducted a prospective analysis of magnesium intake in relation to the incidence of CRC. Magnesium, as the authors indicated, is essential for maintenance of genomic stability and for DNA repair in modulating cell proliferation.[1] In addition, magnesium increases insulin sensitivity in healthy individuals and patients with type 2 diabetes mellitus. The latter group has an increased risk for CRC.[2,3] The authors found a significant inverse dose-response relationship between magnesium intake and risk of CRC, thus suggesting that in women high magnesium intake may reduce the risk of CRC. We should therefore emphasize intake of a healthy diet consisting of fruits, vegetables, whole-grain foods, and beans. Perhaps our mothers were always correct regarding our diet.

J. S. Barkin, MD

References

1. Hartwig A: Role of magnesium in genomic stability. *Mutat Res* 475:113-121, 2001.
2. Paolisso G, Sgambato S, Pizza G, et al: Improved insulin response and action by chronic magnesium administration in aged NIDDM subjects. *Diabetes Care* 12:265-269, 1989.
3. Sjogren A, Floren CH, Nilsson A: Oral administration of magnesium hydroxide to subjects with insulin dependent-diabetes mellitus. Effects of magnesium and potassium levels and on insulin requirements. *Magnesium* 7:117-122, 1988.

Calcium From Diet and Supplements Is Associated With Reduced Risk of Colorectal Cancer in a Prospective Cohort of Women

Flood A, Peters U, Chatterjee N, et al (Univ of Minnesota, Minneapolis; Natl Cancer Inst, Bethesda, Md)

Cancer Epidemiol Biomarkers Prev 14:126-32, 2005 50–10

Introduction.—We investigated the association between calcium intake and colorectal cancer in a prospective cohort of 45,354 women without a history of colorectal cancer who successfully completed a 62-item National Cancer Institute/Block food-frequency questionnaire. Women were followed for an average of 8.5 years, during which time 482 subjects developed colorectal cancer. We used Cox proportional hazards models, with age as the underlying time metric, to estimate risk of colorectal cancer. Cut points between quintiles of energy-adjusted dietary calcium were 412, 529, 656, and 831 mg/day. We created categories for calcium from supplements as follows: 0 mg/day (n = 25,441), 0 to 400 mg/day (n = 9,452), 401 to 800 mg/day (n = 4,176), and >800 mg/day (n = 6,285). Risk ratios and confidence intervals (95% CI) for increasing quintiles of dietary calcium relative to the lowest quintile were 0.79 (0.60-1.04), 0.77 (0.59-1.02), 0.78 (0.60-1.03), and 0.74 (0.56-0.98), $P_{trend} = 0.05$. For increasing categories of calcium from supplements, the risk ratios (and 95% CI) relative to no supplement use were 1.08 (0.87-1.34), 0.96 (0.70-1.32), and 0.76 (0.56-1.02), $P_{trend} = 0.09$. Simultaneously high consumption of calcium from diet and calcium from supplements resulted in even further risk reduction, RR = 0.54 (95% CI, 0.37-0.79) compared with low consumption of both sources of calcium. These data indicate that a difference of < 400 to > 800 mg of calcium per day was associated with an approximately 25% reduction in risk of colorectal cancer, and this reduction in risk occurred regardless of the source of the calcium (i.e., diet or supplements).

► Calcium intake reduces the rate of colonic adenoma recurrence over 3 to 4 years of follow-up in patients with a history of colonic adenomas.[1,2] The potential mechanisms of calcium intake and possible prevention of CRC may be caused by its effects on secondary bile acids or on cell differentiation and apoptosis. Flood et al presented a prospective study of diet and CRC in a cohort of women selected from participants during their breast cancer screening program. This study found that a high intake of dietary and supplemental calcium—greater than 800 mg of calcium every day—resulted in an approximately 25% decrease in risk. Risk reduction was higher (approximately 45%), with simultaneous high consumption of both dietary (>830) and supplemental (> 800) calcium. The effect of both sources of calcium suggests that it was the calcium per se, not the dairy food, that accounted for the risk reduction. Peters et al[3] compared supplemental and dietary calcium intakes of approximately 4000 participants with distal colon adenomas, with calcium intake of approximately 3500 sigmoidoscopy-negative control participants. They found that high calcium (>1200 mg daily) resulted in a 27% decrease in adenoma risk. Thus, we should encourage calcium intake in all our patients, but especially those who are in a high-risk group for development of CRC.

J. S. Barkin, MD

References

1. Baron JA, Beach M, Mandel JS, et al: Calcium supplements for the prevention of colorectal adenoma. Calcium Polyp Prevention Study Group. *N Engl J Med* 340:101-107, 1999.
2. Bonithon-Kopp C, Kronborg O, Giacosa A, et al: Calcium and fiber supplementation and prevention of colorectal adenoma recurrence: A randomized intervention trial. European Cancer Prevention Organization Study Group. *Lancet* 356:1300-1306, 2000.
3. Peters U, Chatterjee N, McGlynn KA, et al: Calcium intake and colorectal adenoma in a US colorectal cancer early detection program. *J Clin Nutr* 80:1358-1365, 2004.

Computed Tomographic Colonography Without Cathartic Preparation for the Detection of Colorectal Polyps

Iannaccone R, Laghi A, Catalano C, et al (Univ of Rome, La Sapienza; Osaka Univ, Japan; Catholic Univ S Cuore, Rome)
Gastroenterology 127:1300-1311, 2004 50–11

Background & Aims.—We prospectively compared the performance of low-dose multidetector computed tomographic colonography (CTC) without cathartic preparation with that of colonoscopy for the detection of colorectal polyps.

Methods.—A total of 203 patients underwent low-dose CTC without cathartic preparation followed by colonoscopy. Before CTC, fecal tagging was achieved by adding diatrizoate meglumine and diatrizoate sodium to regular meals. No subtraction of tagged feces was performed. Colonoscopy was performed 3–7 days after CTC. Three readers interpreted the CTC examinations separately and independently using a primary 2-dimensional approach using multiplanar reconstructions and 3-dimensional images for further characterization. Colonoscopy with segmental unblinding was used as reference standard. The sensitivity of CTC was calculated both on a per-polyp and a per-patient basis. For the latter, specificity, positive predictive values, and negative predictive values were also calculated.

Results.—CTC had an average sensitivity of 95.5% (95% confidence interval [CI], 92.1%–99%) for the identification of colorectal polyps ≥8 mm. With regard to per-patient analysis, CTC yielded an average sensitivity of 89.9% (95% CI, 86%–93.7%), an average specificity of 92.2% (95% CI, 89.5%–94.9%), an average positive predictive value of 88% (95% CI, 83.3%–91.5%), and an average negative predictive value of 93.5% (95% CI, 90.9%–96%). Interobserver agreement was high on a per-polyp basis (κ statistic range, .61–.74) and high to excellent on a per-patient basis (κ statistic range, .79–.91).

Conclusions.—Low-dose multidetector CTC without cathartic preparation compares favorably with colonoscopy for the detection of colorectal polyps.

► Colonoscopy and CT colonography (CTC) require bowel preparation. An aversion to bowel preparation may deter patients from entering a screening program. Therefore, the possibility of labeling the stool during CTC allows differentiation of fecal material from colonic mucosa negates the need for bowel preparation cleansing for CTC. Iannaccone et al prospectively compared the performance of low-dose multidetector CTC without bowel cathartic preparation with that of optical colonoscopy for detection of colorectal polyps. They found that low-dose multidetector CTC without cathartic bowel preparation detected colorectal polyps ≥8 mm with an average sensitivity of 95.5%. The performance of CTC is substantially decreased for smaller polyp detection. Labeling of fecal material decreases false-positive and false-negative errors related to fecal material with an increase in specificity. This study utilized hyoscine-*N*-butylbromide, which is unavailable in the United States; therefore, before embracing this new technique, a US study with a similar drug needs to be performed. In addition, ingestion of the fecal preparation resulted in diarrhea in 6.4% of patients, another similarity to preparation for optical colonoscopy. The population questionnaire was filled out after the optical colonoscopy and, as the authors point out, there may be bias in favor of the fecal tagging regime versus bowel preparation. This preliminary study may be an initial step to a new advance in CTC for screening.

J. S. Barkin, MD

51 Pancreas

Cigarette Smoking Accelerates Progression of Alcoholic Chronic Pancreatitis

Maisonneuve P, Lowenfels AB, Müllhaupt B, et al (European Inst of Oncology, Milan, Italy; New York Med College, Valhalla; Univ Hosp, Zurich, Switzerland; et al)

Gut 54:510-514, 2004 51–1

Background.—Smoking is a recognised risk factor for pancreatic cancer and has been associated with chronic pancreatitis and also with type II diabetes.

Aims.—The aim of this study was to investigate the effect of tobacco on the age of diagnosis of pancreatitis and progression of disease, as measured by the appearance of calcification and diabetes.

Patients.—We used data from a retrospective cohort of 934 patients with chronic alcoholic pancreatitis where information on smoking was available, who were diagnosed and followed in clinical centres in five countries.

Methods.—We compared age at diagnosis of pancreatitis in smokers versus non-smokers, and used the Cox proportional hazards model to evaluate the effects of tobacco on the development of calcification and diabetes, after adjustment for age, sex, centre, and alcohol consumption.

Results.—The diagnosis of pancreatitis was made, on average, 4.7 years earlier in smokers than in non-smokers ($p = 0.001$). Tobacco smoking increased significantly the risk of pancreatic calcifications (hazard ratio (HR) 4.9 (95% confidence interval (CI) 2.3–10.5) for smokers *v* non-smokers) and to a lesser extent the risk of diabetes (HR 2.3 (95% CI 1.2–4.2)) during the course of pancreatitis.

Conclusions.—In this study, tobacco smoking was associated with earlier diagnosis of chronic alcoholic pancreatitis and with the appearance of calcifications and diabetes, independent of alcohol consumption.

▶ Our concepts of diagnosing chronic pancreatitis are evolving. Initially, as clinicians need to, we distinguished the causes of pancreatic insufficiency, which include chronic pancreatitis, usually from alcohol intake, pancreatic surgery with resection, interruption of the vagus nerve, which stimulates the pancreas, and radiation to the abdomen for lymphoma. The most recently described cause of pancreatic insufficiency is autoimmune chronic pancreatitis, whose clinical presentation emulates pancreatic cancer. Our role in treating patients with chronic pancreatitis is to treat the pancreatic insufficiency with pancreatic enzyme and to inhibit its progression. Therefore, for the latter we emphasized the importance of patients discontinuing toxic ingestion if alcoholic pancreatitis is present. Maisonneuve et al reported on the role of tobacco in the progression of alcoholic pancreatitis. We know that cigarette smoking is an important environmental etiological agent of pancreatic carcinoma. In addition, we have learned that chronic pancreatitis predisposes to the development of pancreatic cancer. It is uncertain as to whether this is caused by chronic pancreatitis alone or is compounded by smoking. This multicenter study shows that smoking contributes to deterioration of chronic pancreatitis as measured by the appearance of calcification and diabetes. Calcification in other organs, such as the coronary arteries, has previously been associated with cigarette smoking. Cigarette smoking increased the risk of impaired fasting glucose and may cause insulin resistance in peripheral tissues. The authors found that exposure to tobacco smoking was associated with an earlier diagnosis of chronic alcoholic pancreatitis by approximately 5 years and predisposed to development of both calcification and diabetes. Thus, we need to emphasize to our patients with chronic pancreatitis that they should make a tough choice to stop cigarette smoking. This will decrease the progression of their chronic pancreatitis; whether it will decrease their risk of developing pancreatic cancer is unknown.

J. S. Barkin, MD

Probability of Pancreatic Cancer Following Diabetes: A Population-Based Study

Chari ST, Leibson CL, Rabe KG, et al (Mayo Clinic, Rochester, Minn)
Gastroenterology 129:504-511, 2005 51–2

Background & Aims.—Although diabetes occurs frequently in pancreatic cancer, the value of new-onset diabetes as a marker of underlying pancreatic cancer is unknown.

Methods.—We assembled a population-based cohort of 2122 Rochester, Minnesota, residents age ≥50 years who first met standardized criteria for diabetes between January 1, 1950, and December 31, 1994, and identified those who developed pancreatic cancer within 3 years of meeting criteria for diabetes. We compared observed rates of pancreatic cancer with expected rates based on the Iowa Surveillance Epidemiology and End Results registry. In a nested case control study, we compared body mass index (BMI) and smoking status in diabetes subjects with and without pancreatic cancer.

Results.—Of 2122 diabetic subjects, 18 (0.85%) were diagnosed with pancreatic cancer within 3 years of meeting criteria for diabetes; 10 of 18 (56%) were diagnosed <6 months after first meeting criteria for diabetes, and 3 were resected. The observed-to-expected ratio of pancreatic cancer in the cohort was 7.94 (95% CI, 4.70–12.55). Compared with subjects without pancreatic cancer, diabetic subjects with pancreatic cancer were more likely to have met diabetes criteria after age 69 (OR = 4.52, 95% CI, 1.61–

12.74) years but did not differ significantly with respect to BMI values (29.2 ± 6.8 vs 26.5 ± 5.0, respectively). A larger proportion of those who developed pancreatic cancer were ever smokers (92% vs 69%, respectively), but this did not reach statistical significance.

Conclusions.—Approximately 1% of diabetes subjects aged ≥50 years will be diagnosed with pancreatic cancer within 3 years of first meeting criteria for diabetes. The usefulness of new-onset diabetes as marker of early pancreatic cancer needs further evaluation.

► Pancreatic carcinoma is often found only at an advanced stage and, thus, as expected its 5-year survival is dismal. Our goal is to find these lesions when they are asymptomatic and when they would amenable to surgical cure. Our initial step is to fulfill the goals of identifying a high-risk population for pancreatic cancer. We know that hereditary pancreatitis has a 40% prevalence of pancreatic carcinoma by age 70 years. In addition, patients with chronic pancreatitis, regardless of its etiology, have an increased risk of pancreatic carcinoma. The diagnostic modalities that should be utilized to screen these patients for development of pancreatic cancer include endoscopic US and endoscopic retrograde cholangiopancreatography. Chari et al reported a potential for utilizing hyperglycemia and diabetes to define a population at high risk for pancreatic cancer. The relationship between diabetes mellitus and pancreatic carcinoma is complex. First, patients with longstanding diabetes have a modest increased risk for pancreatic carcinoma. Second, new-onset diabetes is a manifestation of pancreatic cancer. This tumor should be especially sought in those patients who do not have a family history of pancreatic carcinoma and who are slender. The duration of diabetes as a risk factor for pancreatic cancer has been previously unknown. They identified 18 (0.85%) of 2122 diabetic subjects who were 50 years of age or older and had pancreatic cancer within 3 years of meeting criteria for diabetes. This incident is 8 times that for the general population. Glucose intolerance is common in patients with pancreatic carcinoma and occurs in approximately two thirds and occurs at an earlier stage of pancreatic carcinoma than the clinical symptoms of pancreatic carcinoma, which include abdominal pain, weight loss, and jaundice. Thus, in patients who develop diabetes mellitus without a positive family history or other risk factors and are 50 years of age or older, especially if slender, pancreatic carcinoma should be considered.

J. S. Barkin, MD

Association of Extent and Infection of Pancreatic Necrosis With Organ Failure and Death in Acute Necrotizing Pancreatitis

Garg PK, Madan K, Pande GK, et al (All India Inst of Med Sciences, New Delhi)

Clin Gastroenterol Hepatol 3:159-166, 2005 51–3

Background & Aims.—Organ failure is the usual cause of death in acute necrotizing pancreatitis. Our objective was to study whether the extent and infection of pancreatic necrosis correlate with organ failure and mortality.

Methods.—All consecutive patients with acute pancreatitis were prospectively studied. They underwent a detailed clinical and investigative evaluation. Pancreatic necrosis, diagnosed on a computed tomography scan, was graded as <30%, 30%–50%, and >50% necrosis and characterized as either sterile or infected. Logistic regression analysis was done to find out the association of the extent and infection of pancreatic necrosis with organ failure and mortality.

Results.—Of 276 patients (mean age, 41.25 years; 172 men), 104 had pancreatic necrosis: 30 had <30% necrosis, 37 had 30%–50% necrosis, and 37 had >50% necrosis; 74 had sterile necrosis, and 30 had infected necrosis. Of them, 37 (35%) patients developed organ failure. Two significant factors were associated with the development of organ failure, the extent of necrosis (<30% necrosis vs 30%–50% necrosis: $P = .03$; odds ratio [OR], 5.82; 95% confidence interval [CI], 1.15–29.45; <30% necrosis vs >50% necrosis: $P = .0004$; OR, 18.86; 95% CI, 3.75–94.92) and infected pancreatic necrosis ($P = .02$; OR, 3.29; 95% CI, 1.17–9.24). The overall mortality was 22%. Infected pancreatic necrosis ($P = .006$; OR, 4.99; 95% CI, 1.56–16.02) and Acute Physiology, Age, and Chronic Healthy Evaluation II score ($P = .004$; OR, 1.28; 95% CI, 1.08–1.52) were 2 independent predictors of mortality.

Conclusions.—Extent of necrosis and infected pancreatic necrosis were associated with the development of organ failure in patients with acute necrotizing pancreatitis. Infected pancreatic necrosis was the most significant predictor of mortality.

► We classify patients with acute pancreatitis as either having interstitial, also called edematous or necrotizing, pancreatitis. Necrotizing pancreatitis occurs in less than 20% of patients with acute pancreatitis, and its course may be complicated by organ system failure resulting in mortality. Garg et al prospectively evaluated whether the extent of necrosis and infections of the pancreas are associated with the development of organ failure and mortality. They found that there is a significant association between the extent of pancreatic necrosis determined by CT, whether sterile or infected, and the development of organ failure. They also found that the extent of pancreatic necrosis correlated with the development of infection. Infected necrosis increases the inflammatory cascade and contributes to organ failure and was found to be a predictor of organ failure. The authors postulated that the initial pancreatic injury determines the extent of pancreatic necrosis, and the magnitude of the pancreatic injury determines the severity of the inflammatory response. We do not have proven pharmacologic means to decrease the systemic inflammatory response. Unfortunately, the role of prophylactic antibiotics has not been entirely evidence proven. However, I still utilize a wide spectrum antibiotic in patients with extensive necrosis greater than 30% and in those who have organ system failure. This is for prevention of pancreatic infection. The use of CT-guided aspiration of necrotic areas remains the mainstay for diagnosis of pancreatic infections, whose treatment still remains surgical debridement.

J. S. Barkin, MD

52 Liver

Sexual Transmission of HCV Between Spouses

Tahan V, Karaca C, Yildirim B, et al (Marmara Univ School of Medicine, Istanbul, Turkey; Istanbul Univ, Turkey)

Am J Gastroenterol 100:821-824, 2005 52–1

Background and Aims.—The sexual transmission of hepatitis C virus (HCV) is debated. By excluding other risk factors, the role of sexual intercourse in the transmission could be detected more accurately. We screened HCV prevalence and risk factors in the spouses of chronic hepatitis C (CHC) patients and followed the seroconversion rate of anti-HCV negative spouses.

Patients and Methods.—Six hundred spouses of CHC patients were recruited. The spouses' HCV risk factors were questioned and the spouses were tested for anti-HCV. The 216 spouses who were anti-HCV negative were checked annually for anti-HCV.

Results.—Anti-HCV was positive in 12 of 600 (2%) of the spouses. Of the 12 anti-HCV positive spouses, 11 were HCV-RNA positive. Of anti-HCV positive and negative spouse groups, mean age was 52.3 ± 9.8 and 49.8 ± 12.4 yr; duration of marriage was 1521 ± 506.7 and 1532.4 ± 670.2 wk ($p > 0.05$); and the number of total sexual intercourse was 434 ± 295 and 307 ± 333 ($p = 0.055$), respectively. In our prospective study, none of the spouses developed anti-HCV seroconversion in mean 35.7 ± 6.3 months and 257.9 ± 72.2 sexual intercourse.

Conclusions.—Anti-HCV was found positive in 2% of the spouses. None of the seronegative spouses developed seroconversion in the 3-yr follow-up period. This is the first study that stresses the importance of the total number of sexual intercourse in sexual transmission ($p = 0.055$). Our results of special monogamous group with very limited risk factors support the role of number of total sexual intercourse in HCV transmission. However, the seroprevalence rate of the spouses was still within the upper limit of our country population.

► HCV transmission is most often associated with blood contact (needle stick, use of illicit drugs, and unknown route) in half of affected patients. A major concern of patients with HCV is transmission to their spouses. Tahan et al assessed the risk of heterosexual HCV transmission in a study of couples. They showed a seroprevalence of 2% between the spouses of patients with chronic HCV, which is no different than the 1.8% rate in the general population. Interestingly, the HCV RNA sequences are not always the same between the spouses, suggesting a different source of HCV infection. Previous studies of monogamous couples by the same authors have shown less than 1% acute HCV positivity,[1] and therefore use of condoms between these couples is not recommended. They did not find that the duration of marriage was connected with the rate of transmission, although this was found in Asian studies. Vandelli et al[2] performed a similar study, monitoring close to 800 monogamous heterosexual partners of patients with chronic HCV for a 10-year period. Similarly, their data showed extremely low or null rates of transmission. In conclusion, the authors feel that the risk of HCV infection by sexual transmission is low to null in monogamous partners and that couples need not change their sexual practices.[3] This does not mean that sexual transmission of HCV does not occur. Indeed, according to Terrault,[3] this is the second most common risk factor for HCV acquisition among those with acute HCV. Those at high risk, including sex workers, gay men, and those attending a clinic for sexually transmitted diseases, have a higher rate of approximately 4% to 6% infection rate than the general population.[4] What do I tell couples who have a monogamous relationship? Do not change your sexual habits. Terrault[3] recommends use of condoms with sexual intercourse during menstruation or sexual practices that result in genital trauma.

J. S. Barkin, MD

References

1. Mert A, Ozaras R, Tabak F, et al: Spouses of HCV carriers are not at serious risk. *Scand J Infect Dis* 30:644, 1998.
2. Vandelli C, Renzo F, Romano L, et al: Lack of evidence of sexual transmission of hepatitis C among monogamous couples: Results of a 10-year prospective follow-up study. *Am J Gastroenterol* 99:855-859, 2004.
3. Terrault NA: Sex and hepatitis C. *Am J Gastroenterol* 100:825-826, 2005.
4. Terrault N: Sexual activity as a risk factor for hepatitis C. *Hepatology* 36:S99-S105, 2002.

Biomarkers for the Prediction of Liver Fibrosis in Patients With Chronic Alcoholic Liver Disease

Naveau S, Raynard B, Ratziu V, et al (Hôopital Antoine Béclèere, Clamart, France; Groupe Hospitalier Pitié-Salpêtrière, Paris)

Clin Gastroenterol Hepatol 3:167-174, 2005 52–2

Background and Aims.—The aim of this study was to determine the diagnostic use of noninvasive markers of fibrosis in patients with chronic alcoholic liver disease.

Methods.—A total of 221 consecutive patients with an alcohol intake of >50 g/day (median, 100 g/day) and available liver biopsy examination and FibroTest FibroSure (FT) results were included prospectively. Fibrosis was assessed blindly on a 5-stage histologic scale similar to that of the

METAVIR scoring system. Hyaluronic acid was measured and used as a standard serum marker of fibrosis.

Results.—Advanced fibrosis (F2–F4) was present at biopsy examination in 63% of patients. The mean FT value (SE) was F0 = .29 (.05); F1 = .29 (.03), F2 = .40 (.03), F3 = .53 (.04); and F4 = 88 (.02) ($P < .05$ between all groups, except between F0 and F1). As opposed to FT, there was no significant difference for hyaluronic acid between F2 and F1 and between F2 and F0. For F2–F4 vs. F0–F1, the FT area under the ROC curves (AUROC) = .84 (.03) and .79 (.03) for hyaluronic acid. For the diagnosis of F4, the AUROC was very high, .95 for FT and .93 for hyaluronic acid. The discordances of the 2 stages were attributed to biopsy failures in 26 cases and to FT failures in 13 cases.

Conclusions.—In heavy drinkers, FT is a simple and noninvasive quantitative estimate of liver fibrosis. The use of FT may decrease the need for liver biopsy examination.

► Up to 40% of patients with chronic alcoholic liver disease develop sequelae of portal hypertension and end-stage liver disease. The highest risk groups are those who have significant hepatic inflammation and fibrosis on liver biopsy.[1-7] Fibrosis is a dynamic process and thus may fluctuate; inflammation is followed by fibrosis, which leads to impaired function and portal hypertension.[8] Our usual method to determine hepatic histology is by liver biopsy. Development of sensitive and specific noninvasive markers for detecting liver fibrosis could allow for accurate staging of fibrosis. Naveau et al utilized the FT and ActiTest (AT), which have previously been studied in patients with hepatitis B and C, to determine hepatic fibrosis and evaluate whether these tests could detect significant histologic lesions in patients with chronic alcoholic liver disease. In patients with viral hepatitis, the FT-AT fibrosis index significantly decreased following a sustained virologic response.[9] There was also concordance between FT-AT and fibrosis stage in patients receiving combination therapy for viral hepatitis by Poynard et al.[9,10] In their study of patients with chronic liver disease, Naveau et al found that as the FT score increased, so did its specificity. FT score of 0.7 had 91% sensitivity and a specificity of 87%. All cirrhotic patients had an FT score ≥70. However, for lesser degrees of fibrosis, an FT score of 0.3 had 84% sensitivity and a 70% negative predictive value. Unfortunately, there is an overlap in the values with the degrees of liver fibrosis. Serum markers reflect more advanced disease and could be used to identify those with alcoholic cirrhosis according to this single study. Serum markers (platelet count at <125,000) or clinical presence of portal hypertensive disease remains the goal standard for diagnosis of cirrhosis. The role of FT-AT for determination of cirrhosis remains best at the extremes of either cirrhosis or minimal fibrosis.

J. S. Barkin, MD

References

1. Arteel G, Marsano L, Mendez C, et al: Advances in alcoholic liver disease. *Best Pract Res Clin Gastroenterol* 17:625-647, 2003.

2. Diehl AM: Liver disease in alcohol abusers; clinical perspective. *Alcohol* 27:7-11, 2002.
3. Gordon H: Detection of alcoholic liver disease. *World J Gastroenterol* 7:297-302, 2001.
4. Sussman S, Dent CW, Skara S, et al: Alcoholic liver disease (ALD): A new domain for prevention efforts. *Subst Use Misuse* 37:1887-1904, 2002.
5. Chikritzhs TN, Jonas HA, Stockwell TR, et al: Mortality and life-years lost due to alcohol: A comparison of acute and chronic causes. *Med J Aust* 174:281-284, 2001.
6. Menon KV, Gores GJ, Shah VH: Pathogenesis, diagnosis, and treatment of alcoholic liver disease. *Mayo Clin Proc* 76:1021-1029, 2001.
7. Friedman SL, Maher JJ, Bissell DM: Mechanisms and therapy of hepatic fibrosis: Report of the AASLD Single Topic Basic Research Conference. *Hepatology* 32:1403-1408, 2000.
8. Dev A, Patel K, Conrad A, et al: Relationship of smoking and fibrosis in patients with chronic hepatitis C. *Clin Gastroenterol Hepatol* 2006. In print.
9. Poynard T, Imbert-Bismut F, Ratziu V, et al: Biochemical markers of liver fibrosis in patients infected by hepatitis C virus. Longitudinal validation in a randomized trial. The GERMED cyt-04 group. *J Viral Hepatol* 9:128-133, 2002.
10. Poynard T, McHutchison J, Manns M, et al: Biochemical surrogate markers of liver fibrosis and activity in a randomized trial of peginterferon alfa-2b and ribavirin. *Hepatology* 38:481-492, 2003.

The Natural History of Nonalcoholic Fatty Liver Disease: A Population-Based Cohort Study

Adams LA, Lymp JF, St Sauver J, et al (Mayo Clinic, Rochester, Minn)
Gastroenterology 129:113-121, 2005 52–3

Background & Aims.—The natural history of nonalcoholic fatty liver disease (NAFLD) in the community remains unknown. We sought to determine survival and liver-related morbidity among community-based NAFLD patients.

Methods.—Four hundred twenty patients diagnosed with NAFLD in Olmsted County, Minnesota, between 1980 and 2000 were identified using the resources of the Rochester Epidemiology Project. Medical records were reviewed to confirm diagnosis and determine outcomes up to 2003. Overall survival was compared with the general Minnesota population of the same age and sex.

Results.—Mean (SD) age at diagnosis was 49 (15) years; 231 (49%) were male. Mean follow-up was 7.6 (4.0) years (range, 0.1–23.5) culminating in 3192 person-years follow-up. Overall, 53 of 420 (12.6%) patients died. Survival was lower than the expected survival for the general population (standardized mortality ratio, 1.34; 95% CI, 1.003–1.76; $P = .03$). Higher mortality was associated with age (hazard ratio per decade, 2.2; 95% CI, 1.7–2.7), impaired fasting glucose (hazard ratio, 2.6; 95% CI, 1.3–5.2), and cirrhosis (hazard ratio, 3.1, 95% CI, 1.2–7.8). Liver disease was the third leading cause of death (as compared with the thirteenth leading cause of death in the general Minnesota population), occurring in 7 (1.7%) subjects. Twenty-one (5%) patients were diagnosed with cirrhosis, and 13 (3.1%) developed liver-related complications, including 1 requiring transplantation and 2 developing hepatocellular carcinoma.

Conclusions.—Mortality among community-diagnosed NAFLD patients is higher than the general population and is associated with older age, impaired fasting glucose, and cirrhosis. Liver-related death is a leading cause of mortality, although the absolute risk is low.

▶ NAFLD is increasing in frequency. NAFLD may occur in up to 30% of patients in the United States and is secondary to an increase in predisposing factors to NAFLD, including obesity, diabetes mellitus, and metabolic syndrome. NAFLD is the most common chronic liver disease, and it may progress to cirrhosis and the complications of portal hypertension, including liver failure and the development of secondary hepatocellular carcinoma.[1-3] Adams et al presented data on the natural history of NAFLD in community-dwelling patients, including its overall mortality rate and its liver-related morbidity and mortality rates. They found that the mortality rate was significantly increased in patients with NAFLD versus the general population and was associated with impaired fasting glucose and diabetes. The latter is recognized as a risk factor for ischemic heart disease, malignancies, and liver disease: the 3 most common causes of death in their population. Liver disease was the third most common cause of death, accounting for approximately 13% of deaths in NAFLD versus less than 1% in the general population. NAFLD may affect up to one third of persons in a community; thus, it is a large public health concern.[4] Patients with NAFLD without evidence of steatohepatitis have a more benign prognosis,[5,6] and this is the mildest form of the disease. Cirrhosis occurred in 3% of their patients (1 in 30) and conferred a 3-fold increased risk of death. In Day's[7] editorial, he points out that it is likely that the liver-related deaths were in the NASH patients with established cirrhosis at entry into trial. Day emphasizes that the natural history of NAFLD depends on the stage of disease. Patients with simple steatorrhea develop cirrhosis at a rate of 1% to 2% over 15 to 20 years, whereas those with NASH and fibrosis progress to cirrhosis of up to 12% at 8 years.[8,9]

J. S. Barkin, MD

References

1. Angulo P: Nonalcoholic fatty liver disease. *N Engl J Med* 346:1221-1231, 2002.
2. Caldwell SH, Oelsner DH, Iezzoni JC, et al: Cryptogenic cirrhosis: Clinical characterization and risk factors for underlying disease. *Hepatology* 29:664-669, 1999.
3. Bugianesi E, Leone N, Vanni E, et al: Expanding the natural history of nonalcoholic steatohepatitis: From cryptogenic cirrhosis to hepatocellular carcinoma. *Gastroenterology* 123:134-140, 2002.
4. Browning JD, Szczepaniak LS, Dobbins R, et al. Prevalence of hepatic steatosis in an urban population in the United States: Impact of ethnicity. *Hepatology* 40:1387-1395, 2004.
5. Teli MR, James OF, Burt AD, et al: The natural history of nonalcoholic fatty liver: A follow-up study. *Hepatology* 22:1714-1719, 1995.
6. Dam-Larsen S, Franzmann M, Andersen IB, et al: Long-term prognosis of fatty liver: Risk of chronic liver disease and death. *Gut* 53:750-755, 2004.

7. Day CP: Natural history of NAFLD: Remarkably benign in the absence of cirrhosis. *Gastroenterology* 129:375-378, 2005.
8. Matteoni CA, Younossi ZM, Gramlich T, et al: Nonalcoholic fatty liver disease: A spectrum of clinical and pathological severity. *Gastroenterology* 116:1413-1419, 1999.
9. Fassio E, Alvarez E, Dominguez N, et al: Natural history of non alcoholic steatohepatitis: A longitudinal study of repeat liver biopsies. *Hepatology* 40:820-826, 2004.

Preoperative Assessment of the Patient With Liver Disease

Keegan MT, Plevak DJ (Mayo Clinic, Rochester, Minn)
Am J Gastroenterol 100:2116-2127, 2005 52–4

Background.—Among the many challenges to clinical medicine are the aging population, the increasing number of patients with hepatic illness, the increasing cost constraints, the availability of new therapies, and the rapid pace of innovation. For example, the success of liver transplantation has resulted in a growing population of posttransplant patients, with varying degrees of liver dysfunction, who may require surgical intervention. It is generally understood that patients with liver disease are at significant risk when undergoing anesthesia and surgery. However, attempts to quantify that risk have been hampered by the diversity of disease states and illness severity among this population, as well as the variety of procedures these patients may undergo. The indications and contraindications for surgery in patients with liver disease were discussed, and specific recommendations for optimizing the clinical status of a patient with hepatic dysfunction before surgery were provided.

Overview.—Patients with asymptomatic biochemical abnormalities and minimal liver insults will generally do well during surgery and should not be overinvestigated at the risk of delaying a necessary procedure. However, it is sometimes difficult to be sure that an abnormal transaminase is not the onset of acute hepatitis, which can result in significant morbidity or mortality after surgery. Patients with decompensated cirrhosis are at risk for perioperative morbidity or death. Among the patients who should not undergo elective surgery are those with acute viral or alcoholic hepatitis, fulminant hepatic failure, severe chronic hepatitis, Child's class C cirrhosis, severe coagulopathy, or severe extrahepatic complications of liver disease including hypoxemia, cardiomyopathy, or acute renal failure. The urgency of the surgery is an obvious factor in optimizing the patient's condition. Emergency procedures, such as repair of a ruptured aortic aneurysm, permit no delay. Urgent or elective procedures, however, do permit some time for evaluation, deliberation, and therapy. Procedures considered urgent would include performance of a mastectomy for breast cancer and coronary artery bypass grafting (CABG) for stable angina. A thorough history may disclose a history of blood transfusion, IV drug abuse, excessive alcohol intake, easy fatigability, and pruritis. Routine preoperative testing of liver function is not recommended. However, if abnormal liver blood tests are coincidentally found in an asymptomatic patient, elective surgery should be postponed in favor of a more extensive workup.

Conclusions.—Patients with liver disease are at risk for perioperative morbidity and mortality. The severity of illness and the degree of invasiveness of the surgical procedure are associated with a higher risk of complications, but the type of anesthesia is not. Specific indications and contraindications for surgery in patients with various types of liver disease were provided.

► One of the most common requests that we receive from surgeons is for clearance of patients with liver disease to undergo elective operative intervention. We are seeing more of these patients because of an aging population and the increase in the number of patients who have hepatic illness. Keegan and Plevak reviewed in depth the preoperative assessment of the patient with liver disease. Routine preoperative testing of liver function is not recommended.[1] If abnormal elevation of liver enzymes is found incidentally in an asymptomatic individual, elective surgery should be deferred until elucidation of the source of the elevated enzymes is determined.[2] In situations of emergent procedures, one weighs the risks and benefits and proceeds. Our initial approach to patients with liver disease should be to classify patients according to whether they have acute liver disease or chronic liver disease. If a patient is thought to have acute hepatitis, elective surgery is contraindicated, as the morbidity and mortality is increased.[3-5] Other contraindications are listed in the Table. Patients with chronic hepatitis with preserved hepatic function usually do well at surgery; however, the risks increase with increasingly abnormal results of liver tests and with increasingly abnormal liver histology. It is critical to divide the group of patients with chronic liver disease into those with cirrhosis and those without clinical or biochemical evidence of cirrhosis. Clues to the presence of cirrhosis include (1) thrombocytopenia with a platelet count less than 125,000, (2) prolonged international normalized ratio (INR), (3) presence of ascites, (4) encephalopathy, and/or (5) evidence of portal hypertension and hypoalbuminemia. Patients with cirrhosis are classified as having severe disease by either Child's score criteria or the Model for End-Stage Liver Disease (MELD) score. The MELD is a numerical scale, ranging from 6 to 40 points, used for liver transplant candidates aged 12 years or older. The number is calculated by a formula using 3 routine lab test results: bilirubin, INR, and creatinine. It gives each patient a "score" based on how urgently a liver transplant is needed within 3

TABLE.—Contraindications for Elective Surgery

- Acute hepatitis
- Fulminant hepatic failure
- Severe chronic hepatitis
- Child's "C" cirrhosis with severe coagulopathy and/or presence of encephalopathy, elevated bilirubin

Perioperative mortality rates correlate with severity of their liver disease.

months. A higher score is associated with an increased patient mortality within 3 months.

J. S. Barkin, MD

References

1. Schemel WH: Unexpected hepatic dysfunction found by multiple laboratory screening. *Anesth Analg* 55:810-812, 1976.
2. Patel T: Surgery in the patient with liver disease. *Mayo Clin Proc* 74:593-599, 1999.
3. Powell-Jackson P, Greenway B, Williams R: Adverse effects of exploratory laparotomy in patients with unsuspected liver disease. *Br J Surg* 69:449-451, 1982.
4. Hardy KJ, Hughes ESR: Laparotomy in viral hepatitis. *Med J Aust* 1:710-712, 1968.
5. Harville DD, Summerskill WH: Surgery in acute hepatitis. Causes and effects. *JAMA* 184:257-261, 1963.

Drug-Induced Liver Injury: An Analysis of 461 Incidences Submitted to the Spanish Registry Over a 10-Year Period

Andrade RJ, for the Spanish Group for the Study of Drug-Induced Liver Disease (Unidad de Hepatología y Grupo de Estudio para las Hepatopatías Asociadas a Medicamentos, Malaga, Spain; et al)

Gastroenterology 129:512-521, 2005 52–5

Background & Aims.—Progress in the understanding of susceptibility factors to drug-induced liver injury (DILI) and outcome predictability are hampered by the lack of systematic programs to detect bona fide cases.

Methods.—A cooperative network was created in 1994 in Spain to identify all suspicions of DILI following a prospective structured report form. The liver damage was characterized according to hepatocellular, cholestatic, and mixed laboratory criteria and to histologic criteria when available. Further evaluation of causality assessment was centrally performed.

Results.—Since April 1994 to August 2004, 461 out of 570 submitted cases, involving 505 drugs, were deemed to be related to DILI. The antiinfective group of drugs was the more frequently incriminated, amoxicillin-clavulanate accounting for the 12.8% of the whole series. The hepatocellular pattern of damage was the most common (58%), was inversely correlated with age ($P < .0001$), and had the worst outcome (Cox regression, $P < .034$). Indeed, the incidence of liver transplantation and death in this group was 11.7% if patients had jaundice at presentation, whereas the corresponding figure was 3.8% in nonjaundiced patients ($P < .04$). Factors associated with the development of fulminant hepatic failure were female sex (OR = 25; 95% CI: 4.1–151; $P < .0001$), hepatocellular damage (OR = 7.9; 95% CI: 1.6–37; $P < .009$), and higher baseline plasma bilirubin value (OR = 1.15; 95% CI: 1.09–1.22; $P < .0001$).

Conclusions.—Patients with drug-induced hepatocellular jaundice have 11.7% chance of progressing to death or transplantation. Amoxicillin-clavulanate stands out as the most common drug related to DILI.

▶ The information on DILI is derived from spontaneous reporting systems and published case reports. Thus, we probably only have information on a fraction of the complications. One study found a 16-fold actual reaction than that reported. Conversely, approximately half of the reactions are unrelated to the incriminated drug with further evaluations.[1] Andrade et al report the results of hepatotoxicity from a registry, which is a rigorous and uniform approach to causality assessment. Hepatotoxicity from drugs is usually detected postmarketing after several thousand patients have taken the drug. DILI is responsible for half of the causes of acute liver failure[2,3] and 15% of liver transplantations.[4] Unfortunately, we do not know the genetic and environmental factors that influence individual susceptibility. We do not know that the male gender predisposes the toxicity from amoxicillin-clavulanate, whereas female gender predisposes to reactions to most other drugs other than amoxicillin-clavulanate. Predisposing patient factors include diabetes mellitus for methotrexate and older individuals for isoniazid and amoxicillin-clavulanate. The 2 most common mechanisms responsible for drug-induced diseases are (1) idiosyncratic immunoallergic reaction, which is associated with the presence of fever, rash, and eosinophilia; and (2) buildup of a toxic metabolite. Thus, we can see early and delayed onset of hepatotoxicity. DILI can manifest as hepatocellular disease, with increased levels of SGOT and SGPT (40%), cholestasis with elevated bilirubin and alkaline phosphatase levels (40%), or a mixed picture. Eosinophilia may be present. Withdrawal of the offending agent in patients before developing acute liver failure usually results in complete recovery. However, up to one third of patients may have evidence of persisting liver damage.[5] The most commonly reported drugs that caused DILI that are available in the United States included amoxicillin-clavulanate (first), isoniazid plus rifampicin and pyrazinamide (second), ibuprofen, flutamide, ticlopidine, diclofenac, and isoniazid alone.

In summary, in patients with new onset of elevated liver enzymes, assume DILI from intake of new drugs or herbal medicine and institute the diagnostic test, which is still drug withdrawal with liver enzymes returning to normal usually within a few months.

J. S. Barkin, MD

References

1. Aithal GP, Rawlins MD, Day CP: Accuracy of hepatic adverse drug reaction reporting in one English health region. *BMJ* 319:1541, 1999.
2. Zimmerman HJ: *Hepatotoxicity. The adverse effects of drugs and other chemicals on the liver*, ed 2, Philadelphia, 1999, Lippincott Williams & Wilkins.
3. Andrade RJ, Lucena MI, Martin-Vivaldi R, et al: Acute liver injury associated with the use of ebrotidine, a new H2-receptor antagonist. *J Hepatol* 31:641-646, 1999.
4. Andrade RJ, Lucena MI, Rodriguez-Mendizabal M: Hepatic injury caused by acarbose. *Ann Intern Med* 124:931, 1996.
5. Aithal PG, Day CP: The natural history of histologically proved drug-induced liver disease. *Gut* 44:731-735, 1999.

Prevention of Hepatitis B With the Hepatitis B Vaccine
Poland GA, Jacobson RM (Mayo Clinic, Rochester, Minn)
N Engl J Med 351:2832-2838, 2004 52–6

Background.—The hepatitis B virus (HBV) is an enveloped, double-stranded DNA virus and the smallest DNA virus known to affect humans. HBV is very infectious in nonimmune persons. Acute HBV infection can be symptomatic or asymptomatic. A case situation was presented involving a decision as to whether to vaccinate a nurse for HBV after she received a positive result on a pregnancy test.

> *Case Report.*—Woman, 25, who was a registered nurse, came for a visit to initiate prenatal care after learning that she was pregnant. A review of her vaccination status determined that she declined HBV vaccination when it was offered by her current employer because she does not draw blood and so does not consider herself to be at risk for infection. Two questions regarding this patient are discussed: Should she receive the vaccine? What are the current recommendations for HBV vaccination?

Discussion.—Persons with a risk of nonresponse to the HBV vaccine (those older than 30 years, obese persons, and persons with immune deficiency) and those at high risk for exposure to blood or bodily fluids should have their antibody response to the HBV vaccine checked 1 to 3 months after receiving the last dose of vaccine. However, the antibody response is frequently tested years after completion of the vaccination series, in which case a true nonresponse (an antibody level <10 mIU/mL after the appropriate vaccination series) must be distinguished from "waning" antibody levels, which are initially protective but become undetectable over time. The use of HBV vaccine has been associated with a dramatic decrease in the incidence of HBV infections as well as a decrease in the incidence of hepatocellular carcinoma in countries in which it is widely used. Clinicians should strive to achieve universal vaccination of infants and children through the age of 18 years and to identify and vaccinate persons at risk for infection. Testing for hepatitis B surface antigen (HbsAg) is warranted for pregnant women, such as the patient presented in this case vignette. In the case of a positive result, the baby would need hepatitis B immune globulin and vaccination at birth, and it would be necessary to determine whether the infant's father and possibly the patient's other sexual partners could be the source of infection. If the patient is not at high risk, she should be tested again in her last trimester. In view of the potential for work-related exposure in this patient, even if she does not draw blood, immunization is recommended because HBV vaccine is not contraindicated during pregnancy.

Antibody Levels and Protection After Hepatitis B Vaccination: Results of a 15-Year Follow-up

McMahon BJ, Bruden DL, Petersen KM, et al (Centers for Disease Control and Prevention, Anchorage, Alaska; Alaska Native Med Ctr, Anchorage, Alaska; Centers for Disease Control and Prevention, Atlanta, Ga)
Ann Intern Med 142:333-341, 2005 52–7

Background.—The duration of protection afforded by hepatitis B vaccination is unknown.

Objective.—To determine antibody persistence and protection from hepatitis B virus (HBV) infection.

Design.—Prospective cohort study.

Setting.—15 villages in southwest Alaska.

Participants.—1578 Alaska Natives vaccinated at age 6 months or older.

Intervention.—During 1981–1982, participants received 3 doses of plasma-derived hepatitis B vaccine. This cohort was followed annually over the first 11 years, and 841 (53%) persons were tested at 15 years.

Measurements.—Antibody to hepatitis B surface antigen (anti-HBs), markers of HBV infection, and testing to identify HBV variants.

Results.—Levels of anti-HBs in the cohort decreased from a geometric mean concentration of 822 mIU/mL after vaccination to 27 mIU/mL at 15 years. Initial anti-HBs level, older age at vaccination, and male sex were associated with persistence of higher anti-HBs levels at 15 years when analyzed by a longitudinal linear mixed model. After adjustment for initial anti-HBs level and sex, those vaccinated at age 6 months to 4 years had the lowest anti-HBs level at 15 years. Asymptomatic breakthrough infections were detected in 16 participants and occurred more frequently in persons who did not respond to vaccination than those who responded ($P = 0.01$). Among infected persons with viremia, 2 were infected with wild-type HBV and 4 had HBV surface glycoprotein variants, generally accompanied by wild-type HBV.

Limitations.—The loss of participants to follow-up at 15 years was 47%. However, characteristics of persons tested were similar to those of persons lost to follow-up.

Conclusions.—Hepatitis B vaccination strongly protected against infection for at least 15 years in all age groups. Antibody levels decreased the most among persons immunized at 4 years of age or younger.

► HB is acquired by exposure to chronically infected persons, and once an individual is exposed, either viral clearance or chronic infection results. There is an inverse relation between age at the time of infection and viral clearance, with up to 90% of infected neonates having chronic infection. Unfortunately, persistent HPV infection contracted in infancy or early childhood has a higher death rate (up to 25% higher) than persistent infection acquired later in life.[1] The rate of HB is increasing in the United States as a result of exposure of infected persons who have emigrated from endemic areas where they have had neonatal exposure. When adults are exposed to HB, usually by sexual intimacy or illicit drug use, they usually clear their virus after acute illness. However, there is an unknown source of exposure that occurs in a large percentage of the patients. Immunization against HBV has dramatically decreased chronic infection and hepatocellular carcinoma. McMahon et al (Abstract 52–7) reported the duration of protection of HB vaccination beyond 10 years. They found that protection remained effective for 15 years, as evidenced by 84% of the populace having anti-HB surface antigen present. This high rate, as the authors suggested, may be attributable to natural boosting by living in households of infected patients. In addition, they found that in immunized persons there was a decrease in infectivity among those who were chronically infected. Thus, immunization lasts for at least 15 years and we await the follow-up information. This information is especially important as there has been an increase in HBV infection from 1990 to 2002 in men aged 20 to 39 years and in both sexes aged 40 years and older.[2] Poland and Jacobson (Abstract 52–6) recommend that the following groups be vaccinated against HBV: (1) all infants and those younger than 18 years; (2) those with occupational risks, including health care workers, public safety workers, and institutional workers; (3) patients on hemodialysis; (4) travelers to areas with high or intermediate levels of endemic disease who will have contact with blood, medical workers, soldiers, or sexual contact with residents; (5) high-risk groups such as gay men, and those using illicit injection of drugs, and long-term inmates of correctional facilities. These are the recommendations from the advisory committee on immunization practices for the Centers for Disease Control and Prevention.[3]

J. S. Barkin, MD

References

1. Hsieh CC, Tzonou A, Zavitsanos X, et al: Age at first establishment of chronic hepatitis B virus infection and hepatocellular carcinoma risk: A birth order study. *Am J Epidemiol* 136:1115-1121, 1992.
2. Incidence of acute hepatitis B—United States. *MMWR* 52:1252-1254, 2004.
3. Centers for Disease Control: Update on adult immunization: Recommendations of the Immunization Practices Advisory Committee (ACIP). *MMWR* 40(RR-12):1-94, 1991.

The Metabolic Syndrome as a Predictor of Nonalcoholic Fatty Liver Disease

Hamaguchi M, Kojima T, Takeda N, et al (Asahi Univ, Gifu, Japan)
Ann Intern Med 143:722-728, 2005 52–8

Background.—The frequent association of nonalcoholic fatty liver disease with components of the metabolic syndrome such as obesity, hyperglycemia, dyslipidemia, and hypertension is well known. However, no prospective study has examined the role of the metabolic syndrome in the development of this disease.

Objective.—To characterize the longitudinal relationship between the metabolic syndrome and nonalcoholic fatty liver disease.

Design.—A prospective observational study.
Setting.—A medical health checkup program in a general hospital.
Participants.—4401 apparently healthy Japanese men and women, 21 to 80 years of age, with a mean body mass index (BMI) of 22.6 kg/m^2 (SD, 3.0).
Measurements.—Alcohol intake was assessed by using a questionnaire. Biochemical tests for liver and metabolic function and abdominal ultrasonography were done. Modified criteria of the National Cholesterol Education Program Adult Treatment Panel III were used to characterize the metabolic syndrome.
Results.—At baseline, 812 of 4401 (18%) participants had nonalcoholic fatty liver disease. During the mean follow-up period of 414 days (SD, 128), the authors observed 308 new cases (10%) of nonalcoholic fatty liver disease among 3147 participants who were disease-free at baseline and who completed a second examination. Regression of nonalcoholic fatty liver disease was found in 113 (16%) of 704 participants who had the disease at baseline and who completed a second examination. Men and women who met the criteria for the metabolic syndrome at baseline were more likely to develop the disease during follow-up (adjusted odds ratio, 4.00 [95% CI, 2.63 to 6.08] and 11.20 [CI, 4.85 to 25.87], respectively). Nonalcoholic fatty liver disease was less likely to regress in those participants with the metabolic syndrome at baseline.
Limitations.—Ultrasonography may lead to an incorrect diagnosis of nonalcoholic fatty liver disease in 10% to 30% of cases and cannot distinguish steatohepatitis from simple steatosis. Self-reported alcohol intake may cause bias. Because all of the participants were Japanese, generalizability to non-Japanese populations is uncertain.
Conclusions.—The metabolic syndrome is a strong predictor of nonalcoholic fatty liver disease.

► The spectrum of nonalcoholic fatty liver disease (NAFLD) ranges from bland steatosis to necroinflammatory changes of steatohepatitis to cirrhosis and its complications. NAFLD may be the most common cause of elevation of liver enzymes. Hamaguchi et al pointed out that NAFLD is often associated with individual components of metabolic syndrome, or insulin resistance syndrome, which is composed of obesity, type 2 diabetes mellitus, dyslipidemia, and hypertension.[1-3] Obviously, these are also contributing factors to cardiovascular disease. Hamaguchi et al, in a prospective cohort study, evaluated whether there is a relationship of NAFLD with the metabolic syndrome and monitored this group, which allowed us to have longitudinal data. They utilized abdominal US as their diagnostic test for NAFLD as opposed to liver biopsy, which may give an incorrect diagnosis in 10% to 15% of cases. They found that persons with metabolic syndrome have a 4 to 11 times higher risk for future NAFLD, and that when the metabolic syndrome is present with NAFLD, disease regression is less likely. The authors agree that insulin resistance plays a central role in the pathophysiology of NAFLD.[4] Therefore, it is important for health care providers to recognize that the metabolic syndrome is not only associated with cardiovascular events, but also NAFLD. The 5 components as recommended by Adult Treatment Panel III for diagnosing the metabolic syndrome are (1) waist circumference, (2) serum triglyceride level, (3) serum high-density lipoprotein cholesterol level, (4) blood pressure, and (5) fasting plasma glucose level. In addition to its recognition, treatment of this high-risk state (metabolic syndrome) is recommended. Orchard et al[5] reported the effects of intensive lifestyle intervention and metformin on metabolic syndrome incidence and its resolution in participants of the Diabetes Prevention Program. They found that individualized, structured, intensive lifestyle changes and metformin reduced the development of the syndrome in the remaining participants.

J. S. Barkin, MD

References

1. Bellentani S, Saccoccio G, Masutti F, et al: Prevalence of and risk factors for hepatic steatosis in northern Italy. *Ann Intern Med* 132:112-127, 2000.
2. Akbar DH, Kawther AH: Nonalcoholic fatty liver disease in Saudi type II diabetic subjects attending a medical outpatient clinic: Prevalence and general characteristics [letter]. *Diabetes Care* 26:3351-3352, 2003.
3. Assy N, Kaita K, Mymin D, et al: Fatty infiltration of liver in hyperlipidemia patients. *Dig Dis Sci* 45:1929-1934, 2000.
4. Angulo P: Nonalcoholic fatty liver disease. *N Engl J Med* 346:121-131, 2002.
5. Orchard TJ, Temprosa M, Goldberg R, et al: The effect of metformin and intensive lifestyle intervention on the metabolic syndrome: The Diabetes Prevention Program randomized trial. *Ann Intern Med* 142:611-619.

Antiviral Therapy for Cirrhotic Hepatitis C: Association With Reduced Hepatocellular Carcinoma Development and Improved Survival

Shiratori Y, for the Tokyo-Chiba Hepatitis Research Group (Univ of Tokyo; et al)
Ann Intern Med 142:105-114, 2005 52–9

Background.—Although cirrhosis is a major risk factor for development of hepatocellular carcinoma, no definitive prospective analyses have assessed the long-term efficacy of antiviral therapy in cirrhotic patients.

Objective.—To elucidate the role of antiviral therapy in the suppression of liver tumors and survival over a long-term follow-up period.

Design.—Prospective cohort study.

Setting.—25 clinical centers.

Patients.—345 patients with chronic hepatitis C and cirrhosis enrolled in previous trials.

Intervention.—271 patients received 6 to 9 million U of interferon 3 times weekly for 26 to 88 weeks; 74 received no treatment.

Measurements.—Blood tests and abdominal ultrasonography were done regularly to detect hepatocellular carcinoma.

Results.—Hepatocellular carcinoma was detected in 119 patients during a 6.8-year follow-up: 84 (31%) in the interferon-treated group and 35 (47%) in the untreated group. Cumulative incidence of hepatocellular carcinoma among interferon-treated patients was significantly lower than in untreated patients (Cox model: age-adjusted hazard ratio, 0.65 [95% CI,

0.43 to 0.97]; *P* = 0.03), especially sustained virologic responders. A total of 69 patients died during follow-up: 45 (17%) in the treated group and 24 (32%) in the untreated group. Interferon-treated patients had a better chance of survival than the untreated group (Cox model: age-adjusted hazard ratio, 0.54 [CI, 0.33 to 0.89]; *P* = 0.02). This was especially evident in sustained virologic responders.

Limitation.—This was not a randomized, controlled study. Patients enrolled in the control group had declined to receive interferon treatment even though they were eligible for treatment.

Conclusion.—Interferon therapy for cirrhotic patients with chronic hepatitis C, especially those in whom the infection had been cured, inhibited the development of hepatocellular carcinoma and improved survival.

► The most dreaded complication of hepatitis C virus (HCV) infection is the development of hepatocellular carcinoma, which occurs in 1.4% to 3.3% of HCV patients with compensated cirrhosis and is much lower in patients without cirrhosis. The risk factors as summarized by Shiratori et al include men aged 50 to 60 years with advanced liver fibrosis and high liver histologic activity score and high alanine aminotransferase levels. This group of investigators reported on a 7-year study that looked at the efficacy of interferon treatment versus control in cirrhotic patients. Cirrhosis is a major risk factor for the development of hepatocellular carcinoma. The patients elected or declined interferon therapy; therefore, this was not a randomized trial. The authors found that the incidence of hepatocellular carcinoma was significantly reduced in the interferon treatment group compared with the untreated group. In addition, the cumulative incidence of hepatocellular carcinoma was markedly decreased, especially in sustained virologic responders compared with nonresponders and untreated patients. They found that the annual incidence of hepatocellular carcinoma in untreated patients was 6% to 8% versus 4% to 5% in the interferon-treated patients and 2.5% in the sustained responders. Interestingly, deaths from liver failure were increased in the untreated versus treated groups (40% vs 20%), and survival was significantly better in the treated versus untreated patients. In summary, antiviral treatment improved the natural course in cirrhotic patients with HCV infection, especially in those with sustained viral eradication. These results should be even better with combination therapies of pegylated interferon-ribavirin therapies. It is therefore almost never too late to initiate effective HCV therapy.

J. S. Barkin, MD

53 Obesity

Obesity Is Associated With Increased Risk of Gastrointestinal Symptoms: A Population-Based Study

Delgado-Aros S, Locke GR III, Camilleri M, et al (Clin Enteric Neuroscience Translational & Epidemiological Research (CENTER) Program; Mayo Clinic, Rochester, Minn)

Am J Gastroenterol 99:1801-1806, 2004 53–1

Objectives.—Perception of sensations arising from the gastrointestinal tract may be diminished in obese subjects and thus facilitate overeating. Alternatively, excess food intake may cause gastrointestinal (GI) symptoms in obese patients. We evaluated the relationship between body mass index (BMI) and specific GI symptoms in the community.

Methods.—Residents of Olmsted County, MN were selected at random to receive by mail one of two validated questionnaires. The association of reported GI symptoms with BMI (kg/m^2) was assessed using a logistic regression analysis adjusting for age, gender, psychosomatic symptom score, and alcohol and tobacco use.

Results.—Response rate was 74% (1,963 of 2,660). The prevalence of obesity (BMI $\geq$ 30 kg/m^2) was 23%. There was a positive relationship between BMI and frequent vomiting ($p = 0.02$), upper abdominal pain ($p = 0.03$), bloating ($p = 0.002$), and diarrhea ($p = 0.01$). The prevalence of frequent lower abdominal pain, nausea, and constipation was increased among obese (BMI $\geq$ 30 kg/m^2) compared to normal weight participants, however, no significant association was found between BMI and these symptoms.

Conclusions.—In the community, increasing BMI is associated with increased upper GI symptoms, bloating, and diarrhea. Clarification of the cause-and-effect relationships and the mechanisms of these associations require further investigation.

► Obesity is defined by an increased BMI. Those with a BMI greater than 25 kg/m^2 are overweight and those with a BMI greater than 30 kg/m^2 are clinically obese. It is estimated that two thirds of the US population is overweight, and 31% are obese. Obesity is associated with development of heart disease, diabetes, hypertension, hyperlipidemia, osteoarthritis, and carcinoma. Delgado-Aros et al reported a relationship between BMI and specific GI symptoms in the community population. The authors point out that previous studies have shown an increased prevalence of different GI symptoms in obese patients seeking therapy at the tertiary care center compared with community controls. They found a positive linear association between BMI and self-reported GI symptoms in a community population. This included frequent vomiting, upper abdominal pain, bloating, and diarrhea. The bloating and upper abdominal pain, as the authors point out, may be related to the delayed gastric emptying, which has been reported in obese patients.[1-5] Previous information from the same group has shown that BMI is an independent risk factor with the presence of self-reported heartburn and regurgitation.[6] Thus, obesity per se is associated with a wide spectrum of GI symptoms. Unfortunately, their mechanisms are unclear.

J. S. Barkin, MD

References

1. Hutson WR, Wald A: Obesity and weight reduction do not influence gastric emptying and antral motility. *Am J Gastroenterol* 88:1405-1409, 1993.
2. Horowitz M, Collins PJ, Cook DJ, et al: Abnormalities of gastric emptying in obese patients. *Int J Obes* 7:415-421, 1983.
3. Horowitz M, Collins PJ, Shearman DJ: Effect of increasing the caloric/osmotic content of the liquid component of a mixed solid and liquid meal on gastric emptying in obese subjects. *Hum Nutr Clin Nutr* 40:51-56, 1986.
4. Maddox A, Horowitz M, Wishart J, et al: Gastric and esophageal emptying in obesity. *Scand J Gastroenterol* 24:593-598, 1989.
5. Portincasa P, Di Ciaula A, Palmieri V, et al: Effects of cholestyramine on gallbladder and gastric emptying in obese and lean subjects. *Eur J Clin Invest* 25:746-753, 1995.
6. Locke GR III, Talley NJ, Fett SL, et al: Risk factors associated with symptoms of gastroesophageal reflux. *Am J Med* 106:642-649, 1999.

54 Miscellaneous

Prevalence and Burden of Fecal Incontinence: A Population-Based Study in Women

Bharucha AE, Zinsmeister AR, Locke GR, et al (Mayo Clinic College of Medicine, Rochester, Minn; Olmsted Med Ctr, Rochester, Minn)

Gastroenterology 129:42-49, 2005 54–1

Background & Aims.—The epidemiology of fecal incontinence (FI) is incompletely understood. We report the prevalence, clinical spectrum, health care–seeking behavior, and quality of life (QOL) in community women with FI.

Methods.—A questionnaire was mailed to an age-stratified random sample of 5300 Olmsted County, Minnesota, women identified by the Rochester Epidemiology Project. Symptom severity was assessed by a validated scale, and impact on QOL was evaluated for subjects who had any FI during the past year. The prevalence of FI was calculated with direct age adjustment to the 2000 US white female population.

Results.—Altogether, 2800 of 5300 women (53%) responded to the survey. The overall age-adjusted prevalence of FI in the past year was 12.1 per 100 (95% confidence interval, 11.0–13.1). The prevalence increased with age from 7 (third decade) to 22 (sixth decade) per 100 and was steady thereafter. Symptoms were mild (45%), moderate (50%), or severe (5%), and symptom severity was related to the impact of FI on QOL and physician-consulting behavior. Moderate to severe impact on ≥1 domain of QOL was reported by 6% with mild, 35% with moderate, and 82% with severe symptoms, whereas 5% with mild, 10% with moderate, and 48% with severe FI had consulted a physician for FI in the past year.

Conclusions.—More than 1 of 10 adult women in the population have FI; almost 1 of 15 have moderate to severe FI. FI significantly impacts QOL and prompts health care utilization predominantly in women with moderate to severe symptoms.

► Only a small percentage of incontinent patients will discuss FI with their physicians. Whether this is because of embarrassment or the false understanding that it is not a treatable condition is unclear. We are, for the most part, aware of its frequency in elder nursing home residents. Bharucha et al utilized a self-report questionnaire to estimate the prevalence and severity of fecal incontinence in the adult female population and determine the relationship between symptom severity and impact on QOL. They found the age-adjusted prevalence of FI in women was 12.1%, with a gradual increase of FI from 7% of subjects aged 20 to 29 years to 22% of subjects aged 50 to 59 years, with a median age of onset of 55 years of age. Interestingly, severity of symptoms was not related to age. FI is associated with anxiety, depression, and a negative impact on QOL, the latter in approximately 23% of patients and related to severity of symptoms. This article again emphasizes that only 10% of women with FI discussed it with a physician in the preceding year, but 48% with severe symptoms had discussed it with their physician. Overall, 1 of 50 women reported that FI significantly affected their QOL. FI may range from urgency with need to empty the bowel to leakage of liquid or solid stool without any warning. Patients' responses may vary from use of protective devices to altering their activities and staying at home (in severe FI patients). We should ask whether FI in any form is present on our initial review of symptoms of our female patients.

J. S. Barkin, MD

PART EIGHT

ENDOCRINOLOGY, DIABETES, AND METABOLISM

ERNEST L. MAZZAFERRI, MD

Introduction

During the past year, many important articles were published concerning the basic science, prevention, diagnosis and treatment of endocrine disorders. The articles for the Endocrinology section of the YEAR BOOK OF MEDICINE were selected from among 240 articles in the YEAR BOOK OF ENDOCRINOLOGY that our editors and I thought would have a substantial impact on our understanding of endocrine disorders and the practice of endocrinology. From this group, 46 articles were chosen that should be of particular importance to internists because they emphasize prevention of important clinical problems such as diabetes mellitus and coronary artery disease, and early diagnosis and treatment of ubiquitous disorders such as osteoporosis, obesity, and thyroid disease. During the past year, new and important information has been added to our growing understanding of subclinical thyroid dysfunction, including new information concerning its prognosis and treatment. Still, there is considerable debate regarding the treatment of subclinical hypothyroidism, which is reflected in the articles in this section that address this subject. The articles, which have been grouped according to several broad categories, are each accompanied by comments from the section editors of the YEAR BOOK OF ENDOCRINOLOGY.

We hope these articles and their accompanying editorial comments give the reader fresh insight into these common endocrine problems encountered in everyday practice.

Ernest L. Mazzaferri, MD

55 Diabetes Mellitus

Comparison of Basal Insulin Added to Oral Agents Versus Twice-Daily Premixed Insulin as Initial Insulin Therapy for Type 2 Diabetes

Janka HU, Kliebe-Frisch C, Plewe G, et al (Zentralkrankenhaus, Bremen, Germany; Oregon Health and Science Univ, Portland; Aventis Pharma Deutschland, Bad Soden, Germany; et al)

Diabetes Care 28:254-259, 2005 55–1

Objective.—To compare the efficacy and safety of adding once-daily basal insulin versus switching to twice-daily premixed insulin in type 2 diabetic patients insufficiently controlled by oral antidiabetic agents (OADs).

Research Design and Methods.—In a 24-week, multinational, multicenter, open, parallel group clinical trial, 371 insulin-naive patients with poor glycemic control (fasting blood glucose [FBG] ≥120 mg/dl, HbA_{1c} 7.5–10.5%) on OADs (sulfonylurea plus metformin) were randomized to once-daily morning insulin glargine plus glimepiride and metformin (glargine plus OAD) or to 30% regular/70% human NPH insulin (70/30) twice daily without OADs. Insulin dosage was titrated to target FBG ≤100 mg/dl (both insulins) and predinner blood glucose ≤100 mg/dl (70/30 only) using a weekly forced-titration algorithm.

Results.—Mean HbA_{1c} decrease from baseline was significantly more pronounced (−1.64 vs. −1.31%, $P = 0.0003$), and more patients reached HbA_{1c} ≤7.0% without confirmed nocturnal hypoglycemia (45.5 vs. 28.6%, $P = 0.0013$) with glargine plus OAD than with 70/30. Similarly, FBG decrease was greater with glargine plus OAD (adjusted mean difference −17 mg/dl [−0.9 mmol/l], $P < 0.0001$), and more patients reached target FBG ≤100 mg/dl with glargine plus OAD than with 70/30 (31.6 vs. 15.0%, $P = 0.0001$). Glargine plus OAD patients had fewer confirmed hypoglycemic episodes than 70/30 patients (mean 4.07 vs. 9.87/patient-year, $P < 0.0001$).

Conclusions.—Initiating insulin treatment by adding basal insulin glargine once daily to glimepiride plus metformin treatment was safer and more effective than beginning twice-daily injections of 70/30 and discontinuing OADs in type 2 diabetic patients inadequately controlled with OADs.

Initiating Insulin Therapy in Type 2 Diabetes: A Comparison of Biphasic and Basal Insulin Analogs

Raskin P, for the INITIATE Study Group (Univ of Texas, Dallas; et al)

Diabetes Care 28:260-265, 2005 55–2

Objective.—Safety and efficacy of biphasic insulin aspart 70/30 (BIAsp 70/30, prebreakfast and presupper) were compared with once-daily insulin glargine in type 2 diabetic subjects inadequately controlled on oral antidiabetic drugs (OADs).

Research Design and Methods.—This 28-week parallel-group study randomized 233 insulin-naive patients with HbA_{1c} values ≥8.0% on >1,000 mg/day metformin alone or in combination with other OADs. Metformin was adjusted up to 2,550 mg/day before insulin therapy was initiated with 5-6 units BIAsp 70/30 twice daily or 10-12 units glargine at bedtime and titrated to target blood glucose (80-110 mg/dl) by algorithm-directed titration.

Results.—A total of 209 subjects completed the study. At study end, the mean HbA_{1c} value was lower in the BIAsp 70/30 group than in the glargine group (6.91 ± 1.17 vs. 7.41 ± 1.24%, $P < 0.01$). The HbA_{1c} reduction was greater in the BIAsp 70/30 group than in the glargine group (−2.79 ± 0.11 vs. −2.36 ± 0.11%, respectively; $P < 0.01$), especially for subjects with baseline HbA_{1c} >8.5% (−3.13 ± 1.63 vs. −2.60 ± 1.50%, respectively; $P < 0.05$). More BIAsp 70/30-treated subjects reached target HbA_{1c} values than glargine-treated subjects HbA_{1c} ≤6.5%: 42 vs. 28%, $P < 0.05$; HbA_{1c} <7.0%: 66 vs. 40%, $P < 0.001$). Minor hypoglycemia (episodes/year) was greater in the BIAsp 70/30 group than in the glargine group (3.4 ± 6.6 and

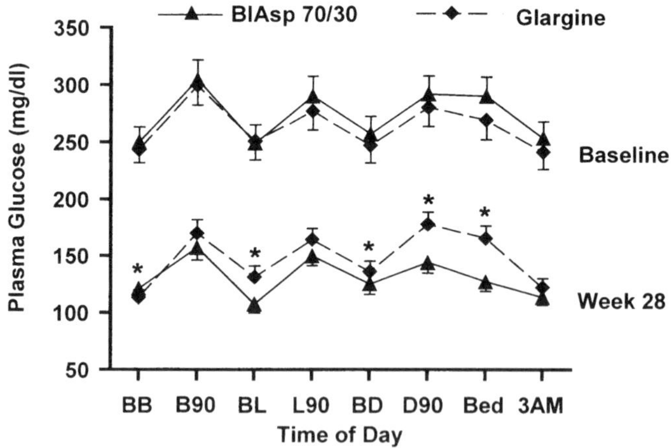

FIGURE 2.—Eight-point SMPG readings before breakfast, lunch, and supper [BB, BL, and BD] and 90 min after breakfast, lunch, and supper [B90, L90, and D90]; at bedtime [Bed]; and at 3:00 A.M. Number of data points at each time point at baseline, 114-116; at week 28, BIAsp 70/30, 97–99; glargine, 105–106. Statistically significant differences ($P < 0.05$) between treatment groups at specific time points are indicated with an asterisk. Error bars represent 2 SE. (Courtesy of Raskin P, Hu P, Allen E, et al: Initiating insulin therapy in type 2 diabetes. *Diabetes Care* 28:260-265, 2005. Copyright 2005 American Diabetes Association. Reprinted with permission from The American Diabetes Association.)

0.7 ± 2.0, respectively; $P < 0.05$). Weight gain and daily insulin dose at study end were greater for BIAsp 70/30-treated subjects than for glargine-treated subjects (weight gain: 5.4 ± 4.8 vs. 3.5 ± 4.5 kg, $P < 0.01$; insulin dose: 78.5 ± 39.5 and 51.3 ± 26.7 units/day, respectively).

Conclusions.—In subjects with type 2 diabetes poorly controlled on OADs, initiating insulin therapy with twice-daily BIAsp 70/30 was more effective in achieving HbA_{1c} targets than once-daily glargine, especially in subjects with HbA_{1c} >8.5% (Fig 2).

► These back-to-back reports (Abstracts 55–1 and 55–2) address the clinically important issue of the best method to start insulin therapy in patients with type 2 diabetes who are not responding to oral agents. A time-honored approach has been to add a long-acting insulin to the existing oral agents, so-called basal insulin therapy. Traditionally, bedtime NPH was used, but there has been a steady switching during the last few years by many practitioners to the analog insulin glargine because of its peak-free effect with less nocturnal hypoglycemia. A second approach has been to begin a twice-daily program of a premixed insulin, with advocates saying the combination of basal and bolus insulins makes for better control in many patients. On the other hand, those who dislike this approach complain about its lack of flexibility because of the fixed ratio of the insulins plus frequent hypoglycemia from the peaking nature of the NPH insulin.

These 2 studies directly compared adding glargine insulin versus a premixture in insulin-naive patients with type 2 diabetes. The study by Janka et al (Abstract 55–1) used twice-daily 70% NPH/30% regular versus morning glargine, with a forced titration schema aimed at achieving a fasting blood glucose 100 mg/dL or less with glargine, and that same value both fasting and predinner with the premix. Baseline HbA1c was 8.8%. The results were clear cut in favor of the glargine: a better improvement of HbA1c to 7.15% with glargine versus 7.49% with the premix, with half the hypoglycemia and a tendency for less weight gain (1.4 kg for glargine vs. 2.1 kg for premix; $P = 0.08$). Furthermore, the findings suggested the reason for the better HgA1c with glargine was an easier ability to optimize FBG values than the premix, one presumes because of the reduced problem with nocturnal hypoglycemia.

This study reinforces my prejudice against the traditional 70/30 premix insulin that combines NPH and regular insulin; my experience with it over the years is that few patients can attain target HbA1c values without unacceptable hypoglycemia or a feeling of being "locked into" their insulin program. I thus reserve it as a last resort. Having said that, it is important to recognize that this study has been criticized somewhat for its design. Patients were enrolled who were failing combination sulfonylurea and metformin therapy: the most common combination oral therapy used in the United States and around the world. In the glargine group, both of these agents were continued, which is the general recommendation for successful basal insulin therapy. However, in the premix group both agents were stopped, which is counter to the belief of most experts that metformin should be continued; many studies have shown benefits for reduced weight gain and better HbA1c values in type 2 diabetes when metformin is combined with insulin, so it is the generally recommended practice to continue it if there is no contraindication. The authors rationalized their protocol by saying that in real-world practice most general practitioners stop all oral agents when premix insulin is added, and that is what they studied. For me, it doesn't matter. As stated above, I see little justification for starting an inflexible twice-daily program over an easier, and I believe safer, once-daily program when starting insulin therapy in type 2 diabetes, and this study does nothing to challenge that.

Analysis of the study by Raskin et al (Abstract 55–2) is more complex. It compared adding bedtime glargine versus a twice-daily analog premix (70% analog NPH-like/30% aspart) to oral agent failures. Again, the study is controversial because of how the oral agents were handled. All patients were on maximal metformin, and prior thiazolidinediones were continued (about 30% of the patients) in both groups. Sulfonylureas were stopped in the premix group as would be expected, but also in the glargine group to make the only treatment difference between the groups the insulin preparations. However, many experts advocate continuation of secretagogues as a fundamental feature of successful basal insulin therapy to optimize prandial blood glucose control. As such, some have argued that its discontinuation in this study provided an advantage to the premix arm.

The results of this study are dramatic and clearly support the power of insulin therapy in patients with type 2 diabetes who are not responding to oral agents. Baseline HbA1c was 9.7%; it fell to 6.9% with the premix and 7.4% with glargine. One can see the reason for the argument over the importance of stopping the secretagogue in the glargine group, as the "better A1C effect of the premix over glargine" has been heavily advertised from this study. The results also showed the problems of a premix: greater weight gain (5.4 vs 3.5 kg over the 30 weeks of the study) and a 5-fold increase in documented blood glucose values less than 56 mg/dL.

Thus, a good news/bad news story. What to do? The first conclusion is again to emphasize the power of starting insulin in patients with type 2 diabetes. I find it frankly amazing that these relatively simple insulin regimens brought the starting HbA1c values of nearly 10% to below (premix) or close to (glargine) the national goal of less than 7%. No oral agent would have near that effect. Stated another way, if your patients need insulin, they need insulin! What about which insulin to start based on the results in this study? To answer that question, one must read the study carefully; there are a few findings that are important to that question but are often little discussed. The overall conclusion of the study is the better HbA1c value in the premix groups, but it turns out that the attained HbA1c values were the same for glargine versus premix when the starting value was up to 8.5%. The authors discount that finding by saying insulin is typically started in the United States after that. Perhaps. My response would be that's a problem that needs fixing. Our national push should be to start insulin earlier, as study after study shows the power of insulin in those who need it, paired with others showing how badly we are doing with diabetes care in this country. Thus, I hope their argument will soon become historic.

A second interesting finding to me is the 8-point profile shown in Fig 2. Note on the bottom part of the figure that blood glucose values are reasonably similar for the 2 groups through the day but then deviate after supper. It suggests those patients could be treated with prandial coverage only at supper—still a twice-daily program—and get equal if not better improvement in HbA1c as the premix program while avoiding the disadvantages. Studies are underway that compare the efficacy of this stepped approach of adding prandial insulin to basal insulin therapy.

For all these reasons, I continue to advocate and use a single injection of basal insulin on top of the patient's oral agents as my starting insulin therapy in patients with type 2 diabetes who do not respond to oral agents.

J. L. Leahy, MD

► The results of this study run counter to the natural prejudices of many "purists" who have an instinctive dislike for premixed (biphasic) insulin; I have to confess that, as a matter of preference, I rarely prescribe premixed insulins. Yet, as in life, in medicine it does us good to confront our prejudices to see how they stand up to objective scrutiny, and this study makes a persuasive case for the use of premixed biphasic insulin analog.

The concern that is most often raised regarding premixed insulin is that as the dose is increased, because the ratio of rapid to longer acting insulin is fixed, there will be a greater risk of hypoglycemia than with either basal insulin alone or with a combination of basal and rapid acting insulin given separately. Significantly more hypoglycemic episodes did indeed occur with the premixed regimen in this report, but, as the authors reasonably point out, none of these was major—major being defined as having neurologic symptoms consistent with hypoglycemia requiring assistance and having a plasma glucose less than 56 mg/dL or reversal of symptoms after food intake, glucagons, or intravenous glucose.

Unlike in Abstract 55–1, there cannot really be argument that the basal insulin (glargine) regimen was not fully implemented; the dosage of glargine achieved was, if anything, slightly greater than in the Treat-to-Target study, and the fasting glucose level virtually identical.[1] It is interesting, though, that the daily insulin dosage reached with the biphasic insulin in the present study was more than 50% greater than the glargine dosage: 78 U versus 51 U. So a potentially valid criticism is that in this study all patients discontinued oral secretagogue, which may have disadvantaged the glargine-treated patients; continuing an oral secretagogue in those patients would have more exactly mimicked the Treat-to-Target study and might have enhanced the postprandial efficacy of the basal insulin regimen. Even that, however, is not certain, because there is still debate as to whether the most commonly used secretagogues, the sulfonylureas, affect postprandial glucose to a greater extent than fasting glucose.

The biphasic insulin used in this study—BIAsp 70/30—is not, at present, the most widely used premixed insulin; the older mixture of regular and NPH is available relatively cheaply in generic form, and for that reason is often preferred by patients for whom cost is a significant issue. One might expect more hypoglycemia to occur with a mixture of regular and NPH, so caution should be exercised in extrapolating the results of this study to those patients.

In an accompanying editorial referring to starting insulin therapy in type 2 patients, Davidson opined that "it probably does not really matter what regimen one initially chooses."[2] The key factor is to continue to intensify the approach until targets are achieved and then to maintain them." In other words, "it does not matter how we get there as long as we do" and "achieving it with the least disruption to patients' lifestyles would seem preferable."[2] I don't think any reasonable person could, or should, disagree with that.

L. Kennedy, MD, FRCP

References

1. Riddle MC, Rosenstock J, Gerich J: The Treat-to-Target trial: Randomized addition of glargine or human NPH insulin to oral therapy of type 2 diabetic patients. *Diabetes Care* 26:3080-3086; 2003.
2. Davidson MB: Starting insulin therapy in type 2 diabetic patients. Does it really matter how? *Diabetes Care* 28:494-495; 2005.

Exenatide Versus Insulin Glargine in Patients With Suboptimally Controlled Type 2 Diabetes: A Randomized Trial

Heine RJ, for the GWAA Study Group (VU Univ, Amsterdam; et al)

Ann Intern Med 143:559-569, 2005 55–3

Background.—Physicians may use either insulin or exenatide injections for patients with type 2 diabetes mellitus who have poor glycemic control despite taking oral blood glucose-lowering drugs.

Objective.—To compare effects of exenatide and insulin glargine on glycemic control in patients with type 2 diabetes mellitus that is suboptimally controlled with metformin and a sulfonylurea.

Design.—26-week multicenter, open-label, randomized, controlled trial.

Setting.—82 outpatient study centers in 13 countries.

Patients.—551 patients with type 2 diabetes and inadequate glycemic control (defined as hemoglobin A_{1c} level ranging from 7.0% to 10.0%) despite combination metformin and sulfonylurea therapy.

Intervention.—Exenatide, 10 μg twice daily, or insulin glargine, 1 daily dose titrated to maintain fasting blood glucose levels of less than 5.6 mmol/L (<100 mg/dL).

Measurements.—Hemoglobin A_{1c} level, fasting plasma glucose level, body weight, 7-point self-monitored blood glucose, standardized test-meal challenge, safety, and tolerability.

Results.—Baseline mean hemoglobin A_{1c} level was 8.2% for patients receiving exenatide and 8.3% for those receiving insulin glargine. At week 26, both exenatide and insulin glargine reduced hemoglobin A_{1c} levels by 1.11% (difference, 0.017 percentage point [95% CI, −0.123 to 0.157 percentage point]). Exenatide reduced postprandial glucose excursions more than insulin glargine, while insulin glargine reduced fasting glucose concentrations more than exenatide (Fig 3). Body weight decreased 2.3 kg with exenatide and increased 1.8 kg with insulin glargine (difference, −4.1 kg [CI, −4.6 to −3.5 kg]). Rates of symptomatic hypoglycemia were similar, but nocturnal hypoglycemia occurred less frequently with exenatide (0.9 event/patient-

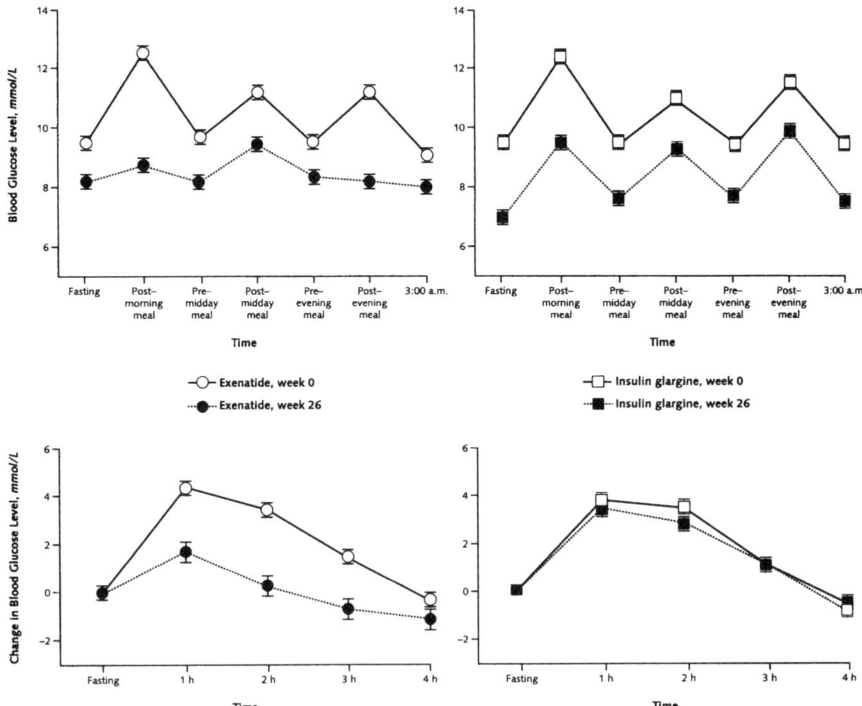

FIGURE 3.—Self-monitored blood glucose profiles (*top*) and postprandial blood glucose concentrations after test meal (*bottom*). Least-square mean (± SE) data for self-monitored glucose concentrations at baseline and week 26 are shown for the exenatide and insulin glargine groups. In a 24-hour period, data were collected just before each meal (fasting, pre-midday meal, pre-evening meal), 2 hours after each meal (post-morning meal, post-midday meal, post-evening meal), and at 3:00 a.m. At week 26, the exenatide group had higher mean values for blood glucose levels at fasting ($P < 0.001$), before lunch ($P = 0.023$), before dinner ($P = 0.006$), and at 3:00 a.m. ($P < 0.001$), but the group had lower glucose levels after morning ($P < 0.001$) and evening ($P < 0.001$) means than the group receiving insulin glargine. Data shown are from the intention-to-treat population. Changes in postprandial blood glucose concentrations from time 0 (fasting) are shown for the subset of patients that underwent the test-meal study. Levels at baseline and at week 26 are shown for exenatide ($n = 41$) and insulin glargine ($n = 37$). Data were collected before the test meal (fasting) and again 1, 2, 3, and 4 hours after the test meal (displayed as mean [± SE]). To convert mmol/L to mg/dL, divide by 0.0555. (Courtesy of Heine RJ, for the GWAA Study Group: Exenatide versus insulin glargine in patients with suboptimally controlled type 2 diabetes: A randomized trial. *Ann Intern Med* 143:559-569, 2005.)

year versus 2.4 events/patient-year; difference, −1.6 events/patient-year [CI, −2.3 to −0.9 event/patient year]). Gastrointestinal symptoms were more common in the exenatide group than in the insulin glargine group, including nausea (57.1% vs. 8.6%), vomiting (17.4% vs. 3.7%) and diarrhea (8.5% vs. 3.0%).

Limitations.—The trial was open-label and did not assess clinical complications related to diabetes. Of the 551 participants, 19.4% of those receiving exenatide and 9.7% of those receiving insulin glargine withdrew from the study. Only 21.6% of the insulin glargine group and 8.6% of the exenatide group achieved the target level for fasting plasma glucose of less than 5.6 mmol/L (<100 mg/dL).

Conclusions.—Exenatide and insulin glargine achieved similar improvements in overall glycemic control in patients with type 2 diabetes that was suboptimally controlled with oral combination therapy. Exenatide was associated with weight reduction and had a higher incidence of gastrointestinal adverse effects than insulin glargine.

► This past year brought us exenatide, which is the first therapy based on a new approach to the treatment of type 2 diabetes through enhanced action of the incretin GLP-1 (glucagon-like peptide-1). Its arrival has been highly anticipated by physicians who look forward to learning how powerful its relatively unique features may be (impaired glucagon secretion, slowed gastric motility, satiety effect, promote beta-cell development or survival) in terms of blood glucose control, weight loss, and whether the natural history of progressive beta-cell dysfunction in this disease could be altered or stopped. Patients quickly became enthused because of its reputation for weight loss. Indeed, many practitioners have had the experience that the previously presumed barrier for starting insulin—the SHOT—seems to have disappeared with exenatide. Many, including myself, have patients who previously avoided insulin at all costs, but have come in requesting exenatide, having heard about the weight loss, and are totally unfazed when told it is a twice-daily injection. Thus, these are the key clinical questions: How good is it? When to use it? What to expect?

I quite like this study. Exenatide is only approved for patients failing sulfonylurea, metformin, or a combination of the 2. The current approach to those patients is often to start a single injection of a long-acting insulin (basal insulin therapy), especially when the HbA_{1c} value is above 8% as it is unlikely a third drug (in this case a thiazolidinedione) will get many of those patients to a value <7%. Now we have exenatide. This study compares head-to head treatment of adding glargine or exenatide to existing therapy. Baseline HbA_{1c} was 8.2%. The results showed equal efficacy for improvement in HbA_{1c}, to 7.1% in both groups so that a little less than 50% in both groups attained <7%. However, there were differences between glargine and exenatide, namely, for weight (−2.3 kg exenatide vs +1.8 kg glargine), and a lot more gastrointestinal side effects with exenatide (nausea 57% vs 9% and vomiting 17% vs 4%), so the dropout rate because of the gastrointestinal side effects was higher in the exenatide-treatment group. None of this is surprising but fits exactly with what would be predicted from the known actions of exenatide from prior trials.

What to do? The answer somewhat is pick your poison—neither therapy is perfect, both have pluses and minuses. Stated another way, this study clearly shows that exenatide is a reasonable substitute for starting basal insulin although the characteristics of the patient group in this study are key to a full interpretation of the results. Prior studies with exenatide have shown modest effects on HbA_{1c}—considerably less than the 1.1% lowering seen in this study—so that I have taught when failing 1 or 2 oral agents, with HbA_{1c} up to 8%, then another oral agent or exenatide can be tried. However, much above 8% then basal insulin should be started. I have not changed that schema based on this study as the starting HbA_{1c} value averaged 8.2%. I continue to expect that basal insulin will be superior in patients with higher starting HbA_{1c} values based on the other published trials. So, no big clinical surprises for me in this study.

However, I love this trial, and the reason is the accompanying figure. It beautifully shows what for me is the key finding of the trial, that the main differentiating feature between exenatide and basal insulin is their modes of action. In other words, glargine and exenatide work *totally differently* for blood glucose control. The panels on the left are exenatide—it hugely improved postmeal glycemia, with only a small improvement in fasting glycemia. In turn, the right panels with glargine show a big improvement in fasting blood glucose, but effectively the same rise and fall at meals. These data show that at this stage of the disease, targeting fasting sugars OR postprandial sugars will both have a big effect on overall glycemia, and that one is not necessarily better than another at this stage of the disease. Moreover, one can easily imagine that combining the 2 would have a spectacular effect on HbA_{1c}. Thus, the data from this study show that GLP-1 drugs primarily control postprandial glycemia, and this is different than basal insulin. As such, it should not be a surprise that trials are underway to critically test combining GLP-1 agents with basal insulin. In my mind, the main power of these drugs will prove to be when used early in the disease (as prevention, monotherapy) or in combination with basal insulin, when attaining postprandial glucose control is the dominate clinical goal.

J. L. Leahy, MD

► It was inevitable that this study would be done. In the last few years, while the "signature trials" of exenatide—in patients with uncontrolled diabetes despite treatment with 1 or 2 oral agents—have been underway (see Abstract –)) the effectiveness of glargine insulin as additional therapy causing less hypoglycemia than other insulins in this situation has been established.[1]

But I want to ask 2 questions. Is this a good study? Is it really sensible to compare exenatide and glargine as alternative treatments?

It is good that the study is randomized; the protocol, involving titration of glargine insulin, precluded the possibility of blinding, but that does not detract from the study in my opinion. Where it seems to fail is in the application of the glargine titration algorithm. From a starting dose of 10 U, glargine was to be increased by 2 U every 3 days to achieve a fasting blood glucose of less than 100 mg/dL. By the end of the study, 26 weeks, the average glargine dosage was just 25 U, but the average fasting glucose was, by my calculation, about 135 mg/dL, far above the stated goal; so one has to ask why the achieved insulin dosage was not higher. In the Treat-to-Target trial the average daily dose of glargine insulin required to achieve a mean A_{1C} of 6.96% and a fasting glucose of about 117 mg/dL over a similar period of time, was 47 units in patients with fairly similar body weight as in this study[1]; adherence to the insulin titration algorithm was encouraged by weekly contact with the patient specifically for that purpose, and a subsequent study (Goal A1C) has reinforced the role that simply contacting patients to remind them to increase the basal insulin dose, if necessary, plays in optimizing this type of therapy.[2] To be fair, Heine et al deal with this to some extent in their discussion, but their conclusion that fixed-dose exenatide achieved similar improvements in overall glycemic control to insulin glargine titration in their patient population would unlikely hold if the glargine treatment algorithm had been more assiduously applied. It may be true, as they say, that the glargine titration schedule and their approach to encouraging patient adherence—with no evidence of any such encouragement after the initial visit—may be more reflective of real-world use. In that case, real-world use has to change.

Turning to my second question, my preceding review hints at why I don't think it is necessarily sensible to compare these as alternative treatment options, except insofar as it illustrates the different effects of the 2 interventions. In my opinion exenatide and basal insulin should not be viewed as competing therapies, but as potentially complementary. Glargine insulin is clearly more effective in reducing fasting glucose, and exenatide is clearly superior in reducing the postprandial glucose excursion. It would have been interesting to combine the therapies in all these patients as an extension to the study, say over another 16 weeks.

I have no doubt that exenatide does represent a truly significant breakthrough in diabetes treatment. Any weight loss, no matter how little, that occurs while improving hyperglycemia and decreasing the calorie loss with glycosuria is a bonus to patients. The effects on postprandial hyperglycemia, particularly important as a contribution to improving overall glycemia in patients whose A_{1C} levels are only modestly elevated, suggest that this drug could make the crucial difference between almost and really normal.

L. Kennedy, MD, FRCP

References

1. Riddle MC, Rosenstock J, Gerich J: The Treat-to-Target trial: Randomized addition of glargine or human NPH insulin to oral therapy of type 2 diabetic patients. *Diabetes Care* 26:3080-3086; 2003.
2. Kennedy L, Hermann W, Strange P, et al: Impact of active versus usual algorithm titration of basal insulin and point-of-care versus laboratory measurement of HbA1c on glycemic control in patients with type 2 diabetes: The Glycemic Optimization with Algorithms and Labs at Point of Care (GOAL A1C) trial. *Diabetes Care* 29:1-8, 2006.

Systematic Review and Meta-analysis of Short-Acting Insulin Analogues in Patients With Diabetes Mellitus

Plank J, Siebenhofer A, Berghold A, et al (Med Univ, Graz, Austria; Inst of Med Technologies and Health Management, Graz, Austria)
Arch Intern Med 165:1337-1344, 2005 55–4

Background.—This article compares the effect of treatment with short-acting insulin (SAI) analogues vs regular insulin on glycemic control, hypoglycemic episodes, quality of life, and diabetes-specific complications.

Methods.—Electronic searches (Cochrane Library, MEDLINE, and EMBASE) and additional searching (pharmaceutical companies, experts, approval agencies, abstracts of diabetology meetings) were performed. Two reviewers independently screened randomized controlled trials to determine inclusion.

Results.—Forty-two randomized controlled trials that assessed the effect of SAI analogues vs regular insulin in 7933 patients with type 1 diabetes mellitus, type 2 diabetes mellitus, and gestational diabetes mellitus were identified. The weighted mean difference between hemoglobin A_{1c} values obtained using SAI analogues and regular insulin was −0.12% (95% confidence interval [CI], −0.17% to −0.07%) for adult patients with type 1 diabetes mellitus and −0.02% (95% CI, −0.10% to 0.07%) for patients with type 2 diabetes mellitus. The standardized mean difference for overall hypoglycemia (episodes per patient per month) was −0.05 (95% CI, −0.22 to 0.11) and −0.04 (95% CI, −0.12 to 0.04) comparing SAI analogues with regular insulin in adult patients with type 1 and type 2 diabetes mellitus, respectively. No differences between treatments were observed in children with type 1 diabetes, pregnant women with type 1 diabetes mellitus, and women with gestational diabetes. Concerning quality of life, improvement was observed only in open-label studies in patients with type 1 diabetes mellitus. No differences were seen in a double-blinded study of patients with type 1 or in the studies of patients with type 2 diabetes mellitus.

Conclusion.—Our analysis suggests only a minor benefit to hemoglobin A_{1c} values in adult patients with type 1 diabetes mellitus but no benefit in the remaining population with type 2 or gestational diabetes from SAI analogue treatment.

► To most endocrinologists, it seems one of the obvious truths in life that insulin analogs are superior to traditional nonanalog insulins. What's not to like. Their actions profiles are much closer to physiologic insulin delivery, the long-acting analogs are more consistent in their day-to-day effect, and anatomic variations in absorption are much less of an issue with analogs than traditional insulins. There is also more flexibility for when the insulin is injected for both the short- and long-acting analogs versus traditional insulins. And I have not even mentioned the well-known reduction in hypoglycemia for both short- and long-acting analogs. I recognize that showing differences in HbA_{1c} values for analogs versus their traditional counterparts has rarely been done. Still, one can lower that value as low as wanted with any insulin, with the only issue being how much hypoglycemia can be tolerated, so the lowered hypoglycemia rates with similar HbA_{1c} values seem all that is needed to prove superiority. This glowing appraisal of analogs is in agreement with my clinical experience plus an excellent review from this year,[1] and a meta-analysis of the long-acting analog, glargine.[2] It was thus a bit disconcerting when this meta-analysis of the short-acting analogs failed to show any real benefit over regular insulin, including lack of a difference in quality of life or hypoglycemia. Indeed, the latter disagrees with a smaller meta-analysis that was published for lispro in 1998.[3]

How to reconcile this result? Importantly, a meta-analysis is a very different scientific way of addressing a question than a regular research study that defines the hypothesis, and then attempts to design the most rigorous and scientifically exact way to test it. We typically judge a study by how well the protocol is designed, and most admire those who get the design right, scientifically and in terms of relevance for patient care. Meta-analysis instead takes all the published studies on a question that meet fairly general criteria—

the good, the bad, and the ugly—and looks for where the preponderant result is. To a nonpractitioner of the science, the technique assumes you will get the right answer if you look at enough studies, as random variables will be canceled out (I apologize to those who do this science, as I know this explanation is incredibly simplistic). Unfortunately, insulin treatment studies are notoriously bad, with few attaining rigorous blood glucose control (ie, the highest risk of hypoglycemia), and most protocols being so contrived as to be irrelevant for normal everyday usage of insulin.

So this study should be looked at for what it is—a running tally of published studies. For insight into insulin therapy, my own practice is to rely on individual research studies that are well designed and rigorously performed.

J. L. Leahy, MD

References

1. Hirsch I: Insulin analogues. *N Engl J Med* 352:174-183, 2005.
2. Rosenstock J, Dailey G, Massi-Benedetti M, et al: Reduced hypoglycemia risk with insulin glargine. A meta-analysis comparing insulin glargine with human NPH insulin in type 2 diabetes. *Diabetes Care* 28:950-955, 2005.
3. Brunelle BL, Llewelyn J, Anderson JH Jr, et al: Meta-analysis of the effect of insulin lispro on severe hypoglycemia in patients with type 1 diabetes. *Diabetes Care* 21:1726-1731, 1998.

Clinical Outcomes in Antihypertensive Treatment of Type 2 Diabetes, Impaired Fasting Glucose Concentration, and Normoglycemia: Antihypertensive and Lipid-Lowering Treatment to Prevent Heart Attack Trial (ALLHAT)

Whelton PK, for the ALLHAT Collaborative Research Group (Tulane Univ, New Orleans, La; et al)

Arch Intern Med 165:1401-1409, 2005 55–5

Background.—Optimal first-step antihypertensive drug therapy in type 2 diabetes mellitus (DM) or impaired fasting glucose levels (IFG) is uncertain. We wished to determine whether treatment with a calcium channel blocker or an angiotensin-converting enzyme inhibitor decreases clinical complications compared with treatment with a thiazide-type diuretic in DM, IFG, and normoglycemia (NG).

Methods.—Active-controlled trial in 31 512 adults, 55 years or older, with hypertension and at least 1 other risk factor for coronary heart disease, stratified into DM (n = 13 101), IFG (n = 1399), and NG (n = 17 012) groups on the basis of national guidelines. Participants were randomly assigned to double-blind first-step treatment with chlorthalidone, 12.5 to 25 mg/d, amlodipine besylate, 2.5 to 10 mg/d, or lisinopril, 10 to 40 mg/d. We conducted an intention-to-treat analysis of fatal coronary heart disease or nonfatal myocardial infarction (primary outcome), total mortality, and other clinical complications.

Results.—There was no significant difference in relative risk (RR) for the primary outcome in DM or NG participants assigned to amlodipine or lisinopril vs chlorthalidone or in IFG participants assigned to lisinopril vs chlorthalidone. A significantly higher RR (95% confidence interval) was noted for the primary outcome in IFG participants assigned to amlodipine vs chlorthalidone (1.73 [1.10-2.72]). Stroke was more common in NG participants assigned to lisinopril vs chlorthalidone (1.31 [1.10-1.57]). Heart failure was more common in DM and NG participants assigned to amlodipine (1.39 [1.22-1.59] and 1.30 [1.12-1.51], respectively) or lisinopril (1.15 [1.00-1.32] and 1.19 [1.02-1.39], respectively) vs chlorthalidone.

Conclusion.—Our results provide no evidence of superiority for treatment with calcium channel blockers or angiotensin-converting enzyme inhibitors compared with a thiazide-type diuretic during first-step antihypertensive therapy in DM, IFG, or NG.

► This is a complex trial that is focused on comparing first-line antihypertensive therapies in person with all degree of glucose tolerance, in terms of cardiovascular outcomes. It included 31,512 adults older than 55 years with hypertension and at least 1 other cardiovascular (CV) risk factor, who were randomly assigned to receive an angiotensin-converting enzyme inhibitor (ACEI) (lisinopril), a calcium channel blocker (CCB) (amlopipine), or a thiazide-type diuretic (chlorthalidone) for an average 5 years. Its strength, and at the same time its curse, is its size, complexity, and diversity of patient populations: 13,101 with DM, 1399 with IFG, and 17,102 with NG. Also, 30% to 38% black subjects, 36% to 60% incidence of known CV disease (CVD), variable use of aspirin, estrogen, and lipid-lowering agents. As such, there is a huge number of subgroup analyses in the article. For our purpose, it is best to look at the "big picture" results to come away with the clinically applicable findings. Also, I will focus on those in the DM group as the most relevant for our purposes.

Chlorthalidone was a little better at lowering blood pressure (BP) in the patients with DM than either of the other agents—from baseline 146/84 to 135/74 with chlorthalidone, 136/75 with amlodipione, and 138/75 with lisinopril (clearly not perfect with any of them, highlighting the need to combine a diuretic with an ACEI or CCB in many patients). Importantly, the better BP with chlorthalidine was most apparent in black patients, with a 4 to 5 mm Hg difference between chlorthalidone and lisinopril, less so with amlodipine. What about CV outcomes? There were no major differences with the 3 drugs, although there were subtleties. There was a small increase in the stroke rate in NG patients who received lisinopril versus chlorthalidone (not in the patients with DM), but this difference was present in all 3 glycemic strata in the black patients. There was also a higher incidence of heart failure with amlodipine versus chlorthalidine.

What to interpret? The authors are quite conservative in their discussion, and conclude "our analysis as failing to demonstrate superiority in protecting against CHD death and nonfatal MI during first-step treatment with an ACEI or a CCB compared with thiazide-type diuretics in those with DM?" Stated another way, you can start with whatever agent you like—the key is to control BP, not how you do that. A similar conclusion was made in an article that surveyed a large number of published trials of various antihypertensive agents in patients with DM that was published in the same issue of the *Archives of Internal Medicine*.[1]

However, one can go a little further with the clinical implications of their results. They go on to point out that chlorthalidine is at least as good, if not better, than the others. It is time honored and cheap, and thus they imply it might be the best choice. Maybe. I am struck that the trial failed to get to national BP goals with any of the agents, and I thus conclude that none alone is enough in most patients as would be predicted by most physicians from their clinical experience. A diuretic combined with 1 of the other agents is likely the best starting program—what, in fact, many primary doctors do using the available combination products. However, there is 1 result in this trial that I am struck by as being important and clinically relevant as well as having been unknown to me before this study—that chlorthalidine was more effective and safer in black patients with diabetes than the other agents. Given the high incidence of both DM and hypertension in black patients, plus the usual standard of care being to use ACEI or angiotensin receptor blocker agents as starting therapy in patients with DM, this observations needs follow-up and confirmation.

J. L. Leahy, MD

Reference

1. Blood Pressure Lowering Treatment Trialists' Collaboration: Effects of different blood pressure-lowering regimens on major cardiovascular events in individuals with and without diabetes mellitus. *Arch Intern Med* 165:1410-1419, 2005.

Lifestyle, Diabetes, and Cardiovascular Risk Factors 10 Years After Bariatric Surgery

Sjöström L, for the Swedish Obese Subjects Study Scientific Group (Sahlgrenska Univ, Göteborg, Sweden; et al)

N Engl J Med 351:2683-2693, 2004 55–6

Background.—Weight loss is associated with short-term amelioration and prevention of metabolic and cardiovascular risk, but whether these benefits persist over time is unknown.

Methods.—The prospective, controlled Swedish Obese Subjects Study involved obese subjects who underwent gastric surgery and contemporaneously matched, conventionally treated obese control subjects. We now report follow-up data for subjects (mean age, 48 years; mean body-mass index, 41) who had been enrolled for at least 2 years (4047 subjects) or 10 years (1703 subjects) before the analysis (January 1, 2004). The follow-up rate for laboratory examinations was 86.6 percent at 2 years and 74.5 percent at 10 years.

Results.—After two years, the weight had increased by 0.1 percent in the control group and had decreased by 23.4 percent in the surgery group (P<0.001) (Table 2). After 10 years, the weight had increased by 1.6 percent

TABLE 2.—Percentage Changes in Weight, Anthropometric Variables, Risk Factors, and Energy Intake at 2 and 10 Years*

Variable	Changes at 2 Yr†			Changes at 10 Yr†			Changes at 10 Yr in Surgery Subgroups		
	Control Group (N=1660)	Surgery Group (N=1845)	Difference (95% CI)	Control Group (N=627)	Surgery Group (N=641)	Difference (95% CI)	Banding (N=156)	Vertical Banded Gastroplasty‡ (N=451)	Gastric Bypass‡ (N=34)
	Percent			Percent			Percent		
Weight	0.1	−23.4	22.2 (21.6 to 22.8)§	1.6	−16.1	16.3 (14.9 to 17.6)§	−13.2	−16.5¶	−25.0§
Height	−0.01	−0.06	0.06 (0.02 to 0.10)¶	−0.3	−0.3	−0.01 (−0.12 to 0.10)	−0.2	−0.3	−0.8§
BMI	0.1	−23.3	22.1 (21.5 to 22.7)§	2.3	−15.7	16.5 (15.1 to 17.8)§	−12.8	−16.0¶	−23.8§
Waist	0.2	−16.9	16.0 (15.4 to 16.5)§	2.8	−10.1	11.3 (10.3 to 12.4)§	−7.6	−10.2¶	−19.3§
Systolic blood pressure	0.5	−4.4	2.8 (2.1 to 3.6)§	4.4	0.5	1.1 (−0.3 to 2.6)	2.1	0.4	−4.7
Diastolic blood pressure	0.3	−5.2	3.2 (2.4 to 3.9)§	−2.0	−2.6	−2.3 (−3.5 to −1.0)§	−1.4	−2.5	−10.4‖
Pulse pressure	3.2	0.6	−0.5 (−2.3 to 1.3)	18.0	10.8	3.5 (0.1 to 6.9)¶	13.8	10.1	6.3
Glucose	5.1	−13.6	16.6 (15.0 to 18.3)§	18.7	−2.5	18.4 (14.7 to 22.1)§	−0.8	−2.5	−10.0
Insulin	10.3	−46.2	51.4 (48.0 to 54.8)§	12.3	−28.2	30.3 (23.9 to 36.6)§	−25.3	−27.2	−54.0§
Uric acid	−0.4	−14.9	13.5 (12.5 to 14.6)§	3.9	−6.2	8.8 (6.4 to 11.1)§	−5.2	−6.1	−12.3
Triglycerides	6.3	−27.2	29.9 (27.4 to 32.5)§	2.2	−16.3	14.8 (10.4 to 19.1)§	−18.0	−14.9	−28.0¶
HDL cholesterol	3.5	22.0	−18.7 (−20.1 to 17.3)§	10.8	24.0	−13.6 (−16.5 to −10.6)§	20.4	23.5	47.5¶
Total cholesterol	0.1	−2.9	1.0 (0.1 to 1.9)¶	−6.0	−5.4	−2.0 (−0.2 to −3.8)¶	−5.0	−5.0	−12.6§
Energy intake	−2.8	−28.6	19.1 (16.0 to 22.2)§	−1.0	−20.7	11.6 (8.1 to 15.0)§	−19.7	−21.6	−12.6

*Data are for all subjects who completed 2 and 10 years of the study and are independent of diagnosis and medications at or after baseline. The changes within each treatment group are unadjusted, whereas the differences between the groups in the changes have been adjusted for sex, age, body mass index (BMI), and the baseline level of the respective variable.

†For values within each group, *minus signs* denote decreases; for differences between the groups, *minus signs* denote smaller reductions or (in the case of HDL cholesterol) larger increases in the surgical group than in the control group.

‡*P* values are for the comparison with the banding subgroup.

§$P < .001$.

¶$P < .05$.

‖$P < .10$.

Abbreviation: CI, Confidence interval.

(Reprinted by permission of *The New England Journal of Medicine* from Sjöström L, for the Swedish Obese Subjects Study Scientific Group: Lifestyle, diabetes, and cardiovascular risk factors 10 years after bariatric surgery. *N Engl J Med* 351:2683-2693, 2004.)

and decreased by 16.1 percent, respectively (P<0.001). Energy intake was lower and the proportion of physically active subjects higher in the surgery group than in the control group throughout the observation period. Two- and 10-year rates of recovery from diabetes, hypertriglyceridemia, low levels of high-density lipoprotein cholesterol, hypertension, and hyperuricemia were more favorable in the surgery group than in the control group, whereas recovery from hypercholesterolemia did not differ between the groups. The surgery group had lower 2- and 10-year incidence rates of diabetes, hypertriglyceridemia, and hyperuricemia than the control group; differences between the groups in the incidence of hypercholesterolemia and hypertension were undetectable.

Conclusions.—As compared with conventional therapy, bariatric surgery appears to be a viable option for the treatment of severe obesity, resulting in long-term weight loss, improved lifestyle, and, except for hypercholesterolemia, amelioration in risk factors that were elevated at baseline.

Laparoscopic Gastric Banding Prevents Type 2 Diabetes and Arterial Hypertension and Induces Their Remission in Morbid Obesity: A 4-Year Case-Controlled Study

Pontiroli AE, Vedani P, Folli F, et al (Università degli Studi di Milano, Milan, Italy; Ospedale San Paolo, Milan, Italy; Ospedale San Raffaele, Milan, Italy; et al)
Diabetes Care 28:2703-2709, 2005 55–7

Objective.—Lifestyle modifications and pharmacological interventions can prevent type 2 diabetes in obese subjects with impaired glucose tolerance. The aim of this study was to compare laparoscopic adjustable gastric banding (LAGB) and conventional diet (No-LAGB) in the prevention (primary intervention study; 56 vs. 29 patients) and remission (secondary intervention study; 17 vs. 20 patients) of type 2 diabetes and hypertension in grade 3 obesity in a 4-year study.

Research Design and Methods.—The subjects (n = 122; age 48.5 ± 1.05 years; BMI 45.7 ± 0.67 kg/m^2) underwent a diagnostic workup, including psychological and psychiatric assessments, in preparation for the LAGB procedure. Of the 122 subjects, 73 had the surgery (LAGB group). The control group (No-LAGB group) consisted of the 49 subjects who refused the surgery but agreed to be followed up; 6 of these subjects dropped out by the 2nd year of the study, so that the final number of patients was 73 and 43 in the LAGB and No-LAGB groups, respectively. All patients had a yearly visit and oral glucose tolerance test.

Results.—From baseline to the end of the 4-year follow-up, BMI decreased from 45.9 ± 0.89 at baseline to 37.7 ± 0.71 kg/m^2 in the LAGB group and remained steady in the No-LAGB group (from 45.2 ± 1.04 to 46.5 ± 1.37 kg/m^2), with no significant differences between the primary and secondary intervention groups. In the primary intervention study, five of the No-LAGB subjects (17.2%) and none of the LAGB subjects (0.0%; P = 0.0001) progressed to type 2 diabetes; in the secondary intervention study, type 2 diabetes remitted in one No-LAGB patient (4.0%) and seven LAGB patients (45.0%; $P = 0.0052$). Hypertension occurred in 11 No-LAGB patients (25.6%) and 1 LAGB patient (1.4%; $P = 0.0001$) and remitted in 1 No-LAGB (2.3%) and 15 LAGB patients (20.5%; $P = 0.0001$). A study of body mass composition revealed a significant reduction of fat mass and a transitory, but not significant, decrease of fat-free mass in LAGB patients.

Conclusions.—In morbid obesity, sustained and long-lasting weight loss obtained through LAGB prevents the occurrence of type 2 diabetes and hypertension and decreases the prevalence of these disorders.

► The average body mass index (BMI) being reported in clinical trials involving type 2 diabetes patients is creeping ever-upwards, and on the western side of the Atlantic I know of some studies where it is just under 35 kg/m^2. The National Institutes of Health guidelines suggest that bariatric surgery is appropriate in morbid obesity when the BMI is greater than 40 in the absence of comorbidities, but greater than 35 in the presence of diabetes or hypertension.[1] So it is not fanciful to think that these studies may in the near future have potential relevance to a majority of patients with, or destined to develop, type 2 diabetes in America. Gastric banding, with or without gastroplasty, is less invasive than gastric bypass surgery, and probably has lower operative morbidity, but the weight reduction is, on average, less, as is apparent in the Sjöström study (Abstract 55–6; Table 2).

I would like to have seen more details of postoperative or surgical complications in both these articles. Sjöström et al report that 0.25% of their surgical patients died postoperatively, while 13% had some postoperative complication, including infection, bleeding, and thromboembolism; in 2.2%, the complications were severe enough to require reoperation. Pontiroli et al (Abstract 55–7) confine themselves to saying that stoma regulation was required in 43 of the 73 patients, reintervention in 8 patients, and removal of the adjustable banding device in 4 (after the study was completed in the case of 2 patients). Neither study gives details of possible longer-term complications such as nutritional deficiency, osteoporosis, and bowel obstruction. Another problem with all studies comparing bariatric surgery with conservative treatment is that they are not randomized, and these two are no exception. However, in both these studies, good efforts were made to match the surgical and nonsurgical patients with respect to important risk factors; in fact, at baseline, the surgical patients in the Sjöström study were slightly, but significantly, more obese, more hypertensive, and more hyperglycemic than the control patients. Comparative data on the occurrence of cardiovascular events and mortality would, of course, be the most compelling evidence of benefit, but this is lacking.[2]

Accepting these caveats, I have to say that the results of both studies are quite impressive. Is it not a sad reflection on modern life that failure to pursue a prudent lifestyle leads to the situation where a surgical intervention could be considered the most successful approach to the prevention and treatment of diabetes and metabolic syndrome?

L. Kennedy, MD, FRCP

References

1. National Institutes of Health: Clinical guidelines on the identification, evaluation, and treatment of overweight and obesity in adults: The evidence report. *Obes Res* 6:51S-209S; 1998.
2. Solomon CG, Dluhy RG: Bariatric surgery: Quick fix or long-term solution? *N Engl J Med* 351:2751-2753, 2004.

Psychoactive Drugs, Alcohol, and Severe Hypoglycemia in Insulin-treated Diabetes: Analysis of 141 Cases

Pedersen-Bjergaard U, Reubsaet JLE, Nielson SL, et al (Hillerød Hosp, Denmark; Univ of Oslo, Norway; Rigshospitalet, Copenhagen; et al)
Am J Med 118:307-310, 2005 55–8

Background.—Alcohol consumption is a well-established risk factor for severe hypoglycemia in patients with insulin-treated diabetes. It has been estimated that alcohol use is involved in up to 19% of severe hypoglycemic episodes. The use of psychoactive drugs has become common and is particularly widespread among young people. As with alcohol, these drugs can also increase the risk of accidents and trauma. Whether the use of psychoactive drugs increases the risk of severe hypoglycemia in patients with insulin-treated diabetes was determined.

Methods.—A prospective case series of adult patients (18 years and older) with known insulin-treated diabetes was assembled to assess and compare the frequency of use of psychoactive drugs and alcohol before episodes of severe hypoglycemia. Severe hypoglycemia was defined as the need of assistance from another person to restore glycemic level. A venous blood sample was drawn from each patient after treatment, and all specimens were screened for 66 of the most commonly used pharmaceutical drugs and 6 illicit drugs that could affect cognitive function and were available in Denmark.

Results.—Psychoactive substances were identified in samples from 31% of patients (Table 2). Alcohol was detected in 17% of samples, with a median plasma ethanol concentration of 50 mg/dL. The most commonly occurring pharmaceutical drugs were antidepressants (5%), benzodiazepines (4%), and opiates (2%). Among the illicit drugs, marijuana was identified in 5% of the samples, and amphetamines were present in 1% of samples. Only 4% of samples were positive for both alcohol and drugs; thus an association between alcohol and drugs was not detected. The identification of illicit drugs was confined to patients younger than 50 years.

Conclusions.—Persons with diabetes are informed of the relationship between alcohol consumption and the risk of severe hypoglycemia and advised to avoid excessive alcohol intake. It is possible that younger patients have been attracted to use psychoactive drugs that were not known to cause hypoglycemia. The increased acceptance of recreational use of these drugs among some segments of the population may be reinforcing this behavior. Health care providers should be cognizant of the possibility of use of psycho-

TABLE 2.—Identification of Psychoactive Drugs and Alcohol in Blood Screens

Drug/Substance	All (n = 141)	Age Group <50 Years (n = 77)	≥50 Years (n = 64)
		Number (%)	
Alcohol	24 (17)	11 (14)	13 (20)
Pharmaceutical drugs			
Antidepressants	7 (5)	3 (4)	4 (6)
Benzodiazepines	5 (4)	2 (3)	3 (5)
Opiates	3 (2)	1 (1)	2 (3)
Neuroleptics	1 (1)	0	1 (2)
Barbiturates	1 (1)	1 (1)	0
All	17 (12)	7 (9)	10 (16)
Illicit drugs			
Marijuana	7 (5)	7 (9)	0
Amphetamine	1 (1)	1 (1)	0
All	8 (6)	8 (10)	0
Overall*	43 (31)	22 (29)	21 (33)

*In 4% of samples, both alcohol and drugs were detected.

(Reprinted from Pedersen-Bjergaard U, Reubsaet JL, Nielsen SL, et al: Psychoactive drugs, alcohol, and severe hypoglycemia in insulin-treated diabetes: Analysis of 141 cases. *Am J Med* 118:307-310, 2005. Copyright 2005, with permission from Elsevier Science.)

active drugs by patients with diabetes and the need to advise these patients to avoid such drugs as diligently as they avoid alcohol. A need exists for additional studies to determine whether a causal relationship is present between recent drug use and severe hypoglycemia.

▶ Inappropriate insulin dose; skipping or delaying a meal; unusual physical exertion—the "usual suspects" rounded up to solve a case of severe hypoglycemia. And, of course, careful examination of the scene nearly always reveals 1, or a combination of 2 or all 3, to be the culprit—as, indeed, it must. This article brings to our attention the potential role of psychoactive drugs as aiding and abetting the commission of the misdemeanor. The evidence, as the authors admit, is purely circumstantial but has more than a ring of truth to it.

The age differences (Table 2) are interesting, though, perhaps, to be expected. Is it really surprising nowadays that 10% of those younger than 50 years tested positive for illicit drug use? Sadly, no. In this respect, I am reminded of an earlier article dealing with the other end of the spectrum, diabetic ketoacidosis[1]; for patients younger than 25 years, invariably, some degree of self-destructive behavior was present—omission of insulin; excessive calorie intake (food and/or alcohol); abuse of other drugs— all contributing to the diabetic emergency. Perhaps, in *any* diabetic emergency, hypoglycemic or hyperglycemic, screening for alcohol and illicit drugs should be standard practice in younger patients (<50 years).

The authors may be correct in saying that people with diabetes "are educated to understand the relation between alcohol consumption and the risk of severe hypoglycemia." However, when I discuss this with patients with long-standing diabetes, it is often news to them that alcohol can increase the risk of hypoglycemia; most seem to assume it is more likely to cause hyperglycemia, and will often cite some personal experience to support this assumption. Clearly, the effects of alcohol on glycemic control are not as straightforward as suggested by these authors, and I cannot go along with their recommendation that diabetic patients are to be advised to avoid alcohol rigorously. (But maybe that's just the Scotch/Irish in me!)

L. Kennedy, MD, FRCP

Reference

1. Thompson CJ, Cummings F, Chalmers J, et al: Abnormal insulin treatment behaviour: A major cause of ketoacidosis in the young adult. *Diabet Med* 12:429-432, 1995.

The Effect of Ruboxistaurin on Nephropathy in Type 2 Diabetes

Tuttle KR, McGill JB, Bakris GL, et al (Heart Inst, Spokane, Wash; Rush Univ, Chicago; Univ of Texas, Dallas; et al)

Diabetes Care 28:2686-2690, 2005 55–9

Background.—Preclinical studies have shown an important role for protein kinase C-β in the pathogenesis of diabetic nephropathy. Ruboxistaurin has been shown to selectively inhibit protein kinase C-β and to ameliorate kidney disease in animal models of diabetes. The effects of ruboxistaurin on diabetic nephropathy in human beings were studied.

Methods.—A randomized, double-blind, placebo-controlled, multicenter pilot study was performed to evaluate the effects of 32 mg/day of ruboxistaurin for 1 year in 123 persons with type 2 diabetes and persistent albuminuria despite therapy with renin-angiotensin system inhibitors. The primary end point was a change in the albumin/creatine ratio (ACR). Estimated glomerular filtration rate (eGFR) was also calculated.

Results.—At baseline, urinary ACR was 764 ± 427 mg/g (mean ± SD) and eGFR was 70 ± 24 mL/min per 1.73 m^2. Systolic and diastolic blood pressures were 135 ± 14 and 75 ± 9 mm Hg, respectively. HbA_{1c} was 8.0% ± 1.2%. After 1 year there was a significant decrease (−24% ± 9%) in urinary ACR in patients treated with ruboxistaurin and a nonsignificant decrease (11%) in the placebo group. The ACR-lowering effect of ruboxistaurin was evident at 1 month. eGFR did not significantly decline in the ruboxistaurin group, whereas the placebo group lost significant eGFR over a 1-year period (Table 3). The between-group differences for changes in ACR and eGFR were not statistically significant, but this pilot study did not have sufficient power to determine such differences.

Conclusions.—In persons with type 2 diabetes and nephropathy, treatment with ruboxistaurin reduced albuminuria and maintained eGFR over a 1-year period. Ruboxistaurin may be a beneficial addition to therapies for diabetic nephropathy.

► There is equal rationale for testing the effect of ruboxistaurin on evolving nephropathy in human diabetes, as in animal studies protein kinase C (PCK)-β

TABLE 3.—Change from Baseline in Urinary ACR and eGFR, Blood Pressure, and A1C at Follow-up Visits

Treatment	*n*	1 Month	3 Months	6 Months	12 Months
Urinary ACR change (%)*					
Placebo	62	−16 ± 7†	−9 ± 8	−9 ± 10	−9 ± 11
RBX	59	−24 ± 7†	−28 ± 6†	−29 ± 8†	−24 ± 9†
Urinary ACR change (mg/g)‡					
Placebo	62	17 (424)	−37 (413)†	21 (661)	26 (896)†
RBX	59	−60 (363)†§	−139 (417)†§	−136 (598)	−121 (481)
eGFR change (ml/min per 1.73 m^2)					
Placebo	62	—	—	−2.7 ± 1.8	−4.8 ± 1.8†
RBX	57	—	—	−0.2 ± 1.9	−2.5 ± 1.9
Systolic blood pressure (mmHg)					
Placebo	62	135 ± 16	135 ± 15	136 ± 16	138 ± 19
RBX	59	135 ± 15	136 ± 15	134 ± 16	134 ± 18
Diastolic blood pressure (mmHg)					
Placebo	62	77 ± 12	76 ± 8	76 ± 10	76 ± 10
RBX	59	74 ± 10	74 ± 9	73 ± 11	74 ± 10
A1C (%)					
Placebo	62	—	—	7.7 ± 1.1	7.7 ± 1.2
RBX	56	—	—	8.0 ± 1.3	7.9 ± 1.3

Data are mean ±SD values unless otherwise indicated.

*ACR change from baseline (%) was calculated from log-transformed values using the ANCOVA model with least-square means (prespecified primary outcome).

†Change from baseline, $P < 0.05$.

‡ACR change from baseline (mg/g) without log transformation reported as median (interquartile range for the middle two quartiles).

§Difference between groups, $P < 0.05$. RBX, 32 mg/day ruboxistaurin.

(Courtesy of Tuttle KR, McGill JB, Bakris GL, et al: The effect of ruboxistaurin on nephropathy in type 2 diabetes. *Diabetes Care* 28:2686-2690, 2005. Copyright 2005 American Diabetes Association. Reprinted with permission from The American Diabetes Association.)

induces a number of processes leading to kidney damage that can be prevented by ruboxistaurin.[1,2] In this pilot study the subjects, despite being treated with stable doses of angiotensin-converting enzyme inhibitor or angiotensin-receptor blocker, or both, for at least 6 months had persistently raised ACR in the range of 200 to 2000 mg/g. Their mean estimated eGFR, calculated by using the equation from the Modification of Diet in Renal Disease study, was 70 mL/min per 1.73m^2.[3] So these were patients in the early stages of nephropathy but already at a stage where steady progression toward end-stage renal disease is the likely outcome despite continuing angiotensin-converting enzyme inhibitor or angiotensin-receptor blocker treatment and close attention to controlling both blood pressure and glycemia.

Table 3 shows the relevant effects of ruboxistaurin: a prompt and significant reduction in urinary ACR occurring as early as 1 month after start of treatment sustained until the end of the study (1 year) and a nonsignificant reduction in eGFR; the placebo-treated patients had a significant reduction in eGFR. Because these effects were relatively small, the study lacked the power to determine statistical difference between the active treatment and placebo groups. This was also the case with serious adverse events, of which there were 9 in 62 placebo-treated patients and 15 in 61 who received ruboxistaurin, including 2 deaths; unfortunately there is precious little detail given about the serious adverse events other than that.

So, cautious optimism seems appropriate, but I would want reassurance about safety in these patients with modest renal impairment. Such reassurance can likely come only from much larger and longer trials, and it would seem worthwhile to investigate the drug in patients with microalbuminuria, not just those with higher levels of albuminuria. I'm sure we are going to hear a lot more about this class of drugs.

L. Kennedy, MD, FRCP

References

1. Ishii H, Jirousek MR, Koya D, et al: Amelioration of vascular dysfunctions in diabetic rats by an oral PKC-β inhibitor. *Science* 272:728-731, 1996.
2. Koya D, Haneda M, Nakagawa H, et al: Amelioration of accelerated diabetic mesangial expansion by treatment with a PKC-β inhibitor in diabetic db/db mice, a rodent model for type 2 diabetes. *FASEB J* 14:439-447, 2000.
3. National Kidney Foundation: National Kidney Foundation Kidney Disease Outcomes Quality Initiative. Available from http://www.kidney.org/professionals/doqi/kdoqi/p5_lab_g4.htm. Accessed 13 Dec 2004.

Prevention of Type 2 Diabetes With Troglitazone in the Diabetes Prevention Program

Knowler WC, for The Diabetes Prevention Program Research Group (George Washington Univ, Rockville, Md)

Diabetes 54:1150-1156, 2005 55–10

Background.—The purpose of the Diabetes Prevention Program (DPP) was to determine whether type 2 diabetes could be prevented or delayed through lifestyle or medication interventions applied to a high-risk population. Troglitazone, an insulin-sensitizing agent, was initially used but was discontinued. Troglitazone therapy was compared with other DPP interventions, in terms of both the short-term, in-trial results and longer term results after troglitazone was discontinued.

Methods.—From 1996 to 1998, study participants were randomly assigned to treatment with metformin (587 participants), troglitazone (585 participants), double placebo (582 participants), or intensive lifestyle intervention (589 participants). Concerns over the liver toxicity of troglitazone and the death of 1 patient in the troglitazone-treated group forced its discontinuation in June 1998.

Results.—During the mean 0.9 year of troglitazone treatment, the diabetes incidence rate was 3.0 cases/100 person-years compared with 12.0, 6.7, and 5.1 cases/100 person-years in the placebo, metformin, and intense lifestyle intervention groups. This effect of troglitazone was attributable in part to improved insulin sensitivity with maintenance of insulin secretion. In the 3 years after troglitazone withdrawal, the diabetes incidence rate was almost identical to that of the placebo group (Fig 3).

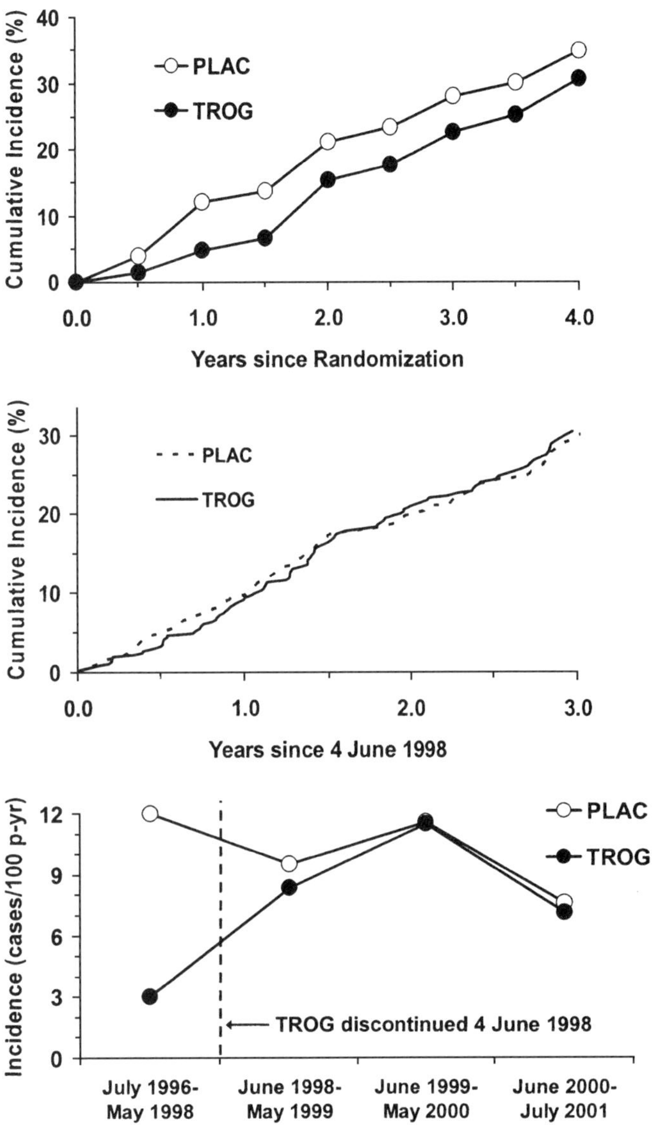

FIGURE 3.—*A*: Cumulative incidence of diabetes (%) from date of randomization in participants assigned to placebo or troglitazone. *B*: Cumulative incidence of diabetes (%) from date of discontinuation of troglitazone (4 June 1998) in participants assigned to placebo or troglitazone. *C*: Diabetes incidence rates (cases/100 person-years) from date of randomization, showing the date of discontinuation of troglitazone (4 June 1998), in participants assigned to placebo or troglitazone. (Courtesy of Knowler WC, Diabetes Prevention Program Research Group: Prevention of type 2 diabetes with troglitazone in the Diabetes Prevention Program. *Diabetes* 54:1150-1156, 2005. Copyright 2005 American Diabetes Association.)

Conclusions.—Troglitazone produced a significant reduction in the incidence of diabetes in the limited period of use, but this effect did not persist after withdrawal of the drug because of concerns about liver toxicity. Additional studies are needed to determine whether other thiazolidinedione drugs used for longer periods can safely prevent diabetes.

► It had been common knowledge for quite a while before this report appeared that the results of the truncated troglitazone arm of the DPP were going to be impressive. The original results had been impressive enough in respect of the effects of intensive lifestyle change and metformin in preventing or delaying the onset of diabetes,[1] but this latest report leads one to wonder just how much more impressive the results with troglitazone might have been had treatment, discontinued for understandable reasons, been of a duration comparable with metformin and lifestyle change.

Perhaps the most interesting aspect of this report, other than the impressive 75% reduction in development of diabetes compared with placebo, is that the preventive effect of troglitazone was not sustained after the drug was discontinued. Another troglitazone study, TRIPOD, in high-risk Hispanic women with a history of gestational diabetes, had suggested the protection against developing diabetes was sustained for about 8 to 9 months after the drug was discontinued.[2] Even so, in the DPP there was no "catch up" in the incidence of diabetes in the troglitazone subjects once it had been discontinued, and the cumulative incidence from time of randomization remained lower than in the placebo group.

As the authors indicate, we can only speculate as to whether the currently available thiazolidinediones, rosiglitazone and pioglitazone, will have similarly spectacular results in reducing the development of diabetes, at least until the results of the diabetes reduction assessment with ramipril and rosiglitazone medication trial become available.

L. Kennedy, MD, FRCP

References

1. The Diabetes Prevention Program Research Group: Reduction in the incidence of type 2 diabetes with lifestyle intervention or metformin. *N Engl J Med* 346:393-403, 2002.
2. Buchanan TA, Xiang AH, Peters RK, et al: preservation of pancreatic β-cell function and prevention of type 2 diabetes by pharmacological treatment of insulin resistance in high-risk Hispanic women. *Diabetes* 51:2796-2803, 2002.

56 Lipoproteins, Atherosclerosis, and Cardiovascular Risk

Reporting Rate of Rhabdomyolysis With Fenofibrate + Statin Versus Gemfibrozil + Any Statin

Jones PH, Davidson MH (Baylor College of Medicine, Houston; Rush Med College, Chicago)

Am J Cardiol 95:120-122, 2005 56–1

Introduction.—There is an increasing trend among physicians to use 3-hydroxy-3-methylglutaryl coenzyme A reductase inhibitors (statins) in combination with other antilipidemic agents. The complementary lipid-altering effects of statins and fibric acid derivatives (fibrates) have led to an increasing use of statin/fibrate combination therapy, particularly for patients who have mixed dyslipidemia. Clinical experience indicates that there may be an increased risk of myotoxicity associated with statin/fibrate combination therapy. However, it is not known whether there are differences in the rate of myotoxicity between the use of fenofibrate and gemfibrozil in combination with statins. To evaluate this question, data from the United States Food and Drug Administration's Adverse Event Reporting System was reviewed to determine how many adverse events were reported for patients who were being treated concomitantly with statins and fibrates. The findings suggest that the use of fenofibrate in combination with statins results in fewer reports of rhabdomyolysis per million prescriptions dispensed than does the use of gemfibrozil.

► The authors determined the reporting rate of statin-associated rhabdomyolysis from January 1, 1998, to March 31, 2002, from the Food and Drug Administration's Adverse Event Reporting System and married this rate with the number of prescriptions for each fibrate and statin dispensed during the same period. To determine the number of prescription for combined statin/fibrate therapy, a study of 28,000 patients was performed (not 280 as stated on the first page of this article; personal communication, PH Jones). Further analysis of these combined data yielded a rate of 140 cases of rhabdomyolysis per million prescriptions for the combination of fenofibrate plus a statin, versus 4600 per million for gemfibrozil plus a statin. The mechanism of this significantly increased rate of rhabdomyolysis when gemfibrozil is used with a statin is thought to be interference with the glucuronidation of the statin by gemfibrozil.[1] The resulting increase in the plasma concentration results in increased myotoxocity. Fenofibrate has no significant effect on the plasma concentration of any statin. Although there are limitations in the Food and Drug Administration's Adverse Event Reporting System that the authors discuss, they conclude that the use of fenofibrate in conjunction with a statin is associated with significantly fewer cases of rhabdomyolysis than the combined use of gemfibrozil and a statin. Personally, this editor feels that it is contraindicated to use a statin with gemfibrozil; whereas, the risk of the combined use of fenofibrate with a statin is acceptable in individuals with mixed dyslipidemia who are at increased risk for a coronary heart disease event.

W. J. Howard, MD

Reference

1. Prueksaritanont T, Zhao JJ, Ma B, et al: Effects of fibrates on metabolism of statins in human hepatocytes. *Drug Metab Dispos* 30:1280-1287, 2002.

Incidence of Hospitalized Rhabdomyolysis in Patients Treated With Lipid-Lowering Drugs

Graham DJ, Staffa JA, Shatin D, et al (Food and Drug Administration, Rockville, Md; Ctr for Health Care Policy and Evaluation, Eden Prairie, Minn; Univ of Massachusetts Med School, Worcester; et al)
JAMA 292:2585-2590, 2004 56–2

Context.—Lipid-lowering agents are widely prescribed in the United States. Reliable estimates of rhabdomyolysis risk with various lipid-lowering agents are not available.

Objective.—To estimate the incidence of rhabdomyolysis in patients treated with different statins and fibrates, alone and in combination, in the ambulatory setting.

Design, Setting, and Patients.—Drug-specific inception cohorts of statin and fibrate users were established using claims data from 11 managed care health plans across the United States. Patients with at least 180 days of prior health plan enrollment were entered into the cohorts between January 1, 1998, and June 30, 2001. Person-time was classified as monotherapy or combined statin-fibrate therapy.

Main Outcome Measure.—Incidence rates of rhabdomyolysis per 10,000 person-years of treatment, number needed to treat, and relative risk of rhabdomyolysis.

Results.—In 252,460 patients treated with lipid-lowering agents, 24 cases of hospitalized rhabdomyolysis occurred during treatment. Average incidence per 10,000 person-years for monotherapy with atorvastatin, pravastatin, or simvastatin was 0.44 (95% confidence interval [CI], 0.20-0.84);

for cerivastatin, 5.34 (95% CI, 1.46-13.68); and for fibrate, 2.82 (95% CI, 0.58-8.24). By comparison, the incidence during unexposed person-time was 0 (95% CI, 0-0.48; *P* = .056). The incidence increased to 5.98 (95% CI, 0.72-216.0) for combined therapy of atorvastatin, pravastatin, or simvastatin with a fibrate, and to 1035 (95% CI, 389-2117) for combined cerivastatin-fibrate use. Per year of therapy, the number needed to treat to observe 1 case of rhabdomyolysis was 22,727 for statin monotherapy, 484 for older patients with diabetes mellitus who were treated with both a statin and fibrate, and ranged from 9.7 to 12.7 for patients who were treated with cerivastatin plus fibrate.

Conclusions.—Rhabdomyolysis risk was similar and low for monotherapy with atorvastatin, pravastatin, and simvastatin; combined statin-fibrate use increased risk, especially in older patients with diabetes mellitus. Cerivastatin combined with fibrate conferred a risk of approximately 1 in 10 treated patients per year.

► The safety of lipid-lowering drug therapy has become of increasing concern over the past several years since cerivastatin was pulled from the market—particularly with regard to muscle toxicity. Using an innovative and seemingly inclusive method, the authors of this study identified 225,640 person-years of monotherapy with either a statin or a fibrate and 7300 person-years of combined statin plus fibrate therapy. An in-depth review of hospitalized cases with possible rhabdomyolysis, using a rigorous definition for this syndrome, revealed 24 cases of rhabdomyolysis. Sixteen cases (13 with a statin and 3 with gemfibrozil) occurred during monotherapy, and 8 cases were documented during combined statin-fibrate therapy. A similar incidence of 0.44 per 10,000 person-years was observed for monotherapy with atorvastatin, simvastatin, and pravastatin, but this increased to 5.34 for cerivastatin. Combined therapy resulted in an incidence of 5.98 for atorvastatin, simvastatin, and pravastatin with a fibrate, and 1035 for cerivastatin and fibrate. Although the authors did not differentiate between fenofibrate and gemfibrozil, a small fraction of the cases of combined therapy were observed for combined fenofibrate-statin treatment. Further analysis indicated that the presence of diabetes mellitis, age greater than 65 years, or both, were risk factors for muscle toxicity. Of more interest to clinicians, the number needed to treat (NNT) per year of therapy to observe 1 case of rhabdomyolysis for statin monotherapy was 22,727, and for the combined use of either atorvastatin, simvastatin, or pravastatin plus a fibrate the NNT was 1672. When a fibrate is combined with cerivastatin, the NNT falls to 9.7 to 12.7. It was further observed that the risk of combination therapy was increased in older patients with diabetes mellitus. The conclusion of this study is supported by the previous article (Abstract 56–1).

W. J. Howard, MD

Intensive Lipid Lowering With Atorvastatin in Patients With Stable Coronary Disease

LaRosa JC, for the Treating to New Targets (TNT) Investigators (State Univ of New York, Brooklyn; et al)

N Engl J Med 352:1425-1435, 2005 56–3

Background.—Previous trials have demonstrated that lowering low-density lipoprotein (LDL) cholesterol levels below currently recommended levels is beneficial in patients with acute coronary syndromes. We prospectively assessed the efficacy and safety of lowering LDL cholesterol levels below 100 mg per deciliter (2.6 mmol per liter) in patients with stable coronary heart disease (CHD).

Methods.—A total of 10,001 patients with clinically evident CHD and LDL cholesterol levels of less than 130 mg per deciliter (3.4 mmol per liter) were randomly assigned to double-blind therapy and received either 10 mg or 80 mg of atorvastatin per day. Patients were followed for a median of 4.9 years. The primary end point was the occurrence of a first major cardiovas-

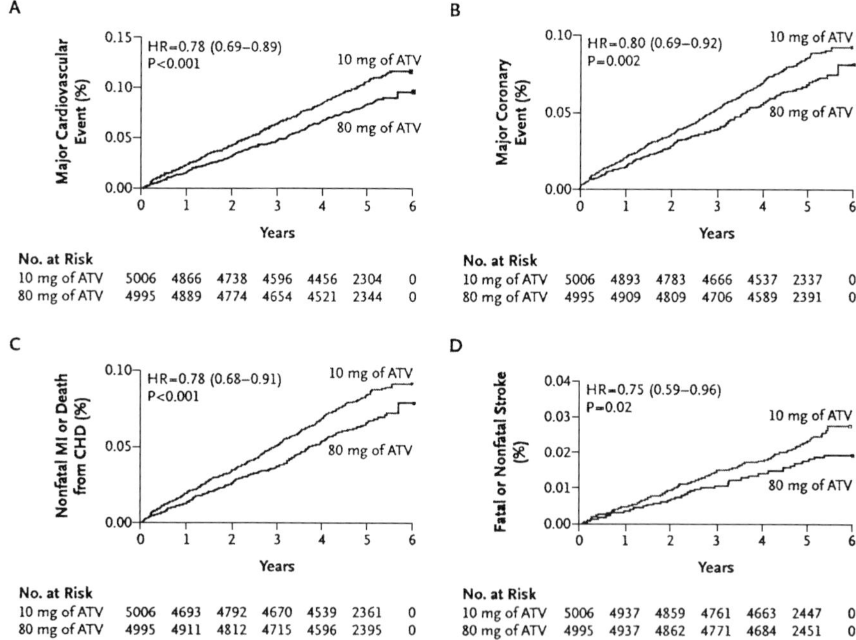

FIGURE 3.—Cumulative incidence of a first major cardiovascular event (A), a first major coronary event (B), nonfatal myocardial infarction (*MI*) or death from coronary heart disease (*CHD*) (C), and a first fatal or nonfatal stroke (D). The primary end point was a first major cardiovascular event, and a first major coronary event was defined as death from CHD, nonfatal non–procedure-related MI, or resuscitation after cardiac arrest. *HR* denotes hazard ratio for the group given 80 mg of atorvastatin (*ATV*) as compared with the group given 10 mg of ATV. (Reprinted by permission of *The New England Journal of Medicine*, from LaRosa JC, for the Treating to New Targets (TNT): Intensive lipid lowering with atorvastatin in patients with stable coronary disease. *N Engl J Med* 352:1425-1435, 2005.)

cular event, defined as death from CHD, nonfatal non–procedure-related myocardial infarction, resuscitation after cardiac arrest, or fatal or nonfatal stroke.

Results.—The mean LDL cholesterol levels were 77 mg per deciliter (2.0 mmol per liter) during treatment with 80 mg of atorvastatin and 101 mg per deciliter (2.6 mmol per liter) during treatment with 10 mg of atorvastatin. The incidence of persistent elevations in liver aminotransferase levels was 0.2 percent in the group given 10 mg of atorvastatin and 1.2 percent in the group given 80 mg of atorvastatin ($P<0.001$). A primary event occurred in 434 patients (8.7 percent) receiving 80 mg of atorvastatin, as compared with 548 patients (10.9 percent) receiving 10 mg of atorvastatin, representing an absolute reduction in the rate of major cardiovascular events of 2.2 percent and a 22 percent relative reduction in risk (hazard ratio, 0.78; 95 percent confidence interval, 0.69 to 0.89; $P<0.001$) (Fig 3). There was no difference between the two treatment groups in overall mortality.

Conclusions.—Intensive lipid-lowering therapy with 80 mg of atorvastatin per day in patients with stable CHD provides significant clinical benefit beyond that afforded by treatment with 10 mg of atorvastatin per day. This occurred with a greater incidence of elevated aminotransferase levels.

► This long-anticipated clinical trial known as TNT for "Treat to New Targets" adds further weight to the recent theme that, with regard to LDL-C, lower is better. Another large study of secondary prevention in 10,001 participants with stable CHD, this trial compared the clinical outcomes of therapy with 10 mg versus 80 mg of atorvastatin for a median of 4.9 years. The results are consistent with the previous trials of moderate versus aggressive LDL-C lowering in patients with an acute coronary syndrome, PROVE-IT and REVERSAL, which were reviewed last year in the Year Book. Although there was only a 24% difference in the on-treatment LDL-C levels between the group treated with 10 mg of atorvastatin versus the group that received 80 mg (LDL-C, 101 mg/dL and 77 mg/dL, respectively), there was a 22% decrease in the primary end point, defined as the occurrence of a major cardiac event (Fig 3). As in PROVE-IT, HDL-C levels were not reduced in the group receiving 80 mg of atorvastatin, which is contrary to previous dose-ranging studies of atorvastatin.

A reassuring aspect of this study was the demonstrated safety of the higher dose of atorvastatin. Although the rate of persistant elevations of alanine aminotransferase with 80 mg of atorvastatin was higher than that seen in the 10-mg group (1.2% vs 0.2%), there was no difference in the occurrence of myalgia (4.8% and 4.2%, respectively) and rhabdomyolysis (2 cases in the group receiving 80 mg of atorvastatin and 3 cases in the group receiving 10 mg of atorvastatin). This demonstrated safety data are of particular importance, given the tendency of many physicians to begin therapy with 80 mg of atorvastatin in patients with CHD, regardless of their LDL-C pretreatment levels. In this editor's opinion, although this therapeutic trend may be safe, current evidence still supports titrating the dose of a statin to achieve the therapeutic goal for LDL-C of less than 100 mg/dL for patients with CHD, with an optional goal of an LDL-C of less than 70 mg/dL in individuals judged to be at very high risk.[1]

W. J. Howard, MD

Reference

1. Grundy SM, for the Coordinating Committee of the National Cholesterol Education Program: Implications of recent clinical trials for the National Cholesterol Education Program Adult Treatment Panel III guidelines. *Circulation* 110:227-239, 2004.

► There is a growing body of data from clinical trials to suggest that lowering of LDL cholesterol below currently recommended levels with higher doses of statins can provide additional benefit on cardiovascular outcomes.[1] Cholesterol reduction with statins appears to benefit patients beyond their effects to prevent atherosclerotic disease.

Despite initial reports that antibiotic therapy against *Chlamydia pneumoniae* might reduce the mortality rate in patients with known coronary disease, recent studies have shown no benefit with this treatment.[2,3]

W. H. Frishman, MD

References

1. Nissen SE, Tuzcu EM, Schoenhagen P, et al: Effect of intensive compared with moderate lipid-lowering therapy on progression of coronary atherosclerosis: A randomized controlled trial. *JAMA* 291:1071-1080, 2004.
2. Grayston JT, for the ACES Investigators: Azithromycin for the secondary prevention of coronary events. *N Engl J Med* 352:1637-1645, 2005.
3. Cannon CP, for the Pravastatin or Atorvastatin Evaluation and Infection Therapy-Thrombolysis in Myocardial Infarction 22 Investigators: Antibiotic treatment of *Chlamydia pneumoniae* after acute coronary syndrome. *N Engl J Med* 352:1646-1654, 2005.

Effects of Long-term Vitamin E Supplementation on Cardiovascular Events and Cancer: A Randomized Controlled Trial

Lonn E, for the HOPE and HOPE-TOO Trial Investigators (McMaster Univ, Hamilton, Ontario, Canada; Univ of Western Ontario, London, Canada; Oxford Univ, England; et al)
JAMA 293:1338-1347, 2005 56–4

Context.—Experimental and epidemiological data suggest that vitamin E supplementation may prevent cancer and cardiovascular events. Clinical trials have generally failed to confirm benefits, possibly due to their relatively short duration.

Objective.—To evaluate whether long-term supplementation with vitamin E decreases the risk of cancer, cancer death, and major cardiovascular events.

Design, Setting, and Patients.—A randomized, double-blind, placebo-controlled international trial (the initial Heart Outcomes Prevention Evaluation [HOPE] trial conducted between December 21, 1993, and April 15, 1999) of patients at least 55 years old with vascular disease or diabetes mellitus was extended (HOPE-The Ongoing Outcomes [HOPE-TOO]) between April 16, 1999, and May 26, 2003. Of the initial 267 HOPE centers that had enrolled 9541 patients, 174 centers participated in the HOPE-TOO trial. Of 7030 patients enrolled at these centers, 916 were deceased at the beginning of the extension, 1382 refused participation, 3994 continued to take the study intervention, and 738 agreed to passive follow-up. Median duration of follow-up was 7.0 years.

Intervention.—Daily dose of natural source vitamin E (400 IU) or matching placebo.

Main Outcome Measures.—Primary outcomes included cancer incidence, cancer deaths, and major cardiovascular events (myocardial infarction, stroke, and cardiovascular death). Secondary outcomes included heart failure, unstable angina, and revascularizations.

Results.—Among all HOPE patients, there were no significant differences in the primary analysis: for cancer incidence, there were 552 patients (11.6%) in the vitamin E group vs 586 (12.3%) in the placebo group (relative risk [RR], 0.94; 95% confidence interval [CI], 0.84-1.06; $P = .30$); for cancer deaths, 156 (3.3%) vs 178 (3.7%), respectively (RR, 0.88; 95% CI, 0.71-1.09; $P = .24$); and for major cardiovascular events, 1022 (21.5%) vs 985 (20.6%), respectively (RR, 1.04; 95% CI, 0.96-1.14; $P = .34$). Patients in the vitamin E group had a higher risk of heart failure (RR, 1.13; 95% CI, 1.01-1.26; $P = .03$) and hospitalization for heart failure (RR, 1.21; 95% CI, 1.00-1.47; $P = .045$). Similarly, among patients enrolled at the centers participating in the HOPE-TOO trial, there were no differences in cancer incidence, cancer deaths, and major cardiovascular events, but higher rates of heart failure and hospitalizations for heart failure.

Conclusion.—In patients with vascular disease or diabetes mellitus, long-term vitamin E supplementation does not prevent cancer or major cardiovascular events and may increase the risk for heart failure.

► The HOPE Trial and the HOPE-TOO extension study followed 9541 participants in the original 5-year study, with 7030 of this original cohort being followed for an additional 4 years on vitamin E (400 IU/d) or placebo. The participants were a high-risk group, as the entry criteria required a history of coronary heart disease (CHD), peripheral vascular disease (PVD), stroke, or diabetes mellitus with an additional risk factor. As with a number of prior studies, vitamin E supplementation had a neutral effect on CHD prevention at the end of 4.5 years. The HOPE-TOO extension study was intended to assess whether longer duration of treatment would prevent cancer and/or cardiovascular disease. At the end of this trial, not only was there no effect on the prevention of CHD or cancer, but there was a significant increase in the risk for congestive heart failure.

Hopefully, the result of HOPE and HOPE-TOO will finally convince the clinical community that vitamin E supplementation is not beneficial and supports the conclusion of the HATS trial that it may be detrimental.[1] The question remains, however, with all of the evidence for the participation of the process of oxidative metabolism in the pathogenics of atherosclerosis, as to why the use of antioxidant therapy has been so disappointing. An accompanying editorial by Greg Brown and John Crowley[2] reviews the prior trials and offers potential explanations for the failure of vitamin E supplementation, plus some hope for the future.

W. J. Howard, MD

References

1. Brown BG, Zhao XQ, Chait A, et al: Simvastatin and niacin, antioxidant vitamins, or the combination for the prevention of coronary disease. *N Engl J Med* 345:1583-1592, 2001.
2. Brown BG, Crowley J: Is there any hope for vitamin E? *JAMA* 293:1387-1390, 2005.

57 Exercise and Obesity

Meta-analysis: Pharmacologic Treatment of Obesity

Li Z, Maglione M, Tu W, et al (RAND Health Division, Santa Monica, Calif; Greater Los Angeles VA Healthcare System; Dept of Veterans Affairs, Cincinnati, Ohio)

Ann Intern Med 142:532-546, 2005 57–1

Background.—In response to the increase in obesity, pharmacologic treatments for weight loss have become more numerous and more commonly used.

Purpose.—To assess the efficacy and safety of weight loss medications approved by the U.S. Food and Drug Administration and other medications that have been used for weight loss.

Data Sources.—Electronic databases, experts in the field, and unpublished information.

Study Selection.—Up-to-date meta-analyses of sibutramine, phentermine, and diethylpropion were identified. The authors assessed in detail 50 studies of orlistat, 13 studies of fluoxetine, 5 studies of bupropion, 9 studies of topiramate, and 1 study each of sertraline and zonisamide. Meta-analysis was performed for all medications except sertraline, zonisamide, and fluoxetine, which are summarized narratively.

Data Extraction.—The authors abstracted information about study design, intervention, co-interventions, population, outcomes, and methodologic quality, as well as weight loss and adverse events from controlled trials of medication.

Data Synthesis.—All pooled weight loss values are reported relative to placebo. A meta-analysis of sibutramine reported a mean difference in weight loss of 4.45 kg (95% CI, 3.62 to 5.29 kg) at 12 months. In the meta-analysis of orlistat, the estimate of the mean weight loss for orlistat-treated patients was 2.89 kg (CI, 2.27 to 3.51 kg) at 12 months. A recent meta-analysis of phentermine and diethylpropion reported pooled mean differences in weight loss at 6 months of 3.6 kg (CI, 0.6 to 6.0 kg) for phentermine-treated patients and 3.0 kg (CI, −1.6 to 11.5 kg) for diethylpropion-treated patients. Weight loss in fluoxetine studies ranged from 14.5 kg of weight lost to 0.4 kg of weight gained at 12 or more months. For bupropion, 2.77 kg (CI, 1.1 to 4.5 kg) of weight was lost at 6 to 12 months. Weight loss due to topiramate at 6 months was 6.5% (CI, 4.8% to 8.3%) of pretreatment weight.

With one exception, long-term studies of health outcomes were lacking. Significant side effects that varied by drug were reported.

Limitations.—Publication bias may exist despite a comprehensive search and despite the lack of statistical evidence for the existence of bias. Evidence of heterogeneity was observed for all meta-analyses.

Conclusions.—Sibutramine, orlistat, phentermine, probably diethylpropion, bupropion, probably fluoxetine, and topiramate promote modest weight loss when given along with recommendations for diet. Sibutramine and orlistat are the 2 most-studied drugs.

► Much skepticism remains about the use of medications to treat obesity. Part of the concern comes from a sense on the part of clinicians that these medications are ineffective and have large numbers of side effects. And yet, there is, simultaneously, a concern that obesity is becoming more and more common and that behavioral treatments are simply providing the kind of weight loss that patients want. It is in this context that the Southern California Evidence-Based Practice Center (which includes the RAND Health Division) performed this extensive meta-analysis of pharmacologic treatments for obesity. This review was contracted by the Agency for Health Care Research and Quality of the US Department of Health and Human Services. This is perhaps the most in-depth review of the literature with regards to pharmacologic treatment for obesity that has been done to date. The analysis identified 1103 articles that related to the topic. They looked broadly at studies that examined a wide range of medications that have been proposed as agents to help people lose weight. Specifically, the article provides an in- depth review of the efficacy and side-effect profile of a large number of medications, including sibutramine, orlistat, phentermine, diethylpropion, fluoxetine, sertraline, bupropion, topiramate, and zonisamide. The core findings of the analysis include a summary of the efficacy of these medications in producing weight loss. These results show that many of these medications appear to produce a statistically significant although relatively small mean change in weight as compared to that produced by placebo. The results of this analysis suggest that sibutramine produces the greatest degree in weight loss, that phentermine produces the next greatest weight loss and that the other medications fall next in line. The article does not conclude that a statistically significant difference exists between the weight loss produced by these medications. A secondary finding of this analysis is the rate of adverse events associated with the commonly used medications in this class. These side effects demonstrate what has been obvious to patients and clinicians for quite some time, that orlistat produces a moderate degree of intestinal side affects, and sibutramine tends to produce an increase in blood pressure and heart rate. The accompanying text of the article goes through an extensive discussion of side effects for many of the medications used for weight loss.

What is not clear from this analysis or from existing literature is whether the degree of weight loss produced by these medications is clinically significant. There are several ways to look at this question. From the patients perspective, the choice would seem to be accepting their weight as it is versus using a medication that has cost and potential side effects and produces a modest weight loss. In some sense, the patient will ultimately be the arbiter of whether the degree of weight loss produced is worth the expense and potential risk of the medication. This is particularly true in this class of medications where insurers rarely pay. Over the long run, though, what are clearly needed are studies that demonstrate the effectiveness of these medications in attenuating meaningful clinical end points, such as cardiovascular events or overall mortality rate. Although evidence is limited that these medications improve intermediate markers, such as blood lipid levels, blood pressure, and measures of insulin sensitivity, it is unclear what clinical meaning should be placed on these changes. Perhaps, the most compelling piece of data comes from the long- term study of orlistat, demonstrating its ability to reduce the risk of type 2 diabetes in a patient.

In summary, a decision about the appropriate use of pharmacologic treatment in obesity remains a matter of opinion. However, this article provides an in-depth and rigorous background on the relevant literature, which at this point is quite extensive. The results of this analysis clearly demonstrate that these medications do produce a degree of weight loss that is likely associated with modest health benefits. In addition, the analysis reassures clinicians as to the relative safety of these medications.

D. H. Bessesen, MD

Meta-analysis: Surgical Treatment of Obesity

Maggard MA, Shugarman LR, Suttorp M, et al (Rand Health Division, Santa Monica, Calif; Greater Los Angeles VA Healthcare System; Univ of Calif, Los Angeles)

Ann Intern Med 142:547-559, 2005 57–2

Background.—Controversy exists regarding the effectiveness of surgery for weight loss and the resulting improvement in health-related outcomes.

Purpose.—To perform a meta-analysis of effectiveness and adverse events associated with surgical treatment of obesity.

Data Sources.—MEDLINE, EMBASE, Cochrane Controlled Trials Register, and systematic reviews.

Study Selection.—Randomized, controlled trials; observational studies; and case series reporting on surgical treatment of obesity.

Data Extraction.—Information about study design, procedure, population, comorbid conditions, and adverse events.

Data Synthesis.—The authors assessed 147 studies. Of these, 89 contributed to the weight loss analysis, 134 contributed to the mortality analysis, and 128 contributed to the complications analysis. The authors identified 1 large, matched cohort analysis that reported greater weight loss with surgery than with medical treatment in individuals with an average body mass index (BMI) of 40 kg/m^2 or greater. Surgery resulted in a weight loss of 20 to 30 kg, which was maintained for up to 10 years and was accompanied by improvements in some comorbid conditions. For BMIs of 35 to 39 kg/m^2, data from case series strongly support superiority of surgery but cannot be considered conclusive. Gastric bypass procedures result in more weight loss than gastroplasty. Bariatric procedures in current use (gastric bypass, laparoscopic adjustable gastric band, vertical banded gastroplasty, and biliopancreatic diversion and switch) have been performed with an overall mortality rate of less than 1%. Adverse events occur in about 20% of cases. A laparoscopic approach results in fewer wound complications than an open approach.

Limitations.—Only a few controlled trials were available for analysis. Heterogeneity was seen among studies, and publication bias is possible.

Conclusions.—Surgery is more effective than nonsurgical treatment for weight loss and control of some comorbid conditions in patients with a BMI of 40 kg/m^2 or greater. More data are needed to determine the efficacy of surgery relative to nonsurgical therapy for less severely obese people. Procedures differ in efficacy and incidence of complications.

► Last year, it was estimated that roughly 150,000 seriously obese people in the United States had gastric bypass surgery in an effort to lose weight. And yet, questions remain in the minds of many clinicians regarding both of the safety and effectiveness of this very aggressive approach to treating obesity. In an effort to comprehensively review the available scientific literature on the effectiveness and morbidity associated with surgical treatments for obesity, the Agency for Health Care Research and Quality of the US Department of Health and Human Services contracted with the Southern California Evidence Based Practice Center to perform this extensive review of existing literature on this topic. The authors evaluated 147 studies of surgical treatment for obesity. A wide range of studies were examined from case-control series to simple case series with 10 or more patients. Small studies were used in an effort to capture more realistic information on adverse events and on the possibility that results were different at centers that performed fewer operations. The analysis highlights in particular, pooled results from controlled trials of weight loss after bariatric surgery. These results suggest that the Roux-en-Y gastric bypass operation (RYGB) produces a substantial amount of weight loss as compared with that seen in control patients. The vertical banded gastroplasty and adjustable gastric banding were found to produce slightly less weight loss.

The article also outlines the effect of weight-loss surgery on a wide range of comorbid conditions, including diabetes, hypertension, dyslipidemia, and sleep apnea. The results across a large number of studies have been consistent in showing that weight-loss surgery provides marked statistically significantly benefits in these conditions. The effects on other coconditions are noted but have been less well studied. Finally, the analysis examines the mortality and morbidity rates associated with weight-loss surgery and finds that, in general, about 1% of patients undergoing these procedures suffer early (within 30 days after operation) mortality, and that late deaths account for another 1%. In addition, surgery appears to be associated with a range of other adverse events, including gastrointestinal symptoms, reflux, vomiting, and other complications. The analysis reviews the evidence that a learning curve is associated with the performance of laparoscopic procedures. The authors review relevant literature concerning the rate of complications that occur with surgeons of relative inexperience as compared with that of those with greater experience and conclude that after a surgeon has performed somewhere between 80 and 150 operations, the incidence of adverse events decreases markedly. However, they highlight, importantly, that the series on which this conclusion is based were done at a time when the technique for performing these operations was new and still under development. They point out that the learning curve may, in fact, be shorter now that the procedure has been well established.

In summary, this is the most comprehensive analysis to date of existing literature on the surgical treatment of obesity. Although much in this article is not new or unexpected, it does provide reassurance that, indeed, gastric bypass surgery provides the highest level of effectiveness in producing weight loss in seriously obese patients, as compared with that of all other treatments. In addition, it highlights how much more we need to know about the long-term effects of this type of surgery on its mortality rate and on the overall cost of care.

D. H. Bessesen, MD

Pharmacologic and Surgical Management of Obesity in Primary Care: A Clinical Practice Guideline From the American College of Physicians

Snow V, for the Clinical Efficacy Assessment Subcommittee of the American College of Physicians (American College of Physicians, Philadelphia; et al)

Ann Intern Med 142:525-531, 2005 57–3

Introduction.—This guideline is based on the evidence report and accompanying background papers developed by the Southern California Evidence-Based Practice Center. The American College of Physicians nominated this topic to the Agency for Healthcare Research and Quality Evidence-Based Practice Center program as part of a concerted effort to complement the guidelines of the US Preventive Services Task Force. The College recommends that all clinicians refer to the Task Force recommendations as part of an overall strategy for managing overweight and obesity, which should always include appropriate diet and exercise for all patients who are overweight or obese. The intent of this guideline is to provide recommendations based on a review of the evidence on pharmacologic and surgical treatments of obesity. The target audience is all clinicians caring for obese patients, defined as a body mass index of 30 kg/m^2 or greater. This guideline is not intended to be used by commercial weight loss centers or for direct-to-consumer marketing by manufacturers and does not apply to patients with body mass indices below 30 kg/m^2.

► Obesity is clearly a major public health problem in the United States, and it is a condition seen by most physicians in their offices every day. And yet, the question of when to intervene and what particular steps to take remains, for many, an issue of practice style. However, this inconsistency of approach is beginning to change with the emergence of a range of clinical practice guidelines from a number of trusted organizations. This particular article outlines the position of the American College of Physicians (ACP) on the pharmacologic and surgical management of obesity and primary care. The ACP represents the specialty of internal medicine and is 1 of the most respected organizations in American medicine. This organization suggested obesity management as a topic to the Agency for Health Care Research and Quality as a complement to the guidelines that were issued last year by the US Preventive Services Task Force. In that previous set of guidelines, it was recommended that all clinicians screen adult patients for obesity and offer counseling and behavioral interventions to promote sustained weight loss when obesity was identified. In this clinical practice guideline, the ACP now provides an algorithm for the management of obesity that they recommend for use in primary care. Specifically, the ACP now recommends that clinicians should counsel obese patients on lifestyle behavioral interventions. They further suggest that when a person has failed to achieve their weight-loss goal through diet and exercise, the clinician should discuss pharmacologic therapy with that patient, including information about the medication's side effects and the lack of long-term safety data. The guideline further recommends that, for obese patients who choose to use medications, the options include sibutramine, orlistat, phentermine, diethylpropion, fluoxetine, and/or bupropion. In particular, they argue that the particular medication chosen would depend on its side-effect profile and the person's tolerance of those side effects. Finally, the guideline suggests that surgery should be considered as an option only for people who have a BMI greater then 40 kg/m^2 and who have tried and failed at an adequate exercise and diet program. Specifically, they encourage the treating physician to consider a range of comorbid conditions, including diabetes, hypertension, hyperlipidemia, and sleep apnea when helping a patient make a decision about weight-loss surgery. They advocate that patients who are sent for surgery be referred to a high- volume center with surgeons who have experience in bariatric surgery. This clinical guideline provides a brief summary of the evidence on which it is based. The evidence is outlined in greater detail in 2 meta-analyses that accompany this article (Abstracts 57–1 and 57–2).

In summary, with a number of respected organizations now developing and promoting clinical guidelines on the management of obesity, primary-care physicians should feel some comfort and confidence that, when they take the time and effort to make suggestions about behavior modification, weight-loss medications, and surgical treatments for obese patients, they are in the mainstream of what expert organizations feel is the standard of clinical practice.

D. H. Bessesen, MD

58 Thyroid Disorders

Thyroid Fine-Needle Aspiration Biopsy in Children and Adolescents: Experience With 218 Aspirates

Amrikachi M, Ponder TB, Wheeler TM, et al (Methodist Hosp, Houston; St Louis Univ; Baylor College of Medicine, Houston; et al)

Diagn Cytopathol 32:189-192, 2005 58–1

Background.—Thyroid nodules are a relatively common finding in adolescents, with a prevalence that ranges from 0.2% to 1.8%. Most of these nodules are benign, but malignant tumors, particularly papillary carcinomas, do occur in this age group. The experience of 1 group with fine-needle aspiration (FNA) of thyroid nodules in adolescents was reviewed to assess the role of FNA biopsy in the management of adolescent thyroid disease and determine its reliability in the identification of candidates for surgical exploration.

Methods.—A review was conducted of thyroid FNA biopsy reports from 4 large university-affiliated teaching hospitals and clinics. These procedures were performed during 16 years, from 1982 to 1998, for a total of 6000 aspirates in all age groups. The follow-up ranged from 1 to 17 years. The present report focused on findings in 218 aspirations from 185 patients in the 10- to 21-year age group. Most (88%) of the patients were female. Cytologic diagnoses were classified as benign, malignant, suggestive of malignancy, or unsatisfactory. The sensitivity and specificity of FNA for diagnosis of thyroid malignancy relative to the final histologic diagnoses were calculated.

TABLE 1.—Cytological Diagnoses of FNA of 218 Thyroid Nodules in the 10- to 21-yr Age Group

Diagnostic Category	Number of Cases (%)
Malignant	17 (8%)
Suspicious	20 (9%)
Benign	119 (54%)
Unsatisfactory	62 (28%)
Total	218

(Courtesy of Amrikachi M, Ponder TB, Wheeler TM, et al: Thyroid fine-needle aspiration biopsy in children and adolescents: experience with 218 aspirates. *Diagn Cytopathol* 32:189-192, 2005.)

TABLE 2.—Cytological Diagnoses of FNA of Thyroid Nodules in the 10- to 15-yr and 15- to 21-yr Old Age Groups

Diagnostic Category	10-15 Yr Old	15-21 Yr Old
Malignant	6%	5%
Suspicious	9%	6%
Benign	52%	54%
Unsatisfactory	33%	35%

(Courtesy of Amrikachi M, Ponder TB, Wheeler TM, et al: Thyroid fine-needle aspiration biopsy in children and adolescents: experience with 218 aspirates. *Diagn Cytopathol* 32:189-192, 2005.)

Results.—Overall, the majority (54%) of cytologic findings in the 10- to 21-year-old group were benign (Table 1). Data were also analyzed for subgroups of patients, 10 to 15 years old, and 15 to 21 years old (Table 2). In these subgroups also, the majority of diagnoses were benign (52% and 54%, respectively). The sensitivity of thyroid FNA in diagnosing thyroid malignancy relative to the final histologic diagnoses was 100%, and the specificity was 65%.

Conclusions.—FNA of thyroid nodules in the pediatric population has high sensitivity and specificity comparable with that in the adult population. Acceptance of this procedure in the routine evaluation of thyroid nodules in children and adolescents should reduce the number of unnecessary surgical procedures for benign thyroid disease.

► Although FNA biopsy (FNAB) is part of the routine evaluation of thyroid nodules in adults, it has for many years been underutilized in the evaluation of children with thyroid nodules, perhaps because thyroid cancer in children has in the past often been viewed as a relatively benign disease. More recent studies, however, now emphasize that pediatric thyroid cancer is a serious disease with major consequences and a high rate of pulmonary metastases.[1-3]

In 1995, Raab et al[4] reported a study of 57 pediatric patients (8 males, 49 females), ranging from 1 to 18 years old, who underwent 66 FNABs. They had only 1 false-negative case of a papillary carcinoma misdiagnosed as a benign nodule. Benign diagnoses included cysts, lymphocytic thyroiditis, granulomatous thyroiditis, follicular hyperplasia, and abscess. Ten (18%) patients had malignant thyroid lesions: 8 with papillary and 2 with follicular thyroid cancer. The malignancy rate of 18% in this study prompted the authors to advise FNAB in the management of children with thyroid nodules.

In 1998, Lugo-Vicente et al[5] performed a study in 24 children to determine whether the management of pediatric thyroid nodules had changed in the era of FNAB cytology. Girls outnumbered boys 5 to 1 in the study, and mean patient age was 14.9 years. Five (26%) of 19 nodules were malignant. Malignant tumors were characterized by localized tenderness of the mass, multinodular appearance of the tumor, and fixation of the nodule to adjacent tissues (all testimony to advanced tumor stage). US and nuclear scans gave no clues for management because the malignant nodules were often cystic, hot or warm on radionuclide scanning (a well known fact to adult endocrinologists). FNAB performed in 18 children achieved an 80% accuracy rate, 60% sensitivity, 90% specificity, and 75% positive and 81% negative predictive values. Physical examination findings, persistence, and growth of the nodule argued for surgery in most children. The authors of this study concluded that "FNA is a safe adjunctive test that plays a *minor role* [emphasis mine] in the decision to withhold surgery and that its greatest strength is to resolve, in cases of suspicious or malignant cytology, that a more radical procedure will be needed." They provided the caveat that "clinical judgment as determined by serial physical findings continues to be the most important factor in the management of thyroid nodules in children."

In what I believe may be the largest study of its kind, Amrikachi et al report their findings in 218 FNABs performed in 4 large university-affiliated hospitals. The 185 patients in the study were from 10 to 21 years old. Most (85%) of the FNABs were done without US guidance by endocrinologists in their offices, and the others were performed by cytopathologists or radiologists. The results of the study are shown in Tables 1 and 2. Eight percent of the children had thyroid malignancies. Table 2 displays the data from children and young adults separately, showing that there is no difference in the accuracy of FNAB in the 2 groups. About half (54%) of the 218 aspirates yielded benign cytology, 80 (67%) of which were categorized as adenomatous or colloid nodules, and 7 (6%) as Hashimoto's thyroiditis. Twenty (9%) of the aspirates were categorized as follicular neoplasms or were described as being suggestive for typical papillary or follicular variant of papillary thyroid carcinoma. Seventeen (8%) patients had malignant tumors, 16 of which were papillary thyroid carcinomas and 1 of which was a medullary thyroid carcinoma. Sixty-two of the aspirates (28%) were inadequate for diagnosis.

The majority (91%) of the 119 patients with a benign cytologic diagnosis were followed up clinically without surgical intervention. Surgery follow-up results were available for only 9 of the 20 patients with suggestive cytology findings and for only 11 of the patients with thyroid cancer. Surgery was performed for benign lesions in 11 (5%) cases, 8 for adenomatous nodules and 3 for follicular adenomas. Only 1 of the 62 patients with unsatisfactory cytology specimens underwent surgery, and the others were followed clinically.

I agree with the authors that the data are comparable to those in adults, except that the rates of thyroid cancer in their children and the other reports mentioned above are about twice the average of 4% that is reported in nearly 13,000 cases from 11 series in a review by Yang et al[6] I would also add that US-FNAB would have improved the high rate of FNAB cytology specimens that were insufficient for diagnosis in this study. The authors concluded that "FNA of thyroid nodules in the pediatric and adolescent population is comparably as sensitive and specific as in the adult population. The acceptance of this procedure in the routine evaluation of young patients' thyroid nodules should reduce the number of unnecessary surgeries for benign thyroid disease." I agree.

I hope the age of long delays in the diagnosis and management of children with thyroid cancer is coming to and end. Seeing only 1 very young pediatric patient with widespread papillary thyroid cancer delayed for years because no one thought about performing an FNAB is enough to make you a firm believer in aggressive management of pediatric thyroid nodules. In my experience, most children younger than 15 years tolerate FNAB with little difficulty, and the procedure should be done without hesitation in children.

E. L. Mazzaferri, MD

References

1. Hung W, Sarlis NJ: Current controversies in the management of pediatric patients with well-differentiated non-medullary thyroid cancer: A review. *Thyroid* 12:683-702, 2002.
2. Bal CS, Padhy AK, Kumar A: Clinical features of differentiated thyroid carcinoma in children and adolescents from a sub-Himalayan iodine-deficient endemic zone. *Nucl Med Commun* 22:881-887, 2001.
3. Bal CS, Kumar A, Chandra P, et al: Is chest x-ray or high-resolution computed tomography scan of the chest sufficient investigation to detect pulmonary metastasis in pediatric differentiated thyroid cancer? *Thyroid* 14:217-225, 2004.
4. Raab SS, Silverman JF, Elsheikh TM, et al: Pediatric thyroid nodules: Disease demographics and clinical management as determined by fine needle aspiration biopsy. *Pediatrics* 95:46-49, 1995.
5. Lugo-Vicente H, Ortiz VN, Irizarry H, et al: Pediatric thyroid nodules: Management in the era of fine needle aspiration. *J Pediatr Surg* 33:1302-1305, 1998.
6. Yang GC, Liebeskind D, Messina AV: Ultrasound-guided fine-needle aspiration of the thyroid assessed by Ultrafast Papanicolaou stain: Data from 1135 biopsies with a two- to six-year follow-up. *Thyroid* 11:581-589, 2001.

Outcome of Radioiodine-131 Therapy in Hyperfunctioning Thyroid Nodules: A 20 Years' Retrospective Study

Ceccarelli C, Bencivelli W, Vitti P, et al (Univ of Pisa, Italy)

Clin Endocrinol (Oxf) 62:331-335, 2005 58–2

Objective.—To investigate the risk of hypothyroidism after radioiodine (^{131}I) treatment for hyperfunctioning thyroid nodules.

Design.—Retrospective analysis of patients treated with ^{131}I for hyperfunctioning thyroid nodules and followed up for a maximum of 20 years.

Patients.—A total of 346 patients treated with ^{131}I in the years 1975-95, for a single hyperfunctioning nodule.

Measurements.—Hypothyroidism was defined as TSH levels > 3.7 mU/l. Kaplan-Meier survival analysis was used to analyse permanence of euthyroidism after ^{131}I. A stepwise Cox proportional hazard model was used to identify factors influencing the progression to hypothyroidism.

Results.—The cumulative incidence of hypothyroidism was 7.6% at 1 year, 28% at 5 years, 46% at 10 years and 60% at 20 years. Age ($P < 0.01$), 24-th ^{131}I uptake ($P < 0.05$) and previous treatment with methimazole (MMI, $P < 0.1$) were associated with a faster progression towards hypothyroidism, while thyroid and nodule size, thyroid status at diagnosis and degree of extranodular thyroid parenchymal suppression had no influence. In hyperthyroid patients with partial parenchymal suppression, however, previous MMI treatment was the most important prognostic factor ($P < 0.01$).

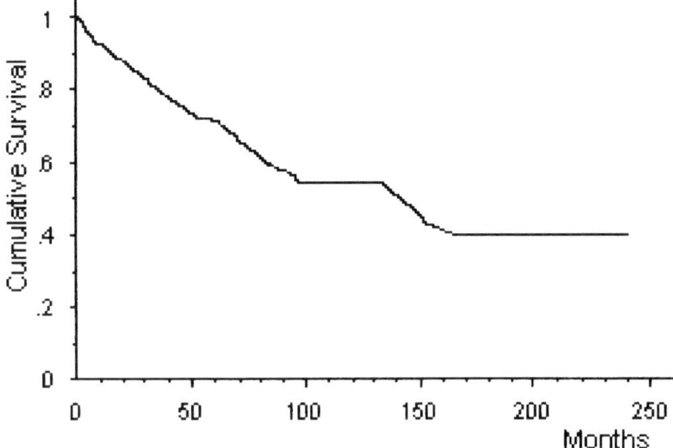

FIGURE 1.—Cumulative permanence in euthyroidism in 346 patients by Kaplan-Meier survival analysis. (Courtesy of Ceccarelli C, Bencivelli W, Vitti P, et al: Outcome of radioiodine-131 therapy in hyperfunctioning thyroid nodules: a 20 years' retrospective study. *Clin Endocrinol (Oxf)* 62:331-335, 2005. Reprinted by permission of Blackwell Publishing.)

Conclusions.—After 20 years of follow-up, 60% of patients treated with ^{131}I for a single hyperfunctioning nodule are hypothyroid. Factors increasing the risk of hypothyroidism are age, ^{131}I uptake and MMI pretreatment. The prognostic value of this last factor, however, depends on the degree of suppression of the extranodular thyroid parenchyma at the scan (Fig 1).

► One would think that the standard approach to treatment of an autonomously functioning thyroid nodule (AFTN) would be ^{131}I therapy, especially when TSH is suppressed and the surrounding normal thyroid parenchyma fails to concentrate ^{131}I, since theoretically this would result in euthyroidism and disappearance of the nodule. This is not the case. Neither is there consensus or solid data that ^{131}I therapy will result in euthyroidism and disappearance of the nodule. Indeed, the opposite is often true.

Surveys carried out in Europe and the United States comparing the diagnostic and therapeutic strategies in patients with solitary thyroid nodules and multinodular goiter show a disparity of recommendations by thyroid experts. Astonishingly, a questionnaire sent in 2000 by Bennedbaek et al[1] to members of the American Thyroid Association found that 37% recommended levothyroxine suppression for patients with a solitary thyroid nodule and a suppressed TSH, whereas only 16% were in favor of ^{131}I therapy, 10% recommended surgery, and the others advocated no therapy. In a previous similar study in 1999, Bennedbaek et al[2] found that 20% of European experts preferred ^{131}I therapy, 32% indicated a preference for levothyroxine therapy, and 32% advised surgery. This wide range of opinions undoubtedly stems from the disparate literature on this subject.

In a study of 23 patients with an AFTN that had been treated with ^{131}I from 4 to 16.5 years earlier (mean, 8.5 years), Goldstein et al[3] found that over half still had palpable thyroid nodules at last follow-up, while about 10% of the nodules had increased in size. Also, 36% of the patients had become hypothyroid, which was not related to nodule size, the level of thyroid function before therapy, or the total amount of ^{131}I that had been administered.

In a similar study of 45 thyrotoxic patients with AFTN reported one year later by Ross et al,[4] 93% were euthyroid 4.9 years (range, 0.5 to 13.5) after being treated with an average of 10.3 mCi of ^{131}I. Three patients developed recurrent hyperthyroidism from 4.5 and 10 years after a single initial treatment, and no patient in their series developed clinical hypothyroidism. Still, 3 had minimal serum TSH elevations of 8.4, 6.2, and 9.6 mIU/L that occurred, respectively, at 1, 4, and 7.5 years after treatment, but all had normal serum T4 levels and were clinically euthyroid. The authors concluded that AFTN may be treated with relatively small amounts of ^{131}I (5 to 15 mCi), and that posttreatment hypothyroidism is very unusual.

About 2 years later, Hegedus et al[5] weighed into the debate, reporting a 1-year follow-up of 27 hyperthyroid patients with AFTN treated with ^{131}I in which all but 2 cases required only one treatment to achieve euthyroidism. In spite of a significant decrease in the size of the contralateral thyroid lobe, none became hypothyroid. They concluded that ^{131}I therapy has an important place in the treatment of AFTN since all their patients became euthyroid within 3 months, only 2 needed more than one ^{131}I treatment, none developed hypothyroidism, and the thyroid volume decreased.

In 1991, Berglund et al[6] reported no recurrences of thyrotoxicosis among patients with AFTN treated with ^{131}I, but 40% developed hypothyroidism over a median of about 9 years (range 0.1 to 8 years). They concluded that patients with AFTN treated with ^{131}I should undergo surveillance for many years, probably for life—a prediction that Ceccarelli et al show was correct.

In the study by Ceccarelli et al, 94% of the patients were euthyroid after one ^{131}I treatment averaging about 14 ± 12 (SD) mCi. (It averaged 17 mCi for those with nodules larger than 4 cm and 13 mCi for patients with smaller nodules.) After 20 years[00bf] follow-up, 60% of the patients were hypothyroid (Fig 1). Univariate analysis identified age over 45 years, higher thyroidal radioiodine uptake (RAIU), and methimazole (MMI) pretreatment as prognostic factors associated with hypothyroidism. Perhaps of most importance, the hazard ratios were 0.45 for age <45 years, 0.63 for RAIU <50%, and 0.67 for MMI pretreatment. The same 3 factors were identified by a stepwise Cox model as affecting the outcome of ^{131}I therapy. Not found to be factors predicting prognosis were the amount of ^{131}I administered, nodule size, and the degree of parenchymal suppression of ^{131}I uptake. In a subset of 148 patients with partial parenchymal suppression, only MMI pretreatment was significant (hazard ratio 0.35%) in predicting hypothyroidism. The adverse effects of treatment were cystic degeneration with a subsequent increase of nodule size in one case, and isolated Graves' disease ophthalmopathy in 2 patients. The development of autoimmune thyrotoxicosis in this setting has been noted by others. For example, a large multicenter survey[7] of patients treated with ^{131}I for hyperthyroidism reported a 0.7% incidence of new Graves' disease after ^{131}I therapy for hyperthyroidism due to causes other than Graves' disease.

Ceccarelli et al report the highest incidence of hypothyroidism found to date following ^{131}I treatment of AFTN. There are 2 likely reasons for this. One is that the diagnosis of hypothyroidism was based on a TSH higher than 3.7 mIU/L, at which levothyroxine treatment was instituted. This was based on the well-reasoned concern about the long-term affects of subclinical hypothyroidism, despite recommendations to the contrary.[8-10] The other reason is that this study reports the longest follow-up of patients with AFTN treated with ^{131}I. Still, the 42% rate of hypothyroidism after 8 years[00bf] follow-up in the Ceccarelli study was similar to rates reported by others after about the same duration of follow-up.[7,11] The amount of ^{131}I did not play a role in the subsequent development of hypothyroidism in the study by Ceccarelli et al, nor has this been the case in most studies[12] The average amount of ^{131}I used to treat AFTN is between 8 and 29 mCi, which is in the range (average 13 mCi) Ceccarelli et al used in their cohort.

As a practical matter, the observations of Ceccarelli et al underscore that life-long surveillance is necessary in patients with AFTN treated with ^{131}I. The fact that subclinical hypothyroidism may go on for some time is particularly worrisome in younger women who are in the child bearing years of life, and in older patients who might experience adverse cardiac events. Whether surgery is a better choice of therapy for AFTN in younger patients looms as a reasonable possibility since their lifetime is likely to be longer than the 20-year follow-up reported by Ceccarelli et al.

E. L. Mazzaferri, MD

References

1. Bennedbaek FN, Hegedus L: Management of the solitary thyroid nodule: Results of a North American survey. *J Clin Endocrinol Metab* 85:2493-2498, 2000.
2. Bennedbaek FN, Perrild H, Hegedus L: Diagnosis and treatment of the solitary thyroid nodule. Results of a European survey. *Clin Endocrinol (Oxf)* 50:357-363, 1999.
3. Goldstein R, Hart IR: Follow-up of solitary autonomous thyroid nodules treated with 131I. *N Engl J Med* 309:1473-1476, 1983.
4. Ross DS, Ridgway EC, Daniels GH: Successful treatment of solitary toxic thyroid nodules with relatively low-dose iodine-131, with low prevalence of hypothyroidism. *Ann Intern Med* 101:488-490, 1984.
5. Hegedus L, Veiergang D, Karstrup S, et al: Compensated 131I-therapy of solitary autonomous thyroid nodules: Effect on thyroid size and early hypothyroidism. *Acta Endocrinol (Copenh)* 113:226-232, 1986.
6. Berglund J, Christensen SB, Dymling JF, et al: The incidence of recurrence and hypothyroidism following treatment with antithyroid drugs, surgery or radioiodine in all patients with thyrotoxicosis in Malmo during the period 1970-1974. *J Intern Med* 229:435-442, 1991.
7. Weiss M, Gorges R, Hirsch C, et al: [Incidence of immunogenic hyperthyroidism after radioiodine therapy of focal thyroid gland autonomy. Results of a multicenter study]. *Med Klin (Munich)* 94:239-244, 1999. German.
8. Col NF, Surks MI, Daniels GH: Subclinical thyroid disease: Clinical applications. *JAMA* 291:239-243, 2004.
9. Surks MI, Ortiz E, Daniels GH, et al: Subclinical thyroid disease: Scientific review and guidelines for diagnosis and management. *JAMA* 291:228-238, 2004.
10. Ringel MD, Mazzaferri EL: Subclinical thyroid dysfunction—can there be a consensus about the consensus? *J Clin Endocrinol Metab* 90:588-590, 2005.
11. Ferrari C, Reschini E, Paracchi A: Treatment of the autonomous thyroid nodule: A review. *Eur J Endocrinol* 135:383-390, 1996.

12. Reiners C, Schneider P: Radioiodine therapy of thyroid autonomy. *Eur J Nucl Med Mol Imaging* 29 Suppl 2:S471-S478, 2002.

Effect of Long-term Continuous Methimazole Treatment of Hyperthyroidism: Comparison With Radioiodine

Azizi F, Ataie L, Hedayati M, et al (Shaheed Beheshti Univ of Med Sciences, Tehran, I.R. Iran)

Eur J Endocrinol 152:695-701, 2005 58–3

Objective.—To investigate the long-term effects of continuous methimazole (MMI) therapy.

Design and Methods.—Five hundred and four patients over 40 years of age with diffuse toxic goiter were treated with MMI for 18 months. Within one year after discontinuation of MMI, hyperthyroidism recurred in 104 patients. They were randomized into 2 groups for continuous antithyroid and radioiodine treatment. Numbers of occurrences of thyroid dysfunction and total costs of management were assessed during 10 years of follow-up. At the end of the study, 26 patients were still on continuous MMI (group 1), and of 41 radioiodine-treated patients (group 2), 16 were euthyroid and 25 became hypothyroid. Serum thyroid and lipid profiles, bone mineral density, and echocardiography data were obtained.

Results.—There was no significant difference in age, sex, duration of symptoms and thyroid function between the two groups. No serious complications occurred in any of the patients. The cost of treatment was lower in group 1 than in group 2. At the end of 10 years, goiter rate was greater and antithyroperoxidase antibody concentration was higher in group 1 than in group 2. Serum cholesterol and low density lipoprotein-cholesterol concentrations were increased in group 2 as compared with group 1; relative risks were 1.8 (1.12-2.95, $P<0.02$) and 1.6 (1.09-2.34, $P<0.02$) respectively. Bone mineral density and echocardiographic measurements were not different between the two groups.

Conclusion.—Long-term continuous treatment of hyperthyroidism with MMI is safe. The complications and the expense of the treatment do not exceed those of radioactive iodine therapy.

▶ The choice of therapy for thyrotoxic Graves' disease differs around the world. In 3 separate questionnaire studies[1] sent to members of the American Thyroid Association (ATA), the European Thyroid Association (ETA), and the Japan Thyroid Association (JTA), ^{131}I was the treatment of choice for 69% of ATA respondents, whereas only 22% of ETA and 11% of JTA respondents chose ^{131}I as their initial therapy. In contrast, only 30.5% of ATA respondents chose antithyroid drugs as first-line therapy compared with 77% of ETA and 88% of JTA respondents. There was, however, consensus on the relative lack of a role for thyroidectomy except for narrow indications, and none suggested long-term antithyroid drug therapy as an alternative treatment. Almost all thyroidologists agree that ^{131}I is the treatment of choice for patients who experience recurrence after antithyroid drug therapy.[2]

The aim of the randomized controlled clinical trial by Azizi et al was to investigate the effectiveness of continuous antithyroid drug therapy over a period of 10 years and to compare the side effects and benefits of this with standard ^{131}I therapy. Although 504 patients were initially enrolled in the study, only 104 (22%) experienced overt symptoms and signs of thyrotoxicosis after 1 year of MMI therapy, and only 34 were randomized to MMI and 51 to ^{131}I therapy. The others opted for different therapy. The mean administered ^{131}I activity was 7.9 mCi (range 5 to 13 mCi). Only 80% returned for follow-up visits. During the 10 years of MMI treatment, most patients were compliant with their medication: only 5.9% of 627 TSH measurements performed in the course of the treatment were higher than 5.0 mIU/L and 7.6% were <0.3 mIU/L. Among those treated with ^{131}I, 989 thyroid function tests were carried out and TSH was >5.0 mIU/L in 12.8% of the tests and <0.3 mIU/L in 9.1% of the tests. As anticipated, the goiter rate was lower in the ^{131}I group (25%) than in the MMI group (50%), and the antithyroperoxidase antibody (TPOAb) titer was significantly higher in the MMI treated group. Total and low-density lipoprotein-cholesterol levels were higher in the ^{131}I group, while mean Z scores were lower in the MMI group.

The cost analysis identified no major differences between the 2 treatments, but the study group was very small, and a major complication in only one of the MMI treated patients would have significantly tilted the balance towards ^{131}I being the least expensive therapy. Also, a quality of life questionnaire was not done as part of the study. Follow-up testing of thyroid function is recommended[2] every 4 to 6 weeks, at least until thyroid function is stable or the patient becomes euthyroid, which may take months and is not factored into the Azizi cost analysis at this frequency and duration. Moreover, the cost of antithyroid drugs in the United States is much higher than quoted in the Azizi study. A 1-year supply of PTU is about $410, and that of MMI is $360 for 15 mg a day and $720 for 30 mg a day.[2]

The authors acknowledge that there are several limitations to this study—namely, the cohort comprised a highly selected group of patients over age 40 years with diffuse toxic goiter who, after initial management with antithyroid drugs for one and a half years, remained thyrotoxic. Second, the drop-out rate was high and might have affected the results. Third, the number of patients available for study was not powered to detect significant differences in cardiovascular, bone, and lipid alterations between the treatment groups. Fourth, immunologic changes were not measured during the study. Fifth, the cost of treatment is based on both groups requiring the same degree of follow-up, but some would argue that the MMI group of patients required more careful follow-up than once every 6 months; moreover, 9 patients required an additional ^{131}I treatment, which was factored into the cost, and may have been alleviated with the administration of larger ^{131}I activities for the initial treatment.

Azizi et al suggest that an alternative approach to the management of Graves' disease is to provide lifelong MMI therapy. Others have shown that long-term treatment with antithyroid drugs offers no additional benefit in terms of improved remission rates of Graves' disease.[3] Moreover, some patients are poor candidates for prolonged antithyroid drug treatment, such as women in their child bearing years, a key group that has a high incidence of Graves' disease, or elderly patients who often have complicating comorbid illnesses. Yet for one reason or other, some patients take antithyroid drugs over many years without complications. As a fledgling faculty member at Ohio State, I saw a gentleman who had been taking propylthiouracil for 25 years (dispensed by his pharmacist brother-in-law), and my advice to the patient was to stop taking it. As one might suspect, he politely left the office, never to return. Some patients opt for long-term antithyroid drug treatment—for years or even decades—and there is no theoretical reason why a patient whose disease is well controlled with a small dose of antithyroid drug could not continue this therapy indefinitely.[2] In fact, in one study,[4] 80 patients were given long-term therapy, averaging 4.4 years (range, 1-14 years) of continuous treatment with a remission rate of 76% and an average follow-up of 7.8 years (1-21 years). Mild reactions occurred in 5 (6%), hypothyroidism in 2 (3%). The authors of the study concluded that antithyroid drug therapy is safe and effective therapy for hyperthyroidism when administered for prolonged periods.

In the final analysis, the choice of therapy resides with the patient. A prospective randomized study comparing antithyroid drugs, ^{131}I therapy and surgery found that patient satisfaction was more than 90% for all three.[5] Still, I doubt that many patients would want to take MMI for the rest of their lives once they know the potential risks of doing this, including agranulocytosis, hepatitis, and vasculitis, or that most physicians would give equal weight to the risks of levothyroxine and MMI therapy, especially over a lifetime. While it is true that the risk of major complications of antithyroid drugs is low, and agranulocytosis risk is highest in the first 90 days of treatment, this and other serious complications may occur a year or more after initiating therapy.[2] MMI-induced vasculitis, jaundice, or thrombocytopenia can occur without much warning at any time during therapy. When the occasional patient opts for long-term MMI therapy, the studies by Azizi et al and Slingerland et al[4] show that this can be done for decades if necessary without obvious deleterious side effects.

E. L. Mazzaferri, MD

References

1. Wartofsky L, Glinoer D, Solomon B, et al: Differences and similarities in the diagnosis and treatment of Graves' disease in Europe, Japan, and the United States. *Thyroid* 1:129-135, 1991.
2. Cooper DS: Antithyroid drugs. *N Engl J Med* 352:905-917, 2005.
3. Maugendre D, Gatel A, Campion L, et al: Antithyroid drugs and Graves' disease—prospective randomized assessment of long-term treatment. *Clin Endocrinol (Oxf)* 50:127-132, 1999.
4. Slingerland DW, Burrows BA: Long-term antithyroid treatment in hyperthyroidism. *JAMA* 242:2408-2410, 1979.
5. Ljunggren JG, Torring O, Wallin G, et al: Quality of life aspects and costs in treatment of Graves' hyperthyroidism with antithyroid drugs, surgery, or radioiodine: Results from a prospective, randomized study. *Thyroid* 8:653-659, 1998.

Thyroid Hormone Replacement Therapy in Primary Hypothyroidism: A Randomized Trial Comparing L-Thyroxine Plus Liothyronine With L-Thyroxine Alone

Escobar-Morreale H, Botella-Carretero J, Gómez-Bueno M, et al (Hosp Ramón y Cajal, Madrid)

Ann Intern Med 142:412-424, 2005 58–4

Background.—Substituting part of the dose of L-thyroxine with small but supraphysiologic doses of liothyronine in hypothyroid patients has yielded conflicting results.

Objective.—To evaluate combinations of L-thyroxine plus liothyronine in hypothyroid patients that match the proportions present in normal secretions of the human thyroid gland.

Design.—Randomized, double-blind, crossover trial.

Setting.—Academic research hospital.

Participants.—28 women with overt primary hypothyroidism.

Intervention.—Crossover trial comparing treatment with L-thyroxine, 100 μg/d (standard treatment), versus treatment with L-thyroxine, 75 μg/d,

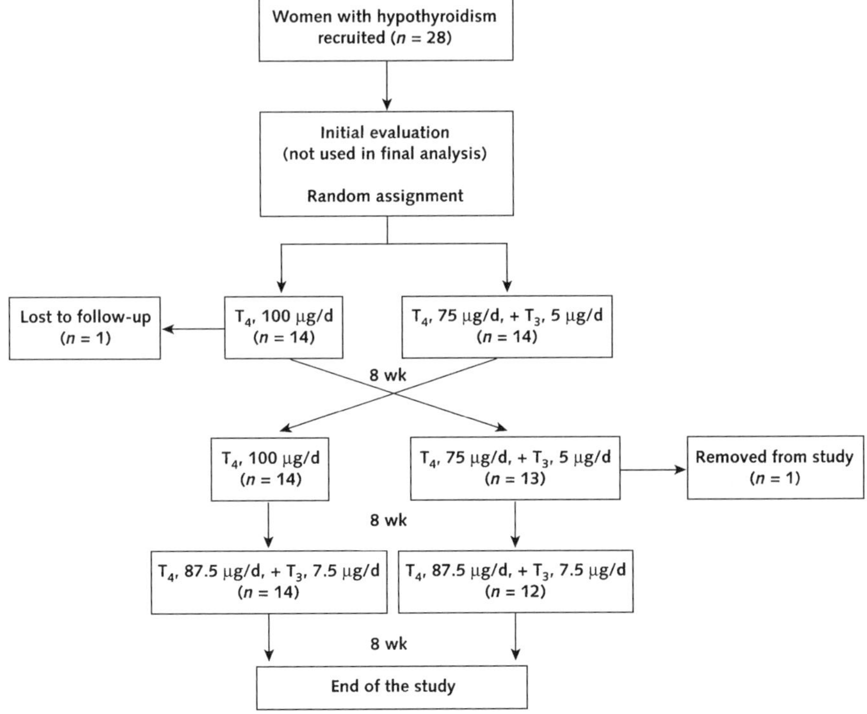

FIGURE 1.—Flow of patients through the study. *Abbreviations: T_3*, Liothyronine (synthetic triiodothyronine); *T_4*, L-thyroxine (synthetic thyroxine). (Courtesy of Escobar-Morreale H, Botella-Carretero J, Gómez-Bueno M, et al: Thyroid hormone replacement therapy in primary hypothyroidism: A randomized trial comparing L-thyroxine plus liothyronine with L-thyroxine alone. *Ann Intern Med* 142:412-424, 2005.)

plus liothyronine, 5 μg/d (combination treatment), for 8-week periods. All patients also received L-thyroxine, 87.5 μg/d, plus liothyronine, 7.5 μg/d (add-on combination treatment), for a final 8-week add-on period.

Measurements.—Primary outcomes included serum thyroid hormone levels, results of quality-of-life and psychometric tests, and patients' preference. Multiple biological thyroid hormone end points were studied as secondary outcomes.

Results.—Compared with standard treatment, combination treatment led to lower free thyroxine levels (decrease, 3.9 pmol/L [95% CI, 2.5 to 5.3 pmol/L]), slightly higher serum levels of thyroid-stimulating hormone (increase, 0.62 mU/L [CI, 0.01 to 1.23 mU/L]), and unchanged free triiodothyronine levels. No improvement was observed in the other primary and secondary end points after combination treatment, with the exception of the Digit Span Test, in which the mean backward score and the mean total score increased slightly (0.6 digit [CI, 0.1 to 1.0 digit] and 0.8 digit [CI, 0.2 to 1.4 digits], respectively). The add-on combination treatment resulted in overreplacement. Levels of thyroid-stimulating hormone decreased by 0.85 mU/L (CI, 0.27 to 1.43 mU/L) and serum free triiodothyronine levels increased by 0.8 pmol/L (CI, 0.1 to 1.5 pmol/L) compared with standard treatment; 10 patients had levels of thyroid-stimulating hormone that were below the normal range. Twelve patients preferred combination treatment, 6 patients preferred the add-on combination treatment, 2 patients preferred standard treatment, and 6 patients had no preference ($P = 0.015$).

Limitations.—Treatment with L-thyroxine, 87.5 μ/d, plus liothyronine, 7.5 μg/d, was an add-on regimen and was not randomized.

Conclusions.—Physiologic combinations of L-thyroxine plus liothyronine do not offer any objective advantage over L-thyroxine alone, yet patients prefer combination treatment (Fig 1).

► Several studies have been provoked by a 1999 article published in *The New England Journal of Medicine* by Bunevicius et al[1] in which 33 hypothyroid Lithuanian patients taking levothyroxine (L-T4) underwent substitution of 50 μg of their usual dose of L-T4 with 12.5 μg of liothyronine (T3), resulting in significantly improved mood and sense of well-being, according to scores on standardized tests, as well as improved cognitive function scores compared with L-T4 therapy alone. In addition, most patients reported that they preferred the combination of L-T4 + T3 therapy.

In 2000, the same authors[2] published a second study in which 26 hypothyroid women, 11 with autoimmune thyroiditis and 15 with treated thyroid cancer, were given either their usual dose of L-T4 or a regimen in which 50 μg of L-T4 was replaced by 12.5 μg of T3. Patients were randomly assigned to one regimen for 5 weeks and then to the second for an additional 5 weeks. After the combined therapy, the patients experienced clear improvements in cognition and mood, with the latter being greater, although the thyroid cancer patients showed more mental improvement than did women with autoimmune thyroiditis. Some mood improvements correlated positively with changes in TSH, whereas others correlated negatively with changes in free T4. The 2 studies from this group have sparked an unusual amount of interest, mainly because if they can be confirmed, then combined L-T4 + T3 treatment would likely become the standard for thyroid hormone replacement therapy. To date, however, no one has been able to confirm these findings.

In a systematic review of the literature on this subject, Escobar-Morreale et al[3] identified 9 controlled clinical trials,[1,2,4-10] including the one selected for the current YEAR BOOK OF ENDOCRINOLOGY, which compared treatment with L-T4 alone and treatment with various combinations of L-T4 + T3 and also included a sufficient number of adult hypothyroid patients to yield meaningful results. Escobar-Morreale et al found that only in the Bunevicius et al studies did combined therapy appear to have beneficial effects on mood, quality of life, and psychometric performance of the patients over that found with L-T4 alone. Moreover, their results have not been confirmed by subsequent studies using T3 substitution protocols or fixed combinations of L-T4 + T3, including those based on the physiological T3 to L-T4 proportions secreted by the human thyroid. Yet in some of these studies, patients preferred L-T4 + T3 combinations, for reasons not explained by changes in the psychological and psychometric tests used.

Why, then, do investigators continue to probe this issue? For one thing, many hypothyroid patients seem to be dissatisfied with their L-T4 replacement therapy. Also, in thyroidectomized rats the combined infusion of L-T4 and T3, as opposed to L-T4 alone, is the only way to restore circulating TSH, T4 and T3 concentrations, as well as the tissue levels of both T4 and T3.[11] Escobar-Morreale et al conclude in their recent review[12] of this subject that, considering the substantial differences in thyroid hormone secretion, transport, and metabolism between rats and humans, it remains an open question whether combined L-T4 + T3 replacement therapy for hypothyroid patients has advantages over treatment with L-T4 alone.

In the latest Escobar-Morreale et al study chosen for the YEAR BOOK, the authors performed a complex crossover trial (Fig 1) that compared L-T4 with a combination of physiologic doses of L-T4 and T3 and found no objective advantages of combined therapy. There were no adverse effects with any of the combined L-T4 + T3 treatments. They concluded that treatment of primary hypothyroidism with L-T4 combinations matching the proportions present in human thyroid secretions does not offer clear advantages over standard L-T4 treatment. For now, there is insufficient evidence to recommend combined L-T4 + T3 therapy for hypothyroid patients, yet why so many patients seem dissatisfied with thyroid hormone replacement therapy remains a major clinical conundrum of our time.

E. L. Mazzaferri, MD

References

1. Bunevicius R, Kazanavicius G, Zalinkevicius R, et al: Effects of thyroxine as compared with thyroxine plus triiodothyronine in patients with hypothyroidism. *N Engl J Med* 340:424-429, 1999.
2. Bunevicius R, Prange AJ: Mental improvement after replacement therapy with thyroxine plus triiodothyronine: Relationship to cause of hypothyroidism. *Int J Neuropsychopharmacol* 3:167-174, 2000.

3. Escobar-Morreale HF, Botella-Carretero JI, Escobar del Rey F, et al: REVIEW: Treatment of hypothyroidism with combinations of levothyroxine plus liothyronine. *J Clin Endocrinol Metab*90:4946-4954, 2005.
4. Appelhof BC, Fliers E, Wekking EM, et al: Combined therapy with levothyroxine and liothyronine in two ratios compared with levothyroxine monotherapy in primary hypothyroidism: A double-blind, randomized, controlled clinical trial. *J Clin Endocrinol Metab*90:2666-2674, 2005.
5. Clyde PW, Harari AE, Getka EJ, et al: Combined levothyroxine plus liothyronine compared with levothyroxine alone in primary hypothyroidism: A randomized controlled trial. *JAMA* 290:2952-2958, 2003.
6. Escobar-Morreale HF, Botella-Carretero JI, Gomez-Bueno M, et al: Thyroid hormone replacement therapy in primary hypothyroidism: A randomized trial comparing L-thyroxine plus liothyronine with L-thyroxine alone. *Ann Intern Med* 142:412-424, 2005.
7. Saravanan P, Simmons DJ, Greenwood R, et al: Partial substitution of thyroxine (T4) with tri-iodothyronine in patients on T4 replacement therapy: Results of a large community-based randomized controlled trial. *J Clin Endocrinol Metab* 90:805-812, 2005.
8. Siegmund W, Spieker K, Weike AI, et al: Replacement therapy with levothyroxine plus triiodothyronine (bioavailable molar ratio 14:1) is not superior to thyroxine alone to improve well-being and cognitive performance in hypothyroidism. *Clin Endocrinol (Oxf)* 60:750-757, 2004.
9. Smith RN, Taylor SA, Massey JC: Controlled clinical trial of combined triiodothyronine and thyroxine in the treatment of hypothyroidism. *Br Med J* 4:145-148, 1970.
10. Walsh JP, Shiels L, Lim EM, et al: Combined thyroxine/liothyronine treatment does not improve well-being, quality of life, or cognitive function compared to thyroxine alone: A randomized controlled trial in patients with primary hypothyroidism. *J Clin Endocrinol Metab* 88:4543-4550, 2003.
11. Escobar-Morreale HF, Obregon MJ, Escobar del Rey F, et al: Replacement therapy for hypothyroidism with thyroxine alone does not ensure euthyroidism in all tissues, as studied in thyroidectomized rats. *J Clin Invest* 96:2828-2838, 1995.
12. Escobar-Morreale HF, Botella-Carretero JI, Escobar del Rey F, et al: REVIEW: Treatment of hypothyroidism with combinations of levothyroxine plus liothyronine. *J Clin Endocrinol Metab* 90:4946-4954, 2005.

The Occurrence of Permanent Thyroid Failure in Patients With Subclinical Postpartum Thyroiditis

Azizi F (Shaheed Beheshti Univ of Med Sciences, Tehran, Islamic Republic of Iran)

Eur J Endocrinol 153:367-371, 2005 58–5

Objective.—The long-term effect of the subclinical form of postpartum thyroid dysfunction (PPTD) has not been well established. This study was conducted to evaluate the outcome of permanent hypothyroidism in a large cohort of women with PPTD.

Design and Methods.—Of 213 women with PPTD, 172 (81%) returned for follow-up. There were 27 (16%) with subclinical (group 1) and 145 (84%) with overt hypothyroidism (group 2). They were all treated with levothyroxine for 23 ± 16 months and followed-up for thyroid function after thyroxine (T_4) withdrawal.

Results.—In group 1, the time of occurrence of PPTD was longer, serum T(4) was higher and TSH was lower than in group 2. After T_4 withdrawal, 59 and 64% of patients became hypothyroid in groups 1 and 2 respectively; however, serum TSH was increased in group 2 as compared with group 1 (29.7 ± 8.4 vs 16.4 ± 15.4 mU/l, $P < 0.002$). The duration of euthyroidism, serum free T_4 and triiodothyronine indices and thyroperoxidase antibodies were not significantly different between the two groups.

Conclusion.—It was concluded that a high percentage of patients with the subclinical form of PPTD proceed to permanent thyroid failure. The timely recognition of mild to severe cases of PPTD is important for the improvement of life for mothers and infants.

► PPTD is an autoimmune disorder characterized by lymphocytic infiltration of the thyroid gland and by thyroid dysfunction, which may be first manifest by thyrotoxicosis followed by a period of euthyroidism that either persists or gives way to hypothyroidism, which may or may not persist.[1] Half or more of the women with PPTD develop permanent hypothyroidism requiring lifelong levothyroxine therapy,[2,3] which is more likely to happen in women aged 30 or older[2] and in those with a TSH levels greater than 20 mIU/L during the postpartum period.[3] Yet whether women with postpartum thyroiditis who develop subclinical hypothyroidism (defined as an elevated serum TSH level with normal serum thyroid hormone concentrations) eventually develop permanent hypothyroidism has, until now, been unknown.

It is this question that Azizi addresses in a study of 213 women with PPTD who presented with hypothyroidism. Women with a past history of thyroid dysfunction were excluded from the study, except when it was associated with PPTD. All the women were 3 to 10 months postpartum and presented with at least one of the following signs or symptoms: thyroid growth, lethargy, fatigue, depression, cold intolerance, dry skin, weight gain, constipation, and sleepiness; 19% had suffered an episode of transient thyrotoxicosis 2 to 4 months after delivery. All patients required treatment, and therapy with levothyroxine (L-T4) was thus begun. Therapy was discontinued 12 to 24 months later, and the patients were carefully followed for thyroid dysfunction.

Of the 213 women, 81% (172) returned for the follow-up study; their mean age was 29.2 ± 4.4 years. There were 27 women (16%) with subclinical and 145 (84%) with overt hypothyroidism. The ultimate rates of developing overt hypothyroidism (59% in group 1 and 64% in group 2) are shown in Fig 1 (see original article).

This study demonstrates that more than half the women with subclinical hypothyroidism develop recurrent thyroid failure after L-T4 withdrawal, although it was subclinical in the majority of cases. Most of the women in this study had palpable goiters, which do not usually occur with PPTD. Goiter was endemic in Iran before iodine was added to the diet in 1995, which might somehow be related to some of the observed changes. Still, there is little question that even the subclinical form of hypothyroidism that occurs with PPTD has a high risk of progressing to permanent hypothyroidism, which might continue throughout the woman's lifetime. This immediately calls into question whether thyroid hormone should ever be discontinued once a woman develops postpartum hypothyroidism that requires therapy.

E. L. Mazzaferri, MD

References

1. Roti E, Uberti E: Post-partum thyroiditis—a clinical update. *Eur J Endocrinol* 146:275-279, 2002.
2. Azizi F: Age as a predictor of recurrent hypothyroidism in patients with postpartum thyroid dysfunction. *J Endocrinol Invest* 27:996-1002, 2004.
3. Premawardhana LDKE, Parkes AB, Ammari F, et al: Postpartum thyroiditis and long-term thyroid status: Prognostic influence of thyroid peroxidase antibodies and ultrasound echogenicity. *J Clin Endocrinol Metab* 85:71-75, 2000.

Propylthiouracil Before ^{131}I Therapy of Hyperthyroid Diseases: Effect on Cure Rate Evaluated by a Randomized Clinical Trial

Bonnema SJ, Bennedbaek FN, Veje A, et al (Odense Univ, Denmark)

J Clin Endocrinol Metab 89:4439-4444, 2004 58–6

Background.—A survey on the management of Graves' disease found that 30% of physicians prefer to render their patients euthyroid with antithyroid drugs before administration of radioactive iodine (^{131}I) therapy. The purpose of this strategy is to avoid an ^{131}I-induced thyroid storm, even though this is a rarely encountered event. The use of pretreatment with antithyroid drugs is called into question if rapid access to ^{131}I is available. Whether pretreatment with propylthiouracil (PTU) before ^{131}I therapy has an effect on the final outcome in patients with hyperthyroid disease was determined.

Methods.—A retrospective review was conducted of outcomes in untreated consecutive hyperthyroid patients with Graves' disease (23 patients) or a toxic nodular goiter (57 patients). The patients were randomly assigned to either PTU or no pretreatment before compensated ^{131}I therapy. The median PTU dose was 100 mg, which was discontinued 4 days before treatment.

Results.—The median ^{131}I activity was 302 MBq. After ^{131}I therapy, the serum free T_4 index increased in the group that received PTU pretreatment. In contrast, there was a significant decrease in the serum free T_4 index in the no-pretreatment group. At 1 year of follow-up, the treatment failure rate in patients with a toxic nodular goiter was 4 times higher in the PTU-pretreated group than in the no-pretreatment group, whereas the difference among patients with Graves' disease was less obvious. Patients in the pretreatment group who were cured had higher serum TSH levels at the time of ^{131}I therapy than those who were not cured. Data analyses showed that only PTU pretreatment had a significant adverse effect on the cure rate in patients with hyperthyroid diseases.

Conclusions.—Pretreatment with PTU reduced the cure rate of ^{131}I therapy in patients with hyperthyroid diseases. However, this adverse effect appeared to be attenuated by a concomitant rise in serum TSH levels.

► Although ^{131}I has been used for decades to treat hyperthyroidism, questions remain about certain details of management. A 1990 survey[1] of American Thyroid Association (ATA) members found that ^{131}I therapy was the treatment of choice for thyrotoxic Graves' disease for nearly 70% of the respondents and that about two thirds tailored the ^{131}I dose to achieve euthyroidism as the goal of therapy, while the other third aimed for hypothyroidism requiring levothyroxine (L-T_4) replacement. In the last 15 years, however, studies have shown that permanent euthyroidism cannot be consistently achieved by tailoring the dose of ^{131}I,[2,3] and that purposefully ablating the thyroid gland and treating the patient with L-T_4 is a more realistic and medically sound therapeutic goal.[4] Even then, 20% to 30% of patients fail to become euthyroid during the first year after the first ^{131}I treatment.[5]

The 1990 ATA survey also found that almost 30% of the respondents routinely used antithyroid drugs (ATDs) for 3 to 7 days before ^{131}I therapy and about 40% used them after ^{131}I therapy. They likely used ATDs with ^{131}I because thyroid hormone levels increase after ^{131}I treatment, exaggerating the symptoms of thyrotoxicosis and rarely precipitating thyroid storm, although using ATDs appears not to prevent this complication.[6] A large number of retrospective studies have shown that PTU pretreatment interferes with ^{131}I therapy.[7-13] Although a few still question whether this radioprotective effect occurs with methimazole, 2 recent randomized trials show that it does not interfere with the final ^{131}I cure rate.[14,15] It is also questionable whether PTU confers any major benefit when given after ^{131}I therapy, although a recent study by Bonnema et al[16] showed that resumption of methimazole after ^{131}I therapy slightly reduced the magnitude of shrinkage of the goiter obtained by ^{131}I, but prevented the temporary thyrotoxicosis in the early period after radiation.

A larger question is whether pretreatment with methimazole should be done at all before ^{131}I therapy, since the rise in serum thyroid hormone concentrations that occurs immediately before ^{131}I therapy results from discontinuing the drug.[17] Burch et al[18] reported that pretreatment with ATDs does not protect against worsening thyrotoxicosis after ^{131}I therapy, but may allow patients to start from a lower baseline level should an aggravation in thyrotoxicosis occur. Nonetheless, when treating seriously thyrotoxic patients with Graves' disease, most thyroidologists seem to be uncomfortable not pretreating them with ATDs, but when this is done, methimazole should be used. Although the 2 increases in serum thyroid hormone concentrations that occur after methimazole withdrawal and after ^{131}I therapy can be prevented by lithium pretreatment,[19] this drug is difficult to use in elderly patients and is largely contraindicated in patients with impaired renal clearance and heart failure.

It is in this setting that Bonnema et al performed a randomized, prospective clinical trial of the effect of PTU treatment before ^{131}I therapy for hyperthyroid patients. The patients in their study comprised a selected cohort for 2 reasons. First, many patients already taking ATDs were not eligible for the study. Second, only patients with recurrent Graves' disease were treated with ^{131}I according to their institutional routine, which is known to represent a more severe form of the disease,[12] and may be a major reason for the ^{131}I failure in their patients with Graves' disease. Although the incidence of hypothyroidism was nearly identical in patients treated or not treated with PTU, the risk of recurrence was more than twice as high among the pretreated patients. Still, the difference in the subgroup with Graves' disease was not statistically significant (Table 2).

There is little question that PTU substantially interferes with the outcome of ^{131}I therapy for hyperthyroid patients and that the drug should not be used for this purpose, especially if ^{131}I therapy might be necessary in the near future, because the effects of PTU last at least 2 months or longer.[11] When ATD pretherapy is necessary—which seems to be a rarely the case—methimazole is the drug of choice except in pregnant women. It seems much safer to pretreat patients with β-blockers before ^{131}I therapy, unless thyrotoxicosis is severe, in which case lithium pretreatment should be considered.

E. L. Mazzaferri, MD

References

1. Solomon B, Glinoer D, Lagasse R, et al: Current trends in the management of Graves' disease. *J Clin Endocrinol Metab* 70:1518-1524, 1990.
2. Catargi B, Leprat F, Guyot M, et al: Optimized radioiodine therapy of Graves' disease: Analysis of the delivered dose and of other possible factors affecting outcome. *Eur J Endocrinol* 141:117-121, 1999.
3. Grosso M, Traino A, Boni G, et al: Comparison of different thyroid committed doses in radioiodine therapy for Graves' hyperthyroidism. *Cancer Biother Radiopharm* 20:218-223, 2005.
4. Franklyn JA, Sheppard MC, Maisonneuve P: Thyroid function and mortality in patients treated for hyperthyroidism. *JAMA* 294:71-80, 2005.
5. Metso S, Jaatinen P, Huhtala H, et al: Long-term follow-up study of radioiodine treatment of hyperthyroidism. *Clin Endocrinol (Oxf)* 61:641-648, 2004.
6. McDermott MT, Kidd GS, Dodson LE Jr, et al: Radioiodine-induced thyroid storm. Case report and literature review. *Am J Med* 75:353-359, 1983.
7. Reynolds LR, Kotchen TA: Antithyroid drugs and radioactive iodine. Fifteen years' experience with Graves' disease. *Arch Intern Med* 139:651-653, 1979.
8. Tuttle RM, Patience T, Budd S: Treatment with propylthiouracil before radioactive iodine therapy is associated with a higher treatment failure rate than therapy with radioactive iodine alone in Graves' disease. *Thyroid* 5:243-247, 1995.
9. Hancock LD, Tuttle RM, LeMar H, et al: The effect of propylthiouracil on subsequent radioactive iodine therapy in Graves' disease. *Clin Endocrinol (Oxf)* 47:425-430, 1997.
10. Turton DB, Silverman ED, Shakir KM: Time interval between the last dose of propylthiouracil and I-131 therapy influences cure rates in hyperthyroidism caused by Graves' disease. *Clin Nucl Med* 23:810-814, 1998.
11. Imseis RE, Vanmiddlesworth L, Massie JD, et al: Pretreatment with propylthiouracil but not methimazole reduces the therapeutic efficacy of iodine-131 in hyperthyroidism. *J Clin Endocrinol Metab* 83:685-687, 1998.
12. Allahabadia A, Daykin J, Sheppard MC, et al: Radioiodine treatment of hyperthyroidism: Prognostic factors for outcome. *J Clin Endocrinol Metab* 86:3611-3617, 2001.
13. Korber C, Schneider P, Korber-Hafner N, et al: Antithyroid drugs as a factor influencing the outcome of radioiodine therapy in Graves' disease and toxic nodular goitre? *Eur J Nucl Med* 28:1360-1364, 2001.
14. Andrade VA, Gross JL, Maia AL: Effect of methimazole pretreatment on serum thyroid hormone levels after radioactive treatment in Graves' hyperthyroidism. *J Clin Endocrinol Metab* 84:4012-4016, 1999.
15. Braga M, Walpert N, Burch HB, et al: The effect of methimazole on cure rates after radioiodine treatment for Graves' hyperthyroidism: A randomized clinical trial. *Thyroid* 12:135-139, 2002.

16. Bonnema SJ, Bennedbaek FN, Gram J, et al: Resumption of methimazole after I therapy of hyperthyroid diseases: Effect on thyroid function and volume evaluated by a randomized clinical trial. *Eur J Endocrinol* 149:485-492, 2003.
17. Burch HB, Solomon BL, Wartofsky L, et al: Discontinuing antithyroid drug therapy before ablation with radioiodine in Graves disease. *Ann Intern Med* 121:553-559, 1994.
18. Burch HB, Solomon BL, Cooper DS, et al: The effect of antithyroid drug pretreatment on acute changes in thyroid hormone levels after 131-I ablation for Graves' disease. *J Clin Endocrinol Metab* 86:3016-3021, 2001.
19. Bogazzi F, Bartalena L, Pinchera A, et al: Adjuvant effect of lithium on radioiodine treatment of hyperthyroidism. *Thyroid* 12:1153-1154, 2002.

59 Parathyroid, Vitamin D, and Bone

Prevalence of Vitamin D Inadequacy Among Postmenopausal North American Women Receiving Osteoporosis Therapy

Holick MF, Siris ES, Binkley N, et al (Boston Univ Med Ctr; Columbia Univ, New York; Univ of Wisconsin, Madison, Wis; et al)

J Clin Endocrinol Metab 90:3215-3224, 2005 59–1

Purpose.—To evaluate serum 25-hydroxyvitamin D [25(OH)D] concentrations and factors related to vitamin D inadequacy in postmenopausal North American women receiving therapy to treat or prevent osteoporosis.

Methods.—Serum 25(OH)D and PTH were obtained in 1536 community-dwelling women between November 2003 and March 2004.

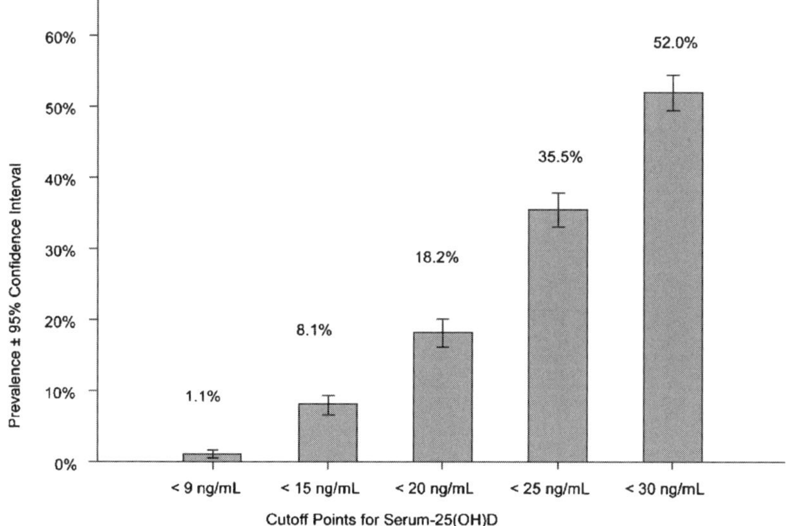

FIGURE 2.—Prevalence of vitamin D inadequacy in all subjects. The percentage of subjects with serum 25(OH)D concentrations below predefined cutoffs of less than 9, less than 15, less than 20, less than 25, and less than 30 ng/ml. (Courtesy of Holick MF, Siris ES, Binkley N, et al: Prevalence of vitamin D inadequacy among postmenopausal North American women receiving osteoporosis therapy. *J Clin Endocrinol Metab* 90:3215-3224, 2005. Copyright 2005 The Endocrine Society.)

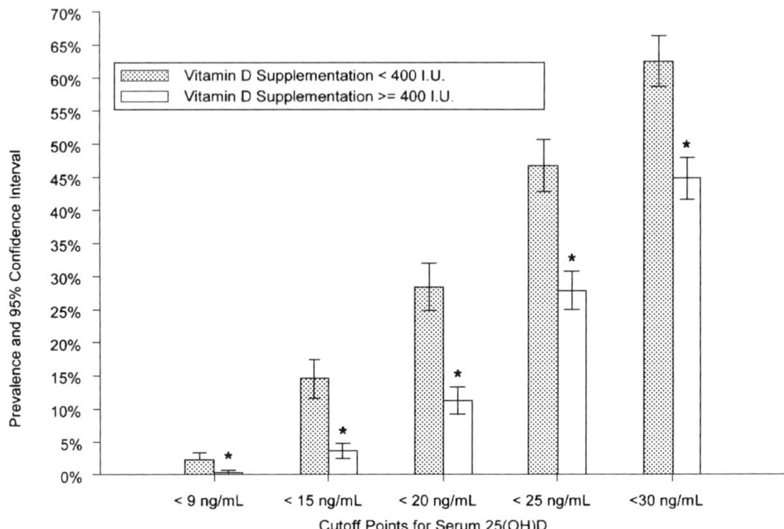

FIGURE 3.—Subgroup analysis of vitamin D inadequacy relative to daily vitamin D supplementation less than 400 IU or 400 IU or more. The percentage of subjects with serum 25(OH)D concentrations below predefined cutoffs of less than 9, less than 15, less than 20, less than 25, and less than 30 ng/ml relative to their daily vitamin D supplementation of either less than 400 IU or 400 IU or more. A *P* value is provided for the difference between subjects with less than 400 IU or 400 IU or more daily vitamin D supplementation at each cutoff. *Asterisk*, $P < 0.001$ for comparison of patients with vitamin D supplementation <400 IU *vs.* ≥400 IU. (Courtesy of Holick MF, Siris ES, Binkley N, et al: Prevalence of vitamin D inadequacy among postmenopausal North American women receiving osteoporosis therapy. *J Clin Endocrinol Metab* 90:3215-3224, 2005. Copyright 2005 The Endocrine Society.)

Multivariate logistic regression was used to assess risk factors for suboptimal (<30 ng/ml) 25(OH)D.

Results.—Ninety-two percent of study subjects were Caucasian, with a mean age of 71 yr. Thirty-five percent resided at or above latitude 42° north, and 24% resided less than 35° north. Mean (SD) serum 25(OH)D was 30.4 (13.2) ng/ml: serum 25(OH)D was less than 20 ng/ml in 18%; less than 25 ng/ml in 36%; and less than 30 ng/ml in 52% (Fig 2). Prevalence of suboptimal 25(OH)D was significantly higher in subjects who took less than 400 *vs.* 400 IU/d or more vitamin D (Fig 3). There was a significant negative correlation between serum PTH concentrations and 25(OH)D. Risk factors related to vitamin D inadequacy included age, race, body mass index, medications known to affect vitamin D metabolism, vitamin D supplementation, exercise, education, and physician counseling regarding vitamin D.

Conclusions.—More than half of North American women receiving therapy to treat or prevent osteoporosis have vitamin D inadequacy, underscoring the need for improved physician and public education regarding optimization of vitamin D status in this population.

► Clinicians have become increasingly aware in recent years of the increased prevalence of vitamin D insufficiency or deficiency in postmenopausal women and older men. Most patients treated for osteoporosis are advised to take adequate vitamin D supplementation appropriate for their age, based on US recommended daily allowances. This study showed that in spite of advice to take vitamin D supplementation, serum 25(OH)D levels remain inadequate in more than half of North American women receiving therapy to treat or prevent osteoporosis.

The authors recruited 1536 community-dwelling women in the fall of 2003 and winter of 2004, and measured their fasting serum 25(OH)D level. The majority of these elderly women were Caucasian, and 35% resided at or above latitude 42° north, and 24% resided at or below 35° north. Their mean serum 25(OH)D level was 30.4 ± 13.2 ng/mL, with 18% having levels less than 20 ng/mL, 36% less than 25 ng/mL, and 52% less than 30 ng/mL (Fig 2). The prevalence of inadequate serum 25(OH)D was higher in subjects taking less than 400 IU/d of vitamin D (Fig 3). There was a significant negative correlation between serum 25(OH)D and serum PTH levels, with the nadir PTH level achieved at a serum 25(OH)D level of 30 ng/mL. The authors concluded that most postmenopausal women receiving therapy for osteoporosis are vitamin D insufficient or deficient.

This study emphasizes that vitamin D status cannot be assumed to be normal in community-dwelling postmenopausal women treated for osteoporosis. Serum 25(OH)D is defined in most studies as being optimal when the level is sufficient to suppress serum PTH levels into the normal range. Some patients may require more than 400 IU/d of vitamin D intake to normalize their serum PTH level.

B. L. Clarke, MD

Hip Fracture in Women Without Osteoporosis

Wainwright SA, for the Study of Osteoporotic Fractures Research Group (Oregon Health and Science Univ, Portland; et al)
J Clin Endocrinol Metab 90:2787-2793, 2005 59–2

Introduction.—The proportion of fractures that occur in women without osteoporosis has not been fully described, and the characteristics of nonosteoporotic women who fracture are not well understood. We measured total hip bone mineral density (BMD) and baseline characteristics including physical activity, falls, and strength for 8065 women aged 65 yr or older participating in the Study of Osteoporotic Fractures and then followed these women for hip fracture for up to 5 yr after BMD measurement. Among all participants, 17% had osteoporosis (total hip BMD T-score ≤ -2.5). Of the 243 women with incident hip fracture, 54% were not osteoporotic at start of follow-up. Nonosteoporotic women who fractured were less likely than osteoporotic women with fracture to have baseline characteristics associated with frailty. Nevertheless, among nonosteoporotic participants, several characteristics increased fracture risk, including advancing age, lack of exercise in the last year, reduced visual contrast sensitivity, falls in the last year, prevalent vertebral fracture, and lower total hip BMD. These findings call attention to the many older women who suffer hip fracture but do not have particularly low antecedent BMD measures and help begin to identify risk factors associated with higher bone density levels.

► Most women with atraumatic or minimally traumatic fractures are thought to have osteoporosis, but the proportion of fractures that occurs in women without osteoporosis, and the characteristics of the nonosteoporotic women who fracture, are not well understood. The recent NORA study demonstrated that the majority of self-reported fractures occurred in women with osteopenia or normal bone density when measured by peripheral dual-energy x-ray absorptiometry or calcaneal US.[1]

The authors of this study evaluated 8065 women aged 65 years and older participating in the Study of Osteoporotic Fractures for baseline hip bone density by dual-energy x-ray absorptiometry, physical activity, falls, and strength, and then followed these women for development of hip fracture for up to 5 years. They found that only 17% of women who fractured had osteoporosis at baseline, defined as T-score less than or equal to −2.5, and that of the 243 women with hip fractures during 5 years of follow-up, more than half were not osteoporotic at baseline. Nonosteoporotic women who developed hip fractures were less likely to have characteristics associated with frailty, but advancing age, lack of exercise in the past year, reduced visual contrast sensitivity, falls in the last year, prevalent vertebral fractures, and lower total hip BMD were associated with fracture risk.

This study confirms that postmenopausal women may sustain hip fractures without meeting current World Health Organization BMD criteria for osteoporosis. These women are characterized by many of the same risk factors as postmenopausal women with osteoporosis who fracture. Risk factors for fracture may play as significant a role as BMD in predicting future fracture risk in some postmenopausal women, and the combination of BMD and risk factors for osteoporosis likely is more predictive of fracture risk than either alone.

B. L. Clarke, MD

References

1. Miller PD, Siris ES, Barrett-Connor E, et al: Prediction of fracture risk in postmenopausal white women with peripheral bone densitometry: Evidence from the National Osteoporosis Risk Assessment. *J Bone Miner Res* 17:2222-2230, 2002.

Relationship Between Osteoporosis and Cardiovascular Disease in Postmenopausal Women

Tankó LB, Christiansen C, Cox DA, et al (Ctr for Clinical and Basic Research, Ballerup, Denmark; Eli Lilly and Company, Indianapolis, Ind; Univ of Calif, San Francisco)

J Bone Miner Res 20:1912-1920, 2005 59–3

Abstract.—In the placebo group of the MORE study, including 2576 postmenopausal women (mean age, 66.5 years), the authors describe a strong linear association between the severity grade of osteoporosis (from

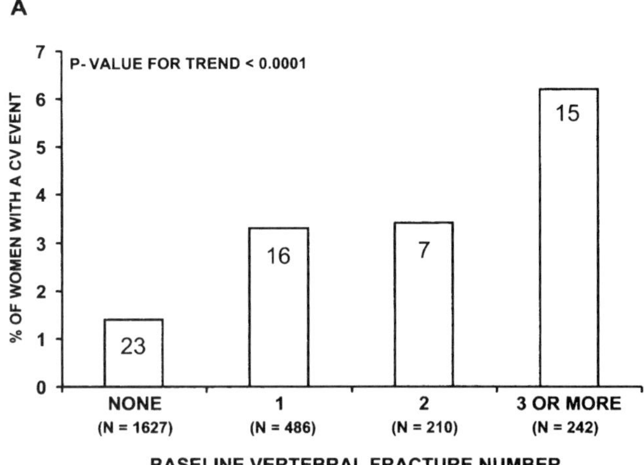

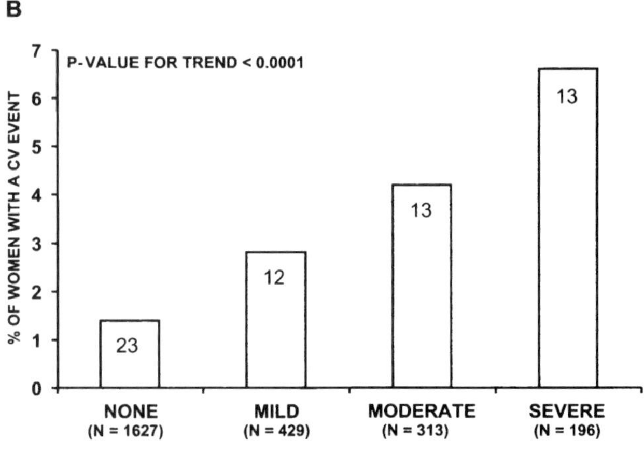

FIGURE 4.—Relationship between the (A) number and (B) severity of osteoporotic vertebral fractures and the risk of cardiovascular events in postmenopausal women. *p* value is from Cochrane-Armitage trend test. Numbers in bars represent number of women with a cardiovascular event. Fracture severity is shown in terms of magnitude of vertebral height reduction. (Courtesy of Tankó LB, Christiansen C, Cox DA, et al: Relationship between osteoporosis and cardiovascular disease in postmenopausal women. *J Bone Min Res* 20:1912-1920, 2005. Reprinted by permission of Blackwell Publishing.)

low BMD to presence of severe vertebral fractures) and the future risk of cardiovascular events. Accordingly, treatment of postmenopausal osteoporosis should include consideration of measures to prevent adverse cardiovascular outcomes.

Introduction.—Observations indicate an inverse association between BMD and the severity of peripheral atherosclerosis in postmenopausal women. The predictive value of osteoporosis and its different severity stages for the risk of acute cardiovascular events remains unknown.

Materials and Methods.—Participants were 2576 women (mean age, 66.5 years) assigned to placebo and followed for 4 years in an osteoporosis treatment trial. Those with at least one vertebral fracture or total hip BMD T score ≤ −2.5 at baseline were defined as having osteoporosis, whereas those without vertebral fracture and total hip BMD T score between −2.5 and −1 were defined as having low bone mass. The primary outcome for these posthoc analyses was the incidence of adjudicated fatal or nonfatal cardiovascular events.

Results.—After adjustment for potential confounders, women with osteoporosis had a 3.9-fold (95% CI, 2.0–7.7; $p < 0.001$) increased risk for cardiovascular events compared with women with low bone mass (Fig 4). Under the same boundaries, a total hip BMD T score ≤ −2.5 versus a T score between −2.5 and −1 was associated with a 2.1-fold (95% CI, 1.2–3.6; $p < 0.01$) increase in risk, whereas presence of at least one vertebral fracture versus no vertebral fracture at baseline was associated with a 3.0-fold (95% CI, 1.8–5.1; $p < 0.001$) increase in risk. The risk of cardiovascular events increased incrementally with the number and increasing severity of baseline vertebral fractures (both $p < 0.001$).

Conclusions.—Postmenopausal women with osteoporosis are at an increased risk for cardiovascular events that is proportional to the severity of osteoporosis at the time of the diagnosis. Treatment of postmenopausal osteoporosis should include consideration of measures to prevent cardiovascular outcomes.

► Postmenopausal women with osteoporosis might be expected to have increased risk of cardiovascular disease based on their age alone. Previous observational studies have suggested an inverse relationship between bone density and cardiovascular disease, but the relationship between postmenopausal osteoporosis and cardiovascular disease has not previously been quantitatively analyzed.

This post-hoc analysis evaluated the risk of cardiovascular events in 2576 reasonably healthy postmenopausal women of mean age 66.5 years followed for 4 years in the placebo group of the MORE (Multiple Outcomes of Raloxifene) clinical trial. Women with osteoporosis at baseline had a 3.9-fold increased risk of cardiovascular events, whereas women with osteopenia had a 3.0-fold increased risk. The risk of cardiovascular events increased with the number and severity of baseline vertebral fractures. The authors concluded that postmenopausal women with osteoporosis are at an increased risk of cardiovascular events that is proportional to the severity of osteoporosis at baseline, independent of age and cardiovascular risk factors.

This study implies that treatment of postmenopausal osteoporosis should include measures to reduce risk of cardiovascular events. This study did not prospectively evaluate whether raloxifene prevents cardiovascular events, which is the subject of ongoing studies.

B. L. Clarke, MD

One Year of Alendronate After One Year of Parathyroid Hormone (1–84) for Osteoporosis

Black DM, for the PaTH Study Investigators (Univ of California, San Francisco; et al)

N Engl J Med 353:555-565, 2005 59–4

Background.—Since the use of parathyroid hormone as a treatment for osteoporosis is limited to two years or less, the question of whether antiresorptive therapy should follow parathyroid hormone therapy is important. We previously reported results after the first year of this randomized trial comparing the use of full-length parathyroid hormone (1–84) alone, alendronate alone, or both combined. In the continuation of this trial, we asked whether antiresorptive therapy is required to maintain gains in bone mineral density after one year of therapy with parathyroid hormone (1–84).

Methods.—In the data reported here, women who had received parathyroid hormone (1–84) monotherapy (100 µg daily) in year 1 were randomly reassigned to one additional year with either placebo (60 subjects) or alendronate (59 subjects). Subjects who had received combination therapy in year 1 received alendronate in year 2; those who had received alendronate monotherapy in year 1 continued with alendronate in year 2. Bone mineral density at the spine and hip was assessed with the use of dual-energy x-ray absorptiometry and quantitative computed tomography (CT).

Results.—Over two years, alendronate therapy after parathyroid hormone therapy led to significant increases in bone mineral density in comparison with the results for placebo after parathyroid hormone therapy, a difference particularly evident for bone mineral density in trabecular bone at the spine on quantitative CT (an increase of 31 percent in the parathyroid hormone–alendronate group as compared with 14 percent in the parathyroid hormone–placebo group). During year 2, subjects receiving placebo lost substantial bone mineral density.

Conclusions.—After one year of parathyroid hormone (1–84), densitometric gains appear to be maintained or increased with alendronate but lost if parathyroid hormone is not followed by an antiresorptive agent. These results have clinical implications for therapeutic choices after the discontinuation of parathyroid hormone.

► In 2002, teriparatide (recombinant human parathyroid hormone [PTH] 1–34) was the first anabolic therapy approved for treatment of postmenopausal osteoporosis in the United States. Additional anabolic agents are being developed and will likely soon be available. Teriparatide was approved for use in postmenopausal women with severe osteoporosis and high risk of fracture for up to 2 years.

It is not yet clear how patients should be treated after they complete 2 years of anabolic therapy with PTH. The authors previously reported the results of 12 months of therapy with PTH 1–84 100 µg/d, alendronate 70 mg once a week, or both combined, in women with postmenopausal osteoporosis.[1] The current study was designed to determine whether anticatabolic therapy is required to preserve gains in bone density achieved with therapy with PTH 1–84 for 1 year.[2] The authors randomized 110 women who completed 1 year of therapy with PTH 1–84 to receive either alendronate 70 mg once a week or placebo. Subjects receiving combination therapy in the first year received alendronate alone in year 2, while women receiving alendronate in year 1 received placebo in year 2. Women receiving alendronate after PTH 1–84 continued to gain significant bone density by dual-energy x-ray absorptiometry or quantitative CT scan measurement during year 2, whereas women receiving placebo after PTH 1–84 lost bone density. The increase in bone mineral density in subjects receiving alendronate after PTH 1–84 was particularly evident at lumbar spine trabecular bone, which increased by 31% during year 2 when assessed by quantitative CT compared with an increase of 14% during year 2 in the PTH 1–84 and placebo group.

The authors concluded that patients with postmenopausal osteoporosis treated with an anabolic agent should be treated with an anticatabolic agent after completing therapy to preserve gains achieved during anabolic therapy. Patients not treated with an anticatabolic agent after anabolic therapy may lose bone density.

B. L. Clarke, MD

References

1. Black DM, Greenspan SL, Ensrud KE, et al: The effects of parathyroid hormone and alendronate alone or in combination in postmenopausal osteoporosis. *N Engl J Med* 349:1207-1215, 2003.
2. Parfitt AM, Riggs BL: Drugs used to treat osteoporosis: The critical need for a uniform nomenclature based on their action on bone remodeling. *J Bone Miner Res* 20:177-184, 2005.

► Individuals with osteoporosis are now fortunate to have available 2 classes of medicine effective in improving bone density: the bisphosphonates, such as alendronate, and parathyroid hormone (PTH) (estrogens, and selective estrogen-receptor modulators, are also available for specific indications). Whereas bisphosphonates act to inhibit bone resorption by osteoclasts, PTH stimulates new bone formation. PTH is the newer kid on the block, and several questions have arisen regarding its use, particularly in conjunction with bisphosphonates. Many of these questions turn on the fact that bone formation in response to PTH is actually a cyclic process that requires periods of bone resorption to go forward. Inhibiting resorption by coadministering a bisphosphonate might therefore block, rather than enhance the effects of PTH, and a study published last year in the *New England Journal of Medicine* (and cited in the 2004 YEAR BOOK OF MEDICINE) indicated that using PTH together with alendronate was no better than using alendronate alone. Another question of interest is what happens after PTH therapy is completed; PTH is currently recommended for no more than 2 years, and in any event, its cost (more than $30,000 per year) would probably make it prohibitive for chronic use.

The present study by Black et al addresses both of these questions. The study used full-length PTH (the agent currently approved by the Food and Drug Administration, teriparatide, is actually a PTH fragment consisting of the first

34 amino acids). Patients with documented osteoporosis were administered either PTH, alendronate, or both for 1 year. Patients who had received PTH were then placed on either alendronate or placebo for an additional year. Patients who had initially received both PTH and alendronate (combination therapy group), or alendronate alone, were continued on their previous regimens during this period. During the course of 2 years, there was no difference in most bone density parameters between the alendronate and PTH plus alendronate groups, supporting the earlier conclusion that PTH is of no value, at least as far as bone density goes, in patients concurrently receiving a bisphosphonate. In contrast, bone density in the PTH-only groups improved significantly during the first year, to a degree equal to, or greater than, alendronate alone. However, bone density in the second year declined in patients whose PTH was simply discontinued. When patients who had taken PTH for 1 year were switched over to alendronate, their improvements in bone density were sustained or even enhanced by the end of the second year.

How would we translate these observations to clinical use? More study is needed, obviously, but most patients completing PTH (or teriparetide) therapy should probably receive a bisphosphonate thereafter, with little downside, and plenty of potential for benefit. On the basis of this study, as well as the previous one, it would also seem that one should initiate PTH therapy without also starting a bisphosphonate. Of course, most physicians don't initially treat their osteoporosis patients with a PTH agent; rather, they turn to PTH only after a bisphonate agent has failed. For that discussion, the reader is referred to Abstract 7–3.

M. H. Pillinger, MD

Comparison of a Single Infusion of Zoledronic Acid With Risedronate for Paget's Disease

Reid IR, Miller P, Lyles K, et al (Univ of Auckland, New Zealand; Colorado Ctr for Bone Research, Lakewood; Duke Univ, Durham, NC; et al)

N Engl J Med 353:898-908, 2005 59–5

Background.—The advent of bisphosphonates advanced therapy for Paget's disease, but more effective and convenient agents are needed to increase adherence. Zoledronic acid, a bisphosphonate administered as a single intravenous infusion, might meet these needs.

Methods.—In two identical, randomized, double-blind, actively controlled trials of 6 months' duration, we compared one 15-minute infusion of 5 mg of zoledronic acid with 60 days of oral risedronate (30 mg per day). The primary efficacy end point was the rate of therapeutic response at six months, defined as a normalization of alkaline phosphatase levels or a reduction of at least 75 percent in the total alkaline phosphatase excess. The results of the studies were pooled.

Results.—At six months, 96.0 percent of patients receiving zoledronic acid had a therapeutic response (169 of 176), as compared with 74.3 percent of patients receiving risedronate (127 of 171, $P<0.001$). Alkaline phosphatase levels normalized in 88.6 percent of patients in the zoledronic acid group and 57.9 percent of patients in the risedronate group (P<0.001) (Fig 2). Zoledronic acid was associated with a shorter median time to a first therapeutic response (64 vs. 89 days, P<0.001). Higher response rates in the

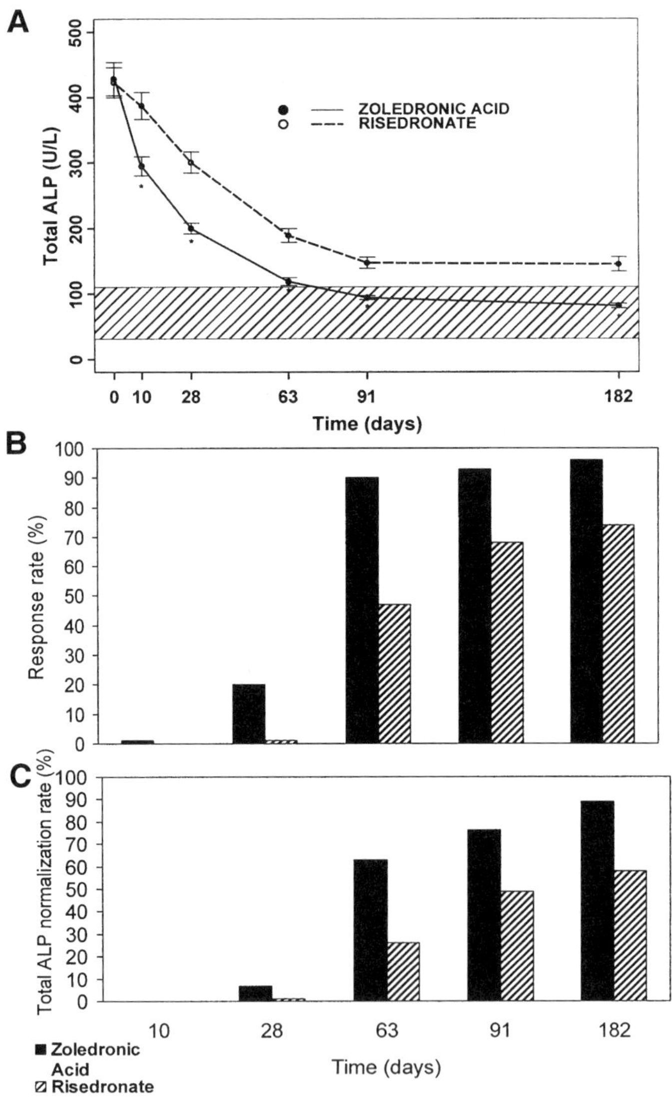

FIGURE 2.—Mean (±SE) levels of serum alkaline phosphatase (Panel A) and percentage of patients with a therapeutic response (Panel B) or normalization of alkaline phosphatase levels (Panel C). The shaded area in Panel A represents the normal range of serum alkaline phosphatase (32 to 110 U per liter) in premenopausal women. (Reprinted by permission of *The New England Journal of Medicine* from Reid IR, Miller P, Lyles K, et al: Comparison of a single infusion of zoledronic acid with risedronate for Paget's disease. *N Engl J Med* 353:898-908, 2005. Copyright 2005, Massachusetts Medical Society. All rights reserved.)

zoledronic acid group were consistent across all demographic, disease-severity, and treatment-history subgroups and with changes in other bone-turnover markers. The physical-component summary score of the Medical Outcomes Study 36-item Short-Form General Health Survey, a measure of the quality of life, increased significantly from baseline at both three and six months in the zoledronic acid group and differed significantly from those in the risedronate group at three months. Pain scores improved in both groups. During post-trial follow-up (median, 190 days), 21 of 82 patients in the risedronate group had a loss of therapeutic response, as compared with 1 of 113 patients in the zoledronic acid group (P<0.001).

Conclusions.—A single infusion of zoledronic acid produces more rapid, more complete, and more sustained responses in Paget's disease than does daily treatment with risedronate.

► Patients with Paget's disease of bone are typically treated with oral bisphosphonates such as alendronate, risedronate, or tiludronate because of their effective suppression of high bone turnover associated with the disease. Regimens involving these agents require high daily oral doses of medication for 6, 2, or 3 months, respectively, and lack of compliance because of side effects or duration of therapy is of concern. More potent agents given less frequently might be as effective at suppressing bone turnover, and more convenient for patients.

In this study, the investigators compared 2 identical, double-blind, actively controlled trials of 6-month duration. In the first study, zoledronic acid 5 mg was infused once over 15 minutes, while in the second study risedronate 30 mg/d was given for 60 days. The primary efficacy end point was rate of therapeutic response at 6 months, defined as normalization of alkaline phosphatase levels or a reduction of at least 75% in the total alkaline phosphatase excess. The study showed that a single infusion of IV zoledronic acid was more effective than daily risedronate for 2 months. Ninety-six percent of patients receiving IV zoledronic acid had a therapeutic response at 6 months, whereas only 74.3% of patients taking oral risedronate had this response, and 88% of patients normalized their alkaline phosphatase levels after zoledronic acid infusion at 6 months, whereas only 57.9% did so after receiving 2 months of oral risedronate. Zoledronic acid caused first therapeutic response at a shorter median interval of 64 days, while risedronate required a median of 89 days.

After completion of the 2 studies, patients were followed for a median of 190 days to determine rate of loss of therapeutic response. Over this interval, 21 of 82 patients receiving risedronate lost their therapeutic response, whereas only 1 of 113 patients receiving IV zoledronic acid lost the response.

This study suggests that IV zoledronic acid may be an effective and long-lasting therapeutic agent for the treatment of Paget's disease. Longer term studies of the effects of zoledronic acid on Paget's disease of bone, as well as renal function and jaw bone health, are underway to assess the safety of this drug.

B. L. Clarke, MD

60 Pituitary

Transsphenoidal Microsurgery for Cushing's Disease: Initial Outcome and Long-term Results

Hammer GD, Tyrrell JB, Lamborn KR, et al (Univ of Michigan, Ann Arbor; Univ of California, San Francisco; Univ of Texas, Dallas; et al)

J Clin Endocrinol Metab 89:6348-6357, 2004 60–1

Introduction.—Untreated Cushing's disease and the resultant chronically elevated glucocorticoid levels lead to severe metabolic disturbances, including diabetes mellitus, obesity, hypertension, muscle wasting, and osteoporosis. Although transsphenoidal resection has become the standard of care for Cushing's disease with high initial success rates, little information is available on the long-term morbidity and mortality of patients in remission compared with patients with recurrent or persistent Cushing's disease after such treatment. We therefore conducted a retrospective study of 289 patients with Cushing's disease who underwent transsphenoidal microsurgery for an ACTH-secreting adenoma at a tertiary care center exclusively by one surgeon (C.B.W.). Postoperative remission was achieved in 82% (n = 236) of patients, with best initial remission rates observed in patients with grade I (86%) and II (83%) or stage 0 (88%), A (94%), and B (100%) tumors. Male gender, larger tumor size, and higher stage predicted poorer initial outcome. Long-term follow-up was obtained on 178 patients, with a median follow-up time of 11.1 yr (range, 0.6–24.1 yr). Thirteen of 150 (9%) of patients in initial remission developed recurrent disease, and 12 patients underwent additional treatment. At last follow-up, only two of these patients had active disease. However, of the 28 patients with initial persistent disease who had follow-up greater than 6 months, 10 patients continued to have active disease at last follow-up. Although overall survival rates in patients with initial remission did not differ significantly from expected compared with the general population based on age and sex distribution, patients with initial persistent disease had a significant increase in mortality compared with the expected mortality. Thus, successful treatment of Cushing's disease is associated with normal long-term survival. These results suggest that patients with persistent Cushing's disease require early and aggressive intervention to attempt to prevent this excess mortality.

► This is yet another update, and perhaps the final one, of the very large surgical series of Dr Charles Wilson at the University of California, San Francisco.

He had an initial surgical remission rate of 82% for patients with intrasellar adenomas (88% for microadenomas). The recurrence rate for those who appeared to be in remission initially was 9%, with a median follow-up of 11.1 years. The median time to recurrence was 4.9 years, so patients need to be followed up carefully for many years for this possibility. Their patients who achieved an initial remission had a long-term mortality rate that was normal, but those who had persistent disease after surgery had an increased mortality rate.

Mancini et al[1] show us why there is such a high mortality rate in patients with Cushing's syndrome by looking at the prevalence of the various components of the metabolic syndrome in such patients. Of the 49 patients with Cushing's syndrome they evaluated, 85% had hypertension, 47% had diabetes, 41% were obese, and 38% had dyslipidemias. The fasting glucose level was the only parameter that correlated with cortisol levels. Clearly, good clinical practice would be to control these cardiovascular risk factors in addition to controlling the Cushing's syndrome.

In a very interesting study, Heald et al[2] report on quality of life scores in patients with Cushing's disease even after the patients had been cured, finding a persistently impaired psychological well-being and psychosocial functioning. These authors postulate that the hypercortisolemia might have long-term adverse effects as a result of the irreversible changes in central nervous system function.

M. E. Molitch, MD

References

1. Mancini T, Kola B, Mantero F, et al: High cardiovascular risk in patients with Cushing's syndrome according to 1999 WHO/ISH guidelines. *Clin Endocrinol* 61:768-777, 2004.
2. Heald AH, Ghosh S, Bray S, et al: Long-term negative impact on quality of life in patients with successfully treated Cushing's disease. *Clin Endocrinol* 61:458-465, 2005.

Anterior Pituitary Dysfunction in Survivors of Traumatic Brain Injury

Agha A, Rogers B, Sherlock M, et al (Beaumont Hosp, Dublin)

J Clin Endocrinol Metab 89:4929-4936, 2004 60–2

Introduction.—Recent data suggest that anterior pituitary dysfunction after traumatic brain injury (TBI) is common. We sought to confirm the results of earlier studies in a larger cohort of patients with dynamic testing of pituitary function. We studied 102 consecutive TBI survivors (85 males; median age 28, range 15-65 yr) who had survived severe or moderate TBI (initial Glasgow Coma Scale score 3–13) at a median of 17 months (range 6–36) post event. GH and ACTH reserves were initially assessed using the glucagon stimulation test (GST). Normative data on GH and cortisol responses to the GST were obtained from 31 matched healthy controls. Patients with subnormal GH or cortisol responses were further evaluated, using the insulin tolerance test (ITT) or arginine + GHRH test for GH assessment and the ITT or 250-μg short synacthen test for the assessment of ACTH reserve. Patients were considered to be GH or ACTH deficient if they failed both the GST and the second provocative test. Baseline thyroid function, prolactin, IGF-I, gonadotropins, testosterone, or estradiol was performed in all patients and compared with local reference ranges. In controls, normal response to the GST was a stimulated GH peak of greater than 5 μg/liter and cortisol peak greater than 450 nmol/liter (16 μg/dl). Eighteen TBI patients (17.6%) had GH response to the GST less than 5 μg/liter, 11 of whom also failed the ITT or the arginine + GHRH tests. GH-deficient patients had significantly higher body mass index ($P = 0.003$), and lower IGF-I concentrations ($P < 0.001$), than GH-sufficient patients. Twenty-three patients (22.5%) had cortisol responses to GST less than 450 nmol/liter, 13 of whom also failed the ITT or short synacthen test. GH or ACTH deficiencies were not related to age, Glasgow Coma Scale score, or the presence of other pituitary hormone abnormalities ($P > 0.05$). Twelve patients (11.8%) had gonadotropin and one (1%) had thyrotrophin deficiencies. Twelve patients (11.8%) had hyperprolactinemia. Twenty-nine patients (28.4%) had at least one anterior pituitary hormone deficiency. This is the largest study, to date, of hypopituitarism after TBI and confirms a high prevalence of undiagnosed anterior pituitary hormone abnormalities in survivors of TBI. Hypopituitarism is a treatable cause of morbidity after TBI. In addition to conventional pituitary hormone

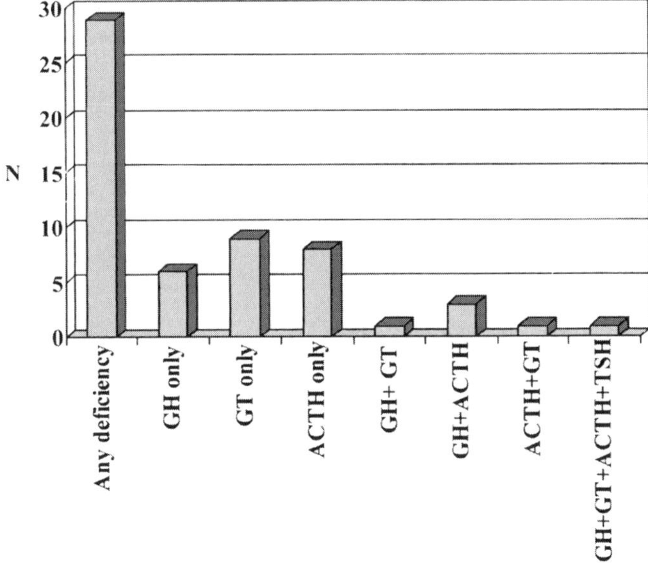

FIGURE 2.—The frequency and pattern of different anterior pituitary hormone deficiency in 102 patients with severe or moderate TBI. GT, Gonadotropins. (Courtesy of Agha A, Rogers B, Sherlock M, et al: Anterior pituitary dysfunction in survivors of traumatic brain injury. *J Clin Endocrinol Metab* 89:4929-4936, 2004. Copyright 2004 The Endocrine Society.)

replacement, the potential of GH treatment to enhance recovery needs to be examined in a prospective study (Fig 2).

► This is a late assessment, that is, a mean of 17 months after the TBI, of pituitary hormone deficiencies in this patient population, and more than 25% had at least 1 hormonal axis deficiency. The tests used to make these assessments leave a little to be desired, and I suspect that this may be an underestimate. On the other hand, Leal-Cerro et al[1] also found that 24.7% of their subjects studied some years after the injury also had at least 1 hormonal axis that was deficient. These are nice data, but I worry about what is happening earlier in the course of these patients. Are they deficient immediately after the injury? Apparently patients with TBI no longer receive high-dose steroids any more.[2] Therefore, those with deficits of their HPA axis are no longer automatically treated with steroids as part of the neurosurgical regimen. How many are acutely acetylcholine deficient? How many die from this? Is there an acute defect caused by brain edema, and so forth, that later resolves? Lots of unanswered questions.

Agha et al[3] also studied posterior pituitary function in this same cohort. Of these 102 patients, 22 had acute diabetes insipidus (DI) and 13 developed inappropriate vasopressin secretion with hyponatremia (all 13 had normal thyroid and adrenal function). They differentiated between inappropriate vasopressin secretion and cerebral salt wasting (1 case). In the later evaluation at 17 months, 7 had permanent DI, with 5 of these being persistent from the acute DI group and 2 developing DI several days later. Thus, 17 of the original patients with acute DI had resolution over time. Two patients had hyponatremia at the late testing, 1 from obstructive hydrocephalus and 1 from the use of citalopram.

M. E. Molitch, MD

References

1. Leal-Cerro A, Flores JM, Rincon M, et al: Prevalence of hypopituitarism and growth hormone deficiency in adults long-term after severe traumatic brain injury. *Clin Endocrinol* 62:525-532, 2005.
2. Roberts I, for the CRASH Trial collaborators: Effect of intravenous corticosteroids on death within 14 days in 10008 adults with clinically significant head injury (MRC CRASH trial): Randomized placebo-controlled trial. *Lancet* 364:1321-1328, 2004.
3. Agha A, Thornton E, O'Kelly P, et al: Posterior pituitary dysfunction after traumatic brain injury. *J Clin Endocrinol Metab* 89:5987-5992, 2004.

Prevalence of Pituitary Deficiency in Patients After Aneurysmal Subarachnoid Hemorrhage

Kreitschmann-Andermahr I, Hoff C, Saller B, et al (Univ Hosp Aachen, Germany; Pfizer GmbH, Karlsruhe, Germany)

J Clin Endocrinol Metab 89:4986-4992, 2004 60–3

Introduction.—After aneurysmal subarachnoid hemorrhage (SAH), patients frequently present with persistent bodily, psychosocial, and cognitive impairments that resemble those of patients with untreated partial or complete pituitary insufficiency. Because of these similarities, the authors hypothesized that aneurysmal SAH may cause pituitary dysfunction. Pituitary function testing was performed in 40 aneurysmal SAH patients between 12 and 72 months after the SAH (Fig 1). A combined TRH-LHRH-arginine test and the insulin tolerance test were performed on two separate days. Only 18 of 40 (45%) of the tested patients had normal pituitary function. Five of 40 exhibited isolated severe GH deficiency (GHD), and an additional three of 40 had severe GHD plus corticotroph deficiency. Isolated corticotroph deficiency was seen in 13 of 40 patients, and one patient showed isolated thyrotroph deficiency. All but one patient with corticotroph insufficiency were female. Patients with severe GHD had gained significantly more weight since their SAH than patients without GHD and exhibited a significantly higher body mass index. None of the clinical parameters indicative of a poor neurological outcome in aneurysmal SAH were related to pituitary insufficiency. In summary, neuroendocrine dysfunction was identified in a substantial portion of patients with previous aneurysmal SAH and should be borne in mind as a potential long-term sequel of the illness.

► Here we have the same thing as with traumatic brain injury. With SAH, 55% of the 40 survivors had normal pituitary function between 1 and 6 years after the bleed. An amazing 16 of 40 had ACTH deficiency and in 13 this was isolated! The authors used an insulin tolerance test for testing and the data look very solid. In a similar evaluation, Dimopoulou et al[1] evaluated 30 patients be-

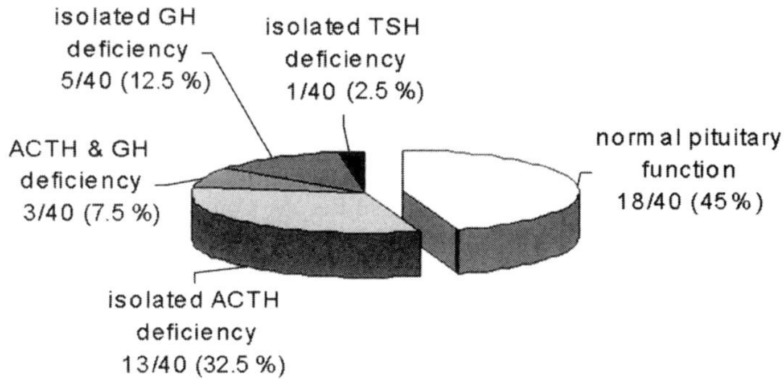

FIGURE 1.—Prevalence of disturbed pituitary function in patients after aneurismal SAH. (Courtesy of Kreitschmann-Andermahr I, Hoff C, Saller B, et al: Prevalence of pituitary deficiency in patients after aneurysmal subarachnoid hemorrhage. *J Clin Endocrinol Metab* 89:4986-4992, 2004. Copyright The Endocrine Society.)

tween 1 and 2 years after SAH. In this article, 47% had some defect but only 10% had ACTH deficiency using the 1 µg $ACTH_{1-24}$ stimulation test.

So, again, these were the survivors. What about those who died in hospital immediately after the hemorrhage? What proportion of those were ACTH deficient? Did that contribute to their demise? For both traumatic brain injury and SAH these are important questions for a young investigator to answer.

M. E. Molitch, MD

Reference

1. Dimopoulou I, Kouyialis AT, Tzanella M, et al: High incidence of neuroendocrine dysfunction in long-term survivors of aneurysmal subarachnoid hemorrhage. *Stroke* 35:2884-2889, 2004.

Acute Management of Pituitary Apoplexy: Surgery or Conservative Management?

Ayuk J, McGregor EJ, Mitchell RD, et al (Queen Elizabeth Hosp, Birmingham, England)

Clin Endocrinol (Oxf) 61:747-752, 2004 60–4

Background.—Pituitary apoplexy is a rare condition that presents with a constellation of acute clinical features, including headache, visual deficits, ophthalmoplegia, and altered mental status resulting from sudden hemorrhage or infarction of a pituitary adenoma. Because pituitary apoplexy is rarely seen, there are no evidence-based standards of optimum care for these patients. The most controversial aspect of management is the role of acute neurosurgical intervention. In recent years, these authors have adopted a conservative approach toward patients with pituitary apoplexy. Whether this less interventional approach affects the long-term clinical outcome in these patients was determined.

Methods.—A retrospective analysis was conducted to evaluate clinical presentation, management, and clinical outcome in patients who were seen acutely with pituitary apoplexy from 1994 to 2004. Data from 33 patients (13 women, 20 men) were included. The patients had a mean age of 52 years. The mean duration of follow-up was 3.7 years.

Results.—The most common presenting symptoms were headache (97%), visual deficits (82%), and nausea/vomiting (78%). Transsphenoidal surgery was performed in 15 patients (46%), and 18 were managed conservatively. Among the indications for surgery were deteriorating visual deficit (13 patients), hemiparesis (1 patient), and altered level of consciousness (1 patient). Of the patients managed neurosurgically, 87% required long-term glucocorticoid replacement, and 60% required long-term thyroid hormone replacement. Among the conservatively managed patients, glucocorticoid replacement was required in 72% of patients, and thyroid hormone replacement was required in 72% of patients. Sex steroid replacement was required in 67% of patients managed neurosurgically and in 83% of patients managed conservatively (Fig 1). At latest follow-up, 1 patient in the conserva-

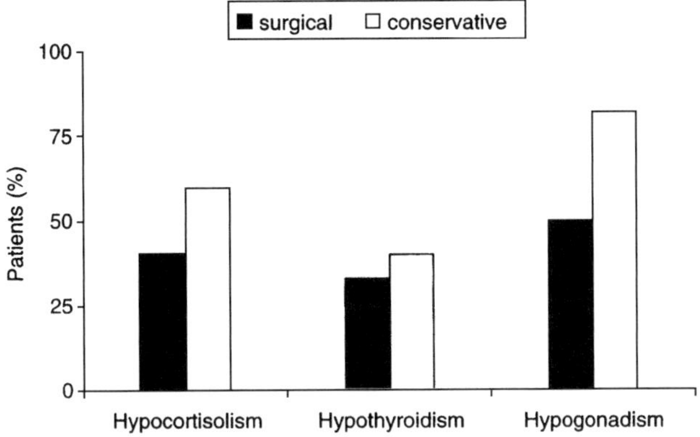

FIGURE 1.—Proportion of patients with hypocortisolism, hypothyroidism and hypogonadism at presentation in the surgically and conservatively managed groups (P = NS). (Courtesy of Ayuk J, McGregor EJ, Mitchell RD, et al: Acute management of pituitary apoplexy: Surgery or conservative management? *Clin Endocrinol (Oxf)* 61:747-752, 2004. Reprinted by permission of Blackwell Publishing.)

tively managed group had required surgery, and 1 patient in the surgically managed group had received pituitary radiotherapy. In both patients, the additional procedures were performed in response to evidence of tumor regrowth on MRI studies.

Conclusions.—Patients with pituitary apoplexy in whom visual deficits are stable or improving may be managed expectantly because there is no identifiable adverse effect on visual or endocrine outcome. Long-term follow-up is important in patients with pituitary apoplexy.

▶ This is a nice retrospective analysis of 33 patients with pituitary apoplexy. I think a few lessons can be learned from this analysis. First, patients who do not have progressive neurologic symptoms but may have ocular symptoms do okay with conservative management, with resolution of their ocular symptoms, but most end up with hypopituitarism. Second, most but not all with progressive neurologic symptoms have resolution of these symptoms, but again, most end up with hypopituitarism. Third, since most patients treated conservatively end up with hypopituitarism anyway, perhaps we endocrinologists should not be so hesitant in sending patients for decompression. This last point, of course, is heavily dependent on having a good neurosurgeon. Fourth, in only 1 patient in each group was there tumor regrowth at follow-up (mean, 3.7 years), so there is no need to resect the tumor remnant, and just MRI follow-up is necessary. This would go against the approach taken by Imboden et al,[1] who decided to remove the remnant tumor in 7 of 8 of their patients 3 to 9 days after the onset of symptoms for symptom relief (headaches primarily). Six of these 7 surgical patients had hypopituitarism on follow-up.

Zayour et al[2] provide an explanation for the hypopituitarism that occurs with apoplexy, finding that intrasellar pressure was very high in all 13 of their patients with apoplexy at the time of surgical decompression. In their series, failure to recover pituitary function correlated with the highest pressures and concomitantly the lowest serum PRL levels, indicating ischemic necrosis of normal pituitary cells. Those patients with normal to elevated PRL levels had return of normal function, indicating the presence of viable pituitary cells.

One of the things we think about with pituitary apoplexy is Sheehan syndrome. Does this still happen much in current practice? Feinberg et al[3] performed a retrospective analysis of 100 patients who had had obstetric hemorrhage, defined as an estimated blood loss of greater than 1000 mL and one of the following: a hemoglobin level less than 7 g/dL, a blood transfusion, a greater than 30% drop in postpartum hematocrit, sustained hypotension secondary to blood loss, or a hysterectomy for intractable bleeding. There were 100 matched controls. Of these 200 patients, 109 responded to a questionnaire asking about symptoms of menstrual dysfunction, lactation difficulty, cold intolerance, fatigue, axillary or pubic hair loss, and infertility, and those with 2 or more symptoms were assessed hormonally. Fourteen of the 55 patients with hemorrhage had 2 or more symptoms, and 8 of the 14 who were tested were normal. Thus, of at least 55 patients with severe obstetric hemorrhage, none had Sheehan syndrome.

M. E. Molitch, MD

References

1. Elasser Imboden PN, de Tribolet N, Lobrinus A, et al: Apoplexy in pituitary macroadenoma. Eight patients presenting in 12 months. *Medicine* 84:188-196, 2005.
2. Zayour DH, Selman WR, Arafah BM: Extreme elevation of intrasellar pressure in patients with pituitary tumor apoplexy: Relation to pituitary function. *J Clin Endocrinol Metab* 89:5649-5654, 2004.
3. Feinberg EC, Molitch ME, Endres LK, et al: The incidence of Sheehan's syndrome after obstetric hemorrhage. *Fertil Steril* 84:975-979, 2005.

Hyponatremia Among Runners in the Boston Marathon

Almond CSD, Shin AY, Fortescue EB, et al (Children's Hosp, Boston; Harvard Med School, Boston; Harvard School of Public Health, Boston)
N Engl J Med 352:1550-1556, 2005 60–5

Background.—The incidence of hyponatremia among marathon runners is unknown, but concerns about this condition have increased with the surge in popularity of marathon running. The death of a 28-year-old woman after her participation in the 2002 Boston Marathon highlighted the seriousness of this illness. The cause of hyponatremia is thought to be excessive fluid intake; however, other risk factors also have been suggested, including the composition of fluids consumed, relatively low body mass index, long racing time, lack of marathon experience, the use of nonsteroidal anti-inflammatory drugs, and female sex. The incidence of hyponatremia among marathon runners was estimated, and the major risk factors involved were identified.

Methods.—Participants in the 2002 Boston Marathon were recruited 1 or 2 days before the race. The study participants were asked to complete a survey regarding demographic information and training history. A blood sample was obtained from each study runner after the race, and each runner completed a questionnaire about their fluid consumption and urine output during the race. Prerace and postrace weights were recorded. Multivariate regression analyses were performed to identify risk factors associated with hyponatremia.

Results.—Of the 766 runners enrolled, 488 runners (64%) provided a usable blood sample after the race. Hyponatremia was present in 13% of the study runners, with 0.6% having critical hyponatremia. Univariate analyses showed that hyponatremia was associated with significant weight gain, consumption of more than 3 L of fluid during the race, a racing time greater than 4 hours, female sex, and low body mass index. On multivariate analysis, hyponatremia was associated with weight gain, a racing time greater than 4 hours, and body mass index extremes.

Conclusions.—A significant proportion of nonelite marathon runners develop hyponatremia, and in some cases the illness can be severe. Factors associated with the development of hyponatremia were considerable weight gain while running, a long racing time (>4 hours), and body mass index extremes.

► This one made the newspapers. So, 13% of the runners tested had serum sodium levels of 135 mEq/L or less, and 0.6% had levels of 120 mEq/L or less. The ones with hyponatremia ended up the race with a weight gain resulting from consumption of more than 3 L of fluids during the race with fluid intake every mile. It is interesting that nowhere in the article is vasopressin mentioned, and none of the authors were endocrinologists or nephrologists. There is no discussion of the physiology of what is going on. These runners were clearly losing salt and water in the form of sweat and then replacing the fluid loss with hypotonic fluids without regard to thirst. If this occurs very rapidly, they can become hyponatremic before their ability to suppress vasopressin allows them to excrete the excess water load. Thirst plays an important role in regulating osmolality, and if people drink hypotonic fluids in large amounts when they are not thirsty, they can get into trouble like this. The fact that these runners actually gained weight shows that they were drinking fluids just to drink fluids and not because they were thirsty. So, drinking 8-oz glasses of water 8 times per day is generally not good for you, and you should just drink when thirsty.

M. E. Molitch, MD

61 Adrenal Disorders

Dexamethasone Infusion Testing in the Diagnosis of Cushing's Syndrome

Tran HA, Petrovsky N (John Hunter Hosp, New South Wales, Australia; Australian Natl Univ, Woden, Australian Capital Territory, Australia)

Endocr J 52:103-109, 2005 61–1

Introduction.—Cushing's syndrome and its various aetiologies is a markedly difficult diagnosis to make given its subtle signs, sometime cyclical nature, and the lack of a single definitive diagnostic test. Although a great variety of diagnostic tests have been developed to assist in the diagnosis, even with the best clinical acumen, biochemistry and medical imaging the diagnosis can remain elusive. The long low and high dose oral dexamethasone suppression test is cumbersome, costly and often requiring an extended inpatient stay. The utility of the dexamethasone suppression test would be greatly enhanced if it could be performed as a short outpatient procedure. In this study we sought to confirm and refine the clinical utility of the high dose 4 mg intravenous dexamethasone suppression test as an alternative diagnostic test for Cushing's syndrome. There were a total of 31 subjects: 8 patients with proven pituitary Cushing's disease, 3 with primary adrenal tumors, 10 with pseudo-Cushing's syndrome and 10 healthy controls. All subjects with pseudo-Cushing's syndrome suppress serum cortisol at +5 and at +24 hours. In subjects with pituitary Cushing's disease, 7 out of 8 (88%) had serum cortisol suppressed at +5 hours but rebounded at +24 hours to at least 70% of the original serum level. Primary adrenal tumors showed a pattern of non-suppression throughout. The 4 mg intravenous dexamethasone suppression test is excellent in ruling out pseudo-Cushing's syndrome. This test is much simpler and more convenient than the *oral* dexamethasone suppression test in confirming clinical suspicion of pituitary Cushing's disease.

Salivary Cortisol Measurement—A Reliable Method for the Diagnosis of Cushing's Syndrome

Trilck M, Flitsch J, Lüdecke DK, et al (Univ Hosp Hamburg-Eppendorf, Germany; Univ Hosp Essen, Germany)

Exp Clin Endocrinol Diabetes 113:225-230, 2005 61–2

Introduction.—The measurement of cortisol in saliva is becoming more widely accepted as a screening test for the diagnosis of hypercortisolism. Since 1986, cortisol measurement in saliva has been continuously used in our department. In this study we compared salivary cortisol profiles from proven Cushing's disease patients with profiles from healthy subjects and obese children. The purpose was to evaluate the predictive value of the method for the diagnosis of hypercortisolism and to define cut-off levels to exclude or identify hypercortisolism. Cortisol in saliva was measured in 150 Cushing's disease patients (30 children, 120 adults, ranging from age 4 – 70), 100 healthy subjects (55 children, 45 adults, ranging from age 6 – 60), and 31 children (age 7 – 15) with an age-related body-mass-index above the 90th percentile. Generally, five saliva samples were taken over the day at 6:00 – 8:00 a.m., 11:00 – 12:00 a.m., 4:00 – 6:00 p.m., 7:00 – 8:00 p.m., and 10:00 p.m. The samples were measured using a radioimmuno-assay (INCSTAR Corporation, Stillwater, Minnesota, USA). For healthy subjects, morning levels of cortisol in saliva between 3-19 µg/l were found. These levels dropped to levels in between <1 – 11 µg/l at 11:00 – 12:00 a.m., <1 – 6 µg/l at 4:00 – 6:00 p.m., <1 – 4.5 µg/l at 7:00 – 8:00 p.m., and <1 – 2.9 µg/l at 10:00 p.m. The measured values showed a correlation with age, height, and weight. In Cushing's disease patients, the circadian salivary cortisol rhythm was missing, compared to healthy subjects. There was no significant difference in salivary cortisol levels or circadian rhythm between healthy or obese children. We found a high sensitivity for the detection of hypercortisolism at the 10:00 p.m. salivary cortisol measurement. The following, age dependent cut-off levels for salivary cortisol at 10:00 p.m. were calculated for the exclusion of hypercortisolism. Age 6 – 10: 1.0 µg/l (specificity 100%, sensitivity 87.5%); age 11 – 15: 1.7 µg/l (specificity 100%, sensitivity 100%); age 16-20: 1.6 µg/l (specificity 100%, sensitivity 76.2%); age 21 – 60: 1.6 µg/l (specificity 100%, sensitivity 90.9%). For the proof of Cushing's syndrome, the following age-dependent cut-off levels at 10:00 p.m. were found: age 6 – 10: 1.9 µg/l (specificity 100%, sensitivity 80%); age 11 – 15: 1.7 µg/l (specificity 100%, sensitivity 100%); age 16 – 20: 2.5 µg/l (specificity 100%, sensitivity 84.2%); age 21 – 60: 1.9 µg/l (specificity 100%, sensitivity 97.6%). The cortisol assessment in saliva is a sensitive and reliable method to discriminate normocortisolemic from hypercortisolemic patients. From our view, the major advantages of this method are the reliability, non-invasiveness, and use in ambulatory patients.

▶ MRI using T1-weighted spin echo with gadolinium contrast has been a standard imaging technique for diagnosing pituitary microadenomas in patients with Cushing's disease. However, up to 50% false-negative studies have been reported with this technique among these patients, and the success may be even lower in the pediatric age population because of smaller tumors and differences in histologic characteristics. To confirm the pituitary origin of the ACTH excess before transsphenoidal surgery, petrosal sinus sampling has been necessary in those cases. Batista et al[1] report that SPGR is a superior variant of MRI for this diagnosis. In a group of 30 children and adolescents studied at the NIH, they compared SPGR-MRI with the standard technique. SPGR-MRI doubled the number of positive diagnoses, especially among microadenomas. Although better, SPGR-MRI only diagnoses 64% of patients, leaving a significant number dependent on other diagnostic methods such as petrosal sinus sampling. Given that the success of surgery depends on the ability to localize the lesion preoperatively, it is clear that further refinements in detection methodology are needed to optimally treat children and adolescents with Cushing's disease.

Cushing's syndrome secondary to pigmented primary nodular adrenocortical hyperplasia (PPNAH) has been well described in adults as a manifestation of Carney complex. Inactivating germline mutations of the regulatory subunit type 1 of protein kinase A (PRKAR1A) have been reported in 40% to 50% of families with this complex. The genetic abnormality causing Carney's complex can be detected in children of affected families, but not many of the reported cases of Cushing's with PPNAH have been reported in this age group. Storr et al[2] report on 6 adolescent patients with this condition. Clinically they presented, like the adults, with ACTH-independent adrenocortical hyperfunction and the medical and surgical management did not differ. The important message is the need to monitor, with appropriate testing, children from families with Carney's complex, especially those who carry the mutation.

The diagnosis of Cushing's syndrome and specifically its etiology may require elaborate testing. Many tests have been validated with high sensitivity and specificity, but the differential diagnosis between Cushing's and pseudo-Cushing's remains problematic. Patients with pseudo-Cushing's exhibit symptoms that overlap with those of true Cushing's syndrome, including depression and obesity, and have elevated urinary free cortisol and borderline overnight dexamethasone suppression. Tran and Petrovsky (Abstract 61–1) have reworked the IV 4 mg dexamethasone suppression test and show very good separation between the response of patients with pituitary Cushing's and those with pseudo-Cushing's who have a normal response. These patients, like normal control subjects, maintain suppression of cortisol levels at 24 hours after the IV infusion of dexamethasone. In contrast, all other types of Cushing's show escape from suppression.

Another test with high sensitivity and specificity is salivary cortisol, especially when measured at 22:00 hours, to assess circadian rhythm. Trilck et al (Abstract 61–2) have standardized cutoff levels according to age. As has been pointed out by others, advantages of salivary cortisol are reliability, noninvasiveness, and use in ambulatory patients.

D. E. Schteingart, MD

References

1. Batista D, Courkoutsakis NA, Oldfield EH, et al: Detection of adrenocorticotropin-secreting pituitary adenomas by magnetic resonance imaging in children and adolescents with Cushing disease. *J Clin Endocrinol Metab* 90:5134-5140, 2005. (2006 YEAR BOOK OF ENDOCRINOLOGY, p 365.)
2. Storr HL, Mitchell H, Swords FM, et al: Clinical features, diagnosis, treatment and molecular studies in paediatric Cushing's syndrome due to primary nodular adrenocortical hyperplasia. *Clin Endocrinol (Oxf)* 61:553-559, 2004. (2006 YEAR BOOK OF ENDOCRINOLOGY, p 363.)

Clinical Review: The Strategy of Immediate Reoperation for Transsphenoidal Surgery for Cushing's Disease

Locatelli M, Vance ML, Laws ER (Ospedale Maggiore Policlinico, Milan, Italy; Univ of Virginia, Charlottesville)

J Clin Endocrinol Metab 90:5478-5482, 2005 61–3

Context.—Transsphenoidal surgery is currently the primary therapeutic option for Cushing's disease. Despite considerable initial success, 10-30% of patients fail to achieve lasting remission.

Evidence Acquisition.—We evaluated a strategy of immediate reoperation in surgical failures judged by plasma cortisol levels that did not fall to 2 µg/dl or less within 72 h of surgery. Of 215 patients with presumed ACTH microadenomas, treated between 1993 and 2004, 12 met inclusion criteria and had prompt (within 15 d) reoperation for residual or missed ACTH microadenoma. These 12 patients represent 28% of those who did not have evidence of postoperative adrenal insufficiency.

Evidence Synthesis.—Based on an outcome measure of sustained subnormal or normal plasma cortisol levels, eight of 12 patients (67%) achieved remission from the two operations. Adjunctive therapies (radiotherapy, gamma knife radiosurgery, and adrenalectomy) led to remission in another three patients. It is recognized that this outcome required either total hypophysectomy (one patient) or postoperative hypopituitarism (all patients in remission).

Conclusion.—Magnetic resonance imaging was not usually helpful in determining therapeutic strategies; however, inferior petrosal sinus sampling was critical in providing confidence that the disease was of pituitary origin. A treatment algorithm is recommended, based on this study.

Characteristics of Recovery of Adrenocortical Function After Treatment for Cushing's Syndrome Due to Pituitary or Adrenal Adenomas

Klose M, Jørgensen K, Kristensen LØ (Herlev Univ Hosp, Denmark)

Clin Endocrinol (Oxf) 61:394-399, 2004 61–4

Objective.—Surgical cure of Cushing's syndrome (CS) is followed by adrenocortical insufficiency, which may be long-lasting. The aim was to elucidate recovery of adrenocortical function, defined as a normal cortisol response to ACTH stimulation, and the relation to ACTH in patients cured for CS due to pituitary Cushing's disease (CD) or adrenal (AA) adenomas.

Design.—A retrospective study including 32 patients considered surgically cured for CS (18 CD, 14 AA).

Results.—Twelve (67%) patients with CD recovered within median 24 months (range 7 months–4½ years) whereas six did not recover within 3-12 years. Plasma ACTH (p-ACTH) at time of recovery was not different from p-ACTH in patients not recovering ($P = 0.9$). Eleven (79%) patients with AA recovered within 24 months (10 months–4 years) whereas three did not recover within 4–10 years. p-ACTH at time of recovery was higher compared to patients not recovering ($P < 0.04$). No differences were observed comparing CD and AA patients concerning preoperative 24-h urinary free cortisol (UFC) excretion, postoperative unstimulated s-cortisol or recovery time. By contrast, p-ACTH measured at time of recovery was higher in AA compared to CD (median 12.3 *vs.* 4.6 pmol/l) ($P < 0.001$), whereas plasma dehydroepiandrosterone sulfate (p-DHEAS) was lower in AA compared to CD (median 300 *vs.* 1500 nmol/l) ($P = 0.02$).

Conclusion.—Recovery of secondary adrenal insufficiency is a slow process in both CD and AA. ACTH measured at time of recovery was significantly higher and DHEAS significantly lower in patients with AA compared to CD, which may suggest different mechanisms of the recovery process and different set points in the glucocorticoid feedback inhibition of ACTH secretion.

Results and Long-term Follow-up After Unilateral Adrenalectomy for ACTH-Independent Hypercortisolism in a Series of Fifty Patients

Iacobone M, Mantero F, Basso SM, et al (Univ of Padua, Italy)
J Endocrinol Invest 28:327-332, 2005 61–5

Introduction.—Untreated hypercortisolism is a fatal state, causing functional disability. Even after successful treatment, clinical recovery is slower than the biochemical one, but data about clinical results, well-being and working capacity after surgery are scarce. This retrospective study aimed at evaluating the long-term outcome of patients after adrenalectomy for ACTH-independent hypercortisolism by the analysis of the clinical results, the survival and the subjective well-being status after surgery. Clinical data in 50 patients suffering from ACTH-independent hypercortisolism and treated between 1980 and 2000 by unilateral adrenalectomy were recorded. At a mean follow-up of 134 months, 3 patients were dead. All the surviving patients were asked to self estimate the physical and psychological recovery after surgery. After surgery, 100% of patients were biochemically cured. A clinical recovery was observed in most cases: obesity in 59.6% and hypertension in 57.5%. Bone mass density (BMD) significantly improved (+20%). The long-term mortality rate did not differ from normal population. Subjectively, a full recovery was confirmed by 95.6% of the surviving patients; it was correlated with the subjective feeling of physical recovery (95.6%) and regained working ability (93.3%). Despite of biochemical and clinical cure, no subjective improvement of the psychological conditions was observed in 26.7% of cases. At long-term follow-up, most objective symptoms of Cushing's syndrome (CS) disappear; subjective health and working ability are often regained, but a psychological impairment could persist in spite of a successful treatment.

Effects of Chronic Administration of PPAR-γ Ligand Rosiglitazone in Cushing's Disease

Ambrosi B, Dall' Asta C, Cannovò S, et al (Univ of Milan, Italy; Univ of Messina, Italy; Opsedale San Giuseppe-Fatebenefratelli, Milan, Italy)
Eur J Endocrinol 151:173-178, 2004 61–6

Objective.—Rosiglitazone, a thiazolidinedione compound with peroxisome proliferator-activated receptor-gamma (PPAR-γ)-binding affinity, is able to suppress adrenocorticotropic hormone (ACTH) secretion in treated mice and in AtT20 pituitary tumor cells. These observations suggested that thiazolidinediones may be effective as therapy for Cushing's disease (CD).

Patients and Methods.—Rosiglitazone (8 mg/day) was administered to 14 patients with active CD (13 women, one man, 18–68 years). Plasma ACTH, serum cortisol (F) and urinary free cortisol (UFC) levels were measured before and then monthly during rosiglitazone administration.

Results.—In six patients a reduction of ACTH and F levels and a normalization of UFC were observed 30–60 days after the beginning of rosiglitazone administration: there was a significant difference between basal and post-treatment values for UFC (1238±211 vs 154±40 nmol/24 h, $P < 0.03$), but not for ACTH (15.9±3.7 vs 7.9±0.9 pmol/l) and F levels (531±73 vs 344±58 nmol/l). Two of six cases, followed up for 7 months, showed a mild clinical improvement. Eight patients were nonresponders after 30–60 days of rosiglitazone treatment: their ACTH, F and UFC levels did not differ before and during drug administration. Immunohistochemical analysis of pituitary tumors removed from two responder and two nonresponder patients showed a similar intense immunoreactivity for PPAR-γ in about 50% of cells.

Conclusions.—The administration of rosiglitazone seems able to normalize cortisol secretion in some patients with CD, at least for short periods. Whether the activation of PPAR-γ by rosiglitazone might be effective as chronic pharmacologic treatment of CD needs a more extensive investigation through a randomized and controlled study.

Use of Radioguided Surgery With [^{111}In]-pentetreotide in the Management of an ACTH-Secreting Bronchial Carcinoid Causing Ectopic Cushing's Syndrome

Grossrubatscher E, Vignati F, Dalino P, et al (Surgery Niguarda Hosp, Milan, Italy; Busto Arsizio Hosp, Milan, Italy)

J Endocrinol Invest 28:72-78, 2005 61–7

Introduction.—Intraoperative [^{111}In]-pentetreotide scintigraphy with a hand-held gamma detector probe has recently been proposed to increase the intraoperative detection rate of small neuroendocrine tumors and their metastases. We report a case of a 28-yr-old woman with ectopic Cushing's syndrome due to an ACTH-secreting bronchial carcinoid, in whom the use of radioguided surgery improved disease management. At presentation, radiolabeled pentetreotide scintigraphy was the only procedure able to detect the ectopic source of ACTH. After radiologic confirmation, the patient underwent removal of a bronchial carcinoid, with disease persistence. After surgery, pentetreotide scintigraphy showed pathologic uptake in the mediastinum not previously detected at surgery and only subsequently confirmed by radiologic studies. Despite a second thoracic exploration, hormonal, scintigraphic, and radiological evidence of residual disease persisted. Radioguided surgery was then performed using a hand-held gamma probe 48 h after iv administration of a tracer dose of radiolabeled [^{111}In-DTPA-D-Phe1]-pentetreotide, which permitted detection and removal of multiple residual mediastinal lymph node metastases. Clinical and radiologic cure, with no evidence of tracer uptake at pentetreotide scintigraphy, was subsequently observed. The use of an intraoperative gamma counter appears a promising procedure in the management of metastatic ACTH-secreting bronchial carcinoids.

Cushing's Syndrome Due to Ectopic Corticotropin Secretion: Twenty Years' Experience at the National Institutes of Health

Ilias I, Torpy DJ, Pacak K, et al (NIH, Bethesda, Md)

J Clin Endocrinol Metab 90:4955-4962, 2005 61–8

Context.—Ectopic ACTH secretion (EAS) is difficult to diagnose and treat. We present our experience with EAS from 1983 to 2004.

Setting.—The study was performed at a tertiary care clinical research center.

Patients.—Ninety patients, aged 8–72 yr, including 48 females were included in the study.

Interventions and Outcome Measures.—Tests included 8 mg dexamethasone suppression, CRH stimulation, inferior petrosal sinus sampling (IPSS), computed tomography, octreotide scan, magnetic resonance imaging, and/or venous sampling. Therapies, pathological examinations, and survival were noted.

Results.—Eighty-six to 94% of patients did not respond to CRH or dexamethasone suppression, whereas 66 of 67 had negative IPSS. To control hypercortisolism, 62 patients received medical treatment, and 33 had bilateral adrenalectomy. Imaging localized tumors in 67 of 90 patients. Surgery confirmed an ACTH-secreting tumor in 59 of 66 patients and cured 65%. Nonthymic carcinoids took longest to localize. Deaths included three of 35 with pulmonary carcinoid, two of five with thymic carcinoid, four of six with gastrinoma, two of 13 with neuroendocrine tumor, two of two with medullary thyroid cancer, one of five with pheochromocytoma, three of three with small-cell lung cancer, and two of 17 with occult tumor. Patients with other carcinoids and esthesioneuroblastoma are alive.

Conclusions.—IPSS best identifies EAS. Initial failed localization is common and suggests pulmonary carcinoid. Although only 47% achieved cure, survival is good except in patients with small-cell lung cancer, medullary thyroid cancer, and gastrinoma.

► Several studies have addressed treatment of Cushing's disease. A hallmark of success with transsphenoidal surgery is immediate suppression of ACTH and cortisol to undetectable levels. In patients who do not show immediate response, recurrence is common and they eventually require repeat TSS, hypophysectomy, pituitary irradiation, medical adrenolytic therapy, or adrenalectomy. Locatelli et al (Abstract 61–3) report on the strategy of immediate reoperation (within 15 days of initial surgery) in 12 patients whose cortisol levels did not fall to less than 2 μg/dL within 72 hours of surgery. After the redo operation, 67% of the patients went into remission. An advantage of this approach is the ease of access to the pituitary while tissues are still healing. The disadvantage is a higher rate of complications, mainly CSF leak.

The other side of this coin is persistent adrenal insufficiency after surgical cure of Cushing's syndrome. Klose et al (Abstract 61–4) report that 67% of patients operated for either pituitary Cushing's or cortisol-secreting adrenal adenomas recover adrenal function within a median of 24 months. However, more than 30% did not recover after many years. At the moment, there is no good way of predicting who will recover and who will not. The reason for lack of recovery is not clear. In this series, plasma ACTH levels were higher in those who recovered than in those who did not. It is possible that persistent inability to recover CRH or ACTH secreting ability determines adrenal recovery in both pituitary Cushing's and adrenal adenomas, but the loss of one of the adrenals in the latter may further jeopardize the capacity to recover.

While most patients with ACTH-dependent Cushing's syndrome require bilateral adrenalectomy for cure, those with ACTH-independent hypercortisolism seemed to do well with unilateral adrenalectomy. Iacobone et al (Abstract 61–5) report on 50 such patients followed up over many years. After surgery, 100% were in biochemical remission and most of them were clinically recovered. Although these patients have bilateral disease they may also exhibit asymmetry of function, and a challenge is deciding which side to remove. The use of iodocholesterol scintigraphy or adrenal venous sampling should be able to determine which side is the most active.

The medical treatment of Cushing's disease is generally directed to the use of adrenal inhibitors such as ketoconazole or adrenolytic drugs such as mitotane. Attempts to use pharmacologic approaches to the pituitary gland have not been successful. Cyproheptadine was proposed by Krieger et al[1] 30 years ago with initial promise but limited long-term response. Rosiglitazone, a thiazolidinedione compound with PPAR-γ, is able to suppress ACTH secretion in mice and in AtT20 pituitary tumor cells. It was logical to try it in patients with pituitary ACTH-dependent Cushing's. Ambrosi et al (Abstract 61–6) reported on 6 patients treated with rosiglitazone 8 mg daily for several months. Almost half of the patients had a decrease in urinary free cortisol and ACTH and cortisol levels, but the changes did not reach statistical significance. Similar inconsistent responses have been found by other investigators. It is possible that some patients may be candidates for this type of treatment, but who and for what reason remains to be determined.

Ectopic ACTH secretion by extrapituitary neoplasms accounts for 10% of cases of Cushing's syndrome. The endocrine diagnosis is not difficult, but detection of the underlying tumor may be time consuming and challenging. Cases of occult bronchial or mediastinal carcinoid tumors may mimic pituitary ACTH-dependent disease. Unfortunately, resection of more malignant lesions is not always curative, and medical treatment not always effective. A series of 90 patients with ectopic ACTH syndrome studied at the NIH over a 20-year period is the basis of a report by Ilias et al (Abstract 61–8). Notable in that report are the following observations: petrosal sinus sampling is the most reliable diagnostic test; initial failed localization suggest pulmonary carcinoid; patients with small cell lung cancer, gastrinomas, and medullary thyroid carcinomas have the worst prognosis; and calcitonin may be a possible biomarker for a variety of tumors (other than medullary thyroid carcinoma) secreting ACTH. The information is not new but the large number of patients represented in this series helps provide more solid concepts concerning ectopic ACTH syndrome.

The surgical treatment of patients with ectopic ACTH-secreting bronchial carcinoids is extremely challenging given the fact that many of these tumors are small and escape detection. A case report by Grossrubatscher et al (Abstract 61–7) describes an interesting approach. Radioguided surgery with a hand-held gamma probe 48 hours after injection of [^{111}In]-pentreotide allowed detection and removal of multiple residual mediastinal lymph node metastases of an ACTH-secreting bronchial carcinoid. Wider experience with this method may be very useful in the treatment of patients with ectopic ACTH syndrome.

D. E. Schteingart, MD

Reference

1. Krieger DT, Amorosa L, Linick F, et al: Cyproheptadine-induced remission of Cushing's disease.*N Engl J Med* 293:893-896, 1975.

62 Developmental Endocrinology

Efficacy and Safety Results of Long-term Growth Hormone Treatment of Idiopathic Short Stature

Kemp SF, Kuntze J, Attie KM, et al (Univ of Arkansas, Little Rock; Burfordville, Mo; Rio de Janeiro, Brazil; et al)

J Clin Endocrinol Metab 90:5247-5253, 2005 62–1

Context.—Small clinical trials of GH treatment of idiopathic short stature (ISS) show variable efficacy.

Objective.—The study was an analysis of a large GH registry for efficacy and safety of GH treatment of ISS. There was also a comparison with a specific clinical trial.

Design.—Up to 7 yr of GH treatment of ISS was evaluated for efficacy and safety in the National Cooperative Growth Study (NCGS).

Setting.—The NCGS study was conducted at Genentech, Inc. and included 47,226 patients.

Patients.—The ISS group included maximum stimulated GH 10 ng/ml or more and/or a report of ISS by investigator (n = 8018; all included for safety). Cohort 1 (n = 2520) was similar to the clinical trial, cohort 2 (n = 283) included subjects younger than 5 yr of age, and cohort 3 (n = 940) was pubertal at GH start.

Intervention.—GH, approximately 0.30 mg/kg·wk, was given.

Main Outcome Measures.—These included growth velocities and height sd (HtSDS). Results: Mean first-year growth velocities in cohorts 1, 2, and 3 increased 4.6, 3.9, and 4.4 cm/yr over pretreatment, respectively. Measures included: baseline mean HtSDS, −2.9, −3.2, and −2.8; mean HtSDS at 1 yr, −2.4, −2.3, and −2.3, respectively. Mean HtSDS after 7 yr in cohorts 1 (n = 303) and 2 (n = 85) and 5 yr in cohort 3 (n = 58) were: −1.2, −1.0, and −1.5, respectively. Cohort 3 shorter treatment time was due to advanced baseline age (mean 13.8 yr) and puberty. Mean HtSDS gain in cohort 1 was comparable with the clinical trial. No new safety signals specific to the NCGS ISS population were observed.

Conclusion.—ISS patients in the GH registry demonstrate a significant increase in HtSDS with the safety profile similar to GH-deficient patients. Results were similar to the clinical trial.

► The power of studies on the basis of GH registries is that large numbers of subjects are evaluated, often overcoming the variability in the necessarily small numbers of subjects in clinical trials. Kemp et al use the large size of the NCGS database to monitor the growth velocities of children treated with GH and compared them with their previously published clinical trial data. Cohort 1 (n = 2520) was similar to the clinical trial, cohort 2 (n = 283) included subjects younger than 5 years, and cohort 3 (n = 940) was pubertal at the start of GH therapy.

The categorization of some of the subjects may be problematic because GH stimulation tests were not standardized or performed on all subjects—if done, neither the stimuli used nor the GH assays were consistent. Subjects were designated as having ISS if their short stature had etiologic factors such as GH neurosecretory dysfunction, bioinactive GH, and other terms commonly applied to patients with ISS. The ISS etiology was established after other known causes of short stature (eg, Turner's syndrome, GH deficiency, small-for-gestational age, Russell-Silver, organic causes, and chronic renal insufficiency) were excluded. The specific criteria used were as follows: (1) maximal stimulated GH greater than 10 ng/mL with or without confirmatory information; and (2) no GH stimulation test result, but text reported on the case report form indicating ISS. These are the compromises that must be made when exploiting the power of the large data bases. In addition, the critical issue of adult height cannot be addressed with these data. No indication of primary IGF-I deficiency (which is prevalent in a cohort of short children) was made.

Primary outcomes were surprisingly consistent for all cohorts, especially in the first few years of therapy, given that the pubertal cohort would attain epiphyseal closure (and a preceding slowing of the growth rate) in the latter years of the study. Mean height velocities increased over the pretreatment velocities by approximately 4 cm/y. Mean height SDS increased approximately 0.5 at 1 year and 1.5 at 5 years with diminishing numbers of subjects at each year. These data are consistent with the previous clinical trial.[1]

Notable also was a greater acceleration in growth velocity in the younger age cohort indicating that more prominent catch-up in growth is possible. There were no new safety signals or any indication of serious side effects. The usual caveats of nonrandom drop out of the less rapidly growing subjects and lack of adult height data are important to acknowledge. However, it is clear that the younger children can accelerate their height velocity, so that during childhood they are more likely to be in the height range of their age peers.

A. D. Rogol, MD, PhD

Reference

1. Hintz RL, Attie KM, Baptista J, Roche A, for the Genentech Collaborative Group: Effect of growth hormone treatment on adult height of children with idiopathic short stature. *N Engl J Med* 340:502-507, 1999.

Primary Hyperparathyroidism in Pediatric Patients

Kollars J, Zarroug AE, van Heerden J, et al (Mayo Clinic and Found, Rochester, Minn)
Pediatrics 115:974-980, 2005 62–2

Background.—Hyperparathyroidism (HPT) is predominantly a disease of adulthood, and is unusual in children, with an incidence of 2 to 5 per 100,000 children. Thus, physicians often fail to check serum calcium and parathyroid hormone (PTH) levels when evaluating children with nonspecific complaints, such as polyuria, fatigue, poor appetite, weight loss, abdominal pain, nausea, and emesis. The result is a delay in recognition and diagnosis of pediatric parathyroid disorders until patients have progressed to significant end-organ disease. The experience with HPT was retrospectively reviewed to better characterize these patients.

Methods.—A retrospective review was conducted of patients younger than 19 years who underwent parathyroid resection for primary HPT from 1970 to 2000 at a single institution.

Results.—The review identified 523 patients. The median age of these patients was 16.8 years, with a range of 4 to 18.9 years. The male-to-female ratio was 3:2. Most of the patients (85%) had an increased PTH level, and 15% had an inappropriately normal PTH level during hypercalcemia. Serum calcium was increased in all patients except for 2 with multiple endocrine neoplasma (MEN)-IIA and 1 patient with familial non-MEN HPT; however, both had increased PTH levels. Alkaline phosphatase levels were significantly higher in children with documented bone involvement. At presentation, 41 (79%) patients were symptomatic, and end-organ damage was present in 23 (44%) patients). A single adenoma was present in 34 (65%) patients; hyperplasia was identified in 16 (27%) patients, and of these cases, 57% occurred in patients diagnosed with MEN-I. Short-term complications included transient hypocalcemia in 29 (56%) patients and transient vocal cord paralysis in 2 (4%) patients. Long-term complications included permanent hypocalcemia in 2 (4%) patients and no recurrent nerve injuries. No parathyroid abnormalities were identified during exploration in 4 (8%) children. Long-term follow up was achieved in 98% of patients for a mean of 13 years. Resolution of hypercalcemia was obtained in 94% of patients.

Conclusions.—Primary HPT is relatively uncommon in children, and therefore, diagnosis is frequently delayed. Primary HPT in children is commonly symptomatic and is associated with significant morbidity. Evaluation of serum calcium and PTH levels is diagnostic in 100% of children in whom primary HPT is suspected. Parathyroid resection is the treatment of choice in children with primary HPT, as it is effective in restoring normal serum calcium levels and has few complications.

► HPT is uncommon in children with an incidence of 2 to 5 per 100,000 children and adolescents. Most are within their adolescent years. Parathyroid adenoma is the most common cause and is usually sporadic; however, HPT may also occur in the setting of MEN-I or -II syndromes or familial non-MEN HPT as a result of multigland disease. Additional familial forms of hypercalcemia include familial hypocalciuric hypercalcemia and neonatal primary HPT. Most children are symptomatic with evidence of nephrocalcinosis, nephrolithiasis, acute pancreatitis, or bone involvement, because the early stages of disease are subtle and not often considered for this rare condition.

Fifty-two patients are described who have fatigue and lethargy; headache, nephrolithiasis, abdominal pain, vomiting and polydipsia being the most common (35%-21%) but not universal signs and symptoms. Hypercalcemia was noted in 89% of all patients and in 100% of those with a parathyroid adenoma or MEN-I as their diagnosis. Median levels of PTH were either increased or, although within the normal range, increased for the degree of hypercalcemia. It should be noted that different PTH assays measure multiple active and inactive fragments of PTH, and it is critical to know what the assay used actually measures. In this review, the phosphate level was often low, the chloride/phosphate ratio was high, and the alkaline phosphatase level was high for age. Operative findings included a single adenoma in 65% of patients. However, it should be clear that the operative findings will reflect the number of subjects (and families) with familial HPT. Most children no longer have hypercalcemia postoperatively. Those that do often have familial disease, and continued surveillance is required.

A. D. Rogol, MD PhD

63 Reproductive Endocrinology

Effects of Estrogen With and Without Progestin on Urinary Incontinence

Hendrix SL, Cochrane BB, Nygaard IE, et al (Wayne State Univ, Detroit; Fred Hutchinson Cancer Research Ctr, Seattle; Univ of Iowa, Iowa City; et al)

JAMA 293:935-948, 2005 63–1

Context.—Menopausal hormone therapy has long been credited with many benefits beyond the indications of relieving hot flashes, night sweats, and vaginal dryness, and it is often prescribed to treat urinary incontinence (UI).

Objective.—To assess the effects of menopausal hormone therapy on the incidence and severity of symptoms of stress, urge, and mixed UI in healthy postmenopausal women.

Design, Setting, and Participants.—Women's Health Initiative multicenter double-blind, placebo-controlled, randomized clinical trials of menopausal hormone therapy in 27,347 postmenopausal women aged 50 to 79 years enrolled between 1993 and 1998, for whom UI symptoms were known in 23,296 participants at baseline and 1 year.

Interventions.—Women were randomized based on hysterectomy status to active treatment or placebo in either the estrogen plus progestin (E + P) or estrogen alone trials. The E + P hormones were 0.625 mg/d of conjugated equine estrogen plus 2.5 mg/d of medroxyprogesterone acetate (CEE + MPA); estrogen alone consisted of 0.625 mg/d of conjugated equine estrogen (CEE). There were 8506 participants who received CEE + MPA (8102 who received placebo) and 5310 who received CEE alone (5429 who received placebo).

Main Outcome Measures.—Incident UI at 1 year among women without UI at baseline and severity of UI at 1 year among women who had UI at baseline.

Results.—Menopausal hormone therapy increased the incidence of all types of UI at 1 year among women who were continent at baseline. The risk was highest for stress UI (CEE + MPA: relative risk [RR], 1.87 [95% confidence interval {CI}, 1.61-2.18]; CEE alone: RR, 2.15 [95% CI, 1.77-2.62]), followed by mixed UI (CEE + MPA: RR, 1.49 [95% CI, 1.10-2.01]; CEE alone: RR, 1.79 [95% CI, 1.26-2.53]). The combination of CEE + MPA had no significant effect on developing urge UI (RR, 1.15; 95% CI, 0.99-1.34), but CEE alone increased the risk (RR, 1.32; 95% CI, 1.10-1.58). Among women experiencing UI at baseline, frequency worsened in both trials (CEE + MPA: RR, 1.38 [95% CI, 1.28-1.49]; CEE alone: RR, 1.47 [95% CI, 1.35-1.61]). Amount of UI worsened at 1 year in both trials (CEE + MPA: RR, 1.20 [95% CI, 1.06-1.36]; CEE alone: RR, 1.59 [95% CI, 1.39-1.82]). Women receiving menopausal hormone therapy were more likely to report that UI limited their daily activities (CEE + MPA: RR, 1.18 [95% CI, 1.06-1.32]; CEE alone: RR, 1.29 [95% CI, 1.15-1.45]) and bothered or disturbed them (CEE + MPA: RR, 1.22 [95% CI, 1.13-1.32]; CEE alone: RR, 1.50 [95% CI, 1.37-1.65]) at 1 year.

Conclusions.—Conjugated equine estrogen alone and CEE + MPA increased the risk of UI among continent women and worsened the characteristics of UI among symptomatic women after 1 year. Conjugated equine estrogen with or without progestin should not be prescribed for the prevention or relief of UI.

▶ Conjugated estrogen with or without progestin does not prevent UI.

A. W. Meikle, MD

Older Men Are as Responsive as Young Men to the Anabolic Effects of Graded Doses of Testosterone on the Skeletal Muscle

Bhasin S, Woodhouse L, Casaburi R, et al (Charles R Drew Univ of Medicine and Science, Los Angeles; Harbor-Univ of California, Torrance; El Camino College, Torrance, Calif; et al)

J Clin Endocrinol Metab 90:678-688, 2005 63–2

Introduction.—Although testosterone levels and muscle mass decline with age, many older men have serum testosterone level in the normal range, leading to speculation about whether older men are less sensitive to testosterone. We determined the responsiveness of androgen-dependent outcomes to graded testosterone doses in older men and compared it to that in young men. The participants in this randomized, double-blind trial were 60 ambulatory, healthy, older men, 60-75 yr of age, who had normal serum testosterone levels. Their responses to graded doses of testosterone were compared with previous data in 61 men, 19-35 yr old. The participants received a long-acting GnRH agonist to suppress endogenous testosterone production and 25, 50, 125, 300, or 600 mg testosterone enanthate weekly for 20 wk. Fat-free mass, fat mass, muscle strength, sexual function, mood, visuospatial cognition, hormone levels, and safety measures were evaluated before, during, and after treatment. Of 60 older men who were randomized, 52 completed the study. After adjusting for testosterone dose, changes in serum total testosterone (change, −6.8, −1.9, +16.1, +49.5, and +101.9 nmol/liter at 25, 50, 125, 300, and 600 mg/wk, respectively) and hemoglobin (change, −3.6, +9.9, +20.9, +12.6, and +29.4 g/liter at 25, 50, 125, 300, and 600 mg/wk, respectively) levels were dose-related in older men and significantly greater in older men than young men (each $P < 0.0001$). The changes in FFM (−0.3, +1.7, +4.2, +5.6, and +7.3 kg, respectively, in five ascending dose groups) and muscle strength in older men were correlated with testosterone dose and concentrations and were not significantly different in young and older men (Fig 4). Changes in fat mass correlated inversely with testosterone dose ($r = -0.54$; $P < 0.001$) and were significantly different in young vs. older men ($P < 0.0001$); young men receiving 25- and 50-mg doses gained more fat mass than older men ($P < 0.0001$). Mood and visuospatial cognition did not change significantly in either group. Frequency of hematocrit greater than 54%, leg edema, and prostate events were numerically higher in older men than in young men. Older men are as responsive as young men to testosterone's anabolic effects; however, older men have lower testosterone clearance rates, higher increments in hemoglobin, and a higher frequency of adverse effects. Although substantial gains in muscle mass and strength can

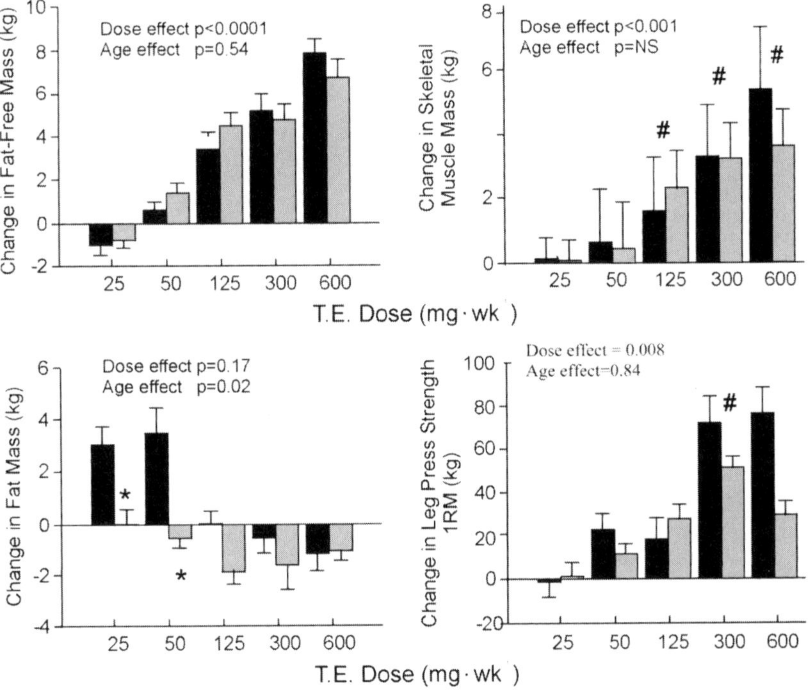

FIGURE 4.—Changes from baseline in FFM, fat mass, leg press strength, and skeletal muscle mass in young (*solid box*) and older (*shaded box*) men in response to graded doses of testosterone enanthate. Healthy, young and older men were randomized to receive a long-acting GnRH agonist plus one of five different doses of testosterone enanthate (25, 50, 125, 300, and 600 mg weekly, im) for 20 wk. Changes in other outcome measures were calculated as the difference between wk 20 and baseline values. Data are the mean ± SEM. If there was a significant age effect, the values for young and older men for each dose were compared using Tukey's multiple comparison procedure. *Significant differences between young and older men receiving that dose ($P < 0.05$). Similarly, if the linear model revealed a significant dose effect, then different dose groups were compared using Tukey's multiple comparison procedure. #Significant difference from 25- and 50-mg doses ($P < 0.05$). (Courtesy of Bhasin S, Woodhouse L, Casaburi R, et al: Older men are as responsive as young men to the anabolic effects of graded doses of testosterone on the skeletal muscle. *J Clin Endocrinol Metab* 90:678-688, 2005. Copyright The Endocrine Society.)

be realized in older men with supraphysiological testosterone doses, these high doses are associated with a high frequency of adverse effects. The best trade-off was achieved with a testosterone dose (125 mg) that was associated with high normal testosterone levels, low frequency of adverse events, and significant gains in fat-free mass and muscle strength.

► As men age, they maintain their responsiveness to testosterone.

A. W. Meikle, MD

Endogenous Sex Hormones and Metabolic Syndrome in Aging Men

Muller M, Grobbee DE, de Tonkelaar I, et al (Univ Med Ctr Utrecht, The Netherlands; Internatl Health Found, Utrecht, The Netherlands; Erasmus Univ, Rotterdam, The Netherlands)

J Clin Endocrinol Metab 90:2618-2623, 2005 63–3

Background.—Sex hormone levels in men change during aging. These changes may be associated with insulin sensitivity and the metabolic syndrome.

Methods.—We studied the association between endogenous sex hormones and characteristics of the metabolic syndrome in 400 independently living men between 40 and 80 yr of age in a cross-sectional study. Serum concentrations of lipids, glucose, insulin, total testosterone (TT), SHBG, estradiol (E2), and dehydroepiandrosterone sulfate (DHEA-S) were measured. Bioavailable testosterone (BT) was calculated using TT and SHBG. Body height, weight, waist-hip circumference, blood pressure, and physical activity were assessed. Smoking and alcohol consumption was estimated from self-report. The metabolic syndrome was defined according to the National Cholesterol Education Program definition, and insulin sensitivity was calculated by use of the quantitative insulin sensitivity check index.

Results.—Multiple logistic regression analyses showed an inverse relationship according to 1 SD increase for circulating TT [odds ratio (OR) = 0.43; 95% confidence interval (CI), 0.32-0.59], BT (OR = 0.62; 95% CI, 0.46-0.83), SHBG (OR = 0.46; 95% CI, 0.33-0.64), and DHEA-S (OR = 0.76; 95% CI, 0.56-1.02) with the metabolic syndrome. Each SD increase in E2 levels was not significantly associated with the metabolic syndrome (OR = 1.16; 95% CI, 0.92-1.45). Linear regression analyses showed that higher TT, BT, and SHBG levels were related to higher insulin sensitivity; β-coefficients (95% CI) were 0.011 (0.008-0.015), 0.005 (0.001-0.009), and 0.013 (0.010-0.017), respectively, whereas no effects were found for DHEA-S and E2. Estimates were adjusted for age, smoking, alcohol consumption, and physical activity score. Further adjustment for insulin levels and body composition measurements attenuated the estimates, and the associations were similar in the group free of cardiovascular disease and diabetes.

Conclusions.—Higher testosterone and SHBG levels in aging males are independently associated with a higher insulin sensitivity and a reduced risk of the metabolic syndrome, independent of insulin levels and body composition measurements, suggesting that these hormones may protect against the development of metabolic syndrome.

▶ Higher serum TT and SHBG concentrations in aging men are independently associated with higher insulin sensitivity and a reduction in risk of the metabolic syndrome.

A. W. Meikle, MD

Subject Index

A

B

D

E

F

G

H

J

K

N

O

P

Q

R

S

T

U

V

W

Y

Z

Author Index

K

L

M

N

O

P

Q

R

S

T

U

V

W

X

Y

Z